# AHA Hospital Statistics™



2005 Edition

AHA Institutional Members $155
Nonmembers $235
AHA Catalog NUMBER 082005
Telephone ORDERS 1-800-AHA-2626

ISSN 0090-6662
ISBN 0-87258-810-6


Printed in the U.S.A.

# Contents

# Acknowledgements & Advisements

## Acknowledgments

The 2005 edition of AHA Hospital Statistics is published by Health Forum an affiliate of the American Hospital Association, Richard J. Davidson, President.

## Advisements

*The data published here should be used with the following advisements: The data are based on replies to an annual survey that seeks a variety of information, not all of which is published in this book. The information gathered by the survey includes specific services, but not all of each hospital's services. Therefore, the data do not reflect an exhaustive list of all services offered by all hospitals. For information on the availability of additional data, please contact Health Forum, (800) 821-2039.*

*Health Forum does not assume responsibility for the accuracy of information voluntarily reported by the individual institutions surveyed. The purpose of this publication is to provide basic data reflecting the delivery of health care in the United States and associated areas, and is not to serve an official and all-inclusive list of services offered by individual hospitals.*

# Trends:

*an overview of 2003*

AHA Hospital Statistics™, *the results of the American Hospital Association's (AHA) Annual Survey of Hospitals, is a comprehensive compilation of data on trends in the hospital field through 2003. But what impact do current events and other trends in the health care field have on hospitals? Taking a look at the events affecting health care in 2003 provides added perspective to these annual survey results. Overall this publication identifies both long-standing and emerging trends and offers insights into what the future may hold for hospitals.*

Caroline Rossi Steinberg
Vice President, Trends Analysis
American Hospital Association

Against a backdrop of a slow economy and the national debate over a Medicare prescription drug benefit, hospitals faced a challenging environment in 2003. Hospitals were in the spotlight on several fronts including the launch of the Quality Initiative—a voluntary effort to publicly report data on key hospital quality indicators; debate over major changes to Medicare hospital payments; increased scrutiny of hospital mergers by the Federal Trade Commission (FTC); and a focus on billing and collection practices by media and lawmakers. Meanwhile, despite a slowdown in health care spending growth[1], health care premiums continued to increase by double-digits making affordable health care coverage a major 2004 campaign issue. Added to the ongoing challenges of the workforce shortage, rising costs to provide care, and difficulty accessing much needed capital, these new pressures made this one of the most difficult health care environments in years.

## The Environment

### Federal Policy Environment

The Medicare Modernization Act (MMA) dominated the federal legislative arena for most of 2003. While a Medicare prescription drug benefit was a central feature of the bill, it also included many important provisions for hospitals. The legislation provided payment relief for hospitals in rural and small urban areas and a full market basket update for the inpatient prospective payment system (PPS) for hospitals submitting quality data to the Centers for Medicaid & Medicare Services (CMS). The legislation also increased federal Medicaid disproportionate share hospital payment allotments to states and provided modest relief from the Medicare indirect medical education cuts of the Balanced Budget Act of 1997 (BBA) and its subsequent refinements. As signed into law, the MMA provided a $25 billion increase in projected Medicare and Medicaid payments to hospitals over a 10-year period.

As Congress debated the MMA, other important hospital issues were under discussion on the regulatory front. In 2002 and 2003, the FTC and the Department of Justice (DOJ) conducted a series of hearings on health care competition law and policy, examining past trends toward greater consolidation among hospitals, physician groups and health care plans—although the focus was predominantly on hospitals. The FTC released its findings and recommendations in its mid-2004 report, "Improving Care: A Dose of Competition," which made a number of recommendations that, if adopted, could have wide-ranging implications for hospitals operating in an already complex and difficult environment. These included changes in how geographic markets are defined in hospital merger cases and various actions that states should take to decrease barriers to competition, such as broadening the membership of state licensing boards, implementing uniform licensing standards and reconsidering certificate of need programs.

Meanwhile, hospitals faced a series of high-profile media stories that raised public and congressional concern about hospital billing and collection practices and how they affect uninsured patients and others unable to pay their hospital bills. Hospitals across the country began reexamining their own practices. The House Energy and Commerce Committee's Subcommittee on Oversight and Investigations (O&I) announced it would hold hearings on hospital billing and collection practices and asked for extensive data from 20 of the largest hospital systems. In December 2003, the AHA released a set of principles and guidelines to help hospitals address this issue. In June 2004, O&I held their hearing on billing and collections the same week that the House Ways and Means Committee held a

1 Center for Studying Health System Change, *Tracking Health Care Costs: Trends Turn Downward in 2003,* Data Bulletin, June 2004· Number 27.

hearing centered around the tax exempt status of hospitals. At about the same time, the hospital field faced a series of related lawsuits.

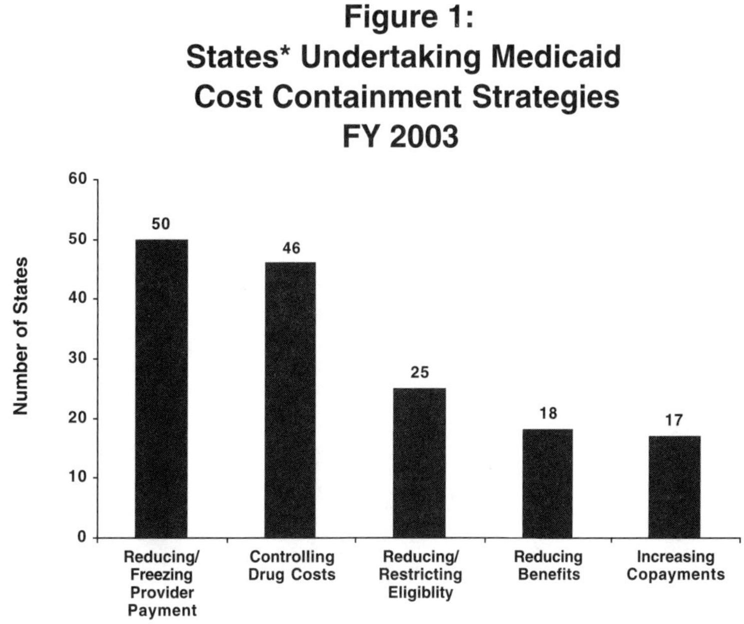


*Includes the District of Columbia

Source: Kaiser Commission on Medicaid and the Uninsured, *States Respond to Fiscal Pressure: A 50-State Update of State Medicaid Spending Growth and Cost Containment Actions*, January 2004.

### State Policy Environment

Fiscal crises dominated state activity. Almost every state faced a budget deficit and turned to Medicaid to help close the gap by trimming program spending. Many governors found provider payments to be a more palatable alternative for budget cuts than reductions in benefits or eligibility, and all but one state reported freezing or reducing provider payments in fiscal year 2003 (Figure 1). In May 2003, Congress passed the Jobs and Growth Tax Relief Reconciliation Act of 2003 and provided $20 billion in temporary fiscal relief to states—with $10 billion provided through an increase in the federal share of Medicaid spending—dampening the need for additional cuts. But this relief expired in June of 2004.

The medical liability insurance crisis also garnered the attention of state officials. Premiums in many states had skyrocketed, leaving some physicians unable to afford coverage. Failure to pass a federal solution spurred 37 states to consider a variety of tort reform measures, including caps on non-economic damages and protections to ensure a provider is only responsible for its share of damages based on an assessment of fault. In 2003, 11 states enacted some measures to change their existing tort system: Arkansas, Florida, Idaho, Montana, Nevada, New Hampshire, New York, Ohio, Texas, Utah and West Virginia.

### Health Care Costs

Health care spending comprised about 15% of the gross domestic product, up from about 9% in 1980. While spending on hospital care remains the largest component of this outlay, the hospital share has fallen by 10 percentage points over the past 20 years. After a period of low growth in the mid-1990s, growth in spending for hospital care recently increased due to more demand for services and rising costs for labor and technology.

Although the growth in health care costs slowed down in 2003, health insurance premiums rose by 13.9%, the largest increase in more than 10 years (Figure 2). Employers continued to shift health insurance costs to employees by raising deductibles and copayments (Figure 3), while health plans enjoyed rising profits.[2]

2 Weiss Ratings, Inc., *HMOs Earn $10.2 Billion in 2003, Nearly Doubling Profits*, Press Release, August 30, 2004.

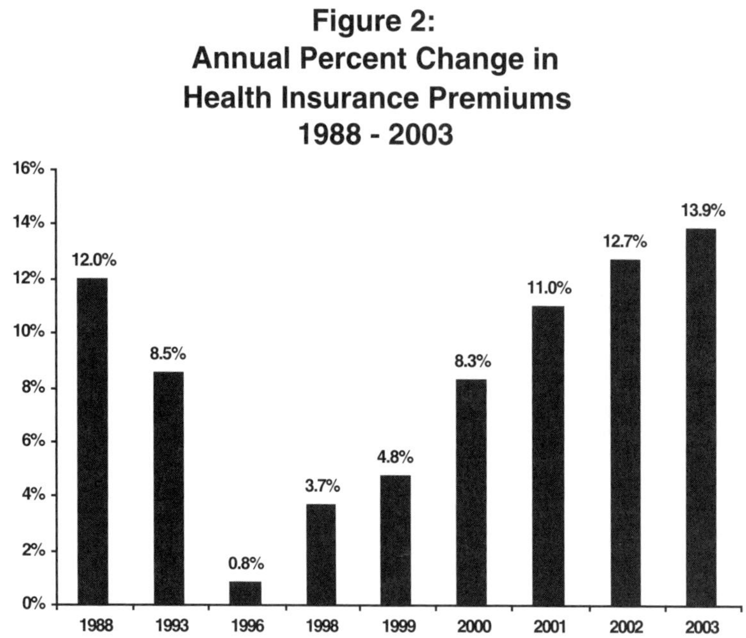


Source: The Kaiser Family Foundation and Health Research and Educational Trust, *Employer Health Benefits*, 1999, 2000, 2001, 2002, 2003.

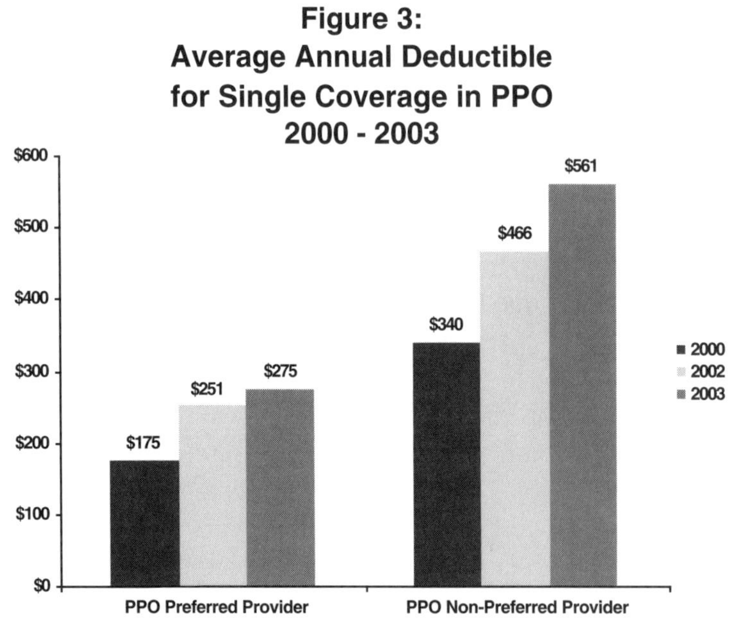


Source: The Kaiser Family Foundation and Health Research and Educational Trust, *Employer Health Benefits*, 2003.

**Coverage and Access**

For most Americans, access to health care is tied to health insurance and, for most non-elderly Americans, access to health insurance is tied to employment. According to the U.S. Census Bureau, 60.4% of Americans receive health coverage through their employer, though the percent of Americans with employer-based coverage has declined over the past decade as Medicaid enrollment has increased and more Americans have joined the ranks of the uninsured.

In 2003, 45 million individuals were without health insurance, an increase of 1.4 million from 2002 (Figure 4). Nationally 15.6% of Americans are without insurance, varying from a low of 8.3% in Minnesota to a high of 25.2% in Texas (Table 1). Although the economic recession officially ended in 2001, the unemployment rate continued to rise in 2003 and probably contributed to the increase in uninsured people. Even so, more than eight out of 10 uninsured individuals are in working families (Figure 5). Research shows that people who go without health insurance are less likely to receive needed care, have poorer health status and die younger than those with coverage.[3] Hospital emergency departments are often the only access point for care for these individuals.

In an effort to contain costs, some employers are experimenting with "consumer-directed plans," hoping to create a financial incentive for employees to be more cost conscious about health care decisions. These plans come in several forms. "Tiered networks" provide different reimbursement levels for different providers based on cost and, in some plans, quality performance. "High deductible plans" seek to encourage employees to spend funds wisely under a deductible of typically $1000 or more. Prior to the passage of the MMA, high deductible plans could be combined with Health Reimbursement Accounts (HRAs). HRAs are funded by employers and can be used toward the deductible or they can be rolled over to the next year but are forfeited if the employee leaves the company. The MMA created Health Savings Accounts (HSAs), a new, more flexible arrangement. In combination with a high-deductible plan that meets specific criteria, HSAs can be funded both by

3 The Kaiser Commission on Medicaid and the Uninsured, *Sicker and Poorer: The Consequences of Being Uninsured,* May 2002.

**Figure 4: Number and Percent Uninsured 1985 - 2003**

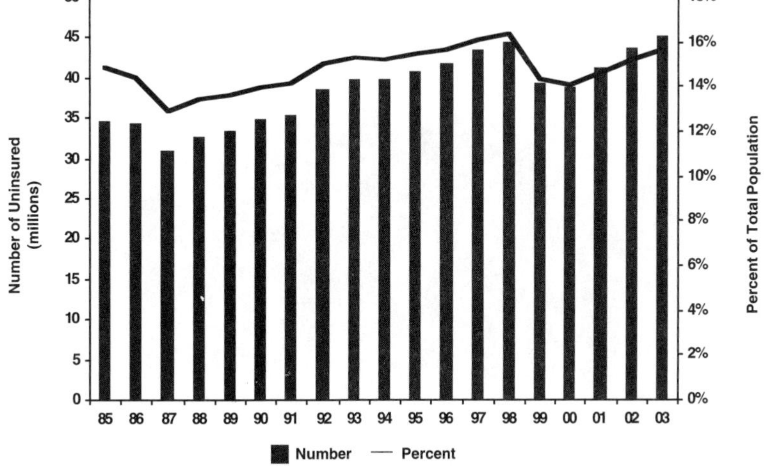


Source: U.S. Census Bureau, *Income, Poverty, and Health Insurance Coverage in the United States: 2003,* August 2004.

**Table 1: Percentage of People Without Health Insurance Coverage by State Using 2-Year Averages: 2002-2003**

| State | Average Percent Uninsured | State | Average Percent Uninsured |
|---|---|---|---|
| Alabama | 13.5 | Montana | 17.3 |
| Alaska | 18.8 | Nebraska | 10.8 |
| Arizona | 16.9 | Nevada | 19.3 |
| Arkansas | 16.9 | New Hampshire | 10.1 |
| California | 18.3 | New Jersey | 14.0 |
| Colorado | 16.7 | New Mexico | 21.6 |
| Connecticut | 10.5 | New York | 15.4 |
| Delaware | 10.5 | North Carolina | 17.0 |
| District of Columbia | 13.6 | North Dakota | 10.9 |
| Florida | 17.7 | Ohio | 12.0 |
| Georgia | 16.3 | Oklahoma | 18.8 |
| Hawaii | 10.1 | Oregon | 15.9 |
| Idaho | 18.3 | Pennsylvania | 11.4 |
| Illinois | 14.3 | Rhode Island | 10.1 |
| Indiana | 13.5 | South Carolina | 13.4 |
| Iowa | 10.4 | South Dakota | 11.8 |
| Kansas | 10.7 | Tennessee | 12.0 |
| Kentucky | 13.8 | Texas | 25.2 |
| Louisiana | 19.5 | Utah | 13.0 |
| Maine | 10.9 | Vermont | 10.1 |
| Maryland | 13.6 | Virginia | 13.3 |
| Massachusetts | 10.3 | Washington | 14.8 |
| Michigan | 11.3 | West Virginia | 15.6 |
| Minnesota | 8.3 | Wisconsin | 10.4 |
| Mississippi | 17.3 | Wyoming | 16.8 |
| Missouri | 11.3 | | |

Source: U.S. Census Bureau, *Income, Poverty, and Health Insurance Coverage in the United States: 2003,* August 2004.

Figure 5:
Working Status of Uninsured Population
2003

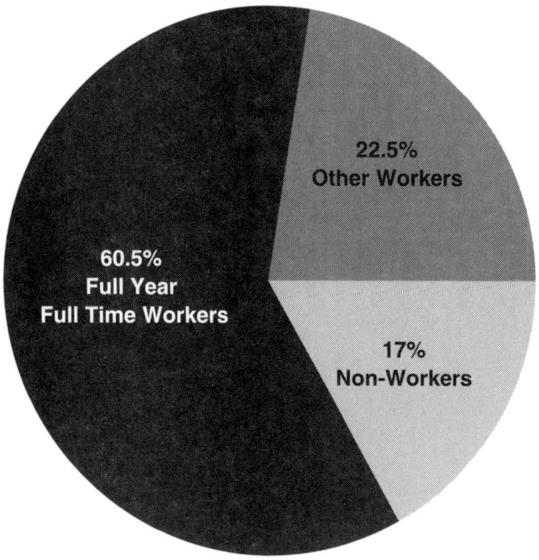


Source: Employee Benefit Research Institute, *Estimates from the March Current Population Survey, 2003 Supplement*, 2004.

employees and employers, rolled over from year to year, used for expenses beyond the deductible, and remain the property of the employee upon departure from the company.

## Pressures Facing Hospitals

Community hospitals continue to face challenges from many fronts. From 2002 to 2003, the 7.5% growth in net patient revenues failed to keep pace with the 8.0% increase in total expenses, resulting in a decline in operating margins from 3.7% to 3.3%. As the economy improved in 2003, however, an increase in non-operating income allowed hospital total margins to increase slightly from 4.4% to 4.8%. Non-operating income includes gains from investments or the sale of other assets (e.g., physician practices, real estate). This type of income has been highly volatile in recent years due to dramatic fluctuations in the stock market and changes in interest rates. This volatility raises the importance of operating margins relative to total margins as an indicator of financial health. In 2003, 30% of hospitals lost money overall while 36% had negative operating margins. The 4.8% total margin for the hospital field compares to 14.3% in after-tax profits for the pharmaceutical industry.[4]

Medicare and Medicaid payment rate increases did not keep pace with growth in costs, further increasing hospital losses for patients covered under these programs. In 2003, Medicare paid hospitals 95 cents on the dollar, while Medicaid paid hospitals 92 cents on the dollar, down considerably from prior years (Figure 6).

### Rising Demand and Increased Costs to Provide Care

The demand for hospital care continued to rise in 2003, though at a somewhat slower pace than in the last several years (Figure 7). Community hospitals admitted about 300,000 more patients in 2003 compared to 2002, an increase of about 1%. Hospitals had 7 million more total outpatient visits. Length of stay remained flat at 5.7 days.

Meanwhile, growth in the cost of providing care continued to increase. Hospital expense per adjusted admission grew by 6.0%, driven by rising labor costs amidst a workforce shortage and rising expenses for pharmaceuticals, new technology and other supplies needed to

4 The Henry J. Kaiser Family Foundation, *Trends and Indicators in the Changing Health Care Marketplace*, April 2004.

provide care. This growth rate is higher than in recent years, but still considerably lower than that experienced in the early 1990s (Figure 8).

### Workforce Shortage

The slowing economy created a temporary dampening of the workforce shortage allowing hospitals to fill some of their vacancies, but pushing payroll costs up by 6.7%. Wage growth for hospitals continued to outpace that of other service fields, but by less than in previous years (Figure 9). The shortage of workers appears to have eased temporarily, but the long-term prognosis remains grim as the registered nurse (RN) workforce is aging rapidly and enrollment in health education programs remains below need. Between 1980 and 2000, RNs under 30 dropped from 30% to 11% of the total RN population.[5] By 2020, the demand for RNs will exceed supply by an estimated 800,000 RNs (Figure 10).

### Growth in Limited-Service Providers

Hospitals face a growing number of physician-owned limited-service providers. These facilities include ambulatory surgery centers, outpatient diagnostic centers, and hospitals that offer only

5 Buerhaus, P.I. et al, " Implications of an Aging Registered Nurse Workforce," *JAMA*: 2000: 283: 2948-2954.

**Figure 6: Payment Relative to Cost for Medicare, Medicaid and Private Payers 1998 - 2003**

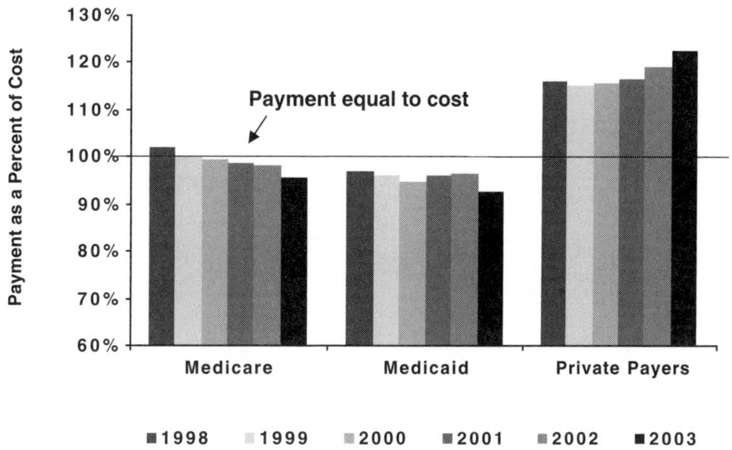


Source: AHA Annual Survey, 1998-2003. Data is for community hospitals.

**Figure 7: Inpatient Admissions and Outpatient Visits 1980 - 2003**

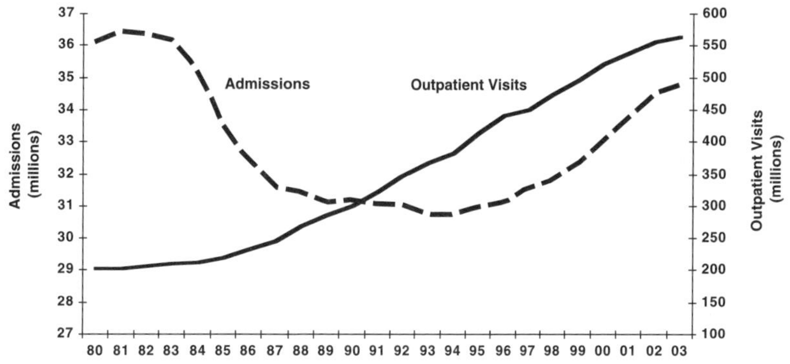


Source: AHA Annual Survey, 1980–2003. Data is for community hospitals.

Figure 8:
Annual Change in Hospital
Expenses per Adjusted Admission
1990 - 2003

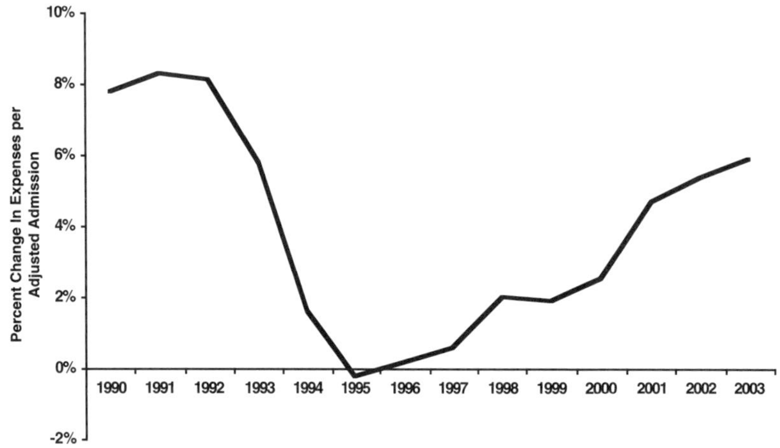


Source: AHA Annual Survey, 1990-2003. Data is for community hospitals.

Figure 9:
Percent Change in Employment Cost Index
Hospitals vs. All Service Industries
2001 - 2003

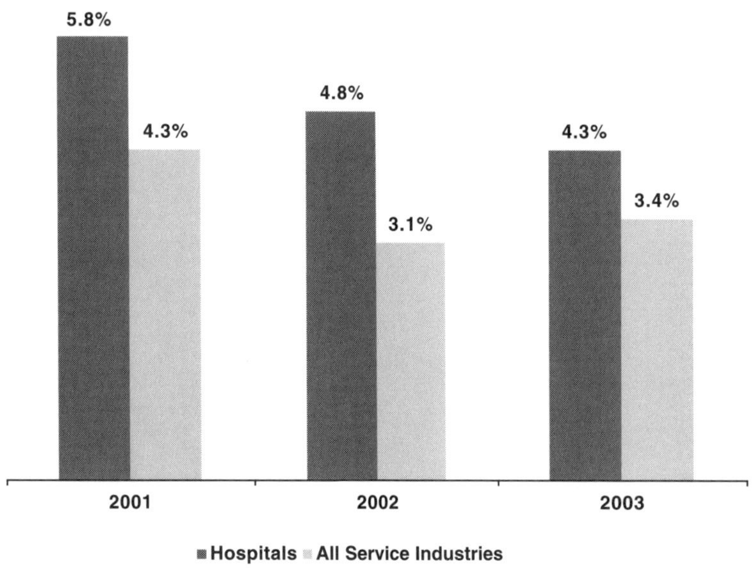


Source: Bureau of Labor Statistics. Data is for total compensation for civilian workers, for 12 months ending with the fourth quarter each year.

a narrow range of services. In particular, the rapid growth of ambulatory surgery centers (Figure 11) has contributed to the first decline in outpatient surgeries for hospitals in more than 20 years.

Although fewer in numbers, physician-owned limited-service hospitals are also a rapidly growing presence in the health care field. The impact of these facilities on the health care delivery system is not yet well understood. Past research in other practice settings indicates that the financial incentives created by physician ownership can lead to higher referral rates for services and potentially unnecessary utilization. The impact on broader access to care for the community is an additional concern. As owners of the facilities to which they refer, physicians have both the ability and the financial incentives to shift the well-reimbursed services and patients to their own facility. This practice can drain essential resources from full-service hospitals that rely on these patients to cross-subsidize money losing but essential community services like burn, emergency and trauma care. Congress recognized these concerns and placed an 18-month moratorium on physician self-referrals of Medicare and Medicaid patients to new limited-service hospitals while CMS and the Medicare Payment Advisory Commission study the issue.

### Access to Capital

Hospitals continually need capital funding to maintain and update facilities, meet the changing needs of patients, and invest in new clinical and information technology. A recent series of studies by the Healthcare Financial Management Association and G. E. Capital documents the increasing needs for capital against declining access to capital. Since 1990, the median age of hospital facilities has increased by about 25%, indicating that investments are not keeping pace with need.[6] According to Standard and Poor's, the number of bond downgrades in 2003 outnumbered upgrades by more than three to one. Since a lower bond rating means higher capital costs, it also leads to less capital access.

### Need to Document and Improve Quality of Care

In the five years since the Institute of Medicine's report, *To Err is Human: Building a Safer Health System*, called for dramatic changes in the health care system, hospitals have redoubled their efforts to

6 Ingenix, *Almanac of Hospital Financial and Operating Indicators*, 2004.

**Figure 10:**
**Forecast of Total Registered Nurse Full Time Equivalents vs. Requirements 2001 - 2020**

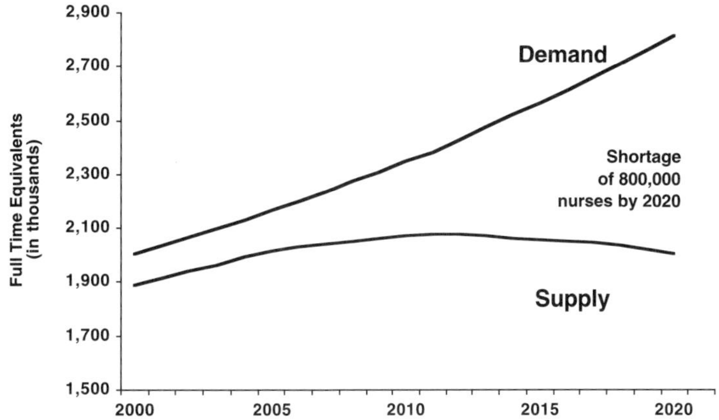


Source: Bureau of Health Professions, National Center for Health Workforce Analysis, *Projected Supply, Demand, and Shortages of Registered Nurses: 2000-2020*, released July 2002.

**Figure 11:**
**Number of Ambulatory Surgery Centers 1997 - 2003**

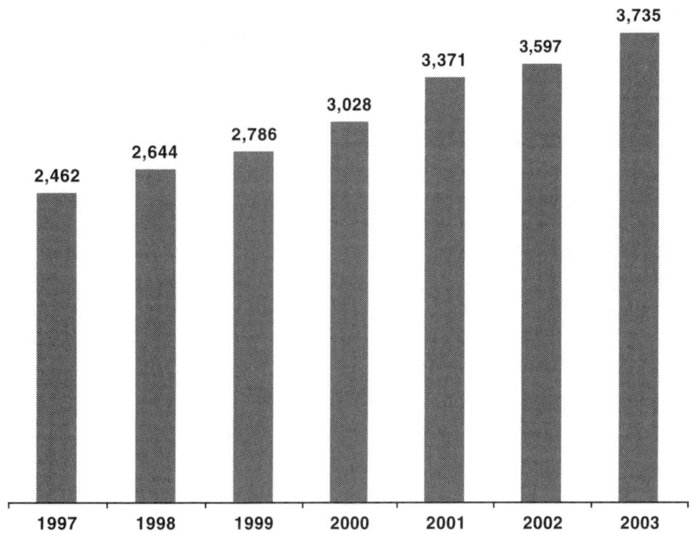


Source: MedPAC, *Report to Congress*, July 2004.

improve systems and processes to provide safer care for patients. Payers increasingly demand accountability, and some are even using quality data as a basis for tiered networks and other pay-for-performance initiatives.

In 2003, The Quality Initiative: A Public Resource on Hospital Performance was launched to develop a national strategy for quality measurement and public accountability. The initiative is a collaborative effort of the American Hospital Association, the Federation of American Hospitals, and the Association of American Medical Colleges with government agencies, professional organizations, purchasers, consumer groups, accrediting bodies, and others. The voluntary initiative calls for hospitals to publicly report data on a series of quality indicators. Congress supported this effort by passing a provision in the MMA that gives a full market basket update to acute care hospitals submitting quality of care data for public display. This represented the first wholesale effort within the Medicare program to link quality to payment. As of September 2004, 98.2% of the acute care hospitals whose payment was affected by this provision of the MMA had met all of CMS's requirements to receive a full payment update for FY 2005.[7] Meanwhile, hospitals continue to invest in system, process and technological changes to further improve quality and patient safety.

## Emerging Strategies

By 2000, hospitals had retrenched after many of the organizational initiatives of the early 1990s—including mergers, development of insurance products, expansion into other levels of care, and various arrangements with physicians—failed to achieve the desired results. Between 2002 and 2003, participation trends were mixed, indicating hospitals are selectively employing various integration strategies—pulling back from some, while increasing participation in others.

**Relationships with Other Hospitals**

In the early to mid-1990s, many hospitals merged, forming networks and systems to take unneeded beds out of the system, seeking efficiencies through consolidation, and forming networks of care that would be attractive to both consumers and payers in the developing managed care environment. As consumer backlash against managed care grew, the attractiveness of tightly managed networks waned. Meanwhile, post-merger integration often proved difficult. In response, the number of hospital mergers declined in the late 1990s—a trend that continued into 2003 (Figure 12).

**Insurance Products**

The number of hospitals offering insurance products showed little change between 2002 and 2003 after considerable volatility in the 1990s. The number of hospitals with HMO insurance products declined slightly, while those with less restrictive products like PPOs increased slightly. Overall trends in the insurance market also show a smaller percentage of employers offering HMO products in 2003.

**Services Beyond Acute Care**

Vertical integration—expanding into services beyond acute care—was a popular strategy in the early 1990s. But hospitals since have pulled back on some of these initiatives. Medicare payment reductions for home health and skilled nursing likely led fewer hospitals to offer these services. Meanwhile, more hospitals are offering hospice, assisted living, and long-term care services.

**Hospital Physician Relations**

Hospitals continue to wrestle with ways to enhance hospital-physician relationships. From 2002 to 2003, more hospitals reported having salaried physicians and physician hospital organizations while fewer participated

7 The Centers for Medicare and Medicaid Services, *Nearly all Eligible Hospitals are Reporting Quality of Care Data*, Press Release, September 2, 2004.

in independent practice associations. Hospital-physician relations will be an area to watch as hospitals respond to the growing trend of physician ownership—extending from office-based diagnostic equipment to freestanding ambulatory surgery centers and limited-service hospitals. As physicians pursue opportunities to increase their income and improve their lifestyle (e.g., reducing emergency department call time), hospitals face challenges maintaining the historical partnership.

**Figure 12: Announced Hospital Mergers and Acquisitions 1998 - 2003**

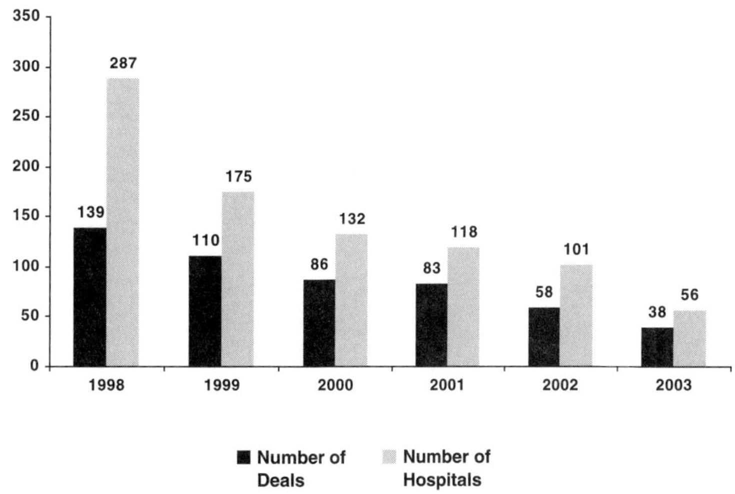


Source: Irving Levin Associates, Inc., *The Health Care Acquisition Report*, Tenth Edition, 2004.

### Community Engagement

The role of hospitals in their communities extends well beyond the delivery of patient care. Hospitals provide an array of community-oriented programs and services, from health screenings to meals-on-wheels, and work with other local providers, government agencies, and community organizations to assess and address community health.

In 2003 the majority of hospitals reported having a long-term plan to improve the health of their communities; working with other providers or public agencies to conduct health status assessments; and using health status indicators to design new or modify existing services.

## Conclusion

At the end of 2003, hospitals faced an unprecedented array of challenges—rising demand, increased costs, a workforce shortage, the need for capital investment, and the threat to community access to care posed by physician-owned limited-service providers. The focus on health care cost containment will be intense in the coming years. Pressures to deal with an increasing federal deficit and a desire to make the federal tax cuts permanent may push legislators to propose reductions in hospital Medicare payments as they did in the Balanced Budget Act of 1997. As states work to get back on a sound financial footing, Medicaid spending will continue to be scrutinized. Meanwhile, many expect employers to intensify their efforts to hold back spending growth for health care coverage, and the number of uninsured Americans is likely to grow. These challenges come at a time when hospitals are trying to improve patient safety, quality and the hospital work environment.

The continually changing landscape requires that hospital leaders become more and more creative. Closely monitoring the policy environment, trends in the insurance industry, and local issues will be critical as hospitals strive to continue delivering quality care in the most cost-effective manner.

# How to Use this Book

For more than five decades, *AHA Hospital Statistics™* has reported aggregate hospital data derived from the AHA Annual Survey and is the definitive source when doing trend analysis with data by bed size category, U.S. Census Divisions, States, and Metropolitan Statistical Areas (MSAs). As the health care delivery system changes, so have the data tracked by the survey and presented in this report. Recent additions include:

- **Community health indicators** that offer readers a connection to the community for their analysis and planning: the data are broken down into beds, admissions, inpatient days, ER outpatient visits, and other indicators per 1000 population, as well as expense per capita.
- **Utilization, personnel and finance** by all MSAs in the United States.
- **Five-year trend data** on physician models, insurance products, and managed care contracts enable you to identify changes in relationships between hospitals and other health care systems and providers.
- **Tables 3 through 6 have been organized** to show breakdowns between inpatient and outpatient care to better reflect market shifts toward outpatient-centered care. Additional clarity is gained by the breakdown between total facility data (which includes nursing home type units under the control of the hospital) and hospital units (which exclude the nursing home data).

**TABLE 6 Sample State**

*U.S. Registered Community Hospitals*
*(Nonfederal, short-term general and other special hospitals)*

**Overview 1999-2003**

| | 2003 | 2002 | 2001 | 2000 | 1999 |
|---|---|---|---|---|---|
| **Physician Models** | | | | | |
| Independent Practice Association | 14 | 17 | 17 | 17 | 14 |
| Group Practice without Walls | 4 | 5 | 5 | 8 | 4 |
| Open Physician-Hospital Organization | 20 | 21 | 24 | 23 | 18 |
| Closed Physician-Hospital Organization | 21 | 17 | 18 | 17 | 11 |
| Management Service Organization | 14 | 18 | 20 | 14 | 9 |
| Integrated Salary Model | 35 | 29 | 30 | 26 | 24 |
| Equity Model | 4 | 3 | 4 | 6 | 3 |
| Foundation | 9 | 8 | 23 | 21 | 19 |
| **Insurance Products** | | | | | |
| Health Maintenance Organization | 20 | 22 | 23 | 24 | 19 |
| Preferred Provider Organization | 39 | 47 | 52 | 53 | 37 |
| Indemnity Fee for Service | 7 | 12 | 14 | 12 | 6 |
| **Managed Care Contracts** | | | | | |
| Health Maintenance Organization | 64 | 67 | 62 | 49 | 42 |
| Preferred Provider Organization | 97 | 93 | 92 | 87 | 72 |

*Example of five-year trend data*

- **Facilities and Services information** on more than 90 categories of hospital facilities and services in Table 7. At a glance, you can determine the number and percentage of hospitals offering a specific service such as Oncology, Angioplasty, Palliative Care Program, Complementary Medicine, Women's Health Services and Tobacco Cessation.
- **Plus, System and Network involvement along with Group Purchasing Organizations** that demonstrate ways in which organizations are linked.

## The survey instrument and the glossary

A good place to begin your analysis is the AHA Annual Survey instrument. Found on page xxx, it includes the instructions, questions, and terms that were used to gather the data for fiscal year 2003. This can be extremely valuable for a clearer understanding of the data we collect and the tables presented in *AHA Hospital Statistics*.

Please also review the glossary in the back of the book. The glossary contains complete definitions for specific terms used in the tables and text of *AHA Hospital Statistics*. These definitions will clarify how terminology is being used.

As mentioned above, it is important to note that the primary focus of the most detailed data contained in *AHA Hospital Statistics* is community hospitals. As defined, community hospitals are all non-federal, short-term general and special hospitals whose facilities and services are available to the public. If the majority of a hospital's patients are admitted to units where the average length of stay is 30 days or less, a hospital may still be classified as short-term even if it includes a nursing- home-type unit. (For a more complete definition of community hospitals, please see the glossary definition, located on page 193.)

**Getting the most out of *Hospital Statistics***
This section of the book provides an introduction for getting the most out of your *AHA Hospital Statistics* 2005 edition. Here, you'll find a guide to the book, with insights into each table.

**Equity model:** An arrangement that allows established practitioners to become shareholders in a professional corporation in exchange for tangible and intangible assets of their existing practices.

**Expenses:** Includes all expenses for the reporting period including payroll, non-payroll, bad debt, and all nonoperating expenses. *Payroll expenses* include all salaries and wages. *Non-payroll expenses* are all professional fees and those salary expenditures excluded from payroll. *Labor related expenses* are defined as payroll expenses plus employee benefits. *Non-labor related expenses* are all other non-payroll expenses. *Bad debt* has been reclassified from a "reduction in revenue" to an expense in accordance with the revised AICPA Audit Guide. However, for purposes of historical consistency, the expense total that appears throughout *AHA Hospital Statistics does not include "bad debt" as an expense item.* Note: Financial data may not add due to rounding.

**Extracorporeal shock wave lithotripter (ESWL):** A medical device used for treating stones in the kidney or ureter. The device disintegrates kidney stones noninvasively through the transmission of acoustic shock waves directed at the stones.

**Fitness center:** Provides exercise, testing, or evaluation programs and fitness activities to the community and hospital employees.

*Example of Glossary definitions.*

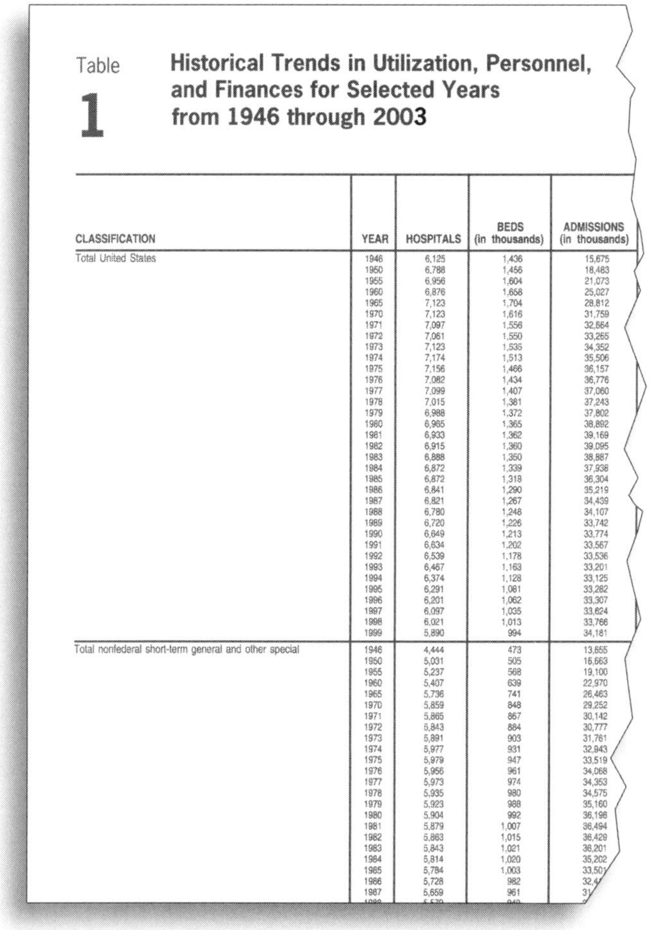

Table **1** **Historical Trends in Utilization, Personnel, and Finances for Selected Years from 1946 through 2003**

| CLASSIFICATION | YEAR | HOSPITALS | BEDS (in thousands) | ADMISSIONS (in thousands) |
|---|---|---|---|---|
| Total United States | 1946 | 6,125 | 1,436 | 15,675 |
| | 1950 | 6,788 | 1,456 | 18,483 |
| | 1955 | 6,956 | 1,604 | 21,073 |
| | 1960 | 6,876 | 1,658 | 25,027 |
| | 1965 | 7,123 | 1,704 | 28,812 |
| | 1970 | 7,123 | 1,616 | 31,759 |
| | 1971 | 7,097 | 1,556 | 32,664 |
| | 1972 | 7,061 | 1,550 | 33,265 |
| | 1973 | 7,123 | 1,535 | 34,352 |
| | 1974 | 7,174 | 1,513 | 35,506 |
| | 1975 | 7,156 | 1,466 | 36,157 |
| | 1976 | 7,082 | 1,434 | 36,776 |
| | 1977 | 7,099 | 1,407 | 37,060 |
| | 1978 | 7,015 | 1,381 | 37,243 |
| | 1979 | 6,988 | 1,372 | 37,802 |
| | 1980 | 6,965 | 1,365 | 38,892 |
| | 1981 | 6,933 | 1,362 | 39,169 |
| | 1982 | 6,915 | 1,360 | 39,095 |
| | 1983 | 6,888 | 1,350 | 38,887 |
| | 1984 | 6,872 | 1,339 | 37,938 |
| | 1985 | 6,872 | 1,318 | 36,304 |
| | 1986 | 6,841 | 1,290 | 35,219 |
| | 1987 | 6,821 | 1,267 | 34,439 |
| | 1988 | 6,780 | 1,248 | 34,107 |
| | 1989 | 6,720 | 1,226 | 33,742 |
| | 1990 | 6,649 | 1,213 | 33,774 |
| | 1991 | 6,634 | 1,202 | 33,567 |
| | 1992 | 6,539 | 1,178 | 33,536 |
| | 1993 | 6,467 | 1,163 | 33,201 |
| | 1994 | 6,374 | 1,128 | 33,125 |
| | 1995 | 6,291 | 1,081 | 33,282 |
| | 1996 | 6,201 | 1,062 | 33,307 |
| | 1997 | 6,097 | 1,035 | 33,624 |
| | 1998 | 6,021 | 1,013 | 33,766 |
| | 1999 | 5,890 | 994 | 34,181 |
| Total nonfederal short-term general and other special | 1946 | 4,444 | 473 | 13,655 |
| | 1950 | 5,031 | 505 | 16,663 |
| | 1955 | 5,237 | 568 | 19,100 |
| | 1960 | 5,407 | 639 | 22,970 |
| | 1965 | 5,736 | 741 | 26,463 |
| | 1970 | 5,859 | 848 | 29,252 |
| | 1971 | 5,865 | 867 | 30,142 |
| | 1972 | 5,843 | 884 | 30,777 |
| | 1973 | 5,891 | 903 | 31,761 |
| | 1974 | 5,977 | 931 | 32,943 |
| | 1975 | 5,979 | 947 | 33,519 |
| | 1976 | 5,956 | 961 | 34,068 |
| | 1977 | 5,973 | 974 | 34,353 |
| | 1978 | 5,935 | 980 | 34,575 |
| | 1979 | 5,923 | 988 | 35,160 |
| | 1980 | 5,904 | 992 | 36,198 |
| | 1981 | 5,879 | 1,007 | 36,494 |
| | 1982 | 5,863 | 1,015 | 36,429 |
| | 1983 | 5,843 | 1,021 | 36,201 |
| | 1984 | 5,814 | 1,020 | 35,202 |
| | 1985 | 5,784 | 1,003 | 33,50 |
| | 1986 | 5,728 | 982 | 32,4 |
| | 1987 | 5,659 | 961 | 31 |

*Example of Table 1*

## Table 1 — Historical Trends in Utilization, Personnel and Finances for Selected Years from 1946 through 2003

**Table 1 at a Glance**

This table is used to evaluate historical data and allows you to examine long-term trends in health care with data dating back more than fifty years. Table 1 reports on all AHA registered hospitals in the United States. One important note: To be considered an AHA-registered hospital, a hospital does not need to be an AHA member. Rather, the hospital must meet particular certification or satisfy a number of requirements. These Registration Requirements immediately follow this section and begin on page (xxvi.)

This table segments the data into various organizational structure categories. Here's a brief look at these different classifications:

- Total United States Hospitals.
- Total Non-Federal Short-term and other special hospitals.
- Community hospitals
- Non-government not-for-profit community hospitals
- Investor-owned (for-profit) community hospitals
- State and local government community hospitals

**Table 1** also provides input on nationwide utilization, personnel and finance trends. You'll find answers to questions such as: *Over the past 25 years, what trends do I see comparing the average length of stay at government and non-government not-for-profit community hospitals and investor-owned for-profit community hospitals?* or *What has been the trend in outpatient visits?*

## Table 2 — 2003 U.S. Registered Hospitals: Utilization, Personnel and Finances

**Table 2 at a Glance**

This table takes a closer look at U.S. Registered Hospitals for 2003. It offers a snapshot of utilization, personnel and finance statistics, and breaks down this information for specialty hospitals. In addition, this is the only table that outlines data on federal hospitals. You'll be able to use this table to better understand the number of beds set-up and staffed, how many personnel and trainees are on the payroll, and what the financial implications of these may be.

# TABLE 3

## TOTAL UNITED STATES

*U.S. Registered Community Hospitals*
*(Nonfederal, short-term general and other special hospitals)*

## Utilization, Personnel, Revenue and Expenses, Community Health Indicators 1999-2003

| | 2003 | 2002 | 2001 | 2000 | 1999 |
|---|---|---|---|---|---|
| **TOTAL FACILITY (Includes Hospital and Nursing Home Units)** | | | | | |
| **Utilization - Inpatient** | | | | | |
| Beds | 839,988 | 853,287 | 862,352 | 872,736 | 902,061 |
| Admissions | 31,811,673 | 31,576,960 | 31,098,959 | 30,945,357 | 30,718,136 |
| Inpatient Days | 191,430,450 | 192,504,015 | 193,747,004 | 199,876,367 | 207,180,278 |
| Average Length of Stay | 6.0 | 6.1 | 6.2 | 6.5 | 6.7 |
| Inpatient Surgeries | 9,735,705 | 9,509,081 | 9,545,612 | 9,700,613 | 9,833,938 |
| Births | 3,726,233 | 3,742,191 | 3,723,871 | 3,764,698 | 3,809,367 |
| **HOSPITAL UNIT (Excludes Separate Nursing Home Units)** | | | | | |
| **Utilization - Inpatient** | | | | | |
| Beds | 758,186 | 769,505 | 782,504 | 794,502 | 824,969 |
| Admissions | 31,265,867 | 31,047,930 | 30,652,820 | 30,577,564 | 30,403,766 |
| Inpatient Days | 165,644,176 | 165,605,620 | 168,189,130 | 174,898,504 | 182,702,882 |
| Average Length of Stay | 5.3 | 5.3 | 5.5 | 5.7 | 6.0 |
| **Personnel** | | | | | |
| Total Full Time | 3,235,153 | 3,183,730 | 3,154,603 | 3,166,729 | 3,147,922 |
| Total Part Time | 1,213,426 | 1,214,232 | 1,153,790 | 1,146,082 | 1,122,957 |
| **Revenue and Expenses - Totals (Includes Inpatient and Outpatient)** | | | | | |
| Total Net Revenue | $333,054,828,642 | $322,459,942,930 | $310,513,291,998 | $298,519,717,355 | $285,858,018,951 |
| Total Expenses | 314,709,758,455 | 301,905,101,393 | 290,128,641,153 | 282,372,557,487 | 272,840,121,437 |

*Example of Table 3. Helps contrast acute and long-term care*

## Table 3 — Total United States

### Table 3 at a Glance

This table provides a look at all U .S. Registered Community Hospitals, in terms of general overview with utilization by inpatient and outpatient, personnel, revenue, expenses and community health indicators. It provides a snapshot of the past five years, allowing you to track emerging trends.

This national information can be compared to local or regional trends, for benchmarking

- Both inpatient and outpatient information is included, for better evaluation of data.
- Reporting by total facility *Includes hospital and Nursing Home Units* and hospital unit only *Excludes Separate Nursing Home Units* helps contrast acute and long-term care.
- Community health indicators can help uncover trends and help determine future facility needs

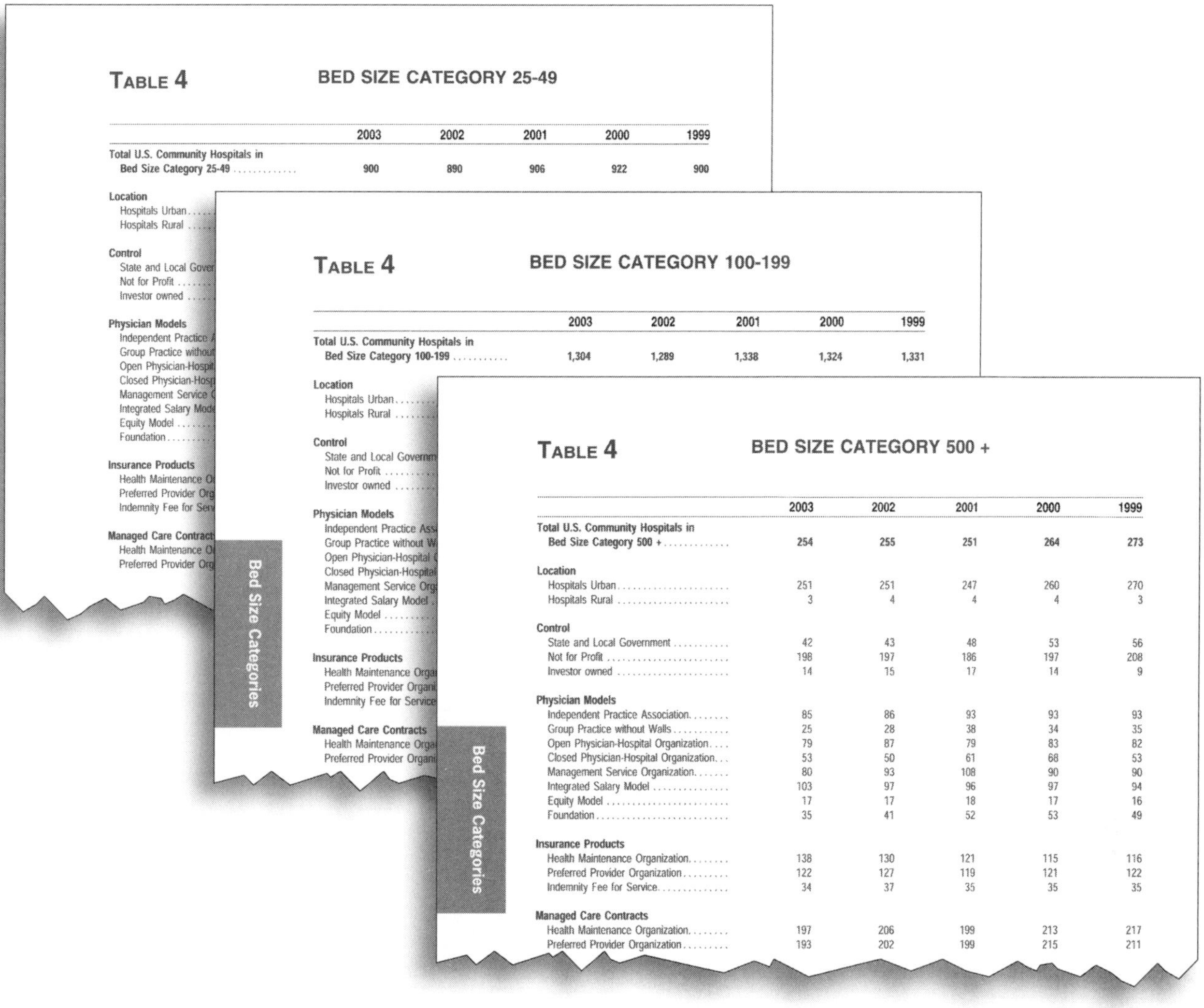
**TABLE 4** BED SIZE CATEGORY 25-49

| | 2003 | 2002 | 2001 | 2000 | 1999 |
|---|---|---|---|---|---|
| **Total U.S. Community Hospitals in Bed Size Category 25-49** | 900 | 890 | 906 | 922 | 900 |

**Location**
Hospitals Urban
Hospitals Rural

**Control**
State and Local Gover
Not for Profit
Investor owned

**Physician Models**
Independent Practice
Group Practice withou
Open Physician-Hospit
Closed Physician-Hosp
Management Service
Integrated Salary Mod
Equity Model
Foundation

**Insurance Products**
Health Maintenance O
Preferred Provider Org
Indemnity Fee for Serv

**Managed Care Contract**
Health Maintenance O
Preferred Provider Org

**TABLE 4** BED SIZE CATEGORY 100-199

| | 2003 | 2002 | 2001 | 2000 | 1999 |
|---|---|---|---|---|---|
| **Total U.S. Community Hospitals in Bed Size Category 100-199** | 1,304 | 1,289 | 1,338 | 1,324 | 1,331 |

**Location**
Hospitals Urban
Hospitals Rural

**Control**
State and Local Governm
Not for Profit
Investor owned

**Physician Models**
Independent Practice Ass
Group Practice without W
Open Physician-Hospital
Closed Physician-Hospital
Management Service Org
Integrated Salary Model
Equity Model
Foundation

**Insurance Products**
Health Maintenance Orga
Preferred Provider Organi
Indemnity Fee for Service

**Managed Care Contracts**
Health Maintenance Orga
Preferred Provider Organi

Bed Size Categories

**TABLE 4** BED SIZE CATEGORY 500 +

| | 2003 | 2002 | 2001 | 2000 | 1999 |
|---|---|---|---|---|---|
| **Total U.S. Community Hospitals in Bed Size Category 500 +** | 254 | 255 | 251 | 264 | 273 |
| **Location** | | | | | |
| Hospitals Urban | 251 | 251 | 247 | 260 | 270 |
| Hospitals Rural | 3 | 4 | 4 | 4 | 3 |
| **Control** | | | | | |
| State and Local Government | 42 | 43 | 48 | 53 | 56 |
| Not for Profit | 198 | 197 | 186 | 197 | 208 |
| Investor owned | 14 | 15 | 17 | 14 | 9 |
| **Physician Models** | | | | | |
| Independent Practice Association | 85 | 86 | 93 | 93 | 93 |
| Group Practice without Walls | 25 | 28 | 38 | 34 | 35 |
| Open Physician-Hospital Organization | 79 | 87 | 79 | 83 | 82 |
| Closed Physician-Hospital Organization | 53 | 50 | 61 | 68 | 53 |
| Management Service Organization | 80 | 93 | 108 | 90 | 90 |
| Integrated Salary Model | 103 | 97 | 96 | 97 | 94 |
| Equity Model | 17 | 17 | 18 | 17 | 16 |
| Foundation | 35 | 41 | 52 | 53 | 49 |
| **Insurance Products** | | | | | |
| Health Maintenance Organization | 138 | 130 | 121 | 115 | 116 |
| Preferred Provider Organization | 122 | 127 | 119 | 121 | 122 |
| Indemnity Fee for Service | 34 | 37 | 35 | 35 | 35 |
| **Managed Care Contracts** | | | | | |
| Health Maintenance Organization | 197 | 206 | 199 | 213 | 217 |
| Preferred Provider Organization | 193 | 202 | 199 | 215 | 211 |

Bed Size Categories

*Example of Table 4. Compares facilities with peers.*

## Table 4 — Bed Size Categories

**Table 4 at a Glance**

This table provides a look at all U.S. Registered Community Hospitals, broken down by bed size. The table includes general overview, utilization, personnel, and revenue and expense information. These categories of bed sizes were developed by the AHA, and have become an industry standard. By categorizing each facility into a peer group, this table provides a snapshot of the past five years allowing you to compare facilities with their peers.

## Table 5

### U.S. CENSUS DIVISION 2: MIDDLE ATLANTIC

*U.S. Registered Community Hospitals*
*(Nonfederal, short-term general and other special hospitals)*

### Utilization, Personnel, Revenue and Expenses, Community Health Indicators 1999-2003

| | 2003 | 2002 | 2001 | 2000 | 1999 |
|---|---|---|---|---|---|
| **COMMUNITY HEALTH INDICATORS PER 1000 POPULATION** | | | | | |
| Total Population (in thousands) | 38,292 | 38,216 | 38,184 | 38,147 | 38,108 |
| **Inpatient** | | | | | |
| Beds | 3.6 | 3.8 | 3.9 | 4.0 | 4.1 |
| Admissions | 135.8 | 136.7 | 136.2 | 138.3 | 137.4 |
| Inpatient Days | 963.5 | 988.8 | 1,019.0 | 1,093.8 | 1,145.0 |
| Inpatient Surgeries | 42.2 | 41.4 | 41.2 | 42.7 | 43.6 |
| Births | 13.0 | 13.2 | 13.6 | 13.7 | 14.3 |
| **Outpatient** | | | | | |
| Emergency Outpatient Visits | 367.7 | 362.0 | 363.4 | 379.5 | 360.1 |
| Other Outpatient Visits | 1,970.9 | 1,802.3 | 1,767.7 | 1,680.3 | 1,573.9 |
| Total Outpatient Visits | 2,338.6 | 2,164.3 | 2,131.1 | 2,059.8 | 1,934.0 |
| Outpatient Surgeries | 67.8 | 62.4 | 59.9 | 55.4 | 53.5 |
| **Expense per Capita (per person)** | $1,494.9 | $1,462.7 | $1,428.6 | $1,429.8 | $1,369.2 |

*Example of Table 5. Uncovers trends to determine future facility needs.*

## Table 5 — U.S. Census Divisions

**Table 5 at a Glance**
This table provides a look at all U.S. Registered Community Hospitals, broken down by Census Division. The table includes general overview, utilization, personnel, and expenses, and community health indicator information. It provides a snapshot of the past five years, allowing you to track trends on a regional level. In addition, this allows you to compare this data to other population based health indicators, offering a more comprehensive look than the survey data alone. Community health indicators can help uncover trends and help determine future facility needs.

## Table 6 — States

**Table 6 at a Glance**
This table provides a look at all U.S. Registered Community Hospitals, broken down by State. The table includes general overview, utilization, personnel, revenue and expenses, and community health indicator information. It provides a snapshot of the past five years, allowing you to track trends on a state level.

**Note:**
You can use the information in tables 3,4,5 and 6 to make accurate comparisons across Total U.S., Bed Size Category, Census Division and State.

## Table 7 — 2003 Facilities and Services in the U.S. Census Divisions and States

### Table 7 at a Glance

This table examines facilities and services by both Census Division and State. A comprehensive alphabetical guide helps make each facility or service easy to find. This table will allow you to better understand what service lines are emerging and how many facilities offer a particular service in a discrete state or region.

**Table7** (Continued)

| CLASSIFICATION | HOSPITALS REPORTING | CASE MANAGEMENT Number | CASE MANAGEMENT Percent | CHILDREN WELLNESS PROGRAM Number | CHILDREN WELLNESS PROGRAM Percent | CHIROPRACTIC SERVICES Number | CHIROPRACTIC SERVICES Percent | COMMUNITY OUTREACH Number | COMMUNITY OUTREACH Percent |
|---|---|---|---|---|---|---|---|---|---|
| UNITED STATES | 4,797 | 2,980 | 62.1 | 783 | 16.3 | 61 | 1.3 | 2,725 | 56.8 |
| COMMUNITY HOSPITALS | 4,113 | 2,620 | 63.7 | 742 | 18.0 | 53 | 1.3 | 2,491 | 60.6 |
| CENSUS DIVISION 1, NEW ENGLAND | 230 | 157 | 68.3 | 63 | 27.4 | 6 | 2.6 | 169 | 73.5 |
| Connecticut | 42 | 32 | 76.2 | 15 | 35.7 | 3 | 7.1 | 32 | 76.2 |
| Maine | 39 | 20 | 51.3 | 9 | 23.1 | 0 | 0.0 | 30 | 76.9 |
| Massachusetts | 85 | 64 | 75.3 | 21 | 24.7 | 2 | 2.4 | 62 | 72.9 |
| New Hampshire | 31 | 20 | 64.5 | 10 | 32.3 | 0 | 0.0 | 23 | 74.2 |
| Rhode Island | 16 | 12 | 75.0 | 4 | 25.0 | 1 | 6.3 | 11 | 68.8 |
| Vermont | 17 | 9 | 52.9 | 4 | 23.5 | 0 | 0.0 | 11 | 64.7 |
| CENSUS DIVISION 2, MIDDLE ATLANTIC | 461 | 344 | 74.6 | 143 | 31.0 | 7 | 1.5 | 345 | 74.8 |
| New Jersey | 71 | 66 | 93.0 | 29 | 40.8 | 2 | 2.8 | 60 | 84.5 |
| New York | 194 | 146 | 75.3 | 61 | 31.4 | 2 | 1.0 | 140 | 72.2 |
| Pennsylvania | 196 | 132 | 67.3 | 53 | 27.0 | 3 | 1.5 | 145 | 74.0 |
| CENSUS DIVISION 3, SOUTH ATLANTIC | 734 | 484 | 66.9 | 123 | 17.0 | 8 | 1.1 | 450 | 62.2 |
| Delaware | 9 | 5 | 55.6 | 4 | 44.4 | 0 | 0.0 | 5 | 55.6 |
| District of Columbia | 17 | 13 | 76.5 | 3 | 17.6 | 2 | 11.8 | 10 | 58.8 |
| Florida | 138 | 117 | 84.8 | 23 | 16.7 | 3 | 2.2 | 89 | 64.5 |
| Georgia | 144 | 87 | 60.4 | 19 | 13.2 | 0 | 0.0 | 75 | 52.1 |
| Maryland | 64 | 47 | 73.4 | 10 | 15.6 | 1 | 1.6 | 46 | 71.9 |
| North Carolina | 119 | 84 | 70.6 | 20 | 16.8 | 1 | 0.8 | 71 | 59.7 |
| South Carolina | 71 | 25 | 35.2 | 25 | 35.2 | 0 | 0.0 | 64 | 90.1 |
| Virginia | 98 | 72 | 73.5 | 9 | 9.2 | 0 | 0.0 | 55 | 56.1 |
| West Virginia | 64 | 34 | 53.1 | 10 | 15.6 | 1 | 1.6 | 35 | 54.7 |
| CENSUS DIVISION 4, EAST NORTH CENTRAL | 741 | 478 | 64.5 | 140 | 18.9 | 15 | 2.0 | 464 | 62.6 |
| Illinois | 193 | 128 | 66.3 | 45 | 23.3 | 5 | 2.6 | 132 | 68.4 |
| Indiana | 110 | 68 | 61.8 | 20 | 18.2 | 1 | 0.9 | 76 | 69.1 |
| Michigan | 148 | 92 | 62.2 | 32 | 21.6 | 0 | 0.0 | 101 | 68.2 |
| Ohio | 156 | 108 | 69.2 | 34 | 21.8 | 9 | 5.8 | 109 | 69.9 |
| Wisconsin | 134 | 82 | 61.2 | 9 | 6.7 | 0 | 0.0 | 46 | 34.3 |
| CENSUS DIVISION 5, EAST SOUTH CENTRAL | 403 | 229 | 56.8 | 26 | 6.5 | 3 | 0.7 | 198 | 49.1 |
| Alabama | 94 | 60 | 63.8 | 5 | 5.3 | 1 | 1.1 | 52 | 55.3 |
| Kentucky | 104 | 64 | 61.5 | 12 | 11.5 | 0 | 0.0 | 49 | 47.1 |
| Mississippi | 106 | 45 | 42.5 | 0 | 0.0 | 0 | 0.0 | 56 | 52.8 |
| Tennessee | 99 | 60 | 60.6 | 9 | 9.1 | 2 | 2.0 | 41 | 41.4 |
| CENSUS DIVISION 6, WEST NORTH CENTRAL | 703 | 308 | 43.8 | 85 | 12.1 | 11 | 1.6 | 370 | 52.6 |
| Iowa | 126 | 68 | 54.0 | 25 | 19.8 | 2 | 1.6 | 68 | 54.0 |
| Kansas | 139 | 48 | 34.5 | 12 | 8.6 | 3 | 2.2 | 46 | 33.1 |
| Minnesota | 115 | 33 | 28.7 | 9 | 7.8 | 1 | 0.9 | 74 | 64.3 |
| Missouri | 151 | 106 | 70.2 | 23 | 15.2 | 4 | 2.6 | 97 | 64.2 |
| Nebraska | 81 | 28 | 34.6 | 5 | 6.2 | 0 | 0.0 | 45 | 55.6 |
| North Dakota | 35 | 7 | 20.0 | 5 | 14.3 | 1 | 2.9 | 16 | 45.7 |
| South Dakota | 56 | 18 | 32.1 | 6 | 10.7 | 0 | 0.0 | 24 | 42.9 |
| CENSUS DIVISION 7, WEST SOUTH CENTRAL | 777 | 492 | 63.3 | 76 | 9.8 | 4 | 0.5 | 316 | 40.7 |
| Arkansas | 65 | 44 | 67.7 | 5 | 7.7 | 0 | 0.0 | 27 | 41.5 |
| Louisiana | 111 | 70 | 63.1 | 18 | 16.2 | 1 | 0.9 | 44 | 39.6 |
| Oklahoma | 115 | 60 | 52.2 | 9 | 7.8 | 1 | 0.9 | 49 | 42.6 |
| Texas | 486 | 318 | 65.4 | 44 | 9.1 | 2 | 0.4 | 196 | 40.3 |
| CENSUS DIVISION 8, MOUNTAIN | 333 | 194 | 58.3 | 47 | 14.1 | 2 | 0.6 | 162 | 48.6 |
| Arizona | 54 | 44 | 81.5 | 8 | 14.8 | 0 | 0.0 | 25 | 46.3 |
| Colorado | 59 | 40 | 67.8 | 10 | 16.9 | 1 | 1.7 | 41 | 69.5 |
| Idaho | 35 | 17 | 48.6 | 5 | 14.3 | 0 | 0.0 | 19 | 54.3 |
| Montana | 54 | 12 | 22.2 | 7 | 13.0 | 0 | 0.0 | 14 | [illegible] |
| Nevada | 20 | 15 | 75.0 | 3 | 15.0 | 0 | 0.0 | 10 | 50.0 |
| New Mexico | 40 | 22 | 55.0 | 7 | 17.5 | 0 | 0.0 | 18 | 45.0 |
| Utah | 44 | 26 | 59.1 | 6 | 13.6 | 1 | 2.3 | 20 | 45.5 |
| Wyoming | 27 | 18 | 66.7 | 1 | 3.7 | 0 | 0.0 | 15 | 55.6 |
| CENSUS DIVISION 9, PACIFIC | 425 | 294 | 69.2 | 80 | 18.8 | 5 | 1.2 | 251 | 59.1 |
| Alaska | 15 | 9 | 60.0 | 1 | 6.7 | 0 | 0.0 | 6 | 40.0 |
| California | 280 | 209 | 74.6 | 55 | 19.6 | 3 | 1.1 | 173 | 61.8 |
| Hawaii | 16 | 10 | 62.5 | 3 | 18.8 | 0 | 0.0 | 8 | 50.0 |
| Oregon | 52 | 28 | 53.8 | 11 | 21.2 | 0 | 0.0 | 31 | [illegible] |
| Washington | 62 | 38 | 61.3 | 10 | 16.1 | 2 | 3.2 | 33 | [illegible] |

*Example of Table 7.*

This collection of facilities and services information data is unique to *AHA Hospital Statistics* and the list is continually growing. Recent additions include:

- Airborne infection isolation room
- Alzheimer center
- Bariatric/weight control services
- Chaplaincy/pastoral care services
- Cardiology services
- Chaplaincy/pastoral care services
- Chemotherapy
- Complementary Medicine (i.e. Alternative Medicine)
- Electron beam computed tomography
- Fertility clinic
- Gamma Knife
- Intensity-modulated Radiation therapy
- Neurological services
- Swing bed
- Genetic Testing/Counseling
- Multislice spiral computed tomography
- Orthopedic service
- Wound management

These new categories reflect the trends as hospitals expand their service lines to mirror the needs of their patients. For example, services such as acupuncture or massage therapy are now accounted for in the Complementary Medicine service item.

This table can answer questions such as: *What percentage of hospitals in the United States offer complementary medicine or wound management?* or *How are these new services distributed by state?*

## Table 8 — Utilization, Personnel and Finances in Community Hospitals by MSAs for 2003.

### Table 8 at a Glance

This table provides a look at all U.S. Registered Community Hospitals, broken down by Metropolitan Statistical Area (MSA). The table includes general overview, utilization, personnel, and finance information. It provides a snapshot of the past year.

### Additional Resources

Again, in the back of the book you will find the comprehensive glossary and the 2003 annual survey questionnaire. The survey itself can be a valuable resource to understanding what was asked in order to gather the data in the book. This survey is also used to produce the *AHA Guide®* and AHA Annual Survey Database™.

# Registration Requirements for Hospitals

## AHA-Registered Hospitals

Any institution that can be classified as a hospital according to the requirements may be registered if it so desires. Membership in the American Hospital Association is not a prerequisite.

The American Hospital Association may, at the sole discretion of the Executive Committee of the Board of Trustees, grant, deny, or withdraw the registration of an institution.

An institution may be registered by the American Hospital Association as a hospital if it is accredited as a hospital by the Joint Commission on Accreditation of Healthcare Organizations or is certified as a provider of acute services under Title 18 of the Social Security Act and has provided the Association with documents verifying the accreditation or certification.

In lieu of the preceding accreditation or certification, an institution licensed as a hospital by the appropriate state agency may be registered by AHA as a hospital by meeting the following alternative requirements:

**Function**: The primary function of the institution is to provide patient services, diagnostic and therapeutic, for particular or general medical conditions.

1. The institution shall maintain at least six inpatient beds, which shall be continuously available for the care of patients who are nonrelated and who stay on the average in excess of 24 hours per admission.

2. The institution shall be constructed, equipped, and maintained to ensure the health and safety of patients and to provide uncrowded, sanitary facilities for the treatment of patients.

3. There shall be an identifiable governing authority legally and morally responsible for the conduct of the hospital.

4. There shall be a chief executive to whom the governing authority delegates the continuous responsibility for the operation of the hospital in accordance with establish policy.

5. There shall be an organized medical staff of fully licensed physicians* that may include other licensed individuals permitted by law and by the hospital to provide patient care services independently in the hospital. The medical staff shall be accountable to the governing authority for maintaining proper standards of medical care, and it shall be governed by bylaws adopted by said staff and approved by the governing authority.

6. Each patient shall be admitted on the authority of a member of the medical staff who has been granted the privilege to admit patients to inpatient services in accordance with state law and criteria for standards of medical care established by the individual medical staff. Each patient's general medical condition is the responsibility of a qualified physician member of the medical staff. When nonphysician members of the medical staff are granted privileges to admit patients, provision is made for prompt medical evaluation of these patients by a qualified physician. Any graduate of a foreign medical school who is permitted to assume responsibilities for patient care shall possess a valid license to practice medicine, or shall be certified by the Educational Commission for Foreign Medical Graduates, or shall have qualified for and have successfully completed an academic year of supervised clinical training under the direction of a medical school approved by the Liaison Committee on GAT Medical Education.

7. Registered nurse supervision and other nursing services are continuous.

8. A current and complete‡ medical record shall be maintained by the institution for each patient and shall be available for reference.

9. Pharmacy service shall be maintained in the institution and shall be supervised by a registered pharmacist.

10. The institution shall provide patients with food service that meets their nutritional and therapeutic requirements; special diets shall also be available.

## Types of Hospitals

In addition to meeting these 10 general registration requirements, hospitals are registered as one of four types of hospitals: general, special, rehabilitation and chronic disease, or psychiatric. The following type of hospital and special requirements for registration are employed:

## General

The primary function of the institution is to provide patient services, diagnostic and therapeutic, for a variety of medical conditions. A general hospital also shall provide:

- diagnostic x-ray services with facilities and staff for a variety of procedures
- clinical laboratory service with facilities and staff for a variety of procedures and with anatomical pathology services regularly and conveniently available
- operating room service with facilities and staff.

## Special

The primary function of the institution is to provide diagnostic and treatment services for patients who have specified medical conditions, both surgical and nonsurgical. A special hospital also shall provide:

- such diagnostic and treatment services as may be determined by the Executive Committee of the Board of Trustees of the American Hospital Association to be appropriate for the specified medical conditions for which medical services are provided shall be maintained in the institution with suitable facilities and staff. If such conditions do not normally require diagnostic x-ray service, laboratory service, or operating room service, and if any such services are therefore not maintained in the institution, there shall be written arrangements to make them available to patients requiring them.
- clinical laboratory services capable of providing tissue diagnosis when offering pregnancy termination services.

## Rehabilitation and Chronic Disease

The primary function of the institution is to provide diagnostic and treatment services to handicapped or disabled individuals requiring restorative and adjustive services. A rehabilitation and chronic disease hospital also shall provide:

- arrangements for diagnostic x-ray services, as required, on a regular and conveniently available basis
- arrangements for clinical laboratory service, as required on a regular and conveniently available basis
- arrangements for operating room service, as required, on a regular and conveniently available basis
- a physical therapy service with suitable facilities and staff in the institution
- an occupational therapy service with suitable facilities and staff in the institution
- arrangements for psychological and social work services on a regular and conveniently available basis

* Physician–Term used to describe an individual with an M.D. or D.O. degree who is fully licensed to practice medicine in all its phases.

‡ The completed records in general shall contain at least the following: the patient's identifying data and consent forms, medical history, record of physical examination, physicians' progress notes, operative notes, nurses' notes, routine x-ray and laboratory reports, doctors' orders, and final diagnosis.

- arrangements for educational and vocational services on a regular and conveniently available basis
- written arrangements with a general hospital for the transfer of patients who require medical, obstetrical, or surgical services not available in the institution.

### Psychiatric

The primary function of the institution is to provide diagnostic and treatment services for patients who have psychiatric-related illnesses. A psychiatric hospital also shall provide:

- arrangements for clinical laboratory service, as required, on a regular and conveniently available basis
- arrangements for diagnostic x-ray services, as required on a regular and conveniently available basis
- psychiatric, psychological, and social work service with facilities and staff in the institution
- arrangements for electroencephalograph services, as required, on a regular and conveniently available basis.
- written arrangements with a general hospital for the transfer of patients who require medical, obstetrical, or surgical services not available in the institution.

The American Hospital Association may, at the sole discretion of the Executive Committee of the Board of Trustees, grant, deny, or withdraw the registration of an institution.

### AOHA-Listed Hospitals

The list of osteopathic hospitals includes both members and nonmembers of the American Osteopathic Healthcare Association.

# Data Comparability

The economic climate, demographic characteristics, personnel issues, and health care financing and payment policies differ by region, state, and city across the country. *Differences in these factors must be taken into account when using the data.* In addition, the profiles of hospitals across comparison groups vary. For example, states will differ in terms of the number and percentage of hospitals by size, ownership, services provided, types of patients treated, and so forth. *Differences in these variables must also be taken into consideration when doing a comparative analysis.*

# Notes on the Survey

The 2005 edition of *AHA Hospital Statistics™* draws its data from the 2003 AHA Annual Survey of Hospitals. It is the statistical complement to the 2005 edition of the *AHA Guide®*, which contains selected data about individual hospitals.

The AHA Survey was mailed to all hospitals, both AHA-registered and nonregistered, in the U.S. and its associated areas: American Samoa, Guam, the Marshall Islands, Puerto Rico, and the Virgin Island. U.S. government hospitals located outside the U.S. were not included. Overall, the average response rate over the past five years has been approximately 85 percent.

## Reporting Period

In completing the survey, hospitals were requested to report data for a full year, in accord with their fiscal year, ending in 2003. The statistical table present data reported or estimated for a 12-month period, except for data on personnel, which represent situations as they existed at the end of the reporting period.

## Respondents

Data for Tables 1 and 2 include 5,764 AHA-registered hospitals in the U.S. Data on community hospitals (nonfederal, short-term general and other special hospitals) only are presented in Tables 3-6, and Table 8.

It is important to note that the AHA-registered hospitals included in *AHA Hospital Statistics* are not necessarily identical to those included in *AHA Guide*. The institutions listed in the 2005 edition of *AHA Guide* include all of those institutions registered as of April 2003. Tables 1-6 in *AHA Hospital Statistics* present data for AHA-registered hospitals that were in operation during the 12-month reporting period ending 2003.

## Estimates

Estimates were made of data for nonreporting hospitals and for reporting hospitals that submitted incomplete AHA Annual Survey questionnaires. Estimates were not made for beds, bassinets and facilities and services. Data for beds and bassinets of nonreporting hospitals were based on the most recent information from those hospitals. (Note that in all statistical tables, whenever bed-size categories are listed, all eight categories appear, whether or not there are hospitals in every category.)

Missing revenue, expenses, admissions, births, inpatient days, surgical operations, outpatient visits, and full-time-equivalent personnel values are estimates from regression models. For all other variables the estimates were based on ratios such as per bed averages derived from data reported by hospitals similar in size, control, major service provided, length of stay, and geographical characteristics to the hospitals that did not report this information.

# Tables 1–2

Table

# 1

## Historical Trends in Utilization, Personnel, and Finances for Selected Years from 1946 through 2003

*Data are for all AHA-registered hospitals in the United States. Data are estimated for nonreporting hospitals with the exception of newborn and outpatient data before 1972. Personnel data exclude residents, interns, and students from 1952 on; personnel data include full-time personnel and full-time equivalents for part-time personnel from 1954 on. As a result of the AHA Annual Survey validation process, the New York state expense data from 1976 were revised after the 1977 edition was published. The revised figures are included below. In order to provide trend data on a consistent basis, the 1970 and 1971 psychiatric and long-term data have been slightly modified. The 1982 FTE figures have updated to provide the most accurate data possible.*

| | | | | | | | | | NEWBORNS | | FTE PERSONNEL | | TOTAL EXPENSES | | |
|---|---|---|---|---|---|---|---|---|---|---|---|---|---|---|---|
| CLASSIFICATION | YEAR | HOSPITALS | BEDS (in thousands) | ADMISSIONS (in thousands) | AVERAGE DAILY CENSUS (in thousands) | ADJUSTED AVERAGE DAILY CENSUS (in thousands) | AVERAGE STAY (days) | OUTPATIENT VISITS (in thousands) | Bassinets | Births | Number (in thousands) | Per 100 Adjusted Census | Amount (In Millions of dollars) | Adjusted per Inpatient Stay (dollars) | Adjusted per Inpatient Day (dollars) |
| Total United States | 1946 | 6,125 | 1,436 | 15,675 | 1,142 | — | — | — | 85,585 | 2,135,327 | 830 | — | $1,963 | — | — |
| | 1950 | 6,788 | 1,456 | 18,483 | 1,253 | — | — | — | 90,101 | 2,742,780 | 1,058 | — | $3,651 | — | — |
| | 1955 | 6,956 | 1,604 | 21,073 | 1,363 | — | — | — | 98,823 | 3,476,753 | 1,301 | — | $5,594 | — | — |
| | 1960 | 6,876 | 1,658 | 25,027 | 1,402 | — | — | — | 102,764 | 3,835,735 | 1,598 | — | $8,421 | — | — |
| | 1965 | 7,123 | 1,704 | 28,812 | 1,403 | — | — | 125,793 | 101,287 | 3,565,344 | 1,952 | — | $12,948 | — | — |
| | 1970 | 7,123 | 1,616 | 31,759 | 1,298 | — | — | 181,370 | 97,128 | 3,537,000 | 2,537 | — | $25,556 | — | — |
| | 1971 | 7,097 | 1,556 | 32,664 | 1,237 | — | — | 199,725 | 94,344 | 3,464,513 | 2,589 | — | $28,812 | — | — |
| | 1972 | 7,061 | 1,550 | 33,265 | 1,209 | — | — | 219,182 | 92,960 | 3,231,875 | 2,671 | — | $32,667 | — | — |
| | 1973 | 7,123 | 1,535 | 34,352 | 1,189 | — | — | 233,555 | 90,071 | 3,087,210 | 2,769 | — | $36,290 | — | — |
| | 1974 | 7,174 | 1,513 | 35,506 | 1,167 | — | — | 250,481 | 88,269 | 3,043,386 | 2,919 | — | $41,406 | — | — |
| | 1975 | 7,156 | 1,466 | 36,157 | 1,125 | — | — | 254,844 | 86,875 | 3,091,629 | 3,023 | — | $48,706 | — | — |
| | 1976 | 7,082 | 1,434 | 36,776 | 1,090 | — | — | 270,951 | 85,284 | 3,067,063 | 3,108 | — | $56,005 | — | — |
| | 1977 | 7,099 | 1,407 | 37,060 | 1,066 | — | — | 263,775 | 83,193 | 3,223,699 | 3,213 | — | $63,630 | — | — |
| | 1978 | 7,015 | 1,381 | 37,243 | 1,042 | — | — | 263,606 | 80,650 | 3,250,373 | 3,280 | — | $70,927 | — | — |
| | 1979 | 6,988 | 1,372 | 37,802 | 1,043 | — | — | 262,009 | 79,720 | 3,376,467 | 3,382 | — | $79,796 | — | — |
| | 1980 | 6,965 | 1,365 | 38,892 | 1,060 | — | — | 262,951 | 79,842 | 3,500,043 | 3,492 | — | $91,886 | — | — |
| | 1981 | 6,933 | 1,362 | 39,169 | 1,061 | — | — | 265,332 | 78,823 | 3,558,274 | 3,661 | — | $107,146 | — | — |
| | 1982 | 6,915 | 1,360 | 39,095 | 1,053 | — | — | 313,667 | 77,998 | 3,615,751 | 3,746 | — | $123,219 | — | — |
| | 1983 | 6,888 | 1,350 | 38,887 | 1,028 | — | — | 273,168 | 77,837 | 3,596,146 | 3,707 | — | $136,315 | — | — |
| | 1984 | 6,872 | 1,339 | 37,938 | 970 | — | — | 276,566 | 77,845 | 3,563,106 | 3,630 | — | $144,114 | — | — |
| | 1985 | 6,872 | 1,318 | 36,304 | 910 | — | — | 282,140 | 77,202 | 3,630,961 | 3,625 | — | $153,327 | — | — |
| | 1986 | 6,841 | 1,290 | 35,219 | 883 | — | — | 294,634 | 76,002 | 3,680,178 | 3,647 | — | $165,194 | — | — |
| | 1987 | 6,821 | 1,267 | 34,439 | 873 | — | — | 310,707 | 74,770 | 3,698,294 | 3,742 | — | $178,662 | — | — |
| | 1988 | 6,780 | 1,248 | 34,107 | 863 | — | — | 336,208 | 72,568 | 3,794,369 | 3,839 | — | $196,704 | — | — |
| | 1989 | 6,720 | 1,226 | 33,742 | 853 | — | — | 352,248 | 71,491 | 3,920,384 | 3,937 | — | $214,886 | — | — |
| | 1990 | 6,649 | 1,213 | 33,774 | 844 | — | — | 368,184 | 70,539 | 4,046,704 | 4,063 | — | $234,870 | — | — |
| | 1991 | 6,634 | 1,202 | 33,567 | 827 | — | — | 387,675 | 69,464 | 4,047,504 | 4,165 | — | $258,508 | — | — |
| | 1992 | 6,539 | 1,178 | 33,536 | 807 | — | — | 417,874 | 69,052 | 4,007,179 | 4,236 | — | $282,531 | — | — |
| | 1993 | 6,467 | 1,163 | 33,201 | 783 | — | — | 435,619 | 67,911 | 3,949,788 | 4,289 | — | $301,538 | — | — |
| | 1994 | 6,374 | 1,128 | 33,125 | 745 | — | — | 453,584 | 67,311 | 3,886,667 | 4,270 | — | $310,834 | — | — |
| | 1995 | 6,291 | 1,081 | 33,282 | 710 | — | — | 483,195 | 66,256 | 3,833,132 | 4,273 | — | $320,252 | — | — |
| | 1996 | 6,201 | 1,062 | 33,307 | 685 | — | — | 505,455 | 65,138 | 3,790,678 | 4,276 | — | $330,531 | — | — |
| | 1997 | 6,097 | 1,035 | 33,624 | 673 | — | — | 520,600 | 64,649 | 3,811,522 | 4,333 | — | $342,334 | — | — |
| | 1998 | 6,021 | 1,013 | 33,766 | 662 | — | — | 545,481 | 63,485 | 3,795,212 | 4,407 | — | $355,450 | — | — |
| | 1999 | 5,890 | 994 | 34,181 | 657 | — | — | 573,461 | 62,714 | 3,829,881 | 4,369 | — | $372,933 | — | — |
| | 2000 | 5,810 | 984 | 34,891 | 650 | — | — | 592,673 | 61,915 | 3,940,017 | 4,454 | — | $395,391 | — | — |
| | 2001 | 5,801 | 987 | 35,644 | 658 | — | — | 612,276 | 61,527 | 3,929,733 | 4,535 | — | $426,849 | — | — |
| | 2002 | 5,794 | 976 | 36,326 | 662 | — | — | 640,515 | 62,151 | 3,934,421 | 4,610 | — | $462,222 | — | — |
| | 2003 | 5,764 | 965 | 36,611 | 657 | — | — | 648,560 | 60,699 | 3,976,886 | 4,651 | — | $498,104 | — | — |

**Table 1** (Continued)

| CLASSIFICATION | YEAR | HOSPITALS | BEDS (in thousands) | ADMISSIONS (in thousands) | AVERAGE DAILY CENSUS (in thousands) | ADJUSTED AVERAGE DAILY CENSUS (in thousands) | AVERAGE LENGTH OF STAY (days) | OUTPATIENT VISITS (in thousands) | NEWBORNS | | FTE PERSONNEL | | EXPENSES | | |
|---|---|---|---|---|---|---|---|---|---|---|---|---|---|---|---|
| | | | | | | | | | Bassinets | Births | Number (in thousands) | Per 100 Adjusted Census | Amount (In Millions of dollars) | Adjusted per Inpatient Stay (dollars) | Adjusted per Inpatient Day (dollars) |
| Total nonfederal short-term general and other special | 1946 | 4,444 | 473 | 13,655 | 341 | — | 9.1 | — | 80,987 | 2,087,503 | 505 | — | $1,169 | — | — |
| | 1950 | 5,031 | 505 | 16,663 | 372 | — | 8.1 | — | 86,019 | 2,660,982 | 662 | — | $2,120 | — | — |
| | 1955 | 5,237 | 568 | 19,100 | 407 | — | 7.8 | — | 93,868 | 3,304,451 | 826 | — | $3,434 | — | — |
| | 1960 | 5,407 | 639 | 22,970 | 477 | — | 7.6 | — | 98,127 | 3,678,051 | 1,080 | — | $5,617 | — | — |
| | 1965 | 5,736 | 741 | 26,463 | 563 | 620 | 7.8 | 92,631 | 96,782 | 3,413,370 | 1,386 | 224 | $9,147 | $316.37 | $40.56 |
| | 1970 | 5,859 | 848 | 29,252 | 662 | 727 | 8.2 | 133,545 | 93,079 | 3,403,064 | 1,929 | 265 | $19,560 | $604.59 | $73.73 |
| | 1971 | 5,865 | 867 | 30,142 | 665 | 736 | 8.0 | 148,423 | 90,444 | 3,337,605 | 1,999 | 272 | $22,400 | $667.44 | $83.43 |
| | 1972 | 5,843 | 884 | 30,777 | 664 | 739 | 7.9 | 166,983 | 89,315 | 3,119,446 | 2,056 | 278 | $25,549 | $747.42 | $94.61 |
| | 1973 | 5,891 | 903 | 31,761 | 681 | 768 | 7.8 | 178,939 | 86,851 | 2,987,089 | 2,149 | 280 | $28,496 | $793.88 | $101.78 |
| | 1974 | 5,977 | 931 | 32,943 | 701 | 793 | 7.8 | 194,838 | 85,208 | 2,947,342 | 2,289 | 289 | $32,751 | $883.04 | $113.21 |
| | 1975 | 5,979 | 947 | 33,519 | 708 | 806 | 7.7 | 196,311 | 83,834 | 2,998,590 | 2,399 | 298 | $39,110 | $1,024.72 | $133.08 |
| | 1976 | 5,956 | 961 | 34,068 | 715 | 816 | 7.7 | 207,725 | 82,307 | 2,962,305 | 2,483 | 304 | $45,402 | $1,172.25 | $152.24 |
| | 1977 | 5,973 | 974 | 34,353 | 717 | 820 | 7.6 | 204,238 | 80,228 | 3,117,756 | 2,581 | 315 | $51,832 | $1,316.70 | $173.25 |
| | 1978 | 5,935 | 980 | 34,575 | 720 | 841 | 7.6 | 204,461 | 78,090 | 3,156,570 | 2,662 | 323 | $58,348 | $1,470.13 | $193.81 |
| | 1979 | 5,923 | 988 | 35,160 | 729 | 841 | 7.6 | 203,873 | 77,277 | 3,287,157 | 2,762 | 328 | $66,184 | $1,631.16 | $215.75 |
| | 1980 | 5,904 | 992 | 36,198 | 748 | 861 | 7.6 | 206,752 | 77,539 | 3,408,699 | 2,879 | 334 | $76,970 | $1,844.19 | $244.44 |
| | 1981 | 5,879 | 1,007 | 36,494 | 764 | 876 | 7.6 | 206,729 | 76,567 | 3,465,683 | 3,039 | 347 | $90,739 | $2,167.70 | $283.94 |
| | 1982 | 5,863 | 1,015 | 36,429 | 763 | 882 | 7.6 | 250,888 | 75,739 | 3,514,761 | 3,110 | 353 | $105,094 | $2,493.09 | $326.68 |
| | 1983 | 5,843 | 1,021 | 36,201 | 750 | 869 | 7.6 | 213,995 | 75,471 | 3,490,629 | 3,102 | 357 | $116,632 | $2,775.55 | $368.01 |
| | 1984 | 5,814 | 1,020 | 35,202 | 703 | 824 | 7.3 | 216,474 | 75,587 | 3,456,467 | 3,023 | 367 | $123,550 | $2,984.00 | $409.85 |
| | 1985 | 5,784 | 1,003 | 33,501 | 650 | 780 | 7.1 | 222,773 | 74,899 | 3,521,296 | 3,003 | 385 | $130,700 | $3,238.94 | $459.57 |
| | 1986 | 5,728 | 982 | 32,410 | 631 | 774 | 7.1 | 234,270 | 73,688 | 3,584,530 | 3,032 | 392 | $140,907 | $3,529.60 | $499.19 |
| | 1987 | 5,659 | 961 | 31,633 | 624 | 780 | 7.2 | 247,704 | 72,516 | 3,602,416 | 3,120 | 400 | $152,909 | $3,848.79 | $536.96 |
| | 1988 | 5,579 | 949 | 31,480 | 622 | 795 | 7.2 | 271,436 | 70,361 | 3,706,748 | 3,209 | 404 | $168,941 | $4,194.39 | $581.08 |
| | 1989 | 5,497 | 936 | 31,141 | 619 | 805 | 7.3 | 287,909 | 69,436 | 3,831,051 | 3,307 | 411 | $185,204 | $4,572.23 | $630.59 |
| | 1990 | 5,420 | 929 | 31,203 | 620 | 820 | 7.3 | 302,691 | 68,443 | 3,958,646 | 3,423 | 417 | $203,927 | $4,929.93 | $681.52 |
| | 1991 | 5,370 | 926 | 31,084 | 612 | 828 | 7.2 | 323,202 | 67,440 | 3,965,489 | 3,539 | 427 | $225,230 | $5,345.63 | $745.37 |
| | 1992 | 5,321 | 923 | 31,053 | 606 | 832 | 7.1 | 349,397 | 67,095 | 3,925,024 | 3,624 | 436 | $248,318 | $5,788.52 | $815.99 |
| | 1993 | 5,289 | 921 | 30,770 | 593 | 834 | 7.0 | 368,358 | 66,060 | 3,870,392 | 3,681 | 441 | $266,382 | $6,120.94 | $874.98 |
| | 1994 | 5,256 | 904 | 30,739 | 569 | 814 | 6.8 | 384,880 | 65,728 | 3,809,367 | 3,697 | 454 | $276,148 | $6,230.33 | $929.65 |
| | 1995 | 5,220 | 874 | 30,966 | 549 | 811 | 6.5 | 415,710 | 64,742 | 3,764,756 | 3,718 | 458 | $286,073 | $6,220.54 | $966.79 |
| | 1996 | 5,160 | 864 | 31,116 | 531 | 800 | 6.2 | 440,845 | 63,646 | 3,723,907 | 3,728 | 466 | $293,920 | $6,225.95 | $1,005.45 |
| | 1997 | 5,082 | 855 | 31,595 | 529 | 813 | 6.1 | 450,907 | 63,247 | 3,742,240 | 3,794 | 467 | $306,088 | $6,266.24 | $1,031.68 |
| | 1998 | 5,039 | 842 | 31,830 | 527 | 821 | 6.0 | 474,366 | 62,162 | 3,726,234 | 3,835 | 467 | $319,035 | $6,387.53 | $1,064.93 |
| | 1999 | 4,977 | 831 | 32,377 | 527 | 835 | 5.9 | 495,850 | 61,534 | 3,760,295 | 3,840 | 460 | $335,405 | $6,512.44 | $1,101.47 |
| | 2000 | 4,934 | 825 | 33,102 | 527 | 850 | 5.8 | 522,970 | 60,845 | 3,880,166 | 3,916 | 461 | $356,757 | $6,650.68 | $1,147.99 |
| | 2001 | 4,927 | 828 | 33,834 | 534 | 866 | 5.8 | 539,316 | 60,454 | 3,873,395 | 3,990 | 461 | $383,911 | $6,979.29 | $1,216.04 |
| | 2002 | 4,949 | 823 | 34,501 | 541 | 887 | 5.7 | 557,336 | 59,974 | 3,870,191 | 4,072 | 459 | $416,791 | $7,353.17 | $1,288.63 |
| | 2003 | 4,918 | 815 | 34,800 | 540 | 895 | 5.7 | 563,804 | 59,662 | 3,915,842 | 4,112 | 459 | $450,403 | $7,798.19 | $1,378.78 |

**Table 1** (Continued)

| CLASSIFICATION | YEAR | HOSPITALS | BEDS (in thousands) | ADMISSIONS (in thousands) | AVERAGE DAILY CENSUS (in thousands) | ADJUSTED AVERAGE DAILY CENSUS (in thousands) | AVERAGE LENGTH OF STAY (days) | OUTPATIENT VISITS (in thousands) | NEWBORNS | | FTE PERSONNEL | | EXPENSES | | |
|---|---|---|---|---|---|---|---|---|---|---|---|---|---|---|---|
| | | | | | | | | | Bassinets | Births | Number (in thousands) | Per 100 Adjusted Census | Amount (In Millions of dollars) | Adjusted per Inpatient Stay (dollars) | Adjusted per Inpatient Day (dollars) |
| Total community hospitals | 1975 | 5,875 | 942 | 33,435 | 706 | 798 | 7.7 | 190,672 | 83,829 | 2,998,552 | 2,392 | 300 | $38,962 | $1,030.34 | $133.81 |
| | 1976 | 5,857 | 956 | 33,979 | 713 | 810 | 7.7 | 201,247 | 82,296 | 2,962,216 | 2,475 | 306 | $45,240 | $1,176.25 | $152.76 |
| | 1979 | 5,842 | 984 | 35,099 | 727 | 833 | 7.6 | 198,778 | 77,266 | 3,287,012 | 2,756 | 331 | $66,004 | $1,641.67 | $217.34 |
| | 1980 | 5,830 | 988 | 36,143 | 747 | 857 | 7.6 | 202,310 | 77,522 | 3,408,482 | 2,873 | 335 | $76,851 | $1,851.04 | $245.12 |
| | 1981 | 5,813 | 1,003 | 36,438 | 763 | 873 | 7.6 | 202,768 | 76,561 | 3,465,401 | 3,033 | 347 | $90,572 | $2,171.20 | $284.33 |
| | 1982 | 5,801 | 1,012 | 36,379 | 762 | 878 | 7.6 | 248,124 | 75,733 | 3,514,457 | 3,103 | 353 | $104,876 | $2,500.52 | $327.37 |
| | 1983 | 5,783 | 1,018 | 36,152 | 749 | 864 | 7.6 | 210,044 | 75,465 | 3,490,254 | 3,096 | 358 | $116,438 | $2,789.18 | $369.49 |
| | 1984 | 5,759 | 1,017 | 35,155 | 702 | 820 | 7.3 | 211,961 | 75,581 | 3,456,308 | 3,017 | 368 | $123,336 | $2,995.38 | $411.10 |
| | 1985 | 5,732 | 1,001 | 33,449 | 649 | 777 | 7.1 | 218,716 | 74,893 | 3,521,135 | 2,997 | 386 | $130,499 | $3,244.74 | $460.19 |
| | 1986 | 5,678 | 978 | 32,379 | 629 | 770 | 7.1 | 231,912 | 73,682 | 3,584,408 | 3,025 | 393 | $140,654 | $3,532.51 | $500.81 |
| | 1987 | 5,611 | 958 | 31,601 | 622 | 776 | 7.2 | 245,524 | 72,510 | 3,602,296 | 3,114 | 401 | $152,585 | $3,850.16 | $538.96 |
| | 1988 | 5,533 | 947 | 31,453 | 620 | 787 | 7.2 | 269,129 | 70,325 | 3,706,402 | 3,205 | 407 | $168,722 | $4,206.73 | $586.33 |
| | 1989 | 5,455 | 933 | 31,116 | 618 | 796 | 7.2 | 285,712 | 69,405 | 3,830,615 | 3,303 | 415 | $184,898 | $4,587.87 | $636.96 |
| | 1990 | 5,384 | 927 | 31,181 | 619 | 813 | 7.2 | 301,329 | 68,412 | 3,958,263 | 3,420 | 421 | $203,693 | $4,946.68 | $686.83 |
| | 1991 | 5,342 | 924 | 31,064 | 611 | 820 | 7.2 | 322,048 | 67,434 | 3,965,396 | 3,535 | 431 | $225,023 | $5,359.56 | $752.10 |
| | 1992 | 5,292 | 921 | 31,034 | 604 | 827 | 7.1 | 348,522 | 67,089 | 3,924,944 | 3,620 | 437 | $248,095 | $5,794.43 | $819.83 |
| | 1993 | 5,261 | 919 | 30,748 | 592 | 828 | 7.0 | 366,885 | 66,054 | 3,870,376 | 3,677 | 444 | $266,089 | $6,132.06 | $880.52 |
| | 1994 | 5,229 | 902 | 30,718 | 568 | 812 | 6.7 | 382,924 | 65,722 | 3,809,367 | 3,692 | 455 | $275,779 | $6,229.83 | $930.71 |
| | 1995 | 5,194 | 873 | 30,945 | 548 | 809 | 6.5 | 414,345 | 64,736 | 3,764,698 | 3,714 | 459 | $285,588 | $6,215.51 | $967.69 |
| | 1996 | 5,134 | 862 | 31,099 | 531 | 799 | 6.2 | 439,863 | 63,640 | 3,723,871 | 3,725 | 466 | $293,755 | $6,224.94 | $1,006.14 |
| | 1997 | 5,057 | 853 | 31,577 | 528 | 811 | 6.1 | 450,140 | 63,241 | 3,742,191 | 3,790 | 467 | $305,763 | $6,261.93 | $1,032.70 |
| | 1998 | 5,015 | 840 | 31,812 | 525 | 819 | 6.0 | 474,193 | 62,156 | 3,726,233 | 3,831 | 468 | $318,834 | $6,385.99 | $1,066.96 |
| | 1999 | 4,956 | 830 | 32,359 | 526 | 833 | 5.9 | 495,346 | 61,528 | 3,760,295 | 3,838 | 461 | $335,246 | $6,511.72 | $1,102.61 |
| | 2000 | 4,915 | 824 | 33,089 | 526 | 849 | 5.8 | 521,404 | 60,839 | 3,880,166 | 3,911 | 461 | $356,564 | $6,648.82 | $1,149.40 |
| | 2001 | 4,908 | 826 | 33,814 | 533 | 865 | 5.7 | 538,480 | 60,448 | 3,873,395 | 3,987 | 461 | $383,735 | $6,979.53 | $1,217.27 |
| | 2002 | 4,927 | 821 | 34,478 | 540 | 886 | 5.7 | 556,404 | 59,974 | 3,870,191 | 4,069 | 459 | $416,591 | $7,354.60 | $1,289.87 |
| | 2003 | 4,895 | 813 | 34,783 | 539 | 894 | 5.7 | 563,186 | 59,662 | 3,915,842 | 4,109 | 460 | $450,124 | $7,796.41 | $1,379.48 |
| Nongovernment not-for-profit community hospitals | 1975 | 3,339 | 658 | 23,722 | 510 | 574 | 7.8 | 131,435 | 57,496 | 2,131,057 | 1,712 | 298 | $27,938 | $1,040.21 | $133.36 |
| | 1976 | 3,345 | 670 | 24,082 | 517 | 586 | 7.9 | 140,914 | 56,442 | 2,100,917 | 1,791 | 306 | $32,764 | $1,208.23 | $152.94 |
| | 1979 | 3,330 | 690 | 24,874 | 528 | 603 | 7.7 | 139,565 | 52,859 | 2,308,548 | 1,999 | 332 | $47,937 | $1,684.40 | $218.06 |
| | 1980 | 3,322 | 692 | 25,566 | 542 | 621 | 7.7 | 142,156 | 52,659 | 2,389,478 | 2,086 | 336 | $55,780 | $1,901.64 | $245.74 |
| | 1981 | 3,340 | 706 | 25,945 | 555 | 636 | 7.8 | 143,380 | 52,302 | 2,455,033 | 2,213 | 399 | $66,267 | $2,225.17 | $285.64 |
| | 1982 | 3,338 | 712 | 25,898 | 553 | 637 | 7.8 | 176,245 | 51,566 | 2,483,345 | 2,265 | 355 | $76,806 | $2,572.93 | $330.41 |
| | 1983 | 3,347 | 718 | 25,827 | 544 | 629 | 7.7 | 150,839 | 51,649 | 2,465,604 | 2,270 | 362 | $85,637 | $2,868.80 | $373.78 |
| | 1984 | 3,351 | 716 | 25,236 | 512 | 598 | 7.4 | 153,281 | 51,491 | 2,446,540 | 2,222 | 372 | $90,814 | $3,072.51 | $415.04 |
| | 1985 | 3,349 | 707 | 24,179 | 476 | 569 | 7.2 | 158,953 | 51,424 | 2,507,288 | 2,216 | 389 | $96,150 | $3,307.41 | $462.69 |
| | 1986 | 3,323 | 689 | 23,483 | 460 | 563 | 7.2 | 167,633 | 50,885 | 2,547,170 | 2,241 | 398 | $103,524 | $3,589.64 | $503.64 |
| | 1987 | 3,274 | 673 | 22,937 | 455 | 566 | 7.2 | 177,413 | 50,133 | 2,557,294 | 2,298 | 406 | $112,325 | $3,914.23 | $543.67 |
| | 1988 | 3,242 | 668 | 22,939 | 456 | 577 | 7.3 | 195,363 | 48,828 | 2,653,794 | 2,373 | 412 | $124,703 | $4,272.95 | $591.13 |
| | 1989 | 3,220 | 661 | 22,792 | 455 | 584 | 7.3 | 209,191 | 48,305 | 2,751,426 | 2,454 | 420 | $136,889 | $4,649.22 | $642.45 |
| | 1990 | 3,191 | 657 | 22,878 | 455 | 596 | 7.3 | 221,073 | 47,441 | 2,833,204 | 2,533 | 424 | $150,673 | $5,001.24 | $692.36 |
| | 1991 | 3,175 | 656 | 22,964 | 451 | 603 | 7.2 | 238,204 | 47,229 | 2,845,995 | 2,624 | 435 | $166,806 | $5,393.30 | $758.21 |
| | 1992 | 3,173 | 656 | 23,056 | 445 | 606 | 7.1 | 257,887 | 47,185 | 2,846,386 | 2,692 | 443 | $183,793 | $5,808.80 | $828.44 |
| | 1993 | 3,154 | 651 | 22,749 | 432 | 602 | 6.9 | 270,138 | 46,214 | 2,802,164 | 2,711 | 451 | $197,187 | $6,177.69 | $897.70 |
| | 1994 | 3,139 | 637 | 22,704 | 413 | 589 | 6.6 | 282,653 | 46,381 | 2,792,116 | 2,719 | 462 | $204,219 | $6,256.72 | $950.31 |
| | 1995 | 3,092 | 610 | 22,557 | 393 | 578 | 6.4 | 303,851 | 45,198 | 2,725,641 | 2,702 | 468 | $209,614 | $6,279.17 | $994.39 |
| | 1996 | 3,045 | 598 | 22,542 | 379 | 567 | 6.1 | 320,746 | 44,650 | 2,683,750 | 2,711 | 478 | $215,950 | $6,344.05 | $1,042.04 |
| | 1997 | 3,000 | 591 | 22,905 | 376 | 575 | 6.0 | 330,215 | 44,484 | 2,698,086 | 2,765 | 481 | $225,287 | $6,392.74 | $1,074.26 |
| | 1998 | 3,026 | 588 | 23,282 | 377 | 587 | 5.9 | 352,114 | 44,087 | 2,715,958 | 2,834 | 483 | $237,978 | $6,525.68 | $1,110.50 |
| | 1999 | 3,012 | 587 | 23,871 | 381 | 605 | 5.8 | 370,784 | 44,172 | 2,746,453 | 2,862 | 473 | $251,534 | $6,607.51 | $1,139.89 |
| | 2000 | 3,003 | 583 | 24,452 | 382 | 618 | 5.7 | 393,168 | 43,655 | 2,833,615 | 2,919 | 472 | $267,051 | $6,717.48 | $1,182.32 |
| | 2001 | 2,998 | 585 | 24,983 | 385 | 628 | 5.6 | 404,901 | 43,640 | 2,829,691 | 2,971 | 473 | $287,250 | $7,051.76 | $1,255.25 |
| | 2002 | 3,025 | 582 | 25,425 | 391 | 646 | 5.6 | 416,910 | 43,241 | 2,820,159 | 3,039 | 471 | $312,726 | $7,457.84 | $1,328.81 |
| | 2003 | 2,984 | 575 | 25,668 | 389 | 647 | 5.5 | 424,215 | 42,965 | 2,854,764 | 3,059 | 473 | $337,696 | $7,904.93 | $1,429.62 |

**Table 1** (Continued)

| CLASSIFICATION | YEAR | HOSPITALS | BEDS (in thousands) | ADMISSIONS (in thousands) | AVERAGE DAILY CENSUS (in thousands) | ADJUSTED AVERAGE DAILY CENSUS (in thousands) | AVERAGE LENGTH OF STAY (days) | OUTPATIENT VISITS (in thousands) | NEWBORNS | | FTE PERSONNEL | | EXPENSES | | |
|---|---|---|---|---|---|---|---|---|---|---|---|---|---|---|---|
| | | | | | | | | | Bassinets | Births | Number (in thousands) | Per 100 Adjusted Census | Amount (In Millions of dollars) | Adjusted per Inpatient Stay (dollars) | Adjusted per Inpatient Day (dollars) |
| Investor-owned (for-profit) community hospitals | 1975 | 775 | 73 | 2,646 | 48 | 53 | 6.6 | 7,713 | 4,062 | 141,392 | 139 | 263 | $2,561 | $876.48 | $132.80 |
| | 1976 | 752 | 76 | 2,734 | 50 | 54 | 6.6 | 8,048 | 4,044 | 144,751 | 147 | 272 | $3,085 | $1,031.91 | $156.35 |
| | 1979 | 727 | 83 | 2,963 | 53 | 59 | 6.6 | 9,289 | 4,110 | 174,843 | 174 | 300 | $4,820 | $1,476.42 | $225.87 |
| | 1980 | 730 | 87 | 3,165 | 57 | 62 | 6.5 | 9,696 | 4,439 | 199,722 | 189 | 304 | $5,847 | $1,675.85 | $257.12 |
| | 1981 | 729 | 88 | 3,239 | 58 | 63 | 6.5 | 9,961 | 4,523 | 207,405 | 203 | 322 | $6,856 | $1,952.56 | $299.02 |
| | 1982 | 748 | 91 | 3,316 | 60 | 66 | 6.6 | 13,193 | 4,736 | 219,675 | 212 | 320 | $8,177 | $2,224.75 | $340.03 |
| | 1983 | 757 | 94 | 3,299 | 59 | 66 | 6.5 | 10,389 | 5,039 | 228,883 | 213 | 323 | $9,208 | $2,517.53 | $385.42 |
| | 1984 | 786 | 100 | 3,314 | 57 | 64 | 6.3 | 11,090 | 5,807 | 242,088 | 214 | 335 | $10,251 | $2,748.51 | $438.30 |
| | 1985 | 805 | 104 | 3,242 | 54 | 63 | 6.1 | 12,378 | 6,117 | 266,839 | 221 | 350 | $11,486 | $3,033.06 | $500.48 |
| | 1986 | 834 | 107 | 3,231 | 54 | 65 | 6.1 | 14,896 | 6,305 | 291,112 | 229 | 354 | $12,987 | $3,341.79 | $552.40 |
| | 1987 | 828 | 106 | 3,157 | 54 | 66 | 6.2 | 16,566 | 6,391 | 306,492 | 242 | 367 | $14,067 | $3,617.19 | $585.01 |
| | 1988 | 790 | 104 | 3,090 | 53 | 66 | 6.2 | 17,926 | 6,254 | 308,828 | 249 | 379 | $15,545 | $4,022.77 | $649.33 |
| | 1989 | 769 | 102 | 3,071 | 53 | 67 | 6.3 | 19,341 | 6,354 | 325,711 | 261 | 390 | $17,240 | $4,406.20 | $707.90 |
| | 1990 | 749 | 101 | 3,066 | 54 | 69 | 6.4 | 20,110 | 6,261 | 340,555 | 273 | 396 | $18,822 | $4,727.27 | $751.55 |
| | 1991 | 738 | 100 | 3,016 | 52 | 69 | 6.3 | 21,174 | 6,358 | 359,115 | 281 | 409 | $20,516 | $5,133.53 | $820.19 |
| | 1992 | 723 | 99 | 2,969 | 51 | 69 | 6.3 | 22,900 | 6,519 | 357,776 | 285 | 412 | $22,496 | $5,548.24 | $888.73 |
| | 1993 | 717 | 99 | 2,946 | 51 | 69 | 6.2 | 24,936 | 6,395 | 363,358 | 289 | 417 | $23,077 | $5,643.21 | $914.39 |
| | 1994 | 719 | 101 | 3,035 | 50 | 70 | 6.1 | 26,443 | 6,329 | 354,477 | 302 | 434 | $23,445 | $5,528.91 | $923.90 |
| | 1995 | 752 | 106 | 3,428 | 55 | 77 | 5.8 | 31,940 | 7,164 | 408,339 | 343 | 443 | $26,653 | $5,425.20 | $946.99 |
| | 1996 | 759 | 109 | 3,684 | 56 | 82 | 5.6 | 37,347 | 7,441 | 444,697 | 359 | 437 | $28,385 | $5,207.44 | $945.49 |
| | 1997 | 797 | 115 | 3,953 | 60 | 89 | 5.5 | 40,919 | 8,026 | 465,919 | 385 | 433 | $31,179 | $5,218.69 | $961.96 |
| | 1998 | 771 | 113 | 3,971 | 60 | 90 | 5.5 | 42,072 | 7,895 | 466,025 | 383 | 425 | $31,732 | $5,262.44 | $968.00 |
| | 1999 | 747 | 107 | 3,905 | 58 | 86 | 5.5 | 39,896 | 7,486 | 467,585 | 362 | 422 | $31,179 | $5,350.07 | $999.03 |
| | 2000 | 749 | 110 | 4,141 | 61 | 90 | 5.4 | 43,378 | 7,792 | 503,497 | 378 | 418 | $34,969 | $5,642.18 | $1,057.32 |
| | 2001 | 754 | 109 | 4,197 | 63 | 92 | 5.4 | 44,706 | 7,413 | 494,669 | 379 | 413 | $37,348 | $5,971.81 | $1,121.31 |
| | 2002 | 766 | 108 | 4,365 | 64 | 93 | 5.3 | 45,215 | 7,467 | 496,988 | 380 | 407 | $40,082 | $6,161.44 | $1,180.83 |
| | 2003 | 790 | 110 | 4,481 | 65 | 95 | 5.3 | 44,246 | 7,491 | 515,693 | 391 | 411 | $43,953 | $6,589.91 | $1,264.50 |
| State and local government community hospitals | 1975 | 1,761 | 210 | 7,067 | 148 | 171 | 7.6 | 51,525 | 22,271 | 726,103 | 540 | 316 | $8,463 | $1,030.86 | $135.64 |
| | 1976 | 1,760 | 210 | 7,163 | 146 | 170 | 7.5 | 52,286 | 21,810 | 716,548 | 537 | 315 | $9,391 | $1,132.50 | $151.00 |
| | 1979 | 1,785 | 211 | 7,262 | 146 | 171 | 7.4 | 49,924 | 20,297 | 803,621 | 583 | 341 | $13,247 | $1,561.04 | $211.89 |
| | 1980 | 1,778 | 209 | 7,413 | 149 | 174 | 7.3 | 50,459 | 20,424 | 819,282 | 598 | 343 | $15,204 | $1,750.13 | $238.63 |
| | 1981 | 1,744 | 210 | 7,255 | 150 | 174 | 7.6 | 49,427 | 19,736 | 802,963 | 618 | 354 | $17,449 | $2,071.57 | $274.25 |
| | 1982 | 1,715 | 210 | 7,165 | 149 | 175 | 7.6 | 58,685 | 19,431 | 811,437 | 627 | 320 | $19,893 | $2,364.09 | $311.56 |
| | 1983 | 1,679 | 207 | 7,025 | 145 | 170 | 7.6 | 48,816 | 18,777 | 795,767 | 613 | 360 | $21,593 | $2,621.28 | $347.56 |
| | 1984 | 1,622 | 201 | 6,606 | 133 | 158 | 7.3 | 47,590 | 18,283 | 767,680 | 581 | 368 | $22,271 | $2,823.13 | $385.17 |
| | 1985 | 1,578 | 189 | 6,028 | 119 | 145 | 7.2 | 47,386 | 17,352 | 747,008 | 561 | 387 | $22,863 | $3,106.14 | $432.84 |
| | 1986 | 1,521 | 182 | 5,665 | 114 | 142 | 7.4 | 49,383 | 16,492 | 746,126 | 555 | 391 | $24,143 | $3,404.69 | $466.17 |
| | 1987 | 1,509 | 180 | 5,507 | 113 | 144 | 7.5 | 51,544 | 15,986 | 738,510 | 573 | 399 | $26,192 | $3,717.77 | $499.33 |
| | 1988 | 1,501 | 175 | 5,424 | 112 | 145 | 7.6 | 55,840 | 15,243 | 743,780 | 583 | 403 | $28,474 | $4,033.67 | $538.63 |
| | 1989 | 1,466 | 170 | 5,253 | 110 | 145 | 7.7 | 57,179 | 14,746 | 753,478 | 589 | 406 | $30,769 | $4,430.12 | $582.15 |
| | 1990 | 1,444 | 169 | 5,236 | 111 | 148 | 7.7 | 60,146 | 14,710 | 784,504 | 614 | 415 | $34,198 | $4,837.76 | $634.45 |
| | 1991 | 1,429 | 168 | 5,084 | 108 | 148 | 7.8 | 62,670 | 13,847 | 760,286 | 630 | 424 | $37,701 | $5,339.75 | $695.89 |
| | 1992 | 1,396 | 166 | 5,008 | 108 | 152 | 7.9 | 67,734 | 13,385 | 720,782 | 643 | 424 | $41,806 | $5,870.76 | $753.92 |
| | 1993 | 1,390 | 169 | 5,054 | 109 | 157 | 7.8 | 71,811 | 13,445 | 704,854 | 676 | 430 | $45,825 | $6,205.52 | $799.73 |
| | 1994 | 1,371 | 164 | 4,979 | 104 | 154 | 7.6 | 73,828 | 13,012 | 662,774 | 672 | 438 | $48,115 | $6,513.39 | $858.62 |
| | 1995 | 1,350 | 157 | 4,961 | 100 | 154 | 7.4 | 78,554 | 12,374 | 630,718 | 670 | 435 | $49,322 | $6,445.18 | $877.85 |
| | 1996 | 1,330 | 155 | 4,873 | 96 | 150 | 7.2 | 81,770 | 11,549 | 595,424 | 654 | 437 | $49,420 | $6,418.65 | $903.41 |
| | 1997 | 1,260 | 148 | 4,720 | 92 | 148 | 7.1 | 79,007 | 10,731 | 578,186 | 640 | 433 | $49,298 | $6,475.07 | $913.62 |
| | 1998 | 1,218 | 139 | 4,559 | 87 | 142 | 7.0 | 80,008 | 10,174 | 544,250 | 614 | 433 | $49,123 | $6,612.23 | $949.36 |
| | 1999 | 1,197 | 136 | 4,583 | 86 | 143 | 6.9 | 84,667 | 9,870 | 546,257 | 614 | 430 | $52,534 | $6,923.35 | $1,006.91 |
| | 2000 | 1,163 | 131 | 4,496 | 83 | 140 | 6.7 | 84,858 | 9,392 | 543,054 | 614 | 438 | $54,544 | $7,106.05 | $1,063.75 |
| | 2001 | 1,156 | 132 | 4,634 | 85 | 145 | 6.7 | 88,873 | 9,395 | 549,035 | 637 | 438 | $59,137 | $7,400.01 | $1,113.79 |
| | 2002 | 1,136 | 130 | 4,688 | 84 | 147 | 6.6 | 94,280 | 9,266 | 553,044 | 651 | 442 | $63,783 | $7,772.93 | $1,188.12 |
| | 2003 | 1,121 | 129 | 4,634 | 84 | 152 | 6.6 | 94,725 | 9,206 | 545,385 | 658 | 434 | $68,475 | $8,205.10 | $1,237.64 |

Table
**2**

# 2003 U.S. Registered Hospitals: Utilization, Personnel, and Finances

*Excludes U.S.-Associated Areas, Puerto Rico, and nonregistered hospitals.*

| CLASSIFICATION | HOSPITALS | BEDS | ADMISSIONS | INPATIENT DAYS | ADJUSTED PATIENT DAYS | AVERAGE DAILY CENSUS | ADJUSTED AVERAGE DAILY CENSUS | AVERAGE STAY (days) | SURGICAL OPERATIONS | OUTPATIENT VISITS | | NEWBORNS | |
|---|---|---|---|---|---|---|---|---|---|---|---|---|---|
| | | | | | | | | | | Emergency | Total | Bassinets | Births |
| UNITED STATES | 5 764 | 965,256 | 36,610,535 | 239,926,018 | — | 657,395 | — | — | 27,884,798 | 115,160,472 | 648,559,904 | 60,699 | 3,976,886 |
| 6-24 Beds | 387 | 6,656 | 188,919 | 820,968 | — | 2,244 | — | — | 221,341 | 1,652,437 | 10,747,344 | 583 | 13,400 |
| 25-49 | 1,073 | 37,509 | 1,182,288 | 6,285,316 | — | 17,230 | — | — | 1,075,247 | 6,717,508 | 36,893,583 | 3,058 | 101,601 |
| 50-99 | 1,297 | 93,258 | 2,903,228 | 20,620,427 | — | 56,567 | — | — | 2,399,208 | 12,522,240 | 66,675,955 | 6,380 | 281,386 |
| 100-199 | 1,373 | 196,222 | 7,309,222 | 46,309,357 | — | 126,880 | — | — | 6,012,039 | 26,472,651 | 138,653,718 | 13,788 | 793,577 |
| 200-299 | 722 | 176,452 | 7,218,249 | 44,378,699 | — | 121,578 | — | — | 5,624,518 | 22,399,158 | 116,553,614 | 12,007 | 780,902 |
| 300-399 | 391 | 134,519 | 5,671,106 | 33,943,937 | — | 92,989 | — | — | 4,045,993 | 16,015,321 | 86,162,424 | 8,798 | 662,053 |
| 400-499 | 199 | 88,678 | 3,679,002 | 23,253,114 | — | 63,700 | — | — | 2,702,051 | 9,625,316 | 64,079,484 | 5,181 | 421,166 |
| 500 or more | 322 | 231,962 | 8,458,521 | 64,314,200 | — | 176,207 | — | — | 5,804,401 | 19,755,841 | 128,793,782 | 10,904 | 922,801 |
| Psychiatric | 487 | 87,980 | 782,579 | 27,359,517 | — | 74,985 | — | — | 3,810 | 123,352 | 10,433,527 | 0 | 0 |
| Hospitals | 475 | 81,688 | 779,566 | 25,531,231 | — | 69,976 | — | — | 3,810 | 121,132 | 10,424,093 | 0 | 0 |
| Institutions for mentally retarded | 12 | 6,292 | 3,013 | 1,828,286 | — | 5,009 | — | — | 0 | 2,220 | 9,434 | 0 | 0 |
| General | 4,940 | 842,351 | 35,230,636 | 203,171,553 | — | 556,664 | — | — | 27,408,662 | 114,310,089 | 625,026,330 | 59,891 | 3,918,306 |
| Hospitals | 4,914 | 839,649 | 35,211,583 | 202,639,314 | — | 555,207 | — | — | 27,397,322 | 114,199,544 | 624,082,795 | 59,891 | 3,918,306 |
| Hospital units of institutions | 26 | 2,702 | 19,053 | 532,239 | — | 1,457 | — | — | 11,340 | 110,545 | 943,535 | 0 | 0 |
| TB and other respiratory diseases | 4 | 222 | 882 | 47,822 | — | 132 | — | — | 0 | 0 | 3,138 | 6 | 0 |
| Obstetrics and gynecology | 18 | 2,305 | 119,665 | 557,638 | — | 1,527 | — | — | 90,498 | 287,620 | 1,830,361 | 709 | 55,315 |
| Eye, ear, nose and throat | 9 | 250 | 6,736 | 22,985 | — | 64 | — | — | 96,437 | 49,941 | 705,314 | 0 | 0 |
| Rehabilitation | 184 | 15,389 | 247,962 | 4,098,550 | — | 11,232 | — | — | 56,540 | 18,555 | 6,379,130 | 0 | 0 |
| Orthopedic | 26 | 1,604 | 59,045 | 309,940 | — | 851 | — | — | 104,216 | 19,034 | 845,665 | 0 | 0 |
| Chronic Disease | 13 | 4,209 | 18,128 | 1,284,830 | — | 3,520 | — | — | 3,333 | 29,309 | 375,656 | 0 | 1 |
| All other | 83 | 10,946 | 144,902 | 3,073,183 | — | 8,420 | — | — | 121,302 | 322,572 | 2,960,783 | 93 | 3,264 |
| Federal | 239 | 47,456 | 973,386 | 11,220,020 | — | 30,742 | — | — | 740,336 | 3,750,933 | 74,240,114 | 993 | 60,970 |
| Psychiatric | 10 | 3,346 | 22,978 | 945,149 | — | 2,588 | — | — | 2,972 | 1,793 | 1,792,016 | 0 | 0 |
| General and other special | 229 | 44,110 | 950,408 | 10,274,871 | — | 28,154 | — | — | 737,364 | 3,749,140 | 72,448,098 | 993 | 60,970 |
| Nonfederal | 5,525 | 917,800 | 35,637,149 | 228,705,998 | — | 626,653 | — | — | 27,144,462 | 111,409,539 | 574,319,790 | 59,706 | 3,915,916 |
| Psychiatric | 477 | 84,634 | 759,601 | 26,414,368 | — | 72,397 | — | — | 838 | 121,559 | 8,641,511 | 0 | 0 |
| Hospitals | 465 | 78,342 | 756,588 | 24,586,082 | — | 67,388 | — | — | 838 | 119,339 | 8,632,077 | 0 | 0 |
| Institutions for mentally retarded | 12 | 6,292 | 3,013 | 1,828,286 | — | 5,009 | — | — | 0 | 2,220 | 9,434 | 0 | 0 |
| TB and other respiratory diseases | 4 | 222 | 882 | 47,822 | — | 132 | — | — | 0 | 0 | 3,138 | 6 | 0 |
| Long-term general and other special | 126 | 17,609 | 76,312 | 5,296,134 | — | 14,511 | — | — | 26,331 | 146,373 | 1,871,261 | 38 | 74 |
| Short-term general and other special | 4,918 | 815,335 | 34,800,354 | 196,947,674 | — | 539,613 | — | — | 27,117,293 | 111,141,607 | 563,803,880 | 59,662 | 3,915,842 |
| Hospital units of institutions | 23 | 2,028 | 17,612 | 297,905 | — | 816 | — | — | 10,755 | 71,736 | 617,834 | 0 | 0 |
| Community Hospitals | 4,895 | 813,307 | 34,782,742 | 196,649,769 | 326,299,942 | 538,797 | 894,019 | 5.7 | 27,106,538 | 111,069,871 | 563,186,046 | 59,662 | 3,915,842 |
| 6-24 Beds | 327 | 5,635 | 162,231 | 658,374 | 2,211,512 | 1,798 | 6,062 | 4.1 | 209,872 | 1,159,015 | 6,512,324 | 489 | 9,347 |
| 25-49 | 965 | 33,613 | 1,098,125 | 5,465,909 | 13,556,517 | 14,986 | 37,138 | 5.0 | 1,038,692 | 6,148,561 | 31,260,985 | 2,860 | 94,761 |
| 50-99 | 1,031 | 74,025 | 2,463,703 | 15,445,684 | 31,549,934 | 42,364 | 86,490 | 6.3 | 2,270,866 | 11,581,730 | 52,959,172 | 6,043 | 264,321 |
| 100-199 | 1,168 | 167,451 | 6,816,567 | 38,281,885 | 69,848,764 | 104,884 | 191,347 | 5.6 | 5,812,028 | 25,687,014 | 119,855,613 | 13,577 | 777,298 |
| 200-299 | 624 | 152,487 | 6,887,304 | 37,271,468 | 60,314,471 | 102,106 | 165,252 | 5.4 | 5,421,403 | 21,701,788 | 100,095,243 | 11,810 | 764,095 |
| 300-399 | 349 | 119,903 | 5,589,833 | 29,998,416 | 46,233,983 | 82,178 | 126,669 | 5.4 | 3,997,560 | 15,897,067 | 80,938,013 | 8,798 | 662,053 |
| 400-499 | 172 | 76,333 | 3,591,216 | 19,709,937 | 30,100,688 | 53,993 | 82,471 | 5.5 | 2,666,350 | 9,497,408 | 57,202,954 | 5,181 | 421,166 |
| 500 or more | 259 | 183,860 | 8,173,763 | 49,818,096 | 72,484,073 | 136,488 | 198,590 | 6.1 | 5,689,767 | 19,397,288 | 114,361,742 | 10,904 | 922,801 |
| Nongovernment not-for-profit | 2,984 | 574,587 | 25,668,173 | 142,041,074 | 236,213,615 | 389,163 | 647,176 | 5.5 | 20,451,183 | 78,574,555 | 424,214,892 | 42,965 | 2,854,764 |
| Investor-owned (for profit) | 790 | 109,671 | 4,480,597 | 23,874,581 | 34,759,393 | 65,400 | 95,221 | 5.3 | 3,405,631 | 14,186,177 | 44,246,062 | 7,491 | 515,693 |
| State and Local Government | 1,121 | 129,049 | 4,633,972 | 30,734,114 | 55,326,934 | 84,234 | 151,622 | 6.6 | 3,249,724 | 18,309,139 | 94,725,092 | 9,206 | 545,385 |

**Table 2** (Continued)

| CLASSIFICATION | FULL-TIME EQUIVALENT PERSONNEL | | | | | FULL-TIME EQUIVALENT TRAINEES | | | EXPENSES | | | | | | |
|---|---|---|---|---|---|---|---|---|---|---|---|---|---|---|---|
| | | | | | | | | | LABOR | | | | TOTAL | | |
| | Physicians and Dentists | Registered Nurses | Licensed Practical Nurses | Other Salaried Personnel | Total Personnel | Medical and Dental Residents | Other Trainees | Total Trainees | Payroll (in thousands) | Employee Benefits (in thousands) | Total (in thousands) | Percent of Total | Amount (in thousands) | Adjusted per Admission | Adjusted per Inpatient Day |
| UNITED STATES | 99,862 | 1,105,251 | 153,722 | 3,292,111 | 4,650,946 | 86,155 | 11,806 | 97,961 | $213,209,680 | $52,125,690 | $265,335,370 | 53.3 | $498,103,754 | — | — |
| 6-24 Beds | 1,458 | 7,587 | 2,382 | 32,255 | 43,682 | 24 | 248 | 272 | $1,700,091 | $396,403 | $2,096,493 | 61.0 | $3,439,436 | — | — |
| 25-49 | 4,348 | 35,780 | 10,714 | 136,310 | 187,152 | 220 | 157 | 377 | $6,899,230 | $1,649,769 | $8,548,999 | 54.6 | $15,649,536 | — | — |
| 50-99 | 7,068 | 80,315 | 19,900 | 277,424 | 384,707 | 704 | 433 | 1,137 | $15,611,549 | $3,803,156 | $19,414,705 | 56.0 | $34,682,480 | — | — |
| 100-199 | 17,132 | 198,910 | 34,668 | 608,409 | 859,119 | 6,036 | 2,702 | 8,738 | $37,437,722 | $9,076,722 | $46,514,444 | 53.9 | $86,219,474 | — | — |
| 200-299 | 17,986 | 208,523 | 27,702 | 599,822 | 854,033 | 8,095 | 1,619 | 9,714 | $38,556,885 | $9,679,276 | $48,236,160 | 53.3 | $90,567,816 | — | — |
| 300-399 | 10,768 | 165,850 | 19,112 | 470,421 | 666,151 | 10,060 | 1,105 | 11,165 | $31,299,104 | $7,446,699 | $38,745,803 | 52.4 | $73,883,724 | — | — |
| 400-499 | 10,212 | 118,901 | 12,180 | 336,123 | 477,416 | 14,361 | 1,795 | 16,156 | $23,135,033 | $5,814,424 | $28,949,458 | 52.4 | $55,196,204 | — | — |
| 500 or more | 30,890 | 289,385 | 27,064 | 831,347 | 1,178,686 | 46,655 | 3,747 | 50,402 | $58,570,066 | $14,259,240 | $72,829,307 | 52.6 | $138,465,085 | — | — |
| Psychiatric | 5,053 | 25,093 | 9,567 | 163,639 | 203,352 | 508 | 957 | 1,465 | $8,040,855 | $2,368,889 | $10,409,743 | 73.2 | $14,223,389 | — | — |
| Hospitals | 4,964 | 24,686 | 9,215 | 151,597 | 190,462 | 508 | 898 | 1,406 | $7,554,977 | $2,223,334 | $9,778,311 | 72.6 | $13,461,353 | — | — |
| Institutions for mentally retarded | 89 | 407 | 352 | 12,042 | 12,890 | 0 | 59 | 59 | $485,878 | $145,555 | $631,433 | 82.9 | $762,036 | — | — |
| General | 92,219 | 1,055,704 | 138,313 | 3,030,914 | 4,317,150 | 84,647 | 10,563 | 95,210 | $199,342,176 | $48,372,975 | $247,715,151 | 52.5 | $471,410,572 | — | — |
| Hospitals | 91,897 | 1,055,233 | 137,963 | 3,026,621 | 4,311,714 | 84,616 | 10,536 | 95,152 | $199,059,498 | $48,318,200 | $247,377,698 | 52.5 | $470,940,022 | — | — |
| Hospital units of institutions | 322 | 471 | 350 | 4,293 | 5,436 | 31 | 27 | 58 | $282,678 | $54,775 | $337,453 | 71.7 | $470,550 | — | — |
| TB and other respiratory diseases | 0 | 95 | 83 | 464 | 642 | 0 | 0 | 0 | $23,549 | $7,634 | $31,182 | 57.6 | $54,101 | — | — |
| Obstetrics and gynecology | 267 | 3,780 | 422 | 9,648 | 14,117 | 128 | 17 | 145 | $662,352 | $152,731 | $815,083 | 57.6 | $1,416,129 | — | — |
| Eye, ear, nose and throat | 108 | 481 | 42 | 2,459 | 3,090 | 103 | 27 | 130 | $124,841 | $33,400 | $158,241 | 46.0 | $343,915 | — | — |
| Rehabilitation | 503 | 8,686 | 2,771 | 41,252 | 53,212 | 104 | 40 | 144 | $2,085,131 | $457,152 | $2,542,283 | 59.4 | $4,277,455 | — | — |
| Orthopedic | 385 | 2,013 | 216 | 7,385 | 9,999 | 63 | 8 | 71 | $533,559 | $130,121 | $663,679 | 50.9 | $1,302,874 | — | — |
| Chronic Disease | 264 | 1,106 | 709 | 6,951 | 9,030 | 21 | 6 | 27 | $412,273 | $111,794 | $524,068 | 65.0 | $805,695 | — | — |
| All other | 1,063 | 8,293 | 1,599 | 29,399 | 40,354 | 581 | 188 | 769 | $1,984,944 | $490,994 | $2,475,938 | 58.0 | $4,269,623 | — | — |
| Federal | 22,724 | 53,993 | 15,180 | 208,272 | 300,169 | 7,751 | 2,755 | 10,506 | $15,888,249 | $3,976,761 | $19,865,010 | 64.4 | $30,865,933 | — | — |
| Psychiatric | 346 | 1,362 | 621 | 7,375 | 9,704 | 1 | 25 | 26 | $616,148 | $145,905 | $762,054 | 70.0 | $1,088,749 | — | — |
| General and other special | 22,378 | 52,631 | 14,559 | 200,897 | 290,465 | 7,750 | 2,730 | 10,480 | $15,272,100 | $3,830,856 | $19,102,956 | 64.2 | $29,777,184 | — | — |
| Nonfederal | 77,138 | 1,051,258 | 138,542 | 3,083,839 | 4,350,777 | 78,404 | 9,051 | 87,455 | $197,321,431 | $48,148,929 | $245,470,360 | 52.5 | $467,237,821 | — | — |
| Psychiatric | 4,707 | 23,731 | 8,946 | 156,264 | 193,648 | 507 | 932 | 1,439 | $7,424,707 | $2,222,983 | $9,647,690 | 73.5 | $13,134,640 | — | — |
| Hospitals | 4,618 | 23,324 | 8,594 | 144,222 | 180,758 | 507 | 873 | 1,380 | $6,938,829 | $2,077,428 | $9,016,257 | 72.9 | $12,372,604 | — | — |
| Institutions for mentally retarded | 89 | 407 | 352 | 12,042 | 12,890 | 0 | 59 | 59 | $485,878 | $145,555 | $631,433 | 82.9 | $762,036 | — | — |
| TB and other respiratory diseases | 0 | 95 | 83 | 464 | 642 | 0 | 0 | 0 | $23,549 | $7,634 | $31,182 | 57.6 | $54,101 | — | — |
| Long-term general and other special | 863 | 5,768 | 2,885 | 35,154 | 44,670 | 53 | 165 | 218 | $1,893,684 | $461,258 | $2,354,942 | 64.6 | $3,646,095 | — | — |
| Short-term general and other special | 71,568 | 1,021,664 | 126,628 | 2,891,957 | 4,111,817 | 77,844 | 7,954 | 85,798 | $187,979,492 | $45,457,053 | $233,436,545 | 51.8 | $450,402,985 | — | — |
| Hospital units of institutions | 233 | 318 | 300 | 2,338 | 3,189 | 31 | 0 | 31 | $156,518 | $18,548 | $175,066 | 62.8 | $278,727 | — | — |
| Community Hospitals | 71,335 | 1,021,346 | 126,328 | 2,889,619 | 4,108,628 | 77,813 | 7,954 | 85,767 | $187,822,974 | $45,438,505 | $233,261,479 | 51.8 | $450,124,257 | $7,796.41 | $1,379.48 |
| 6-24 Beds | 490 | 5,930 | 2,097 | 21,044 | 29,561 | 6 | 15 | 21 | $1,029,790 | $231,516 | $1,261,307 | 51.3 | $2,456,994 | $4,371.97 | $1,111.00 |
| 25-49 | 2,922 | 32,542 | 9,766 | 118,383 | 163,613 | 132 | 47 | 179 | $5,982,560 | $1,396,120 | $7,378,681 | 52.8 | $13,984,834 | $5,005.25 | $1,031.59 |
| 50-99 | 3,168 | 67,988 | 15,401 | 216,103 | 302,660 | 196 | 109 | 305 | $12,065,748 | $3,005,188 | $15,070,936 | 53.5 | $28,189,310 | $5,553.05 | $893.48 |
| 100-199 | 11,420 | 179,434 | 28,999 | 523,044 | 742,897 | 4,180 | 1,618 | 5,798 | $32,113,015 | $7,721,236 | $39,834,251 | 52.7 | $75,609,452 | $6,190.89 | $1,082.47 |
| 200-299 | 10,114 | 189,744 | 22,675 | 525,786 | 748,319 | 5,598 | 413 | 6,011 | $34,006,991 | $8,313,881 | $42,320,872 | 52.2 | $81,020,518 | $7,316.97 | $1,343.30 |
| 300-399 | 9,120 | 160,500 | 17,251 | 440,968 | 627,839 | 9,950 | 971 | 10,921 | $29,253,939 | $6,934,026 | $36,187,965 | 51.4 | $70,380,925 | $8,184.43 | $1,522.28 |
| 400-499 | 8,430 | 113,192 | 10,042 | 306,535 | 438,199 | 13,158 | 1,671 | 14,829 | $21,237,694 | $5,288,468 | $26,526,162 | 51.4 | $51,603,684 | $9,395.72 | $1,714.37 |
| 500 or more | 25,671 | 272,016 | 20,097 | 737,756 | 1,055,540 | 44,593 | 3,110 | 47,703 | $52,133,237 | $12,548,070 | $64,681,307 | 51.0 | $126,878,540 | $10,639.82 | $1,750.43 |
| Nongovernment not-for-profit | 57,411 | 756,821 | 80,196 | 2,164,358 | 3,058,786 | 56,718 | 5,288 | 62,006 | $141,577,393 | $34,365,443 | $175,942,836 | 52.1 | $337,696,001 | $7,904.93 | $1,429.62 |
| Investor-owned (for profit) | 1,594 | 111,095 | 20,140 | 258,521 | 391,350 | 1,143 | 181 | 1,324 | $17,124,214 | $3,694,194 | $20,818,409 | 47.4 | $43,953,346 | $6,589.91 | $1,264.50 |
| State and Local Government | 12,330 | 153,430 | 25,992 | 466,740 | 658,492 | 19,952 | 2,485 | 22,437 | $29,121,367 | $7,378,868 | $36,500,235 | 53.3 | $68,474,910 | $8,205.10 | $1,237.64 |

# Tables 3–6

# TABLE 3

# TOTAL UNITED STATES

*U.S. Registered Community Hospitals*
*(Nonfederal, short-term general and other special hospitals)*

## Overview 1999–2003

Total U.S.

| | 2003 | 2002 | 2001 | 2000 | 1999 |
|---|---|---|---|---|---|
| **TOTAL U.S. Community Hospitals** | **4,895** | **4,927** | **4,908** | **4,915** | **4,956** |
| **Bed Size Category** | | | | | |
| 6-24 | 327 | 321 | 281 | 288 | 299 |
| 25-49 | 965 | 931 | 916 | 910 | 887 |
| 50-99 | 1,031 | 1,072 | 1,070 | 1,055 | 1,082 |
| 100-199 | 1,168 | 1,190 | 1,218 | 1,236 | 1,266 |
| 200-299 | 624 | 625 | 635 | 656 | 642 |
| 300-399 | 349 | 358 | 348 | 341 | 365 |
| 400-499 | 172 | 174 | 191 | 182 | 161 |
| 500 + | 259 | 256 | 249 | 247 | 254 |
| **Location** | | | | | |
| Hospitals Urban | 2,729 | 2,749 | 2,741 | 2,740 | 2,767 |
| Hospitals Rural | 2,166 | 2,178 | 2,167 | 2,175 | 2,189 |
| **Control** | | | | | |
| State and Local Government | 1,121 | 1,136 | 1,156 | 1,163 | 1,197 |
| Not for Profit | 2,984 | 3,025 | 2,998 | 3,003 | 3,012 |
| Investor owned | 790 | 766 | 754 | 749 | 747 |
| **Physician Models** | | | | | |
| Independent Practice Association | 777 | 771 | 770 | 831 | 874 |
| Group Practice without Walls | 188 | 193 | 195 | 211 | 198 |
| Open Physician-Hospital Organization | 791 | 820 | 849 | 939 | 975 |
| Closed Physician-Hospital Organization | 279 | 294 | 316 | 360 | 414 |
| Management Service Organization | 480 | 519 | 545 | 655 | 770 |
| Integrated Salary Model | 1,334 | 1,224 | 1,122 | 1,126 | 1,106 |
| Equity Model | 58 | 67 | 58 | 91 | 103 |
| Foundation | 197 | 202 | 212 | 252 | 290 |
| **Insurance Products** | | | | | |
| Health Maintenance Organization | 693 | 698 | 715 | 870 | 1,009 |
| Preferred Provider Organization | 937 | 923 | 873 | 1,028 | 1,156 |
| Indemnity Fee for Service | 288 | 265 | 247 | 286 | 303 |
| **Managed Care Contracts** | | | | | |
| Health Maintenance Organization | 2,743 | 2,740 | 2,738 | 2,804 | 2,916 |
| Preferred Provider Organization | 3,227 | 3,218 | 3,217 | 3,233 | 3,310 |
| **Affiliations** | | | | | |
| Hospitals in a System* | 2,626 | 2,606 | 2,580 | 2,542 | 2,524 |
| Hospitals in a Network | 1,393 | 1,343 | 1,341 | 1,327 | 1,310 |
| Hospitals in a Group Purchasing Organization | 3,650 | 3,495 | 3,495 | 3,344 | 3,080 |

* Please note that system affiliate information for hospitals is derived from AHA membership. In years prior to 2003 the affiliation was derived from a question on the AHA Annual Survey of hospitals; therefore, non-responding hospitals were not included in the system affiliation counts. Years prior to 2003 have been updated to reflect this change, which now include affiliation for non-reporting hospitals.

# TABLE 3

## TOTAL UNITED STATES

*U.S. Registered Community Hospitals*
*(Nonfederal, short-term general and other special hospitals)*

## Utilization, Personnel, Revenue and Expenses, Community Health Indicators 1999–2003

| | 2003 | 2002 | 2001 | 2000 | 1999 |
|---|---|---|---|---|---|
| **TOTAL FACILITY (Includes Hospital and Nursing Home Units)** | | | | | |
| **Utilization - Inpatient** | | | | | |
| Beds | 813,307 | 820,653 | 825,966 | 823,560 | 829,575 |
| Admissions | 34,782,742 | 34,478,280 | 33,813,589 | 33,089,467 | 32,359,042 |
| Inpatient Days | 196,649,769 | 196,690,099 | 194,106,316 | 192,420,368 | 191,884,270 |
| Average Length of Stay | 5.7 | 5.7 | 5.7 | 5.8 | 5.9 |
| Inpatient Surgeries | 9,940,922 | 10,105,010 | 9,779,583 | 9,729,336 | 9,539,593 |
| Births | 3,915,842 | 3,870,191 | 3,873,395 | 3,890,166 | 3,760,295 |
| **Utilization - Outpatient** | | | | | |
| Emergency Outpatient Visits | 111,069,871 | 109,951,738 | 105,957,778 | 103,144,030 | 99,484,462 |
| Other Outpatient Visits | 452,116,175 | 446,452,474 | 432,522,600 | 418,260,946 | 395,861,824 |
| Total Outpatient Visits | 563,186,046 | 556,404,212 | 538,480,378 | 521,404,976 | 495,346,286 |
| Outpatient Surgeries | 17,165,616 | 17,361,176 | 16,684,726 | 16,383,374 | 15,845,492 |
| **Personnel** | | | | | |
| Full Time RNs | 796,715 | 772,479 | 751,095 | 745,113 | 739,086 |
| Full Time LPNs | 103,635 | 104,058 | 104,534 | 101,683 | 106,739 |
| Part Time RNs | 449,340 | 431,274 | 413,832 | 424,801 | 397,950 |
| Part Time LPNs | 45,367 | 43,600 | 43,446 | 45,011 | 45,561 |
| Total Full Time | 3,512,182 | 3,489,190 | 3,428,159 | 3,332,232 | 3,297,689 |
| Total Part Time | 1,364,483 | 1,328,930 | 1,285,207 | 1,320,696 | 1,246,661 |
| **Revenue - Inpatient** | | | | | |
| Gross Inpatient Revenue | $721,919,505,541 | $622,963,195,767 | $544,087,612,104 | $481,753,558,221 | $436,802,516,912 |
| **Revenue - Outpatient** | | | | | |
| Gross Outpatient Revenue | $392,059,642,209 | $338,185,339,792 | $289,605,612,366 | $255,130,109,523 | $224,677,472,092 |
| **Revenue and Expenses - Totals (Includes Inpatient and Outpatient)** | | | | | |
| Total Gross Revenue | $1,113,979,147,750 | $961,148,535,559 | $833,693,224,470 | $736,883,667,744 | $661,439,989,004 |
| Deductions from Revenue | 676,289,161,428 | 553,855,167,351 | 463,168,133,776 | 394,634,720,840 | 340,074,141,264 |
| Net Patient Revenue | 437,689,986,322 | 407,293,368,208 | 370,525,090,694 | 342,248,946,904 | 321,365,847,740 |
| Other Operating Revenue | 27,914,540,848 | 25,253,169,830 | 23,816,314,195 | 21,691,829,666 | 20,954,555,617 |
| Other Nonoperating Revenue | 7,094,210,853 | 3,333,738,368 | 6,353,280,081 | 9,649,649,680 | 9,207,219,318 |
| Total Net Revenue | 472,698,738,023 | 435,880,276,406 | 400,694,684,970 | 373,590,426,250 | 351,527,622,675 |
| Total Expenses | 450,124,257,375 | 416,591,058,927 | 383,734,757,143 | 356,563,789,627 | 335,197,410,905 |
| **HOSPITAL UNIT (Excludes Separate Nursing Home Units)** | | | | | |
| **Utilization - Inpatient** | | | | | |
| Beds | 744,153 | 749,058 | 753,592 | 746,918 | 746,638 |
| Admissions | 34,424,735 | 34,096,173 | 33,408,199 | 32,639,620 | 31,814,468 |
| Inpatient Days | 174,691,978 | 174,148,040 | 171,049,431 | 168,133,112 | 165,919,000 |
| Average Length of Stay | 5.1 | 5.1 | 5.1 | 5.2 | 5.2 |
| **Personnel** | | | | | |
| Total Full Time | 3,460,507 | 3,440,069 | 3,376,958 | 3,274,082 | 3,239,743 |
| Total Part Time | 1,336,141 | 1,304,545 | 1,259,927 | 1,291,840 | 1,218,813 |
| **Revenue and Expenses - Totals (Includes Inpatient and Outpatient)** | | | | | |
| Total Net Revenue | $467,647,023,673 | $431,242,102,280 | $396,133,790,471 | $368,509,487,402 | $346,323,409,701 |
| Total Expenses | 445,704,797,515 | 412,517,083,689 | 380,087,229,391 | 353,070,652,573 | 331,217,766,222 |
| **COMMUNITY HEALTH INDICATORS PER 1000 POPULATION** | | | | | |
| Total Population (in thousands) | 290,810 | 287,974 | 285,094 | 282,178 | 279,040 |
| **Inpatient** | | | | | |
| Beds | 2.8 | 2.8 | 2.9 | 2.9 | 3.0 |
| Admissions | 119.6 | 119.7 | 118.6 | 117.3 | 116.0 |
| Inpatient Days | 676.2 | 683.0 | 680.9 | 681.9 | 687.7 |
| Inpatient Surgeries | 34.2 | 35.1 | 34.3 | 34.5 | 34.2 |
| Births | 13.5 | 13.4 | 13.6 | 13.8 | 13.5 |
| **Outpatient** | | | | | |
| Emergency Outpatient Visits | 381.9 | 381.8 | 371.7 | 365.5 | 356.5 |
| Other Outpatient Visits | 1,554.7 | 1,550.3 | 1,517.1 | 1,482.3 | 1,418.7 |
| Total Outpatient Visits | 1,936.6 | 1,932.1 | 1,888.8 | 1,847.8 | 1,775.2 |
| Outpatient Surgeries | 59.0 | 60.3 | 58.5 | 58.1 | 56.8 |
| **Expense per Capita (per person)** | $1,547.8 | $1,446.6 | $1,346.0 | $1,263.6 | $1,201.3 |

# TABLE 4

# BED SIZE CATEGORY 6-24

*U.S. Registered Community Hospitals*
*(Nonfederal, short-term general and other special hospitals)*

## Overview 1999–2003

| | 2003 | 2002 | 2001 | 2000 | 1999 |
|---|---|---|---|---|---|
| **Total Community Hospitals in** | | | | | |
| **Bed Size Category 6-24** | **327** | **321** | **281** | **288** | **299** |
| **Location** | | | | | |
| Hospitals Urban | 67 | 66 | 56 | 57 | 64 |
| Hospitals Rural | 260 | 255 | 225 | 231 | 235 |
| **Control** | | | | | |
| State and Local Government | 149 | 146 | 135 | 143 | 151 |
| Not for Profit | 149 | 149 | 122 | 126 | 127 |
| Investor owned | 29 | 26 | 24 | 19 | 21 |
| **Physician Models** | | | | | |
| Independent Practice Association | 39 | 42 | 36 | 31 | 25 |
| Group Practice without Walls | 13 | 14 | 10 | 12 | 9 |
| Open Physician-Hospital Organization | 25 | 21 | 17 | 20 | 21 |
| Closed Physician-Hospital Organization | 9 | 11 | 9 | 6 | 8 |
| Management Service Organization | 12 | 20 | 14 | 12 | 15 |
| Integrated Salary Model | 86 | 85 | 73 | 64 | 65 |
| Equity Model | 1 | 4 | 3 | 3 | 5 |
| Foundation | 6 | 13 | 9 | 7 | 13 |
| **Insurance Products** | | | | | |
| Health Maintenance Organization | 30 | 35 | 30 | 34 | 30 |
| Preferred Provider Organization | 48 | 53 | 35 | 42 | 40 |
| Indemnity Fee for Service | 11 | 18 | 11 | 10 | 5 |
| **Managed Care Contracts** | | | | | |
| Health Maintenance Organization | 122 | 124 | 100 | 101 | 120 |
| Preferred Provider Organization | 177 | 181 | 160 | 164 | 175 |
| **Affiliations** | | | | | |
| Hospitals in a System* | 119 | 114 | 88 | 83 | 86 |
| Hospitals in a Network | 94 | 97 | 79 | 77 | 67 |
| Hospitals in a Group Purchasing Organization | 214 | 212 | 192 | 178 | 169 |

* Please note that system affiliate information for hospitals is derived from AHA membership. In years prior to 2003 the affiliation was derived from a question on the AHA Annual Survey of hospitals; therefore, non-responding hospitals were not included in the system affiliation counts. Years prior to 2003 have been updated to reflect this change, which now include affiliation for non-reporting hospitals.

Bed Size Categories

# TABLE 4

# BED SIZE CATEGORY 6-24

*U.S. Registered Community Hospitals*
*(Nonfederal, short-term general and other special hospitals)*

## Utilization, Personnel, Revenue and Expenses 1999–2003

| | 2003 | 2002 | 2001 | 2000 | 1999 |
|---|---|---|---|---|---|
| **TOTAL FACILITY (Includes Hospital and Nursing Home Units)** | | | | | |
| **Utilization - Inpatient** | | | | | |
| Beds | 5,635 | 5,629 | 4,964 | 5,156 | 5,442 |
| Admissions | 162,231 | 161,716 | 140,467 | 140,735 | 145,418 |
| Inpatient Days | 658,374 | 666,858 | 566,345 | 601,199 | 651,124 |
| Average Length of Stay | 4.1 | 4.1 | 4.0 | 4.3 | 4.5 |
| Inpatient Surgeries | 33,263 | 26,172 | 23,655 | 21,084 | 22,445 |
| Births | 9,347 | 10,297 | 9,300 | 9,836 | 11,283 |
| **Utilization - Outpatient** | | | | | |
| Emergency Outpatient Visits | 1,159,015 | 1,053,994 | 796,297 | 743,260 | 676,879 |
| Other Outpatient Visits | 5,353,309 | 4,875,803 | 3,759,485 | 3,812,179 | 3,973,601 |
| Total Outpatient Visits | 6,512,324 | 5,929,797 | 4,555,782 | 4,555,439 | 4,650,480 |
| Outpatient Surgeries | 176,609 | 160,854 | 120,783 | 111,263 | 117,592 |
| **Personnel** | | | | | |
| Full Time RNs | 4,612 | 4,451 | 3,684 | 3,744 | 3,935 |
| Full Time LPNs | 1,710 | 1,677 | 1,468 | 1,363 | 1,469 |
| Part Time RNs | 2,647 | 2,498 | 2,069 | 2,443 | 2,369 |
| Part Time LPNs | 779 | 709 | 669 | 713 | 752 |
| Total Full Time | 24,113 | 23,058 | 18,993 | 18,944 | 20,593 |
| Total Part Time | 10,942 | 10,753 | 9,128 | 10,287 | 10,026 |
| **Revenue - Inpatient** | | | | | |
| Gross Inpatient Revenue | $1,238,430,927 | $1,187,061,180 | $865,976,268 | $785,583,707 | $803,992,451 |
| **Revenue - Outpatient** | | | | | |
| Gross Outpatient Revenue | $2,945,148,175 | $2,471,688,778 | $1,560,963,930 | $1,539,812,867 | $1,377,204,771 |
| **Revenue and Expenses - Totals (Includes Inpatient and Outpatient)** | | | | | |
| Total Gross Revenue | $4,183,579,102 | $3,658,749,958 | $2,426,940,198 | $2,325,396,574 | $2,181,197,222 |
| Deductions from Revenue | 1,799,934,162 | 1,513,681,706 | 951,093,256 | 907,556,076 | 782,264,529 |
| Net Patient Revenue | 2,383,644,940 | 2,145,068,252 | 1,475,846,942 | 1,417,840,498 | 1,398,932,693 |
| Other Operating Revenue | 198,380,153 | 162,911,063 | 154,437,602 | 115,552,533 | 170,916,578 |
| Other Nonoperating Revenue | 36,877,876 | 28,315,990 | 33,912,311 | 38,248,611 | 87,134,276 |
| Total Net Revenue | 2,618,902,969 | 2,336,295,305 | 1,664,196,855 | 1,571,641,642 | 1,656,983,547 |
| Total Expenses | 2,456,994,289 | 2,235,953,879 | 1,613,936,534 | 1,549,776,034 | 1,658,451,372 |
| **HOSPITAL UNIT (Excludes Separate Nursing Home Units)** | | | | | |
| **Utilization - Inpatient** | | | | | |
| Beds | 5,569 | 5,470 | 4,864 | 5,063 | 5,352 |
| Admissions | 162,101 | 161,090 | 140,181 | 140,230 | 144,893 |
| Inpatient Days | 639,363 | 619,452 | 528,596 | 568,533 | 623,695 |
| Average Length of Stay | 3.9 | 3.8 | 3.8 | 4.1 | 4.3 |
| **Personnel** | | | | | |
| Total Full Time | 23,964 | 22,960 | 18,929 | 18,716 | 20,537 |
| Total Part Time | 10,854 | 10,689 | 9,066 | 10,074 | 9,985 |
| **Revenue and Expenses - Totals (Includes Inpatient and Outpatient)** | | | | | |
| Total Net Revenue | $2,612,681,706 | $2,324,685,737 | $1,654,040,740 | $1,564,960,209 | $1,650,222,760 |
| Total Expenses | 2,454,449,892 | 2,230,173,614 | 1,608,501,142 | 1,543,940,406 | 1,653,276,803 |

# TABLE 4

# BED SIZE CATEGORY 25-49

*U.S. Registered Community Hospitals*
*(Nonfederal, short-term general and other special hospitals)*

## Overview 1999–2003

| | 2003 | 2002 | 2001 | 2000 | 1999 |
|---|---|---|---|---|---|
| **Total Community Hospitals in Bed Size Category 25-49** | **965** | **931** | **916** | **910** | **887** |
| **Location** | | | | | |
| Hospitals Urban | 225 | 220 | 214 | 201 | 192 |
| Hospitals Rural | 740 | 711 | 702 | 709 | 695 |
| **Control** | | | | | |
| State and Local Government | 371 | 363 | 374 | 375 | 374 |
| Not for Profit | 475 | 461 | 442 | 440 | 423 |
| Investor owned | 119 | 107 | 100 | 95 | 90 |
| **Physician Models** | | | | | |
| Independent Practice Association | 130 | 128 | 113 | 106 | 114 |
| Group Practice without Walls | 28 | 27 | 35 | 29 | 17 |
| Open Physician-Hospital Organization | 88 | 87 | 83 | 102 | 96 |
| Closed Physician-Hospital Organization | 32 | 33 | 33 | 39 | 40 |
| Management Service Organization | 55 | 56 | 53 | 62 | 64 |
| Integrated Salary Model | 252 | 212 | 200 | 183 | 169 |
| Equity Model | 7 | 6 | 4 | 10 | 9 |
| Foundation | 23 | 19 | 23 | 26 | 31 |
| **Insurance Products** | | | | | |
| Health Maintenance Organization | 86 | 78 | 87 | 89 | 110 |
| Preferred Provider Organization | 171 | 152 | 133 | 143 | 153 |
| Indemnity Fee for Service | 53 | 41 | 45 | 45 | 48 |
| **Managed Care Contracts** | | | | | |
| Health Maintenance Organization | 424 | 421 | 416 | 406 | 436 |
| Preferred Provider Organization | 591 | 578 | 557 | 561 | 571 |
| **Affiliations** | | | | | |
| Hospitals in a System* | 428 | 393 | 385 | 383 | 364 |
| Hospitals in a Network | 249 | 221 | 219 | 216 | 208 |
| Hospitals in a Group Purchasing Organization | 699 | 643 | 639 | 612 | 584 |

* Please note that system affiliate information for hospitals is derived from AHA membership. In years prior to 2003 the affiliation was derived from a question on the AHA Annual Survey of hospitals; therefore, non-responding hospitals were not included in the system affiliation counts. Years prior to 2003 have been updated to reflect this change, which now include affiliation for non-reporting hospitals.

# TABLE 4

## BED SIZE CATEGORY 25-49

*U.S. Registered Community Hospitals*
*(Nonfederal, short-term general and other special hospitals)*

## Utilization, Personnel, Revenue and Expenses 1999–2003

| | 2003 | 2002 | 2001 | 2000 | 1999 |
|---|---|---|---|---|---|
| **TOTAL FACILITY (Includes Hospital and Nursing Home Units)** | | | | | |
| **Utilization - Inpatient** | | | | | |
| Beds | 33,613 | 33,200 | 33,263 | 33,333 | 32,816 |
| Admissions | 1,098,125 | 1,062,147 | 1,030,375 | 994,641 | 959,482 |
| Inpatient Days | 5,465,909 | 5,313,229 | 5,159,467 | 5,031,151 | 4,957,792 |
| Average Length of Stay | 5.0 | 5.0 | 5.0 | 5.1 | 5.2 |
| Inpatient Surgeries | 220,545 | 224,701 | 205,619 | 206,859 | 197,717 |
| Births | 94,761 | 90,518 | 87,770 | 88,275 | 84,491 |
| **Utilization - Outpatient** | | | | | |
| Emergency Outpatient Visits | 6,148,561 | 5,851,427 | 5,346,064 | 5,195,946 | 5,055,140 |
| Other Outpatient Visits | 25,112,424 | 23,874,930 | 22,594,571 | 21,811,383 | 18,814,467 |
| Total Outpatient Visits | 31,260,985 | 29,726,357 | 27,940,635 | 27,007,329 | 23,869,607 |
| Outpatient Surgeries | 818,147 | 772,158 | 747,613 | 676,172 | 610,784 |
| **Personnel** | | | | | |
| Full Time RNs | 25,073 | 23,627 | 22,343 | 22,830 | 21,305 |
| Full Time LPNs | 8,085 | 7,654 | 7,400 | 7,333 | 6,978 |
| Part Time RNs | 14,926 | 13,569 | 13,038 | 14,072 | 13,333 |
| Part Time LPNs | 3,375 | 3,221 | 3,132 | 3,424 | 3,191 |
| Total Full Time | 134,252 | 126,569 | 120,976 | 116,462 | 110,210 |
| Total Part Time | 59,079 | 54,844 | 51,639 | 54,820 | 50,931 |
| **Revenue - Inpatient** | | | | | |
| Gross Inpatient Revenue | $10,355,433,556 | $9,424,112,207 | $7,883,987,594 | $7,196,766,831 | $6,561,005,229 |
| **Revenue - Outpatient** | | | | | |
| Gross Outpatient Revenue | $14,642,949,853 | $12,499,434,007 | $10,608,878,116 | $9,410,834,420 | $7,991,583,099 |
| **Revenue and Expenses - Totals (Includes Inpatient and Outpatient)** | | | | | |
| Total Gross Revenue | $24,998,383,409 | $21,923,546,214 | $18,492,865,710 | $16,607,601,251 | $14,552,588,328 |
| Deductions from Revenue | 11,978,398,999 | 10,327,317,002 | 8,222,555,507 | 7,231,526,571 | 6,067,585,675 |
| Net Patient Revenue | 13,019,984,410 | 11,596,229,212 | 10,270,310,203 | 9,376,074,680 | 8,485,002,653 |
| Other Operating Revenue | 1,326,340,570 | 1,245,298,074 | 1,134,586,636 | 959,276,038 | 826,240,928 |
| Other Nonoperating Revenue | 202,900,746 | 135,373,750 | 212,155,156 | 312,430,036 | 217,293,330 |
| Total Net Revenue | 14,549,225,726 | 12,976,901,036 | 11,617,051,995 | 10,647,780,754 | 9,528,536,911 |
| Total Expenses | 13,984,833,741 | 12,594,583,292 | 11,381,539,275 | 10,391,935,057 | 9,283,978,476 |
| **HOSPITAL UNIT (Excludes Separate Nursing Home Units)** | | | | | |
| **Utilization - Inpatient** | | | | | |
| Beds | 31,309 | 31,025 | 31,189 | 31,299 | 30,763 |
| Admissions | 1,092,499 | 1,056,128 | 1,023,053 | 987,780 | 952,964 |
| Inpatient Days | 4,742,669 | 4,637,216 | 4,511,675 | 4,419,903 | 4,319,613 |
| Average Length of Stay | 4.3 | 4.4 | 4.4 | 4.5 | 4.5 |
| **Personnel** | | | | | |
| Total Full Time | 132,280 | 124,998 | 119,566 | 115,277 | 109,069 |
| Total Part Time | 57,909 | 54,116 | 50,898 | 54,115 | 50,264 |
| **Revenue and Expenses - Totals (Includes Inpatient and Outpatient)** | | | | | |
| Total Net Revenue | $14,428,934,219 | $12,864,807,992 | $11,521,210,710 | $10,559,902,580 | $9,428,841,798 |
| Total Expenses | 13,887,155,639 | 12,509,264,997 | 11,315,045,682 | 10,335,837,413 | 9,223,711,698 |

# TABLE 4

## BED SIZE CATEGORY 50-99

*U.S. Registered Community Hospitals*
*(Nonfederal, short-term general and other special hospitals)*

## Overview 1999–2003

| | 2003 | 2002 | 2001 | 2000 | 1999 |
|---|---|---|---|---|---|
| **Total Community Hospitals in Bed Size Category 50-99** | **1,031** | **1,072** | **1,070** | **1,055** | **1,082** |
| **Location** | | | | | |
| Hospitals Urban | 418 | 417 | 407 | 400 | 414 |
| Hospitals Rural | 613 | 655 | 663 | 655 | 668 |
| **Control** | | | | | |
| State and Local Government | 253 | 273 | 278 | 279 | 285 |
| Not for Profit | 565 | 590 | 593 | 581 | 584 |
| Investor owned | 213 | 209 | 199 | 195 | 213 |
| **Physician Models** | | | | | |
| Independent Practice Association | 147 | 137 | 138 | 153 | 158 |
| Group Practice without Walls | 38 | 34 | 37 | 38 | 36 |
| Open Physician-Hospital Organization | 139 | 162 | 158 | 168 | 177 |
| Closed Physician-Hospital Organization | 47 | 45 | 45 | 54 | 61 |
| Management Service Organization | 67 | 64 | 70 | 85 | 114 |
| Integrated Salary Model | 245 | 221 | 196 | 191 | 195 |
| Equity Model | 11 | 9 | 3 | 9 | 14 |
| Foundation | 33 | 34 | 29 | 49 | 50 |
| **Insurance Products** | | | | | |
| Health Maintenance Organization | 101 | 108 | 105 | 121 | 154 |
| Preferred Provider Organization | 183 | 170 | 149 | 178 | 226 |
| Indemnity Fee for Service | 52 | 55 | 42 | 54 | 61 |
| **Managed Care Contracts** | | | | | |
| Health Maintenance Organization | 495 | 499 | 509 | 511 | 541 |
| Preferred Provider Organization | 656 | 649 | 660 | 644 | 662 |
| **Affiliations** | | | | | |
| Hospitals in a System* | 529 | 552 | 545 | 527 | 550 |
| Hospitals in a Network | 268 | 260 | 267 | 264 | 269 |
| Hospitals in a Group Purchasing Organization | 766 | 753 | 751 | 697 | 637 |

* Please note that system affiliate information for hospitals is derived from AHA membership. In years prior to 2003 the affiliation was derived from a question on the AHA Annual Survey of hospitals; therefore, non-responding hospitals were not included in the system affiliation counts. Years prior to 2003 have been updated to reflect this change, which now include affiliation for non-reporting hospitals.

# BED SIZE CATEGORY 50-99

*U.S. Registered Community Hospitals*
*(Nonfederal, short-term general and other special hospitals)*

## Utilization, Personnel, Revenue and Expenses 1999–2003

| | 2003 | 2002 | 2001 | 2000 | 1999 |
|---|---|---|---|---|---|
| **TOTAL FACILITY (Includes Hospital and Nursing Home Units)** | | | | | |
| **Utilization - Inpatient** | | | | | |
| Beds | 74,025 | 76,882 | 76,924 | 75,865 | 78,121 |
| Admissions | 2,463,703 | 2,471,386 | 2,421,938 | 2,354,896 | 2,316,862 |
| Inpatient Days | 15,445,684 | 15,874,178 | 15,461,340 | 15,195,600 | 15,548,467 |
| Average Length of Stay | 6.3 | 6.4 | 6.4 | 6.5 | 6.7 |
| Inpatient Surgeries | 611,190 | 610,705 | 588,354 | 580,886 | 568,696 |
| Births | 264,321 | 262,390 | 262,605 | 276,308 | 266,469 |
| **Utilization - Outpatient** | | | | | |
| Emergency Outpatient Visits | 11,581,730 | 11,669,278 | 11,093,357 | 10,601,048 | 10,292,153 |
| Other Outpatient Visits | 41,377,442 | 41,672,959 | 40,237,990 | 38,783,686 | 35,863,458 |
| Total Outpatient Visits | 52,959,172 | 53,342,237 | 51,331,347 | 49,384,734 | 46,155,611 |
| Outpatient Surgeries | 1,659,676 | 1,613,367 | 1,485,774 | 1,448,514 | 1,385,596 |
| **Personnel** | | | | | |
| Full Time RNs | 51,823 | 51,193 | 49,209 | 48,531 | 48,609 |
| Full Time LPNs | 12,490 | 13,012 | 12,956 | 12,749 | 13,349 |
| Part Time RNs | 32,371 | 31,630 | 29,477 | 31,250 | 30,651 |
| Part Time LPNs | 5,846 | 6,137 | 5,747 | 6,141 | 6,460 |
| Total Full Time | 244,695 | 247,846 | 244,068 | 233,169 | 233,659 |
| Total Part Time | 116,518 | 114,178 | 110,165 | 115,307 | 110,546 |
| **Revenue - Inpatient** | | | | | |
| Gross Inpatient Revenue | $32,333,642,062 | $28,405,320,827 | $24,513,608,917 | $22,750,944,141 | $21,097,563,298 |
| **Revenue - Outpatient** | | | | | |
| Gross Outpatient Revenue | $29,770,749,660 | $25,936,635,813 | $22,106,129,277 | $19,990,370,027 | $17,597,291,726 |
| **Revenue and Expenses - Totals (Includes Inpatient and Outpatient)** | | | | | |
| Total Gross Revenue | $62,104,391,722 | $54,341,956,640 | $46,619,738,194 | $42,741,314,168 | $38,694,855,024 |
| Deductions from Revenue | 34,407,137,154 | 28,088,461,303 | 23,028,290,004 | 21,022,033,394 | 18,058,805,944 |
| Net Patient Revenue | 27,697,254,568 | 26,253,495,337 | 23,591,448,190 | 21,719,280,774 | 20,636,049,080 |
| Other Operating Revenue | 1,469,952,946 | 1,036,671,212 | 1,028,923,986 | 992,807,456 | 1,007,752,277 |
| Other Nonoperating Revenue | 386,699,226 | 260,065,744 | 683,658,777 | 657,785,910 | 448,107,493 |
| Total Net Revenue | 29,553,906,740 | 27,550,232,293 | 25,304,030,953 | 23,369,874,140 | 22,091,908,850 |
| Total Expenses | 28,189,310,174 | 26,141,500,525 | 24,030,935,779 | 22,322,022,731 | 20,967,397,999 |
| **HOSPITAL UNIT (Excludes Separate Nursing Home Units)** | | | | | |
| **Utilization - Inpatient** | | | | | |
| Beds | 61,716 | 64,086 | 64,717 | 63,189 | 65,129 |
| Admissions | 2,429,002 | 2,431,740 | 2,384,021 | 2,315,942 | 2,269,013 |
| Inpatient Days | 11,488,717 | 11,846,603 | 11,602,606 | 11,205,030 | 11,512,534 |
| Average Length of Stay | 4.7 | 4.9 | 4.9 | 4.8 | 5.1 |
| **Personnel** | | | | | |
| Total Full Time | 236,652 | 240,319 | 237,000 | 224,763 | 226,412 |
| Total Part Time | 111,367 | 109,200 | 105,562 | 110,426 | 106,029 |
| **Revenue and Expenses - Totals (Includes Inpatient and Outpatient)** | | | | | |
| Total Net Revenue | $28,977,815,508 | $26,950,192,407 | $24,745,283,010 | $22,858,172,678 | $21,542,991,451 |
| Total Expenses | 27,720,675,559 | 25,675,955,624 | 23,602,034,845 | 21,923,794,277 | 20,558,590,538 |

# TABLE 4

## BED SIZE CATEGORY 100-199

*U.S. Registered Community Hospitals*
*(Nonfederal, short-term general and other special hospitals)*

## Overview 1999–2003

| | 2003 | 2002 | 2001 | 2000 | 1999 |
|---|---|---|---|---|---|
| **Total Community Hospitals in Bed Size Category 100-199** | **1,168** | **1,190** | **1,218** | **1,236** | **1,266** |
| **Location** | | | | | |
| Hospitals Urban | 752 | 766 | 783 | 795 | 816 |
| Hospitals Rural | 416 | 424 | 435 | 441 | 450 |
| **Control** | | | | | |
| State and Local Government | 178 | 181 | 198 | 196 | 214 |
| Not for Profit | 729 | 750 | 757 | 769 | 791 |
| Investor owned | 261 | 259 | 263 | 271 | 261 |
| **Physician Models** | | | | | |
| Independent Practice Association | 186 | 193 | 198 | 229 | 222 |
| Group Practice without Walls | 39 | 48 | 50 | 55 | 50 |
| Open Physician-Hospital Organization | 201 | 220 | 242 | 274 | 294 |
| Closed Physician-Hospital Organization | 66 | 78 | 82 | 87 | 100 |
| Management Service Organization | 104 | 130 | 143 | 178 | 213 |
| Integrated Salary Model | 267 | 261 | 241 | 265 | 269 |
| Equity Model | 16 | 15 | 16 | 26 | 21 |
| Foundation | 45 | 43 | 46 | 60 | 66 |
| **Insurance Products** | | | | | |
| Health Maintenance Organization | 147 | 150 | 151 | 196 | 243 |
| Preferred Provider Organization | 198 | 196 | 208 | 247 | 286 |
| Indemnity Fee for Service | 60 | 53 | 51 | 59 | 79 |
| **Managed Care Contracts** | | | | | |
| Health Maintenance Organization | 663 | 691 | 706 | 752 | 776 |
| Preferred Provider Organization | 744 | 776 | 805 | 820 | 849 |
| **Affiliations** | | | | | |
| Hospitals in a System* | 669 | 676 | 691 | 693 | 694 |
| Hospitals in a Network | 312 | 313 | 325 | 315 | 315 |
| Hospitals in a Group Purchasing Organization | 846 | 837 | 858 | 850 | 763 |

* Please note that system affiliate information for hospitals is derived from AHA membership. In years prior to 2003 the affiliation was derived from a question on the AHA Annual Survey of hospitals; therefore, non-responding hospitals were not included in the system affiliation counts. Years prior to 2003 have been updated to reflect this change, which now include affiliation for non-reporting hospitals.

# TABLE 4

## BED SIZE CATEGORY 100-199

*U.S. Registered Community Hospitals*
*(Nonfederal, short-term general and other special hospitals)*

## Utilization, Personnel, Revenue and Expenses 1999–2003

| | 2003 | 2002 | 2001 | 2000 | 1999 |
|---|---|---|---|---|---|
| **TOTAL FACILITY (Includes Hospital and Nursing Home Units)** | | | | | |
| **Utilization - Inpatient** | | | | | |
| Beds | 167,451 | 171,625 | 174,024 | 175,778 | 181,115 |
| Admissions | 6,816,567 | 6,826,388 | 6,777,542 | 6,734,707 | 6,683,621 |
| Inpatient Days | 38,281,885 | 38,569,069 | 38,508,731 | 38,624,802 | 39,220,552 |
| Average Length of Stay | 5.6 | 5.6 | 5.7 | 5.7 | 5.9 |
| Inpatient Surgeries | 1,879,739 | 1,975,373 | 1,907,604 | 1,857,378 | 1,855,847 |
| Births | 777,298 | 786,784 | 804,377 | 811,163 | 799,904 |
| **Utilization - Outpatient** | | | | | |
| Emergency Outpatient Visits | 25,687,014 | 25,708,579 | 25,605,993 | 25,135,121 | 24,700,172 |
| Other Outpatient Visits | 94,168,599 | 91,864,503 | 89,314,524 | 89,047,867 | 85,635,833 |
| Total Outpatient Visits | 119,855,613 | 117,573,082 | 114,920,517 | 114,182,988 | 110,336,005 |
| Outpatient Surgeries | 3,932,289 | 3,960,322 | 3,897,374 | 3,921,040 | 3,798,060 |
| **Personnel** | | | | | |
| Full Time RNs | 136,785 | 133,870 | 132,993 | 134,882 | 135,087 |
| Full Time LPNs | 23,626 | 23,445 | 23,871 | 23,104 | 24,310 |
| Part Time RNs | 85,328 | 86,030 | 84,269 | 89,261 | 87,233 |
| Part Time LPNs | 10,708 | 10,416 | 10,859 | 11,416 | 11,576 |
| Total Full Time | 613,056 | 617,804 | 612,894 | 601,589 | 607,315 |
| Total Part Time | 271,318 | 274,304 | 270,898 | 285,929 | 281,113 |
| **Revenue - Inpatient** | | | | | |
| Gross Inpatient Revenue | $115,221,061,460 | $101,757,585,465 | $88,826,998,928 | $81,494,205,969 | $73,304,767,289 |
| **Revenue - Outpatient** | | | | | |
| Gross Outpatient Revenue | $77,984,208,408 | $67,393,901,996 | $59,081,658,626 | $55,132,963,490 | $48,727,503,116 |
| **Revenue and Expenses - Totals (Includes Inpatient and Outpatient)** | | | | | |
| Total Gross Revenue | $193,205,269,868 | $169,151,487,461 | $147,908,657,554 | $136,627,169,459 | $122,032,270,405 |
| Deductions from Revenue | 117,286,043,669 | 97,607,890,820 | 81,506,420,194 | 73,520,588,504 | 61,736,298,969 |
| Net Patient Revenue | 75,919,226,199 | 71,543,596,641 | 66,402,237,360 | 63,106,580,955 | 60,295,971,436 |
| Other Operating Revenue | 3,017,184,270 | 2,890,345,556 | 2,813,935,425 | 2,769,788,344 | 2,772,654,915 |
| Other Nonoperating Revenue | 1,043,280,208 | 793,439,831 | 1,064,678,719 | 1,377,282,079 | 1,366,384,506 |
| Total Net Revenue | 79,979,690,677 | 75,227,382,028 | 70,280,851,504 | 67,253,651,378 | 64,435,010,857 |
| Total Expenses | 75,609,452,071 | 71,359,095,546 | 66,360,396,087 | 63,358,364,315 | 60,794,792,716 |
| **HOSPITAL UNIT (Excludes Separate Nursing Home Units)** | | | | | |
| **Utilization - Inpatient** | | | | | |
| Beds | 146,593 | 150,384 | 152,541 | 153,990 | 156,820 |
| Admissions | 6,720,086 | 6,725,794 | 6,672,956 | 6,618,001 | 6,539,049 |
| Inpatient Days | 31,606,046 | 31,911,182 | 31,662,149 | 31,797,892 | 31,621,341 |
| Average Length of Stay | 4.7 | 4.7 | 4.7 | 4.8 | 4.8 |
| **Personnel** | | | | | |
| Total Full Time | 599,180 | 604,557 | 599,785 | 587,721 | 591,911 |
| Total Part Time | 262,755 | 266,592 | 263,165 | 277,067 | 272,228 |
| **Revenue and Expenses - Totals (Includes Inpatient and Outpatient)** | | | | | |
| Total Net Revenue | $78,847,746,301 | $74,065,919,906 | $69,200,831,169 | $66,041,517,516 | $63,158,997,513 |
| Total Expenses | 74,610,675,288 | 70,382,713,681 | 65,492,148,426 | 62,568,627,003 | 59,804,230,111 |

# TABLE 4

# BED SIZE CATEGORY 200-299

*U.S. Registered Community Hospitals*
*(Nonfederal, short-term general and other special hospitals)*

## Overview 1999–2003

| | 2003 | 2002 | 2001 | 2000 | 1999 |
|---|---|---|---|---|---|
| **Total Community Hospitals in Bed Size Category 200-299** | **624** | **625** | **635** | **656** | **642** |
| **Location** | | | | | |
| Hospitals Urban | 523 | 529 | 526 | 551 | 534 |
| Hospitals Rural | 101 | 96 | 109 | 105 | 108 |
| **Control** | | | | | |
| State and Local Government | 62 | 69 | 69 | 71 | 71 |
| Not for Profit | 462 | 462 | 467 | 488 | 480 |
| Investor owned | 100 | 94 | 99 | 97 | 91 |
| **Physician Models** | | | | | |
| Independent Practice Association | 100 | 90 | 103 | 127 | 136 |
| Group Practice without Walls | 30 | 27 | 24 | 31 | 36 |
| Open Physician-Hospital Organization | 151 | 140 | 143 | 171 | 178 |
| Closed Physician-Hospital Organization | 47 | 45 | 56 | 61 | 71 |
| Management Service Organization | 86 | 86 | 92 | 118 | 152 |
| Integrated Salary Model | 180 | 159 | 154 | 167 | 151 |
| Equity Model | 10 | 11 | 10 | 20 | 23 |
| Foundation | 28 | 29 | 34 | 43 | 49 |
| **Insurance Products** | | | | | |
| Health Maintenance Organization | 114 | 105 | 113 | 151 | 146 |
| Preferred Provider Organization | 123 | 125 | 123 | 154 | 160 |
| Indemnity Fee for Service | 51 | 43 | 41 | 46 | 42 |
| **Managed Care Contracts** | | | | | |
| Health Maintenance Organization | 439 | 422 | 424 | 454 | 456 |
| Preferred Provider Organization | 459 | 442 | 435 | 460 | 466 |
| **Affiliations** | | | | | |
| Hospitals in a System* | 382 | 370 | 374 | 382 | 355 |
| Hospitals in a Network | 192 | 179 | 173 | 195 | 189 |
| Hospitals in a Group Purchasing Organization | 493 | 462 | 459 | 461 | 418 |

Bed Size Categories

* Please note that system affiliate information for hospitals is derived from AHA membership. In years prior to 2003 the affiliation was derived from a question on the AHA Annual Survey of hospitals; therefore, non-responding hospitals were not included in the system affiliation counts. Years prior to 2003 have been updated to reflect this change, which now include affiliation for non-reporting hospitals.

# TABLE 4

# BED SIZE CATEGORY 200-299

*U.S. Registered Community Hospitals*
*(Nonfederal, short-term general and other special hospitals)*

## Utilization, Personnel, Revenue and Expenses 1999–2003

| | 2003 | 2002 | 2001 | 2000 | 1999 |
|---|---|---|---|---|---|
| **TOTAL FACILITY (Includes Hospital and Nursing Home Units)** | | | | | |
| **Utilization - Inpatient** | | | | | |
| Beds | 152,487 | 152,682 | 154,420 | 159,807 | 155,831 |
| Admissions | 6,887,304 | 6,799,664 | 6,630,307 | 6,702,478 | 6,389,172 |
| Inpatient Days | 37,271,468 | 37,122,247 | 36,923,111 | 37,942,444 | 36,493,064 |
| Average Length of Stay | 5.4 | 5.5 | 5.6 | 5.7 | 5.7 |
| Inpatient Surgeries | 1,985,604 | 1,957,651 | 1,910,132 | 1,992,966 | 1,883,032 |
| Births | 764,095 | 753,559 | 733,456 | 788,352 | 755,274 |
| **Utilization - Outpatient** | | | | | |
| Emergency Outpatient Visits | 21,701,788 | 21,513,390 | 20,309,391 | 20,436,782 | 19,533,629 |
| Other Outpatient Visits | 78,393,455 | 80,910,560 | 79,286,800 | 78,811,142 | 71,343,993 |
| Total Outpatient Visits | 100,095,243 | 102,423,950 | 99,596,191 | 99,247,924 | 90,877,622 |
| Outpatient Surgeries | 3,435,799 | 3,394,622 | 3,265,812 | 3,358,516 | 3,163,861 |
| **Personnel** | | | | | |
| Full Time RNs | 146,013 | 141,467 | 136,338 | 137,548 | 132,812 |
| Full Time LPNs | 18,329 | 18,402 | 18,036 | 18,703 | 20,192 |
| Part Time RNs | 87,456 | 85,147 | 80,856 | 86,744 | 80,212 |
| Part Time LPNs | 8,691 | 8,442 | 8,752 | 9,181 | 9,349 |
| Total Full Time | 618,665 | 616,865 | 600,028 | 614,344 | 588,843 |
| Total Part Time | 271,315 | 260,312 | 247,526 | 265,162 | 249,790 |
| **Revenue - Inpatient** | | | | | |
| Gross Inpatient Revenue | $138,068,942,960 | $119,690,492,836 | $103,904,499,291 | $92,657,723,538 | $84,461,242,677 |
| **Revenue - Outpatient** | | | | | |
| Gross Outpatient Revenue | $72,993,639,658 | $64,425,216,711 | $54,235,790,743 | $47,912,514,899 | $42,225,301,889 |
| **Revenue and Expenses - Totals (Includes Inpatient and Outpatient)** | | | | | |
| Total Gross Revenue | $211,062,582,618 | $184,115,709,547 | $158,140,290,034 | $140,570,238,437 | $126,686,544,566 |
| Deductions from Revenue | 130,733,370,398 | 108,902,937,426 | 90,371,126,069 | 75,560,084,371 | 67,487,466,289 |
| Net Patient Revenue | 80,329,212,220 | 75,212,772,121 | 67,769,163,965 | 65,010,154,066 | 59,199,078,277 |
| Other Operating Revenue | 3,686,516,113 | 3,204,222,444 | 3,278,654,426 | 3,511,441,863 | 3,261,463,827 |
| Other Nonoperating Revenue | 1,211,869,399 | 836,318,819 | 1,301,236,089 | 1,789,700,386 | 2,038,058,222 |
| Total Net Revenue | 85,227,597,732 | 79,253,313,384 | 72,349,054,480 | 70,311,296,315 | 64,498,600,326 |
| Total Expenses | 81,020,518,283 | 75,580,360,702 | 68,913,526,440 | 67,057,555,091 | 61,099,993,147 |
| **HOSPITAL UNIT (Excludes Separate Nursing Home Units)** | | | | | |
| **Utilization - Inpatient** | | | | | |
| Beds | 140,386 | 140,310 | 141,629 | 145,501 | 140,318 |
| Admissions | 6,798,001 | 6,706,901 | 6,530,211 | 6,592,395 | 6,261,091 |
| Inpatient Days | 33,411,165 | 33,216,134 | 32,784,136 | 33,230,080 | 31,689,032 |
| Average Length of Stay | 4.9 | 5.0 | 5.0 | 5.0 | 5.1 |
| **Personnel** | | | | | |
| Total Full Time | 609,113 | 608,134 | 591,000 | 602,872 | 577,378 |
| Total Part Time | 266,160 | 256,082 | 242,702 | 259,423 | 244,444 |
| **Revenue and Expenses - Totals (Includes Inpatient and Outpatient)** | | | | | |
| Total Net Revenue | $84,316,957,990 | $78,446,952,108 | $71,458,934,077 | $69,473,697,175 | $63,481,487,264 |
| Total Expenses | 80,276,845,970 | 74,919,598,886 | 68,260,569,539 | 66,366,724,426 | 60,356,593,743 |

# TABLE 4

## BED SIZE CATEGORY 300-399

*U.S. Registered Community Hospitals*
*(Nonfederal, short-term general and other special hospitals)*

## Overview 1999–2003

| | 2003 | 2002 | 2001 | 2000 | 1999 |
|---|---|---|---|---|---|
| **Total Community Hospitals in Bed Size Category 300-399** | **349** | **358** | **348** | **341** | **365** |
| **Location** | | | | | |
| Hospitals Urban | 320 | 328 | 324 | 314 | 339 |
| Hospitals Rural | 29 | 30 | 24 | 27 | 26 |
| **Control** | | | | | |
| State and Local Government | 43 | 41 | 38 | 38 | 43 |
| Not for Profit | 263 | 270 | 269 | 255 | 274 |
| Investor owned | 43 | 47 | 41 | 48 | 48 |
| **Physician Models** | | | | | |
| Independent Practice Association | 72 | 81 | 76 | 68 | 89 |
| Group Practice without Walls | 10 | 14 | 11 | 11 | 15 |
| Open Physician-Hospital Organization | 78 | 89 | 100 | 94 | 96 |
| Closed Physician-Hospital Organization | 38 | 38 | 40 | 49 | 62 |
| Management Service Organization | 59 | 65 | 72 | 79 | 93 |
| Integrated Salary Model | 119 | 108 | 96 | 90 | 103 |
| Equity Model | 4 | 6 | 9 | 5 | 13 |
| Foundation | 22 | 20 | 29 | 27 | 33 |
| **Insurance Products** | | | | | |
| Health Maintenance Organization | 79 | 80 | 83 | 94 | 128 |
| Preferred Provider Organization | 83 | 88 | 87 | 96 | 121 |
| Indemnity Fee for Service | 23 | 19 | 24 | 30 | 33 |
| **Managed Care Contracts** | | | | | |
| Health Maintenance Organization | 255 | 257 | 251 | 237 | 261 |
| Preferred Provider Organization | 257 | 263 | 262 | 243 | 262 |
| **Affiliations** | | | | | |
| Hospitals in a System* | 221 | 224 | 218 | 214 | 220 |
| Hospitals in a Network | 113 | 122 | 118 | 101 | 107 |
| Hospitals in a Group Purchasing Organization | 285 | 270 | 263 | 235 | 229 |

Bed Size Categories

* Please note that system affiliate information for hospitals is derived from AHA membership. In years prior to 2003 the affiliation was derived from a question on the AHA Annual Survey of hospitals; therefore, non-responding hospitals were not included in the system affiliation counts. Years prior to 2003 have been updated to reflect this change, which now include affiliation for non-reporting hospitals.

# TABLE 4

## BED SIZE CATEGORY 300-399

*U.S. Registered Community Hospitals*
*(Nonfederal, short-term general and other special hospitals)*

## Utilization, Personnel, Revenue and Expenses 1999–2003

| | 2003 | 2002 | 2001 | 2000 | 1999 |
|---|---|---|---|---|---|
| **TOTAL FACILITY (Includes Hospital and Nursing Home Units)** | | | | | |
| **Utilization - Inpatient** | | | | | |
| Beds | 119,903 | 123,399 | 119,753 | 117,220 | 126,259 |
| Admissions | 5,589,833 | 5,606,593 | 5,328,441 | 5,135,313 | 5,419,172 |
| Inpatient Days | 29,998,416 | 30,625,907 | 28,949,110 | 28,175,816 | 30,446,266 |
| Average Length of Stay | 5.4 | 5.5 | 5.4 | 5.5 | 5.6 |
| Inpatient Surgeries | 1,596,627 | 1,670,246 | 1,575,266 | 1,548,365 | 1,633,543 |
| Births | 662,053 | 634,624 | 628,124 | 608,029 | 635,465 |
| **Utilization - Outpatient** | | | | | |
| Emergency Outpatient Visits | 15,897,067 | 16,337,980 | 15,412,370 | 14,679,081 | 14,883,092 |
| Other Outpatient Visits | 65,040,946 | 62,754,461 | 59,829,649 | 58,764,729 | 60,965,514 |
| Total Outpatient Visits | 80,938,013 | 79,092,441 | 75,242,019 | 73,443,810 | 75,848,606 |
| Outpatient Surgeries | 2,400,933 | 2,501,205 | 2,398,395 | 2,380,845 | 2,453,087 |
| **Personnel** | | | | | |
| Full Time RNs | 124,882 | 124,773 | 119,926 | 115,123 | 122,695 |
| Full Time LPNs | 14,381 | 15,634 | 14,521 | 12,961 | 13,849 |
| Part Time RNs | 71,225 | 66,826 | 63,220 | 64,123 | 65,952 |
| Part Time LPNs | 5,717 | 5,895 | 5,187 | 5,663 | 5,658 |
| Total Full Time | 534,706 | 546,123 | 523,968 | 501,162 | 532,328 |
| Total Part Time | 208,123 | 198,483 | 192,906 | 195,777 | 194,111 |
| **Revenue - Inpatient** | | | | | |
| Gross Inpatient Revenue | $122,641,223,447 | $104,931,029,759 | $90,736,055,640 | $79,128,945,312 | $76,331,193,232 |
| **Revenue - Outpatient** | | | | | |
| Gross Outpatient Revenue | $59,808,208,882 | $52,506,396,042 | $43,966,846,914 | $37,931,362,986 | $36,396,156,547 |
| **Revenue and Expenses - Totals (Includes Inpatient and Outpatient)** | | | | | |
| Total Gross Revenue | $182,449,432,329 | $157,437,425,801 | $134,702,902,554 | $117,060,308,298 | $112,727,349,779 |
| Deductions from Revenue | 114,079,609,997 | 92,566,575,914 | 77,014,066,878 | 63,980,293,228 | 58,693,834,397 |
| Net Patient Revenue | 68,369,822,332 | 64,870,849,887 | 57,688,835,676 | 53,080,015,070 | 54,033,515,382 |
| Other Operating Revenue | 4,730,386,954 | 3,898,682,632 | 3,334,900,779 | 2,688,378,669 | 2,807,882,430 |
| Other Nonoperating Revenue | 1,184,335,242 | 518,357,079 | 858,386,079 | 1,305,643,872 | 1,555,611,944 |
| Total Net Revenue | 74,284,544,528 | 69,287,889,598 | 61,882,122,534 | 57,074,037,611 | 58,397,009,756 |
| Total Expenses | 70,380,924,713 | 66,128,522,671 | 59,027,238,261 | 54,273,518,296 | 55,544,241,173 |
| **HOSPITAL UNIT (Excludes Separate Nursing Home Units)** | | | | | |
| **Utilization - Inpatient** | | | | | |
| Beds | 113,798 | 116,100 | 112,537 | 110,180 | 117,501 |
| Admissions | 5,542,090 | 5,547,159 | 5,269,008 | 5,074,369 | 5,343,133 |
| Inpatient Days | 28,032,233 | 28,315,464 | 26,728,772 | 25,970,657 | 27,715,550 |
| Average Length of Stay | 5.1 | 5.1 | 5.1 | 5.1 | 5.2 |
| **Personnel** | | | | | |
| Total Full Time | 529,334 | 539,889 | 517,844 | 494,730 | 525,524 |
| Total Part Time | 205,408 | 195,895 | 190,500 | 193,029 | 190,991 |
| **Revenue and Expenses - Totals (Includes Inpatient and Outpatient)** | | | | | |
| Total Net Revenue | $73,673,285,779 | $68,590,373,760 | $61,250,007,293 | $56,555,661,812 | $57,738,046,612 |
| Total Expenses | 69,826,896,240 | 65,561,221,517 | 58,607,498,709 | 53,867,071,704 | 55,030,932,464 |

# Table 4

# BED SIZE CATEGORY 400-499

*U.S. Registered Community Hospitals*
*(Nonfederal, short-term general and other special hospitals)*

## Overview 1999–2003

| | 2003 | 2002 | 2001 | 2000 | 1999 |
|---|---|---|---|---|---|
| **Total Community Hospitals in Bed Size Category 400-499** | **172** | **174** | **191** | **182** | **161** |
| **Location** | | | | | |
| Hospitals Urban | 168 | 170 | 186 | 178 | 157 |
| Hospitals Rural | 4 | 4 | 5 | 4 | 4 |
| **Control** | | | | | |
| State and Local Government | 22 | 27 | 27 | 25 | 19 |
| Not for Profit | 141 | 139 | 153 | 147 | 132 |
| Investor owned | 9 | 8 | 11 | 10 | 10 |
| **Physician Models** | | | | | |
| Independent Practice Association | 40 | 34 | 38 | 41 | 45 |
| Group Practice without Walls | 10 | 6 | 5 | 9 | 11 |
| Open Physician-Hospital Organization | 41 | 37 | 36 | 41 | 38 |
| Closed Physician-Hospital Organization | 15 | 19 | 20 | 22 | 24 |
| Management Service Organization | 38 | 34 | 37 | 41 | 42 |
| Integrated Salary Model | 58 | 63 | 59 | 61 | 53 |
| Equity Model | 3 | 5 | 3 | 5 | 5 |
| Foundation | 19 | 17 | 17 | 13 | 17 |
| **Insurance Products** | | | | | |
| Health Maintenance Organization | 46 | 54 | 60 | 69 | 70 |
| Preferred Provider Organization | 50 | 54 | 53 | 63 | 55 |
| Indemnity Fee for Service | 12 | 17 | 11 | 16 | 11 |
| **Managed Care Contracts** | | | | | |
| Health Maintenance Organization | 136 | 131 | 137 | 138 | 121 |
| Preferred Provider Organization | 136 | 135 | 143 | 139 | 125 |
| **Affiliations** | | | | | |
| Hospitals in a System* | 99 | 103 | 115 | 109 | 99 |
| Hospitals in a Network | 62 | 52 | 66 | 62 | 52 |
| Hospitals in a Group Purchasing Organization | 138 | 127 | 141 | 131 | 107 |

* Please note that system affiliate information for hospitals is derived from AHA membership. In years prior to 2003 the affiliation was derived from a question on the AHA Annual Survey of hospitals; therefore, non-responding hospitals were not included in the system affiliation counts. Years prior to 2003 have been updated to reflect this change, which now include affiliation for non-reporting hospitals.

# TABLE 4

## BED SIZE CATEGORY 400-499

*U.S. Registered Community Hospitals*
*(Nonfederal, short-term general and other special hospitals)*

## Utilization, Personnel, Revenue and Expenses 1999–2003

| | 2003 | 2002 | 2001 | 2000 | 1999 |
|---|---|---|---|---|---|
| **TOTAL FACILITY (Includes Hospital and Nursing Home Units)** | | | | | |
| **Utilization - Inpatient** | | | | | |
| Beds | 76,333 | 77,145 | 84,745 | 80,763 | 71,580 |
| Admissions | 3,591,216 | 3,592,594 | 3,778,746 | 3,616,530 | 3,045,448 |
| Inpatient Days | 19,709,937 | 19,862,987 | 21,312,743 | 20,509,972 | 17,853,905 |
| Average Length of Stay | 5.5 | 5.5 | 5.6 | 5.7 | 5.9 |
| Inpatient Surgeries | 1,090,817 | 1,126,781 | 1,143,813 | 1,102,058 | 904,289 |
| Births | 421,166 | 435,738 | 462,372 | 439,821 | 357,548 |
| **Utilization - Outpatient** | | | | | |
| Emergency Outpatient Visits | 9,497,408 | 9,056,989 | 9,345,972 | 9,488,926 | 7,263,184 |
| Other Outpatient Visits | 47,705,546 | 48,784,217 | 50,233,673 | 42,716,283 | 36,604,300 |
| Total Outpatient Visits | 57,202,954 | 57,841,206 | 59,579,645 | 52,205,209 | 43,867,484 |
| Outpatient Surgeries | 1,575,533 | 1,593,516 | 1,642,696 | 1,578,111 | 1,366,726 |
| **Personnel** | | | | | |
| Full Time RNs | 88,447 | 84,885 | 87,244 | 82,895 | 72,380 |
| Full Time LPNs | 8,010 | 8,147 | 9,335 | 8,237 | 8,563 |
| Part Time RNs | 49,498 | 48,158 | 50,157 | 49,484 | 35,968 |
| Part Time LPNs | 4,063 | 3,431 | 3,334 | 3,052 | 3,315 |
| Total Full Time | 385,375 | 384,050 | 398,066 | 367,265 | 320,457 |
| Total Part Time | 135,326 | 134,897 | 140,706 | 139,517 | 106,306 |
| **Revenue - Inpatient** | | | | | |
| Gross Inpatient Revenue | $86,492,048,000 | $76,255,983,382 | $70,893,560,813 | $59,609,190,161 | $47,414,569,510 |
| **Revenue - Outpatient** | | | | | |
| Gross Outpatient Revenue | $42,384,600,302 | $36,410,066,420 | $32,818,521,002 | $28,221,840,088 | $20,680,259,396 |
| **Revenue and Expenses - Totals (Includes Inpatient and Outpatient)** | | | | | |
| Total Gross Revenue | $128,876,648,302 | $112,666,049,802 | $103,712,081,815 | $87,831,030,249 | $68,094,828,906 |
| Deductions from Revenue | 79,457,940,352 | 66,486,965,120 | 58,861,160,338 | 48,605,733,601 | 36,254,726,963 |
| Net Patient Revenue | 49,418,707,950 | 46,179,084,682 | 44,850,921,477 | 39,225,296,648 | 31,840,101,943 |
| Other Operating Revenue | 3,773,263,993 | 3,352,108,431 | 3,212,320,490 | 2,780,992,924 | 2,533,086,920 |
| Other Nonoperating Revenue | 706,372,733 | 335,957,588 | 906,755,338 | 1,176,559,766 | 923,857,533 |
| Total Net Revenue | 53,898,344,676 | 49,867,150,701 | 48,969,997,305 | 43,182,849,338 | 35,297,046,396 |
| Total Expenses | 51,603,683,919 | 47,419,293,980 | 47,321,475,681 | 41,299,819,174 | 33,866,308,713 |
| **HOSPITAL UNIT (Excludes Separate Nursing Home Units)** | | | | | |
| **Utilization - Inpatient** | | | | | |
| Beds | 71,539 | 73,121 | 79,957 | 76,238 | 65,996 |
| Admissions | 3,558,390 | 3,561,076 | 3,739,662 | 3,573,245 | 2,995,719 |
| Inpatient Days | 18,222,561 | 18,643,835 | 19,847,882 | 19,084,886 | 16,114,892 |
| Average Length of Stay | 5.1 | 5.2 | 5.3 | 5.3 | 5.4 |
| **Personnel** | | | | | |
| Total Full Time | 381,347 | 381,097 | 394,265 | 362,720 | 316,695 |
| Total Part Time | 133,586 | 133,611 | 139,265 | 137,566 | 104,747 |
| **Revenue and Expenses - Totals (Includes Inpatient and Outpatient)** | | | | | |
| Total Net Revenue | $53,233,188,699 | $49,559,582,082 | $48,644,983,381 | $42,890,966,938 | $34,714,064,245 |
| Total Expenses | 50,974,060,344 | 47,151,005,398 | 46,998,302,690 | 41,054,265,159 | 33,528,138,196 |

# TABLE 4

## BED SIZE CATEGORY 500 +

*U.S. Registered Community Hospitals*
*(Nonfederal, short-term general and other special hospitals)*

## Overview 1999–2003

| | 2003 | 2002 | 2001 | 2000 | 1999 |
|---|---|---|---|---|---|
| **Total Community Hospitals in Bed Size Category 500 +** | **259** | **256** | **249** | **247** | **254** |
| **Location** | | | | | |
| Hospitals Urban | 256 | 253 | 245 | 244 | 251 |
| Hospitals Rural | 3 | 3 | 4 | 3 | 3 |
| **Control** | | | | | |
| State and Local Government | 43 | 36 | 37 | 36 | 40 |
| Not for Profit | 200 | 204 | 195 | 197 | 201 |
| Investor owned | 16 | 16 | 17 | 14 | 13 |
| **Physician Models** | | | | | |
| Independent Practice Association | 63 | 66 | 68 | 76 | 85 |
| Group Practice without Walls | 20 | 23 | 23 | 26 | 24 |
| Open Physician-Hospital Organization | 68 | 64 | 70 | 69 | 75 |
| Closed Physician-Hospital Organization | 25 | 25 | 31 | 42 | 48 |
| Management Service Organization | 59 | 64 | 64 | 80 | 77 |
| Integrated Salary Model | 127 | 115 | 103 | 105 | 101 |
| Equity Model | 6 | 11 | 10 | 13 | 13 |
| Foundation | 21 | 27 | 25 | 27 | 31 |
| **Insurance Products** | | | | | |
| Health Maintenance Organization | 90 | 88 | 86 | 116 | 128 |
| Preferred Provider Organization | 81 | 85 | 85 | 105 | 115 |
| Indemnity Fee for Service | 26 | 19 | 22 | 26 | 24 |
| **Managed Care Contracts** | | | | | |
| Health Maintenance Organization | 209 | 195 | 195 | 205 | 205 |
| Preferred Provider Organization | 207 | 194 | 195 | 202 | 200 |
| **Affiliations** | | | | | |
| Hospitals in a System* | 179 | 174 | 164 | 151 | 156 |
| Hospitals in a Network | 103 | 99 | 94 | 97 | 103 |
| Hospitals in a Group Purchasing Organization | 209 | 191 | 192 | 180 | 173 |

* Please note that system affiliate information for hospitals is derived from AHA membership. In years prior to 2003 the affiliation was derived from a question on the AHA Annual Survey of hospitals; therefore, non-responding hospitals were not included in the system affiliation counts. Years prior to 2003 have been updated to reflect this change, which now include affiliation for non-reporting hospitals.

# Table 4

# BED SIZE CATEGORY 500 +

*U.S. Registered Community Hospitals*
*(Nonfederal, short-term general and other special hospitals)*

## Utilization, Personnel, Revenue and Expenses 1999–2003

| | 2003 | 2002 | 2001 | 2000 | 1999 |
|---|---|---|---|---|---|
| **TOTAL FACILITY (Includes Hospital and Nursing Home Units)** | | | | | |
| **Utilization - Inpatient** | | | | | |
| Beds | 183,860 | 180,091 | 177,873 | 175,638 | 178,411 |
| Admissions | 8,173,763 | 7,957,792 | 7,705,773 | 7,410,167 | 7,399,867 |
| Inpatient Days | 49,818,096 | 48,655,624 | 47,225,469 | 46,339,384 | 46,713,100 |
| Average Length of Stay | 6.1 | 6.1 | 6.1 | 6.3 | 6.3 |
| Inpatient Surgeries | 2,523,137 | 2,513,381 | 2,425,140 | 2,419,740 | 2,474,024 |
| Births | 922,801 | 896,281 | 885,391 | 868,382 | 849,861 |
| **Utilization - Outpatient** | | | | | |
| Emergency Outpatient Visits | 19,397,288 | 18,760,101 | 18,048,334 | 16,863,866 | 17,080,213 |
| Other Outpatient Visits | 94,964,454 | 91,715,041 | 87,265,908 | 84,513,677 | 82,660,658 |
| Total Outpatient Visits | 114,361,742 | 110,475,142 | 105,314,242 | 101,377,543 | 99,740,871 |
| Outpatient Surgeries | 3,166,630 | 3,365,132 | 3,126,279 | 2,908,913 | 2,949,786 |
| **Personnel** | | | | | |
| Full Time RNs | 219,080 | 208,213 | 199,358 | 199,560 | 202,263 |
| Full Time LPNs | 17,004 | 16,087 | 16,947 | 17,233 | 18,029 |
| Part Time RNs | 105,889 | 97,416 | 90,746 | 87,424 | 82,232 |
| Part Time LPNs | 6,188 | 5,349 | 5,766 | 5,421 | 5,260 |
| Total Full Time | 957,320 | 926,875 | 909,166 | 879,297 | 884,284 |
| Total Part Time | 291,862 | 281,159 | 262,239 | 253,897 | 243,838 |
| **Revenue - Inpatient** | | | | | |
| Gross Inpatient Revenue | $215,568,723,129 | $181,311,610,111 | $156,462,924,653 | $138,130,198,562 | $126,828,183,226 |
| **Revenue - Outpatient** | | | | | |
| Gross Outpatient Revenue | $91,530,137,271 | $76,542,000,025 | $65,226,823,758 | $54,990,410,746 | $49,682,171,548 |
| **Revenue and Expenses - Totals (Includes Inpatient and Outpatient)** | | | | | |
| Total Gross Revenue | $307,098,860,400 | $257,853,610,136 | $221,689,748,411 | $193,120,609,308 | $176,470,354,774 |
| Deductions from Revenue | 186,546,726,697 | 148,361,338,060 | 123,213,421,530 | 103,806,905,095 | 90,993,158,498 |
| Net Patient Revenue | 120,552,133,703 | 109,492,272,076 | 98,476,326,881 | 89,313,704,213 | 85,477,196,276 |
| Other Operating Revenue | 9,712,515,849 | 9,462,930,418 | 8,858,554,851 | 7,873,591,839 | 7,574,557,742 |
| Other Nonoperating Revenue | 2,321,875,423 | 425,909,567 | 1,292,497,612 | 2,991,999,020 | 2,570,772,014 |
| Total Net Revenue | 132,586,524,975 | 119,381,112,061 | 108,627,379,344 | 100,179,295,072 | 95,622,526,032 |
| Total Expenses | 126,878,540,185 | 115,131,748,332 | 105,085,709,086 | 96,310,798,929 | 91,982,247,309 |
| **HOSPITAL UNIT (Excludes Separate Nursing Home Units)** | | | | | |
| **Utilization - Inpatient** | | | | | |
| Beds | 173,243 | 168,562 | 166,158 | 161,458 | 164,759 |
| Admissions | 8,122,566 | 7,906,285 | 7,649,107 | 7,337,658 | 7,308,606 |
| Inpatient Days | 46,549,224 | 44,958,154 | 43,383,615 | 41,856,131 | 42,322,343 |
| Average Length of Stay | 5.7 | 5.7 | 5.7 | 5.7 | 5.8 |
| **Personnel** | | | | | |
| Total Full Time | 948,637 | 918,115 | 898,569 | 867,283 | 872,217 |
| Total Part Time | 288,102 | 278,360 | 258,769 | 250,140 | 240,125 |
| **Revenue and Expenses - Totals (Includes Inpatient and Outpatient)** | | | | | |
| Total Net Revenue | $131,556,413,469 | $118,439,588,288 | $107,658,500,091 | $98,564,608,494 | $94,608,758,058 |
| Total Expenses | 125,954,038,585 | 114,087,149,972 | 104,203,128,358 | 95,410,392,185 | 91,062,292,669 |

# Census Divisions

| | |
|---|---|
| **Census Division 1** | **New England**<br>Connecticut, Maine, Massachusetts, New Hampshire, Rhode Island, Vermont |
| **Census Division 2** | **Middle Atlantic**<br>New Jersey, New York, Pennsylvania |
| **Census Division 3** | **South Atlantic**<br>Delaware, District of Columbia, Florida, Georgia, Maryland, North Carolina, South Carolina, Virginia, West Virginia |
| **Census Division 4** | **East North Central**<br>Illinois, Indiana, Michigan, Ohio, Wisconsin |
| **Census Division 5** | **East South Central**<br>Alabama, Kentucky, Mississippi, Tennessee |
| **Census Division 6** | **West North Central**<br>Iowa, Kansas, Minnesota, Missouri, Nebraska, North Dakota, South Dakota |
| **Census Division 7** | **West South Central**<br>Arkansas, Louisiana, Oklahoma, Texas |
| **Census Division 8** | **Mountain**<br>Arizona, Colorado, Idaho, Montana, Nevada, New Mexico, Utah, Wyoming |
| **Census Division 9** | **Pacific**<br>Alaska, California, Hawaii, Oregon, Washington |

# TABLE 5

# U.S. CENSUS DIVISION 1: NEW ENGLAND

*U.S. Registered Community Hospitals*
*(Nonfederal, short-term general and other special hospitals)*

## Overview 1999–2003

| | 2003 | 2002 | 2001 | 2000 | 1999 |
|---|---|---|---|---|---|
| **Total Community Hospitals in Census Division 1, New England** | **203** | **203** | **205** | **205** | **204** |
| **Bed Size Category** | | | | | |
| 6-24 | 6 | 8 | 3 | 4 | 5 |
| 25-49 | 36 | 32 | 39 | 38 | 35 |
| 50-99 | 46 | 46 | 44 | 44 | 46 |
| 100-199 | 61 | 58 | 60 | 61 | 62 |
| 200-299 | 28 | 30 | 28 | 26 | 25 |
| 300-399 | 12 | 15 | 16 | 17 | 16 |
| 400-499 | 2 | 1 | 2 | 2 | 2 |
| 500 + | 12 | 13 | 13 | 13 | 13 |
| **Location** | | | | | |
| Hospitals Urban | 126 | 126 | 128 | 128 | 127 |
| Hospitals Rural | 77 | 77 | 77 | 77 | 77 |
| **Control** | | | | | |
| State and Local Government | 6 | 7 | 8 | 8 | 9 |
| Not for Profit | 183 | 185 | 186 | 185 | 184 |
| Investor owned | 14 | 11 | 11 | 12 | 11 |
| **Physician Models** | | | | | |
| Independent Practice Association | 58 | 58 | 57 | 52 | 61 |
| Group Practice without Walls | 13 | 16 | 18 | 15 | 18 |
| Open Physician-Hospital Organization | 63 | 66 | 71 | 71 | 78 |
| Closed Physician-Hospital Organization | 15 | 18 | 20 | 21 | 21 |
| Management Service Organization | 26 | 33 | 36 | 36 | 48 |
| Integrated Salary Model | 82 | 73 | 71 | 67 | 71 |
| Equity Model | 6 | 6 | 4 | 4 | 4 |
| Foundation | 11 | 13 | 15 | 13 | 18 |
| **Insurance Products** | | | | | |
| Health Maintenance Organization | 22 | 23 | 28 | 31 | 37 |
| Preferred Provider Organization | 26 | 22 | 19 | 18 | 22 |
| Indemnity Fee for Service | 9 | 5 | 5 | 5 | 5 |
| **Managed Care Contracts** | | | | | |
| Health Maintenance Organization | 153 | 156 | 163 | 161 | 169 |
| Preferred Provider Organization | 150 | 143 | 149 | 148 | 151 |
| **Affiliations** | | | | | |
| Hospitals in a System* | 71 | 71 | 76 | 74 | 70 |
| Hospitals in a Network | 63 | 60 | 61 | 66 | 60 |
| Hospitals in a Group Purchasing Organization | 171 | 161 | 164 | 155 | 153 |

* Please note that system affiliate information for hospitals is derived from AHA membership. In years prior to 2003 the affiliation was derived from a question on the AHA Annual Survey of hospitals; therefore, non-responding hospitals were not included in the system affiliation counts. Years prior to 2003 have been updated to reflect this change, which now include affiliation for non-reporting hospitals.

U.S. Census Divisions

# TABLE 5

# U.S. CENSUS DIVISION 1: NEW ENGLAND

*U.S. Registered Community Hospitals*
*(Nonfederal, short-term general and other special hospitals)*

## Utilization, Personnel, Revenue and Expenses, Community Health Indicators 1999–2003

| | 2003 | 2002 | 2001 | 2000 | 1999 |
|---|---|---|---|---|---|
| **TOTAL FACILITY (Includes Hospital and Nursing Home Units)** | | | | | |
| **Utilization - Inpatient** | | | | | |
| Beds | 33,600 | 34,324 | 35,385 | 34,944 | 34,915 |
| Admissions | 1,598,123 | 1,580,396 | 1,567,000 | 1,519,012 | 1,500,667 |
| Inpatient Days | 8,854,347 | 9,120,976 | 9,144,828 | 8,917,327 | 8,771,404 |
| Average Length of Stay | 5.5 | 5.8 | 5.8 | 5.9 | 5.8 |
| Inpatient Surgeries | 454,152 | 459,541 | 444,897 | 448,066 | 447,135 |
| Births | 169,753 | 168,792 | 169,198 | 170,638 | 169,142 |
| **Utilization - Outpatient** | | | | | |
| Emergency Outpatient Visits | 6,275,074 | 6,233,520 | 5,973,441 | 5,916,202 | 5,784,739 |
| Other Outpatient Visits | 31,540,633 | 29,869,397 | 29,179,090 | 26,862,517 | 25,245,873 |
| Total Outpatient Visits | 37,815,707 | 36,102,917 | 35,152,531 | 32,778,719 | 31,030,612 |
| Outpatient Surgeries | 1,036,806 | 1,004,499 | 987,409 | 956,844 | 903,825 |
| **Personnel** | | | | | |
| Full Time RNs | 35,156 | 33,504 | 34,016 | 32,203 | 30,186 |
| Full Time LPNs | 2,189 | 2,408 | 2,390 | 2,391 | 2,078 |
| Part Time RNs | 34,385 | 33,457 | 33,183 | 33,845 | 33,145 |
| Part Time LPNs | 2,083 | 2,160 | 2,219 | 2,321 | 2,272 |
| Total Full Time | 186,008 | 186,629 | 186,757 | 173,630 | 165,298 |
| Total Part Time | 108,478 | 105,969 | 105,157 | 107,014 | 105,196 |
| **Revenue - Inpatient** | | | | | |
| Gross Inpatient Revenue | $28,271,467,530 | $25,243,211,994 | $23,006,462,654 | $21,145,777,686 | $19,052,712,630 |
| **Revenue - Outpatient** | | | | | |
| Gross Outpatient Revenue | $24,060,068,236 | $20,277,289,066 | $17,354,624,925 | $15,014,223,925 | $13,647,875,340 |
| **Revenue and Expenses - Totals (Includes Inpatient and Outpatient)** | | | | | |
| Total Gross Revenue | $52,331,535,766 | $45,520,501,060 | $40,361,087,579 | $36,160,001,611 | $32,700,587,970 |
| Deductions from Revenue | 27,574,266,243 | 22,938,130,804 | 19,755,206,105 | 17,289,206,287 | 15,008,365,053 |
| Net Patient Revenue | 24,757,269,523 | 22,582,370,256 | 20,605,881,474 | 18,870,795,324 | 17,692,222,917 |
| Other Operating Revenue | 3,069,276,617 | 2,275,478,442 | 2,061,229,915 | 1,644,812,612 | 1,737,545,613 |
| Other Nonoperating Revenue | 210,317,295 | 69,173,336 | 256,835,969 | 706,498,132 | 665,388,606 |
| Total Net Revenue | 28,036,863,435 | 24,927,022,034 | 22,923,947,358 | 21,222,106,068 | 20,095,157,136 |
| Total Expenses | 26,783,737,017 | 24,762,701,274 | 22,650,945,919 | 20,923,125,622 | 19,745,944,243 |
| **HOSPITAL UNIT (Excludes Separate Nursing Home Units)** | | | | | |
| **Utilization - Inpatient** | | | | | |
| Beds | 31,720 | 32,069 | 32,730 | 32,263 | 32,117 |
| Admissions | 1,577,277 | 1,563,633 | 1,550,961 | 1,498,475 | 1,477,023 |
| Inpatient Days | 8,217,257 | 8,350,064 | 8,190,799 | 8,007,120 | 7,885,831 |
| Average Length of Stay | 5.2 | 5.3 | 5.3 | 5.3 | 5.3 |
| **Personnel** | | | | | |
| Total Full Time | 183,960 | 185,430 | 184,640 | 171,537 | 163,198 |
| Total Part Time | 106,700 | 104,927 | 103,487 | 105,170 | 103,333 |
| **Revenue and Expenses - Totals (Includes Inpatient and Outpatient)** | | | | | |
| Total Net Revenue | $27,883,105,011 | $24,763,704,581 | $22,729,636,795 | $21,051,443,144 | $19,894,763,328 |
| Total Expenses | 26,640,736,159 | 24,599,025,809 | 22,469,904,390 | 20,769,362,219 | 19,578,964,509 |
| **COMMUNITY HEALTH INDICATORS PER 1000 POPULATION** | | | | | |
| Total Population (in thousands) | 14,205 | 14,134 | 14,048 | 13,952 | 13,838 |
| **Inpatient** | | | | | |
| Beds | 2.4 | 2.4 | 2.5 | 2.5 | 2.5 |
| Admissions | 112.5 | 111.8 | 111.5 | 108.9 | 108.4 |
| Inpatient Days | 623.3 | 645.3 | 651.0 | 639.1 | 633.9 |
| Inpatient Surgeries | 32.0 | 32.5 | 31.7 | 32.1 | 32.3 |
| Births | 11.9 | 11.9 | 12.0 | 12.2 | 12.2 |
| **Outpatient** | | | | | |
| Emergency Outpatient Visits | 441.7 | 441.0 | 425.2 | 424.0 | 418.0 |
| Other Outpatient Visits | 2,220.3 | 2,113.2 | 2,077.1 | 1,925.3 | 1,824.4 |
| Total Outpatient Visits | 2,662.1 | 2,554.3 | 2,502.3 | 2,349.4 | 2,242.5 |
| Outpatient Surgeries | 73.0 | 71.1 | 70.3 | 68.6 | 65.3 |
| **Expense per Capita (per person)** | $1,885.5 | $1,751.9 | $1,612.4 | $1,499.6 | $1,427.0 |

# TABLE 5

## U.S. CENSUS DIVISION 2: MIDDLE ATLANTIC

*U.S. Registered Community Hospitals*
*(Nonfederal, short-term general and other special hospitals)*

## Overview 1999–2003

| | 2003 | 2002 | 2001 | 2000 | 1999 |
|---|---|---|---|---|---|
| **Total Community Hospitals** | | | | | |
| **in Census Division 2, Middle Atlantic** | **486** | **493** | **495** | **502** | **509** |
| **Bed Size Category** | | | | | |
| 6-24 | 9 | 8 | 7 | 8 | 7 |
| 25-49 | 22 | 21 | 22 | 20 | 25 |
| 50-99 | 61 | 64 | 61 | 64 | 59 |
| 100-199 | 144 | 148 | 145 | 152 | 151 |
| 200-299 | 107 | 103 | 111 | 112 | 116 |
| 300-399 | 51 | 55 | 52 | 47 | 52 |
| 400-499 | 39 | 40 | 42 | 46 | 41 |
| 500 + | 53 | 54 | 55 | 53 | 58 |
| **Location** | | | | | |
| Hospitals Urban | 406 | 412 | 415 | 423 | 428 |
| Hospitals Rural | 80 | 81 | 80 | 79 | 81 |
| **Control** | | | | | |
| State and Local Government | 29 | 30 | 29 | 28 | 28 |
| Not for Profit | 429 | 441 | 444 | 453 | 461 |
| Investor owned | 28 | 22 | 22 | 21 | 20 |
| **Physician Models** | | | | | |
| Independent Practice Association | 92 | 99 | 98 | 120 | 126 |
| Group Practice without Walls | 22 | 21 | 20 | 26 | 20 |
| Open Physician-Hospital Organization | 70 | 76 | 81 | 104 | 101 |
| Closed Physician-Hospital Organization | 19 | 26 | 25 | 33 | 44 |
| Management Service Organization | 56 | 64 | 72 | 89 | 96 |
| Integrated Salary Model | 132 | 118 | 99 | 112 | 93 |
| Equity Model | 9 | 9 | 6 | 14 | 13 |
| Foundation | 12 | 11 | 9 | 14 | 17 |
| **Insurance Products** | | | | | |
| Health Maintenance Organization | 87 | 82 | 70 | 97 | 101 |
| Preferred Provider Organization | 85 | 79 | 79 | 98 | 97 |
| Indemnity Fee for Service | 24 | 17 | 17 | 15 | 15 |
| **Managed Care Contracts** | | | | | |
| Health Maintenance Organization | 319 | 317 | 330 | 351 | 351 |
| Preferred Provider Organization | 304 | 300 | 315 | 332 | 321 |
| **Affiliations** | | | | | |
| Hospitals in a System* | 220 | 215 | 211 | 211 | 201 |
| Hospitals in a Network | 147 | 152 | 148 | 155 | 146 |
| Hospitals in a Group Purchasing Organization | 351 | 350 | 350 | 334 | 289 |

* Please note that system affiliate information for hospitals is derived from AHA membership. In years prior to 2003 the affiliation was derived from a question on the AHA Annual Survey of hospitals; therefore, non-responding hospitals were not included in the system affiliation counts. Years prior to 2003 have been updated to reflect this change, which now include affiliation for non-reporting hospitals.

# TABLE 5

## U.S. CENSUS DIVISION 2: MIDDLE ATLANTIC

*U.S. Registered Community Hospitals*
*(Nonfederal, short-term general and other special hospitals)*

## Utilization, Personnel, Revenue and Expenses, Community Health Indicators 1999–2003

| | 2003 | 2002 | 2001 | 2000 | 1999 |
|---|---|---|---|---|---|
| **TOTAL FACILITY (Includes Hospital and Nursing Home Units)** | | | | | |
| **Utilization - Inpatient** | | | | | |
| Beds | 128,420 | 130,198 | 134,007 | 134,044 | 136,493 |
| Admissions | 5,430,928 | 5,356,471 | 5,303,235 | 5,285,812 | 5,230,020 |
| Inpatient Days | 34,910,712 | 34,925,191 | 35,582,339 | 35,972,872 | 36,152,830 |
| Average Length of Stay | 6.4 | 6.5 | 6.7 | 6.8 | 6.9 |
| Inpatient Surgeries | 1,491,422 | 1,540,104 | 1,530,873 | 1,570,780 | 1,573,521 |
| Births | 504,382 | 503,700 | 502,368 | 504,630 | 506,591 |
| **Utilization - Outpatient** | | | | | |
| Emergency Outpatient Visits | 15,567,144 | 15,474,182 | 15,262,789 | 14,855,507 | 14,638,689 |
| Other Outpatient Visits | 80,640,481 | 79,593,390 | 80,890,968 | 79,672,796 | 76,499,179 |
| Total Outpatient Visits | 96,207,625 | 95,067,572 | 96,153,757 | 94,528,303 | 91,137,868 |
| Outpatient Surgeries | 2,717,736 | 2,779,831 | 2,688,679 | 2,673,923 | 2,560,005 |
| **Personnel** | | | | | |
| Full Time RNs | 128,214 | 124,834 | 125,764 | 125,727 | 124,392 |
| Full Time LPNs | 13,474 | 14,200 | 14,431 | 14,326 | 14,634 |
| Part Time RNs | 59,196 | 58,048 | 55,226 | 57,785 | 56,507 |
| Part Time LPNs | 5,444 | 5,567 | 5,408 | 5,704 | 5,939 |
| Total Full Time | 589,789 | 591,456 | 587,752 | 580,514 | 578,915 |
| Total Part Time | 185,751 | 182,720 | 179,456 | 182,798 | 179,758 |
| **Revenue - Inpatient** | | | | | |
| Gross Inpatient Revenue | $139,643,847,699 | $114,499,007,759 | $102,755,097,357 | $88,555,896,320 | $79,559,155,616 |
| **Revenue - Outpatient** | | | | | |
| Gross Outpatient Revenue | $62,623,808,550 | $53,178,962,709 | $45,742,770,658 | $39,791,596,044 | $35,350,638,604 |
| **Revenue and Expenses - Totals (Includes Inpatient and Outpatient)** | | | | | |
| Total Gross Revenue | $202,267,656,249 | $167,677,970,468 | $148,497,868,015 | $128,347,492,364 | $114,909,794,220 |
| Deductions from Revenue | 131,171,564,551 | 101,832,776,300 | 87,693,668,174 | 71,418,197,617 | 61,003,893,361 |
| Net Patient Revenue | 71,096,091,698 | 65,845,194,168 | 60,804,199,841 | 56,929,294,747 | 53,905,900,859 |
| Other Operating Revenue | 5,043,277,779 | 4,945,663,508 | 4,858,174,712 | 4,373,128,371 | 4,158,957,000 |
| Other Nonoperating Revenue | 1,180,634,845 | 473,985,594 | 879,603,162 | 1,200,687,387 | 1,229,111,646 |
| Total Net Revenue | 77,320,004,322 | 71,264,843,270 | 66,541,977,715 | 62,503,110,505 | 59,293,969,505 |
| Total Expenses | 76,052,322,704 | 70,060,852,900 | 65,738,326,638 | 61,666,014,763 | 58,864,243,581 |
| **HOSPITAL UNIT (Excludes Separate Nursing Home Units)** | | | | | |
| **Utilization - Inpatient** | | | | | |
| Beds | 118,319 | 118,462 | 122,977 | 121,947 | 123,387 |
| Admissions | 5,382,414 | 5,305,173 | 5,251,290 | 5,228,518 | 5,165,103 |
| Inpatient Days | 31,572,094 | 30,977,155 | 31,838,056 | 31,790,693 | 31,784,098 |
| Average Length of Stay | 5.9 | 5.8 | 6.1 | 6.1 | 6.2 |
| **Personnel** | | | | | |
| Total Full Time | 581,806 | 582,279 | 579,127 | 569,721 | 570,193 |
| Total Part Time | 181,832 | 178,921 | 175,863 | 178,618 | 176,154 |
| **Revenue and Expenses - Totals (Includes Inpatient and Outpatient)** | | | | | |
| Total Net Revenue | $76,454,812,926 | $70,357,276,445 | $65,632,075,736 | $61,678,553,426 | $58,381,802,745 |
| Total Expenses | 75,242,014,798 | 69,170,940,306 | 65,050,830,005 | 61,035,255,854 | 58,149,232,081 |
| **COMMUNITY HEALTH INDICATORS PER 1000 POPULATION** | | | | | |
| Total Population (in thousands) | 40,194 | 40,038 | 39,877 | 39,715 | 39,506 |
| **Inpatient** | | | | | |
| Beds | 3.2 | 3.3 | 3.4 | 3.4 | 3.5 |
| Admissions | 135.1 | 133.8 | 133.0 | 133.1 | 132.4 |
| Inpatient Days | 868.6 | 872.3 | 892.3 | 905.8 | 915.1 |
| Inpatient Surgeries | 37.1 | 38.5 | 38.4 | 39.6 | 39.8 |
| Births | 12.5 | 12.6 | 12.6 | 12.7 | 12.8 |
| **Outpatient** | | | | | |
| Emergency Outpatient Visits | 387.3 | 386.5 | 382.7 | 374.1 | 370.5 |
| Other Outpatient Visits | 2,006.3 | 1,987.9 | 2,028.5 | 2,006.1 | 1,936.4 |
| Total Outpatient Visits | 2,393.6 | 2,374.4 | 2,411.2 | 2,380.2 | 2,306.9 |
| Outpatient Surgeries | 67.6 | 69.4 | 67.4 | 67.3 | 64.8 |
| **Expense per Capita (per person)** | $1,892.1 | $1,749.8 | $1,648.5 | $1,552.7 | $1,490.0 |

# TABLE 5

## U.S. CENSUS DIVISION 3: SOUTH ATLANTIC

*U.S. Registered Community Hospitals*
*(Nonfederal, short-term general and other special hospitals)*

## Overview 1999–2003

| | 2003 | 2002 | 2001 | 2000 | 1999 |
|---|---|---|---|---|---|
| **Total Community Hospitals in Census Division 3, South Atlantic** | **731** | **731** | **730** | **739** | **749** |
| **Bed Size Category** | | | | | |
| 6-24 | 23 | 21 | 14 | 17 | 15 |
| 25-49 | 94 | 97 | 101 | 104 | 100 |
| 50-99 | 137 | 135 | 134 | 128 | 131 |
| 100-199 | 207 | 200 | 201 | 212 | 225 |
| 200-299 | 111 | 116 | 121 | 122 | 119 |
| 300-399 | 70 | 73 | 66 | 66 | 76 |
| 400-499 | 30 | 30 | 34 | 35 | 29 |
| 500 + | 59 | 59 | 59 | 55 | 54 |
| **Location** | | | | | |
| Hospitals Urban | 442 | 442 | 442 | 449 | 456 |
| Hospitals Rural | 289 | 289 | 288 | 290 | 293 |
| **Control** | | | | | |
| State and Local Government | 138 | 138 | 142 | 145 | 152 |
| Not for Profit | 403 | 407 | 398 | 400 | 404 |
| Investor owned | 190 | 186 | 190 | 194 | 193 |
| **Physician Models** | | | | | |
| Independent Practice Association | 66 | 54 | 69 | 82 | 90 |
| Group Practice without Walls | 23 | 11 | 16 | 23 | 25 |
| Open Physician-Hospital Organization | 114 | 119 | 127 | 136 | 149 |
| Closed Physician-Hospital Organization | 41 | 39 | 47 | 59 | 68 |
| Management Service Organization | 58 | 64 | 73 | 95 | 114 |
| Integrated Salary Model | 187 | 175 | 158 | 162 | 157 |
| Equity Model | 17 | 15 | 9 | 20 | 23 |
| Foundation | 17 | 20 | 17 | 18 | 27 |
| **Insurance Products** | | | | | |
| Health Maintenance Organization | 85 | 85 | 97 | 122 | 145 |
| Preferred Provider Organization | 126 | 136 | 137 | 158 | 193 |
| Indemnity Fee for Service | 47 | 39 | 37 | 48 | 47 |
| **Managed Care Contracts** | | | | | |
| Health Maintenance Organization | 375 | 391 | 385 | 407 | 412 |
| Preferred Provider Organization | 451 | 475 | 462 | 476 | 492 |
| **Affiliations** | | | | | |
| Hospitals in a System* | 425 | 432 | 426 | 434 | 430 |
| Hospitals in a Network | 225 | 228 | 228 | 224 | 235 |
| Hospitals in a Group Purchasing Organization | 502 | 471 | 460 | 447 | 438 |

* Please note that system affiliate information for hospitals is derived from AHA membership. In years prior to 2003 the affiliation was derived from a question on the AHA Annual Survey of hospitals; therefore, non-responding hospitals were not included in the system affiliation counts. Years prior to 2003 have been updated to reflect this change, which now include affiliation for non-reporting hospitals.

# Table 5

# U.S. CENSUS DIVISION 3: SOUTH ATLANTIC

*U.S. Registered Community Hospitals*
*(Nonfederal, short-term general and other special hospitals)*

## Utilization, Personnel, Revenue and Expenses, Community Health Indicators 1999–2003

| | 2003 | 2002 | 2001 | 2000 | 1999 |
|---|---|---|---|---|---|
| **TOTAL FACILITY (Includes Hospital and Nursing Home Units)** | | | | | |
| **Utilization - Inpatient** | | | | | |
| Beds | 151,754 | 152,236 | 152,052 | 150,851 | 151,812 |
| Admissions | 6,646,826 | 6,587,288 | 6,453,744 | 6,262,051 | 6,069,521 |
| Inpatient Days | 37,810,333 | 37,509,493 | 36,338,028 | 35,935,189 | 35,729,929 |
| Average Length of Stay | 5.7 | 5.7 | 5.6 | 5.7 | 5.9 |
| Inpatient Surgeries | 1,967,152 | 2,024,048 | 1,975,208 | 1,890,490 | 1,838,331 |
| Births | 695,242 | 695,805 | 694,845 | 682,848 | 644,602 |
| **Utilization - Outpatient** | | | | | |
| Emergency Outpatient Visits | 22,063,587 | 21,281,267 | 20,100,193 | 19,803,910 | 18,439,689 |
| Other Outpatient Visits | 61,832,573 | 61,195,587 | 58,426,774 | 56,939,217 | 52,499,260 |
| Total Outpatient Visits | 83,896,160 | 82,476,854 | 78,526,967 | 76,743,127 | 70,938,949 |
| Outpatient Surgeries | 3,348,605 | 3,403,716 | 3,193,345 | 3,038,185 | 2,975,263 |
| **Personnel** | | | | | |
| Full Time RNs | 158,536 | 154,257 | 149,286 | 148,599 | 145,609 |
| Full Time LPNs | 19,070 | 19,491 | 19,553 | 19,172 | 20,456 |
| Part Time RNs | 72,088 | 68,654 | 66,294 | 66,561 | 58,528 |
| Part Time LPNs | 7,195 | 6,084 | 5,903 | 6,265 | 6,674 |
| Total Full Time | 647,733 | 646,894 | 632,576 | 616,500 | 600,721 |
| Total Part Time | 206,568 | 196,385 | 189,909 | 197,464 | 180,821 |
| **Revenue - Inpatient** | | | | | |
| Gross Inpatient Revenue | $122,068,281,181 | $109,659,179,223 | $94,782,493,433 | $86,421,077,582 | $77,252,538,734 |
| **Revenue - Outpatient** | | | | | |
| Gross Outpatient Revenue | $65,980,405,893 | $59,025,023,880 | $49,302,316,636 | $44,278,693,852 | $38,501,572,608 |
| **Revenue and Expenses - Totals (Includes Inpatient and Outpatient)** | | | | | |
| Total Gross Revenue | $188,048,687,074 | $168,684,203,103 | $144,084,810,069 | $130,699,771,434 | $115,754,111,342 |
| Deductions from Revenue | 109,766,909,281 | 95,540,558,726 | 77,834,582,485 | 69,108,825,847 | 58,573,353,779 |
| Net Patient Revenue | 78,281,777,793 | 73,143,644,377 | 66,250,227,584 | 61,590,945,587 | 57,180,757,563 |
| Other Operating Revenue | 3,910,102,561 | 3,729,711,113 | 3,560,755,143 | 3,203,398,523 | 3,141,920,126 |
| Other Nonoperating Revenue | 1,393,458,811 | 271,679,355 | 1,030,898,593 | 1,593,464,950 | 1,555,718,488 |
| Total Net Revenue | 83,585,339,165 | 77,145,034,845 | 70,841,881,320 | 66,387,809,060 | 61,878,396,177 |
| Total Expenses | 78,776,238,107 | 73,497,910,915 | 66,532,756,720 | 62,074,155,739 | 57,070,729,065 |
| **HOSPITAL UNIT (Excludes Separate Nursing Home Units)** | | | | | |
| **Utilization - Inpatient** | | | | | |
| Beds | 138,905 | 139,408 | 139,864 | 137,102 | 137,364 |
| Admissions | 6,592,950 | 6,530,617 | 6,395,710 | 6,192,854 | 5,997,119 |
| Inpatient Days | 33,500,043 | 33,321,870 | 32,356,811 | 31,455,354 | 30,973,296 |
| Average Length of Stay | 5.1 | 5.1 | 5.1 | 5.1 | 5.2 |
| **Personnel** | | | | | |
| Total Full Time | 636,985 | 636,583 | 622,774 | 605,040 | 589,107 |
| Total Part Time | 202,824 | 192,884 | 186,585 | 193,201 | 176,916 |
| **Revenue and Expenses - Totals (Includes Inpatient and Outpatient)** | | | | | |
| Total Net Revenue | $82,539,369,201 | $76,360,437,261 | $70,107,007,948 | $64,887,088,976 | $61,054,258,380 |
| Total Expenses | 77,834,105,235 | 72,794,408,670 | 65,904,113,552 | 61,442,541,205 | 56,365,852,982 |
| **COMMUNITY HEALTH INDICATORS PER 1000 POPULATION** | | | | | |
| Total Population (in thousands) | 54,345 | 53,564 | 52,751 | 51,960 | 51,141 |
| **Inpatient** | | | | | |
| Beds | 2.8 | 2.8 | 2.9 | 2.9 | 3.0 |
| Admissions | 122.3 | 123.0 | 122.3 | 120.5 | 118.7 |
| Inpatient Days | 695.8 | 700.3 | 688.9 | 691.6 | 698.7 |
| Inpatient Surgeries | 36.2 | 37.8 | 37.4 | 36.4 | 35.9 |
| Births | 12.8 | 13.0 | 13.2 | 13.1 | 12.6 |
| **Outpatient** | | | | | |
| Emergency Outpatient Visits | 406.0 | 397.3 | 381.0 | 381.1 | 360.6 |
| Other Outpatient Visits | 1,137.8 | 1,142.5 | 1,107.6 | 1,095.8 | 1,026.6 |
| Total Outpatient Visits | 1,543.8 | 1,539.8 | 1,488.6 | 1,477.0 | 1,387.1 |
| Outpatient Surgeries | 61.6 | 63.5 | 60.5 | 58.5 | 58.2 |
| **Expense per Capita (per person)** | $1,449.6 | $1,372.2 | $1,261.3 | $1,194.6 | $1,115.9 |

**TABLE 5**

# U.S. CENSUS DIVISION 4: EAST NORTH CENTRAL

*U.S. Registered Community Hospitals*
*(Nonfederal, short-term general and other special hospitals)*

## Overview 1999–2003

| | 2003 | 2002 | 2001 | 2000 | 1999 |
|---|---|---|---|---|---|
| **Total Community Hospitals in Census Division 4, East North Central....** | **732** | **737** | **734** | **732** | **744** |
| **Bed Size Category** | | | | | |
| 6-24 | 25 | 28 | 22 | 22 | 27 |
| 25-49 | 128 | 121 | 114 | 108 | 107 |
| 50-99 | 170 | 173 | 178 | 171 | 180 |
| 100-199 | 184 | 189 | 193 | 200 | 200 |
| 200-299 | 99 | 101 | 100 | 104 | 103 |
| 300-399 | 60 | 59 | 58 | 56 | 54 |
| 400-499 | 28 | 26 | 30 | 29 | 30 |
| 500 + | 38 | 40 | 39 | 42 | 43 |
| **Location** | | | | | |
| Hospitals Urban | 442 | 444 | 440 | 443 | 448 |
| Hospitals Rural | 290 | 293 | 294 | 289 | 296 |
| **Control** | | | | | |
| State and Local Government | 109 | 113 | 114 | 112 | 119 |
| Not for Profit | 588 | 592 | 592 | 591 | 596 |
| Investor owned | 35 | 32 | 28 | 29 | 29 |
| **Physician Models** | | | | | |
| Independent Practice Association | 107 | 102 | 108 | 111 | 110 |
| Group Practice without Walls | 41 | 43 | 47 | 41 | 36 |
| Open Physician-Hospital Organization | 182 | 189 | 195 | 206 | 203 |
| Closed Physician-Hospital Organization | 80 | 72 | 74 | 82 | 88 |
| Management Service Organization | 109 | 106 | 120 | 136 | 141 |
| Integrated Salary Model | 256 | 235 | 229 | 244 | 247 |
| Equity Model | 6 | 12 | 16 | 18 | 18 |
| Foundation | 45 | 33 | 38 | 41 | 43 |
| **Insurance Products** | | | | | |
| Health Maintenance Organization | 149 | 142 | 154 | 179 | 199 |
| Preferred Provider Organization | 177 | 164 | 165 | 207 | 225 |
| Indemnity Fee for Service | 56 | 43 | 46 | 62 | 58 |
| **Managed Care Contracts** | | | | | |
| Health Maintenance Organization | 543 | 503 | 515 | 530 | 545 |
| Preferred Provider Organization | 596 | 554 | 565 | 575 | 602 |
| **Affiliations** | | | | | |
| Hospitals in a System* | 378 | 370 | 369 | 354 | 356 |
| Hospitals in a Network | 249 | 223 | 225 | 218 | 211 |
| Hospitals in a Group Purchasing Organization | 635 | 592 | 593 | 593 | 550 |

* Please note that system affiliate information for hospitals is derived from AHA membership. In years prior to 2003 the affiliation was derived from a question on the AHA Annual Survey of hospitals; therefore, non-responding hospitals were not included in the system affiliation counts. Years prior to 2003 have been updated to reflect this change, which now include affiliation for non-reporting hospitals.

# TABLE 5

## U.S. CENSUS DIVISION 4: EAST NORTH CENTRAL

*U.S. Registered Community Hospitals*
*(Nonfederal, short-term general and other special hospitals)*

## Utilization, Personnel, Revenue and Expenses, Community Health Indicators 1999–2003

| | 2003 | 2002 | 2001 | 2000 | 1999 |
|---|---|---|---|---|---|
| **TOTAL FACILITY (Includes Hospital and Nursing Home Units)** | | | | | |
| **Utilization - Inpatient** | | | | | |
| Beds | 127,610 | 129,716 | 130,407 | 131,722 | 133,061 |
| Admissions | 5,520,916 | 5,549,822 | 5,418,071 | 5,299,180 | 5,188,356 |
| Inpatient Days | 29,253,281 | 29,754,022 | 29,208,239 | 29,197,099 | 29,318,858 |
| Average Length of Stay | 5.3 | 5.4 | 5.4 | 5.5 | 5.7 |
| Inpatient Surgeries | 1,583,427 | 1,588,289 | 1,532,612 | 1,536,652 | 1,471,103 |
| Births | 600,200 | 594,899 | 600,441 | 607,172 | 593,698 |
| **Utilization - Outpatient** | | | | | |
| Emergency Outpatient Visits | 18,517,606 | 18,125,078 | 17,712,357 | 17,307,818 | 16,699,402 |
| Other Outpatient Visits | 92,718,085 | 88,307,662 | 87,341,487 | 84,498,586 | 78,099,894 |
| Total Outpatient Visits | 111,235,691 | 106,432,740 | 105,053,844 | 101,806,404 | 94,799,296 |
| Outpatient Surgeries | 3,170,597 | 3,101,230 | 2,952,188 | 2,876,537 | 2,818,860 |
| **Personnel** | | | | | |
| Full Time RNs | 126,117 | 120,224 | 118,745 | 120,794 | 121,346 |
| Full Time LPNs | 12,233 | 12,113 | 12,747 | 12,183 | 12,823 |
| Part Time RNs | 93,802 | 91,896 | 88,913 | 86,191 | 81,180 |
| Part Time LPNs | 7,637 | 7,846 | 8,117 | 7,573 | 7,764 |
| Total Full Time | 582,922 | 573,239 | 568,559 | 560,718 | 554,898 |
| Total Part Time | 289,862 | 288,607 | 277,406 | 267,821 | 258,605 |
| **Revenue - Inpatient** | | | | | |
| Gross Inpatient Revenue | $96,047,624,484 | $87,407,038,737 | $77,251,473,672 | $69,620,488,497 | $63,685,574,779 |
| **Revenue - Outpatient** | | | | | |
| Gross Outpatient Revenue | $68,892,199,155 | $59,494,801,802 | $51,950,625,736 | $45,806,914,434 | $40,204,948,871 |
| **Revenue and Expenses - Totals (Includes Inpatient and Outpatient)** | | | | | |
| Total Gross Revenue | $164,939,823,639 | $146,901,840,539 | $129,202,099,408 | $115,427,402,931 | $103,890,523,650 |
| Deductions from Revenue | 90,427,903,676 | 77,136,739,719 | 65,676,992,538 | 56,498,399,187 | 48,691,629,504 |
| Net Patient Revenue | 74,511,919,963 | 69,765,100,820 | 63,525,106,870 | 58,929,003,744 | 55,198,894,146 |
| Other Operating Revenue | 4,093,763,516 | 3,815,440,330 | 3,607,534,822 | 3,175,250,858 | 3,010,491,498 |
| Other Nonoperating Revenue | 972,806,700 | 293,313,105 | 917,722,672 | 2,618,184,368 | 2,339,165,296 |
| Total Net Revenue | 79,578,490,179 | 73,873,854,255 | 68,050,364,364 | 64,722,438,970 | 60,548,550,940 |
| Total Expenses | 76,040,358,335 | 71,241,901,629 | 65,691,365,693 | 60,750,436,230 | 57,553,715,808 |
| **HOSPITAL UNIT (Excludes Separate Nursing Home Units)** | | | | | |
| **Utilization - Inpatient** | | | | | |
| Beds | 118,053 | 120,239 | 119,618 | 119,146 | 119,021 |
| Admissions | 5,458,596 | 5,486,852 | 5,346,426 | 5,218,146 | 5,091,228 |
| Inpatient Days | 26,320,238 | 26,833,806 | 25,943,340 | 25,392,256 | 25,194,957 |
| Average Length of Stay | 4.8 | 4.9 | 4.9 | 4.9 | 4.9 |
| **Personnel** | | | | | |
| Total Full Time | 576,932 | 567,494 | 561,829 | 551,564 | 545,069 |
| Total Part Time | 285,379 | 284,867 | 273,564 | 262,824 | 253,308 |
| **Revenue and Expenses - Totals (Includes Inpatient and Outpatient)** | | | | | |
| Total Net Revenue | $78,947,912,790 | $73,267,139,602 | $67,427,818,977 | $64,122,423,465 | $59,695,796,166 |
| Total Expenses | 75,500,191,134 | 70,722,664,220 | 65,195,547,192 | 60,219,162,173 | 56,849,086,779 |
| **COMMUNITY HEALTH INDICATORS PER 1000 POPULATION** | | | | | |
| Total Population (in thousands) | 45,837 | 45,635 | 45,440 | 45,223 | 44,969 |
| **Inpatient** | | | | | |
| Beds | 2.8 | 2.8 | 2.9 | 2.9 | 3.0 |
| Admissions | 120.4 | 121.6 | 119.2 | 117.2 | 115.4 |
| Inpatient Days | 638.2 | 652.0 | 642.8 | 645.6 | 652.0 |
| Inpatient Surgeries | 34.5 | 34.8 | 33.7 | 34.0 | 32.7 |
| Births | 13.1 | 13.0 | 13.2 | 13.4 | 13.2 |
| **Outpatient** | | | | | |
| Emergency Outpatient Visits | 404.0 | 397.2 | 389.8 | 382.7 | 371.4 |
| Other Outpatient Visits | 2,022.8 | 1,935.1 | 1,922.1 | 1,868.5 | 1,736.7 |
| Total Outpatient Visits | 2,426.8 | 2,332.3 | 2,311.9 | 2,251.2 | 2,108.1 |
| Outpatient Surgeries | 69.2 | 68.0 | 65.0 | 63.6 | 62.7 |
| **Expense per Capita (per person)** | $1,658.9 | $1,561.1 | $1,445.7 | $1,343.3 | $1,279.8 |

# TABLE 5

## U.S. CENSUS DIVISION 5: EAST SOUTH CENTRAL

*U.S. Registered Community Hospitals*
*(Nonfederal, short-term general and other special hospitals)*

## Overview 1999–2003

| | 2003 | 2002 | 2001 | 2000 | 1999 |
|---|---|---|---|---|---|
| **Total Community Hospitals** | | | | | |
| **in Census Division 5, East South Central . . .** | **427** | **426** | **429** | **429** | **431** |
| **Bed Size Category** | | | | | |
| 6-24 | 14 | 15 | 8 | 8 | 7 |
| 25-49 | 96 | 83 | 81 | 79 | 77 |
| 50-99 | 108 | 118 | 118 | 120 | 131 |
| 100-199 | 112 | 113 | 125 | 126 | 120 |
| 200-299 | 41 | 41 | 42 | 45 | 44 |
| 300-399 | 22 | 23 | 21 | 21 | 24 |
| 400-499 | 12 | 12 | 16 | 12 | 8 |
| 500 + | 22 | 21 | 18 | 18 | 20 |
| **Location** | | | | | |
| Hospitals Urban | 169 | 168 | 169 | 167 | 168 |
| Hospitals Rural | 258 | 258 | 260 | 262 | 263 |
| **Control** | | | | | |
| State and Local Government | 117 | 118 | 125 | 127 | 130 |
| Not for Profit | 197 | 197 | 196 | 194 | 197 |
| Investor owned | 113 | 111 | 108 | 108 | 104 |
| **Physician Models** | | | | | |
| Independent Practice Association | 44 | 50 | 39 | 47 | 54 |
| Group Practice without Walls | 9 | 17 | 8 | 16 | 13 |
| Open Physician-Hospital Organization | 55 | 58 | 58 | 56 | 68 |
| Closed Physician-Hospital Organization | 15 | 15 | 12 | 16 | 20 |
| Management Service Organization | 46 | 53 | 48 | 53 | 61 |
| Integrated Salary Model | 81 | 81 | 69 | 62 | 58 |
| Equity Model | 1 | 2 | 5 | 6 | 7 |
| Foundation | 23 | 28 | 28 | 33 | 29 |
| **Insurance Products** | | | | | |
| Health Maintenance Organization | 53 | 56 | 54 | 60 | 73 |
| Preferred Provider Organization | 116 | 130 | 113 | 103 | 132 |
| Indemnity Fee for Service | 29 | 32 | 30 | 26 | 32 |
| **Managed Care Contracts** | | | | | |
| Health Maintenance Organization | 178 | 184 | 169 | 150 | 166 |
| Preferred Provider Organization | 215 | 244 | 244 | 183 | 200 |
| **Affiliations** | | | | | |
| Hospitals in a System* | 262 | 254 | 259 | 263 | 255 |
| Hospitals in a Network | 103 | 99 | 96 | 81 | 86 |
| Hospitals in a Group Purchasing Organization | 252 | 222 | 219 | 190 | 190 |

* Please note that system affiliate information for hospitals is derived from AHA membership. In years prior to 2003 the affiliation was derived from a question on the AHA Annual Survey of hospitals; therefore, non-responding hospitals were not included in the system affiliation counts. Years prior to 2003 have been updated to reflect this change, which now include affiliation for non-reporting hospitals.

# Table 5

## U.S. CENSUS DIVISION 5: EAST SOUTH CENTRAL

*U.S. Registered Community Hospitals*
*(Nonfederal, short-term general and other special hospitals)*

## Utilization, Personnel, Revenue and Expenses, Community Health Indicators 1999–2003

| | 2003 | 2002 | 2001 | 2000 | 1999 |
|---|---|---|---|---|---|
| **TOTAL FACILITY (Includes Hospital and Nursing Home Units)** | | | | | |
| **Utilization - Inpatient** | | | | | |
| Beds | 63,959 | 64,591 | 65,898 | 65,356 | 65,106 |
| Admissions | 2,538,273 | 2,492,114 | 2,467,417 | 2,424,100 | 2,407,150 |
| Inpatient Days | 14,171,337 | 13,856,950 | 13,998,816 | 14,074,178 | 14,113,317 |
| Average Length of Stay | 5.6 | 5.6 | 5.7 | 5.8 | 5.9 |
| Inpatient Surgeries | 736,740 | 727,890 | 713,144 | 721,871 | 717,980 |
| Births | 228,955 | 224,418 | 227,383 | 225,101 | 226,028 |
| **Utilization - Outpatient** | | | | | |
| Emergency Outpatient Visits | 8,827,897 | 8,643,710 | 8,156,784 | 8,104,971 | 7,978,531 |
| Other Outpatient Visits | 22,769,805 | 23,996,038 | 21,946,093 | 22,539,023 | 20,776,140 |
| Total Outpatient Visits | 31,597,702 | 32,639,748 | 30,102,877 | 30,643,994 | 28,754,671 |
| Outpatient Surgeries | 1,231,214 | 1,226,607 | 1,213,146 | 1,188,571 | 1,137,417 |
| **Personnel** | | | | | |
| Full Time RNs | 58,601 | 55,716 | 53,990 | 55,378 | 56,988 |
| Full Time LPNs | 11,555 | 10,859 | 11,156 | 10,173 | 10,980 |
| Part Time RNs | 23,463 | 23,303 | 20,347 | 19,888 | 17,267 |
| Part Time LPNs | 3,101 | 3,233 | 2,953 | 2,788 | 2,706 |
| Total Full Time | 242,696 | 237,483 | 240,670 | 234,318 | 235,391 |
| Total Part Time | 68,463 | 70,708 | 61,263 | 63,007 | 54,327 |
| **Revenue - Inpatient** | | | | | |
| Gross Inpatient Revenue | $42,807,554,660 | $37,236,405,608 | $33,763,537,509 | $30,460,414,643 | $28,522,093,205 |
| **Revenue - Outpatient** | | | | | |
| Gross Outpatient Revenue | $24,877,139,678 | $21,335,998,517 | $18,799,075,976 | $16,791,511,923 | $14,755,549,582 |
| **Revenue and Expenses - Totals (Includes Inpatient and Outpatient)** | | | | | |
| Total Gross Revenue | $67,684,694,338 | $58,572,404,125 | $52,562,613,485 | $47,251,926,566 | $43,277,642,787 |
| Deductions from Revenue | 41,532,647,725 | 33,820,962,603 | 29,633,078,052 | 26,118,962,696 | 23,230,987,570 |
| Net Patient Revenue | 26,152,046,613 | 24,751,441,522 | 22,929,535,433 | 21,132,963,870 | 20,046,655,217 |
| Other Operating Revenue | 1,382,136,450 | 1,112,863,364 | 1,079,038,669 | 1,196,170,102 | 1,213,648,825 |
| Other Nonoperating Revenue | 392,950,942 | 246,155,552 | 537,095,911 | 626,610,283 | 460,092,660 |
| Total Net Revenue | 27,927,134,005 | 26,110,460,438 | 24,545,670,013 | 22,955,744,255 | 21,720,396,702 |
| Total Expenses | 26,377,671,189 | 24,262,441,941 | 23,153,845,874 | 21,606,133,823 | 20,621,277,359 |
| **HOSPITAL UNIT (Excludes Separate Nursing Home Units)** | | | | | |
| **Utilization - Inpatient** | | | | | |
| Beds | 58,436 | 59,825 | 60,461 | 59,945 | 58,914 |
| Admissions | 2,509,212 | 2,464,015 | 2,440,081 | 2,396,395 | 2,374,559 |
| Inpatient Days | 12,442,021 | 12,297,077 | 12,160,748 | 12,269,882 | 12,083,301 |
| Average Length of Stay | 5.0 | 5.0 | 5.0 | 5.1 | 5.1 |
| **Personnel** | | | | | |
| Total Full Time | 238,017 | 233,711 | 236,531 | 230,035 | 229,862 |
| Total Part Time | 67,226 | 69,573 | 60,176 | 61,799 | 52,946 |
| **Revenue and Expenses - Totals (Includes Inpatient and Outpatient)** | | | | | |
| Total Net Revenue | $27,597,631,434 | $25,813,696,396 | $24,261,954,693 | $22,629,453,822 | $21,349,301,577 |
| Total Expenses | 26,092,562,236 | 24,024,754,092 | 22,927,686,517 | 21,350,689,942 | 20,365,677,195 |
| **COMMUNITY HEALTH INDICATORS PER 1000 POPULATION** | | | | | |
| Total Population (in thousands) | 17,342 | 17,225 | 17,137 | 17,051 | 16,915 |
| **Inpatient** | | | | | |
| Beds | 3.7 | 3.7 | 3.8 | 3.8 | 3.8 |
| Admissions | 146.4 | 144.7 | 144.0 | 142.2 | 142.3 |
| Inpatient Days | 817.2 | 804.5 | 816.9 | 825.4 | 834.4 |
| Inpatient Surgeries | 42.5 | 42.3 | 41.6 | 42.3 | 42.4 |
| Births | 13.2 | 13.0 | 13.3 | 13.2 | 13.4 |
| **Outpatient** | | | | | |
| Emergency Outpatient Visits | 509.1 | 501.8 | 476.0 | 475.3 | 471.7 |
| Other Outpatient Visits | 1,313.0 | 1,393.1 | 1,280.6 | 1,321.8 | 1,228.2 |
| Total Outpatient Visits | 1,822.1 | 1,894.9 | 1,756.6 | 1,797.2 | 1,699.9 |
| Outpatient Surgeries | 71.0 | 71.2 | 70.8 | 69.7 | 67.2 |
| **Expense per Capita (per person)** | $1,521.1 | $1,408.5 | $1,351.1 | $1,267.1 | $1,219.1 |

U.S. Census Divisions

# TABLE 5

# U.S. CENSUS DIVISION 6: WEST NORTH CENTRAL

*U.S. Registered Community Hospitals*
*(Nonfederal, short-term general and other special hospitals)*

## Overview 1999–2003

| | 2003 | 2002 | 2001 | 2000 | 1999 |
|---|---|---|---|---|---|
| **Total Community Hospitals in Census Division 6, West North Central** . . . | **675** | **679** | **673** | **673** | **672** |
| **Bed Size Category** | | | | | |
| 6-24 | 91 | 89 | 85 | 87 | 85 |
| 25-49 | 196 | 192 | 188 | 186 | 183 |
| 50-99 | 181 | 186 | 185 | 182 | 185 |
| 100-199 | 109 | 111 | 112 | 113 | 116 |
| 200-299 | 42 | 46 | 48 | 48 | 44 |
| 300-399 | 23 | 22 | 22 | 25 | 31 |
| 400-499 | 15 | 15 | 14 | 13 | 7 |
| 500 + | 18 | 18 | 19 | 19 | 21 |
| **Location** | | | | | |
| Hospitals Urban | 179 | 180 | 181 | 176 | 175 |
| Hospitals Rural | 496 | 499 | 492 | 497 | 497 |
| **Control** | | | | | |
| State and Local Government | 243 | 247 | 245 | 250 | 248 |
| Not for Profit | 400 | 404 | 402 | 403 | 402 |
| Investor owned | 32 | 28 | 26 | 20 | 22 |
| **Physician Models** | | | | | |
| Independent Practice Association | 103 | 96 | 95 | 95 | 83 |
| Group Practice without Walls | 26 | 18 | 22 | 24 | 23 |
| Open Physician-Hospital Organization | 84 | 86 | 97 | 99 | 103 |
| Closed Physician-Hospital Organization | 44 | 45 | 46 | 50 | 62 |
| Management Service Organization | 30 | 33 | 35 | 37 | 57 |
| Integrated Salary Model | 269 | 240 | 230 | 221 | 219 |
| Equity Model | 4 | 8 | 5 | 7 | 5 |
| Foundation | 11 | 13 | 16 | 17 | 31 |
| **Insurance Products** | | | | | |
| Health Maintenance Organization | 80 | 84 | 90 | 119 | 139 |
| Preferred Provider Organization | 142 | 137 | 130 | 152 | 162 |
| Indemnity Fee for Service | 35 | 39 | 37 | 41 | 45 |
| **Managed Care Contracts** | | | | | |
| Health Maintenance Organization | 327 | 321 | 338 | 337 | 338 |
| Preferred Provider Organization | 500 | 485 | 501 | 508 | 491 |
| **Affiliations** | | | | | |
| Hospitals in a System* | 321 | 319 | 300 | 286 | 288 |
| Hospitals in a Network | 266 | 257 | 262 | 262 | 239 |
| Hospitals in a Group Purchasing Organization | 584 | 551 | 577 | 570 | 527 |

U.S. Census Divisions

* Please note that system affiliate information for hospitals is derived from AHA membership. In years prior to 2003 the affiliation was derived from a question on the AHA Annual Survey of hospitals; therefore, non-responding hospitals were not included in the system affiliation counts. Years prior to 2003 have been updated to reflect this change, which now include affiliation for non-reporting hospitals.

**TABLE 5**

# U.S. CENSUS DIVISION 6: WEST NORTH CENTRAL

*U.S. Registered Community Hospitals*
*(Nonfederal, short-term general and other special hospitals)*

## Utilization, Personnel, Revenue and Expenses, Community Health Indicators 1999–2003

| | 2003 | 2002 | 2001 | 2000 | 1999 |
|---|---|---|---|---|---|
| **TOTAL FACILITY (Includes Hospital and Nursing Home Units)** | | | | | |
| **Utilization - Inpatient** | | | | | |
| Beds | 72,821 | 74,277 | 75,020 | 75,842 | 76,718 |
| Admissions | 2,543,012 | 2,509,141 | 2,481,753 | 2,411,096 | 2,346,771 |
| Inpatient Days | 16,336,089 | 16,581,836 | 16,650,444 | 16,570,765 | 16,752,113 |
| Average Length of Stay | 6.4 | 6.6 | 6.7 | 6.9 | 7.1 |
| Inpatient Surgeries | 707,127 | 720,434 | 702,686 | 686,916 | 685,775 |
| Births | 269,860 | 261,872 | 261,796 | 256,291 | 256,899 |
| **Utilization - Outpatient** | | | | | |
| Emergency Outpatient Visits | 7,227,615 | 7,108,385 | 6,937,436 | 6,666,448 | 6,682,798 |
| Other Outpatient Visits | 40,336,692 | 38,591,201 | 37,737,290 | 36,706,774 | 34,185,839 |
| Total Outpatient Visits | 47,564,307 | 45,699,586 | 44,674,726 | 43,373,222 | 40,868,637 |
| Outpatient Surgeries | 1,347,067 | 1,359,578 | 1,329,461 | 1,309,685 | 1,289,568 |
| **Personnel** | | | | | |
| Full Time RNs | 54,159 | 54,055 | 51,206 | 51,850 | 52,237 |
| Full Time LPNs | 8,314 | 8,391 | 8,162 | 8,099 | 8,358 |
| Part Time RNs | 50,492 | 49,543 | 49,074 | 46,048 | 45,113 |
| Part Time LPNs | 6,510 | 6,403 | 6,465 | 6,384 | 6,904 |
| Total Full Time | 255,790 | 255,451 | 247,196 | 241,470 | 240,530 |
| Total Part Time | 163,150 | 161,431 | 160,957 | 152,362 | 145,649 |
| **Revenue - Inpatient** | | | | | |
| Gross Inpatient Revenue | $43,068,295,116 | $38,854,088,608 | $34,125,326,110 | $30,690,964,864 | $27,978,962,967 |
| **Revenue - Outpatient** | | | | | |
| Gross Outpatient Revenue | $28,711,176,583 | $24,929,041,928 | $21,796,597,517 | $18,954,856,055 | $16,696,279,258 |
| **Revenue and Expenses - Totals (Includes Inpatient and Outpatient)** | | | | | |
| Total Gross Revenue | $71,779,471,699 | $63,783,130,536 | $55,921,923,627 | $49,645,820,919 | $44,675,242,225 |
| Deductions from Revenue | 38,464,014,644 | 33,035,135,970 | 27,904,622,957 | 23,918,824,972 | 20,629,836,841 |
| Net Patient Revenue | 33,315,457,055 | 30,747,994,566 | 28,017,300,670 | 25,726,995,947 | 24,045,405,384 |
| Other Operating Revenue | 1,991,615,171 | 1,794,417,297 | 1,614,130,546 | 1,472,106,386 | 1,441,566,383 |
| Other Nonoperating Revenue | 475,289,837 | 239,434,505 | 447,993,850 | 654,168,860 | 576,521,233 |
| Total Net Revenue | 35,782,362,063 | 32,781,846,368 | 30,079,425,066 | 27,853,271,193 | 26,063,493,000 |
| Total Expenses | 33,732,351,628 | 31,131,081,814 | 28,645,889,268 | 26,440,620,590 | 24,629,816,297 |
| **HOSPITAL UNIT (Excludes Separate Nursing Home Units)** | | | | | |
| **Utilization - Inpatient** | | | | | |
| Beds | 58,746 | 60,750 | 60,574 | 60,766 | 61,370 |
| Admissions | 2,498,473 | 2,461,630 | 2,428,943 | 2,348,985 | 2,275,386 |
| Inpatient Days | 11,824,025 | 12,331,933 | 12,028,176 | 11,854,940 | 11,875,181 |
| Average Length of Stay | 4.7 | 5.0 | 5.0 | 5.0 | 5.2 |
| **Personnel** | | | | | |
| Total Full Time | 247,353 | 248,644 | 239,190 | 232,906 | 232,075 |
| Total Part Time | 154,976 | 154,831 | 153,653 | 144,687 | 138,530 |
| **Revenue and Expenses - Totals (Includes Inpatient and Outpatient)** | | | | | |
| Total Net Revenue | $35,041,868,383 | $32,099,995,655 | $29,384,362,820 | $27,176,111,952 | $25,386,846,064 |
| Total Expenses | 33,067,542,356 | 30,539,871,194 | 28,042,574,090 | 25,851,000,854 | 24,051,512,537 |
| **COMMUNITY HEALTH INDICATORS PER 1000 POPULATION** | | | | | |
| Total Population (in thousands) | 19,569 | 19,464 | 19,368 | 19,271 | 19,131 |
| **Inpatient** | | | | | |
| Beds | 3.7 | 3.8 | 3.9 | 3.9 | 4.0 |
| Admissions | 130.0 | 128.9 | 128.1 | 125.1 | 122.7 |
| Inpatient Days | 834.8 | 851.9 | 859.7 | 859.9 | 875.7 |
| Inpatient Surgeries | 36.1 | 37.0 | 36.3 | 35.6 | 35.8 |
| Births | 13.8 | 13.5 | 13.5 | 13.3 | 13.4 |
| **Outpatient** | | | | | |
| Emergency Outpatient Visits | 369.3 | 365.2 | 358.2 | 345.9 | 349.3 |
| Other Outpatient Visits | 2,061.3 | 1,982.7 | 1,948.5 | 1,904.8 | 1,786.9 |
| Total Outpatient Visits | 2,430.6 | 2,347.9 | 2,306.7 | 2,250.7 | 2,136.3 |
| Outpatient Surgeries | 68.8 | 69.9 | 68.6 | 68.0 | 67.4 |
| **Expense per Capita (per person)** | $1,723.8 | $1,599.4 | $1,479.1 | $1,372.1 | $1,287.4 |

# TABLE 5

## U.S. CENSUS DIVISION 7: WEST SOUTH CENTRAL

*U.S. Registered Community Hospitals*
*(Nonfederal, short-term general and other special hospitals)*

## Overview 1999–2003

| | 2003 | 2002 | 2001 | 2000 | 1999 |
|---|---|---|---|---|---|
| **Total Community Hospitals in Census Division 7, West South Central...** | **737** | **736** | **727** | **717** | **722** |
| **Bed Size Category** | | | | | |
| 6-24 | 84 | 82 | 80 | 73 | 78 |
| 25-49 | 212 | 199 | 195 | 196 | 187 |
| 50-99 | 148 | 160 | 153 | 151 | 151 |
| 100-199 | 144 | 151 | 155 | 146 | 159 |
| 200-299 | 65 | 58 | 58 | 68 | 63 |
| 300-399 | 42 | 44 | 44 | 41 | 44 |
| 400-499 | 14 | 16 | 15 | 14 | 14 |
| 500 + | 28 | 26 | 27 | 28 | 26 |
| **Location** | | | | | |
| Hospitals Urban | 404 | 401 | 394 | 384 | 388 |
| Hospitals Rural | 333 | 335 | 333 | 333 | 334 |
| **Control** | | | | | |
| State and Local Government | 241 | 240 | 243 | 245 | 252 |
| Not for Profit | 284 | 287 | 276 | 271 | 265 |
| Investor owned | 212 | 209 | 208 | 201 | 205 |
| **Physician Models** | | | | | |
| Independent Practice Association | 135 | 124 | 117 | 124 | 137 |
| Group Practice without Walls | 28 | 28 | 25 | 30 | 26 |
| Open Physician-Hospital Organization | 152 | 152 | 151 | 181 | 176 |
| Closed Physician-Hospital Organization | 35 | 45 | 52 | 50 | 60 |
| Management Service Organization | 86 | 90 | 86 | 119 | 142 |
| Integrated Salary Model | 138 | 118 | 101 | 100 | 104 |
| Equity Model | 11 | 10 | 9 | 18 | 24 |
| Foundation | 43 | 43 | 51 | 60 | 67 |
| **Insurance Products** | | | | | |
| Health Maintenance Organization | 92 | 99 | 104 | 129 | 160 |
| Preferred Provider Organization | 152 | 146 | 131 | 170 | 196 |
| Indemnity Fee for Service | 33 | 40 | 32 | 43 | 56 |
| **Managed Care Contracts** | | | | | |
| Health Maintenance Organization | 446 | 447 | 452 | 454 | 478 |
| Preferred Provider Organization | 551 | 541 | 550 | 553 | 578 |
| **Affiliations** | | | | | |
| Hospitals in a System* | 417 | 412 | 413 | 397 | 393 |
| Hospitals in a Network | 163 | 157 | 153 | 171 | 185 |
| Hospitals in a Group Purchasing Organization | 580 | 553 | 547 | 521 | 417 |

* Please note that system affiliate information for hospitals is derived from AHA membership. In years prior to 2003 the affiliation was derived from a question on the AHA Annual Survey of hospitals; therefore, non-responding hospitals were not included in the system affiliation counts. Years prior to 2003 have been updated to reflect this change, which now include affiliation for non-reporting hospitals.

**TABLE 5**

# U.S. CENSUS DIVISION 7: WEST SOUTH CENTRAL

*U.S. Registered Community Hospitals*
*(Nonfederal, short-term general and other special hospitals)*

## Utilization, Personnel, Revenue and Expenses, Community Health Indicators 1999–2003

| | 2003 | 2002 | 2001 | 2000 | 1999 |
|---|---|---|---|---|---|
| **TOTAL FACILITY (Includes Hospital and Nursing Home Units)** | | | | | |
| **Utilization - Inpatient** | | | | | |
| Beds | 96,130 | 95,764 | 95,071 | 94,317 | 94,732 |
| Admissions | 4,078,542 | 4,055,293 | 3,949,513 | 3,818,189 | 3,716,015 |
| Inpatient Days | 21,638,131 | 21,541,966 | 20,782,167 | 20,064,215 | 19,957,836 |
| Average Length of Stay | 5.3 | 5.3 | 5.3 | 5.3 | 5.4 |
| Inpatient Surgeries | 1,175,915 | 1,161,699 | 1,128,483 | 1,125,604 | 1,097,488 |
| Births | 518,123 | 510,996 | 509,537 | 503,994 | 483,514 |
| **Utilization - Outpatient** | | | | | |
| Emergency Outpatient Visits | 13,452,657 | 13,229,179 | 12,453,535 | 11,823,842 | 11,499,044 |
| Other Outpatient Visits | 40,138,468 | 40,646,350 | 38,124,472 | 36,704,726 | 34,854,535 |
| Total Outpatient Visits | 53,591,125 | 53,875,529 | 50,578,007 | 48,528,568 | 46,353,579 |
| Outpatient Surgeries | 1,681,169 | 1,714,003 | 1,661,253 | 1,659,492 | 1,647,551 |
| **Personnel** | | | | | |
| Full Time RNs | 93,754 | 90,845 | 86,746 | 85,534 | 85,777 |
| Full Time LPNs | 20,978 | 20,342 | 20,274 | 20,174 | 21,987 |
| Part Time RNs | 30,242 | 31,644 | 31,071 | 29,440 | 27,595 |
| Part Time LPNs | 6,063 | 5,984 | 6,264 | 5,767 | 5,806 |
| Total Full Time | 401,709 | 391,498 | 382,735 | 375,496 | 378,422 |
| Total Part Time | 98,693 | 103,037 | 100,545 | 94,690 | 91,406 |
| **Revenue - Inpatient** | | | | | |
| Gross Inpatient Revenue | $81,205,887,599 | $71,476,469,794 | $61,419,028,742 | $53,960,636,392 | $48,750,503,268 |
| **Revenue - Outpatient** | | | | | |
| Gross Outpatient Revenue | $41,590,646,664 | $36,305,540,752 | $31,134,758,847 | $26,985,710,323 | $24,048,411,053 |
| **Revenue and Expenses - Totals (Includes Inpatient and Outpatient)** | | | | | |
| Total Gross Revenue | $122,796,534,263 | $107,782,010,546 | $92,553,787,589 | $80,946,346,715 | $72,758,914,321 |
| Deductions from Revenue | 77,614,278,554 | 64,781,749,664 | 54,100,450,992 | 46,520,754,796 | 39,647,718,729 |
| Net Patient Revenue | 45,182,255,709 | 43,000,260,882 | 38,453,336,597 | 34,425,591,919 | 33,111,195,592 |
| Other Operating Revenue | 3,693,991,228 | 3,420,018,355 | 3,072,362,313 | 2,917,928,679 | 2,836,835,943 |
| Other Nonoperating Revenue | 791,266,808 | 273,239,612 | 598,918,958 | 687,359,457 | 688,647,700 |
| Total Net Revenue | 49,667,513,745 | 46,693,518,849 | 42,124,617,868 | 38,030,880,055 | 36,636,679,235 |
| Total Expenses | 46,189,639,214 | 42,808,056,150 | 39,110,488,373 | 36,305,621,658 | 33,769,783,746 |
| **HOSPITAL UNIT (Excludes Separate Nursing Home Units)** | | | | | |
| **Utilization - Inpatient** | | | | | |
| Beds | 92,827 | 92,331 | 91,100 | 89,865 | 89,550 |
| Admissions | 4,045,462 | 4,019,877 | 3,903,804 | 3,757,331 | 3,641,325 |
| Inpatient Days | 20,745,917 | 20,607,960 | 19,699,547 | 18,867,455 | 18,527,824 |
| Average Length of Stay | 5.1 | 5.1 | 5.0 | 5.0 | 5.1 |
| **Personnel** | | | | | |
| Total Full Time | 398,271 | 388,745 | 379,354 | 371,015 | 374,262 |
| Total Part Time | 97,522 | 102,090 | 99,685 | 93,749 | 90,326 |
| **Revenue and Expenses - Totals (Includes Inpatient and Outpatient)** | | | | | |
| Total Net Revenue | $49,379,694,810 | $46,432,845,269 | $41,800,329,627 | $37,720,612,218 | $36,016,882,393 |
| Total Expenses | 45,925,560,145 | 42,603,810,235 | 38,889,779,063 | 36,104,024,942 | 33,477,930,476 |
| **COMMUNITY HEALTH INDICATORS PER 1000 POPULATION** | | | | | |
| Total Population (in thousands) | 32,852 | 32,409 | 31,966 | 31,551 | 31,108 |
| **Inpatient** | | | | | |
| Beds | 2.9 | 3.0 | 3.0 | 3.0 | 3.0 |
| Admissions | 124.1 | 125.1 | 123.6 | 121.0 | 119.5 |
| Inpatient Days | 658.7 | 664.7 | 650.1 | 635.9 | 641.6 |
| Inpatient Surgeries | 35.8 | 35.8 | 35.3 | 35.7 | 35.3 |
| Births | 15.8 | 15.8 | 15.9 | 16.0 | 15.5 |
| **Outpatient** | | | | | |
| Emergency Outpatient Visits | 409.5 | 408.2 | 389.6 | 374.8 | 369.6 |
| Other Outpatient Visits | 1,221.8 | 1,254.2 | 1,192.7 | 1,163.4 | 1,120.4 |
| Total Outpatient Visits | 1,631.3 | 1,662.4 | 1,582.3 | 1,538.1 | 1,490.1 |
| Outpatient Surgeries | 51.2 | 52.9 | 52.0 | 52.6 | 53.0 |
| **Expense per Capita (per person)** | $1,406.0 | $1,320.9 | $1,223.5 | $1,150.7 | $1,085.6 |

# TABLE 5

## U.S. CENSUS DIVISION 8: MOUNTAIN

*U.S. Registered Community Hospitals*
*(Nonfederal, short-term general and other special hospitals)*

## Overview 1999–2003

| | 2003 | 2002 | 2001 | 2000 | 1999 |
|---|---|---|---|---|---|
| **Total Community Hospitals in Census Division 8, Mountain** | **348** | **349** | **345** | **347** | **346** |
| **Bed Size Category** | | | | | |
| 6-24 | 43 | 38 | 35 | 38 | 39 |
| 25-49 | 83 | 90 | 86 | 88 | 82 |
| 50-99 | 88 | 85 | 87 | 87 | 91 |
| 100-199 | 63 | 67 | 69 | 67 | 71 |
| 200-299 | 35 | 35 | 33 | 34 | 32 |
| 300-399 | 19 | 19 | 20 | 18 | 17 |
| 400-499 | 10 | 9 | 9 | 10 | 9 |
| 500 + | 7 | 6 | 6 | 5 | 5 |
| **Location** | | | | | |
| Hospitals Urban | 143 | 143 | 140 | 136 | 136 |
| Hospitals Rural | 205 | 206 | 205 | 211 | 210 |
| **Control** | | | | | |
| State and Local Government | 103 | 103 | 108 | 110 | 116 |
| Not for Profit | 181 | 180 | 175 | 176 | 175 |
| Investor owned | 64 | 66 | 62 | 61 | 55 |
| **Physician Models** | | | | | |
| Independent Practice Association | 49 | 46 | 45 | 60 | 67 |
| Group Practice without Walls | 8 | 12 | 11 | 11 | 13 |
| Open Physician-Hospital Organization | 43 | 41 | 36 | 49 | 58 |
| Closed Physician-Hospital Organization | 12 | 17 | 15 | 22 | 23 |
| Management Service Organization | 22 | 20 | 20 | 26 | 33 |
| Integrated Salary Model | 102 | 84 | 87 | 78 | 77 |
| Equity Model | 4 | 4 | 2 | 1 | 3 |
| Foundation | 3 | 8 | 9 | 13 | 16 |
| **Insurance Products** | | | | | |
| Health Maintenance Organization | 54 | 51 | 56 | 61 | 55 |
| Preferred Provider Organization | 57 | 51 | 55 | 70 | 57 |
| Indemnity Fee for Service | 29 | 27 | 27 | 31 | 25 |
| **Managed Care Contracts** | | | | | |
| Health Maintenance Organization | 155 | 146 | 143 | 154 | 172 |
| Preferred Provider Organization | 189 | 176 | 176 | 188 | 185 |
| **Affiliations** | | | | | |
| Hospitals in a System* | 196 | 191 | 187 | 186 | 186 |
| Hospitals in a Network | 101 | 87 | 88 | 85 | 80 |
| Hospitals in a Group Purchasing Organization | 248 | 236 | 252 | 239 | 215 |

* Please note that system affiliate information for hospitals is derived from AHA membership. In years prior to 2003 the affiliation was derived from a question on the AHA Annual Survey of hospitals; therefore, non-responding hospitals were not included in the system affiliation counts. Years prior to 2003 have been updated to reflect this change, which now include affiliation for non-reporting hospitals.

# TABLE 5

## U.S. CENSUS DIVISION 8: MOUNTAIN

*U.S. Registered Community Hospitals*
*(Nonfederal, short-term general and other special hospitals)*

## Utilization, Personnel, Revenue and Expenses, Community Health Indicators 1999–2003

| | 2003 | 2002 | 2001 | 2000 | 1999 |
|---|---|---|---|---|---|
| **TOTAL FACILITY (Includes Hospital and Nursing Home Units)** | | | | | |
| **Utilization - Inpatient** | | | | | |
| Beds | 42,159 | 42,499 | 42,116 | 41,536 | 41,168 |
| Admissions | 1,936,327 | 1,894,701 | 1,825,214 | 1,773,119 | 1,708,013 |
| Inpatient Days | 9,825,461 | 9,643,564 | 9,432,684 | 9,198,430 | 9,134,857 |
| Average Length of Stay | 5.1 | 5.1 | 5.2 | 5.2 | 5.3 |
| Inpatient Surgeries | 570,828 | 573,886 | 551,364 | 551,078 | 554,791 |
| Births | 298,539 | 292,890 | 277,576 | 273,536 | 264,003 |
| **Utilization - Outpatient** | | | | | |
| Emergency Outpatient Visits | 6,191,190 | 6,124,812 | 5,444,391 | 5,579,598 | 5,254,445 |
| Other Outpatient Visits | 25,210,413 | 23,424,496 | 22,599,897 | 21,879,555 | 21,342,609 |
| Total Outpatient Visits | 31,401,603 | 29,549,308 | 28,044,288 | 27,459,153 | 26,597,054 |
| Outpatient Surgeries | 824,022 | 868,934 | 813,341 | 838,426 | 849,404 |
| **Personnel** | | | | | |
| Full Time RNs | 44,847 | 42,583 | 38,561 | 38,435 | 37,953 |
| Full Time LPNs | 4,688 | 4,955 | 4,809 | 4,412 | 4,718 |
| Part Time RNs | 22,105 | 20,935 | 18,430 | 20,841 | 18,639 |
| Part Time LPNs | 2,130 | 2,112 | 1,965 | 2,185 | 1,990 |
| Total Full Time | 186,346 | 179,836 | 170,748 | 162,370 | 163,460 |
| Total Part Time | 67,402 | 65,555 | 60,208 | 65,617 | 59,319 |
| **Revenue - Inpatient** | | | | | |
| Gross Inpatient Revenue | $37,659,338,009 | $33,651,462,085 | $27,813,469,466 | $25,420,640,854 | $22,802,959,773 |
| **Revenue - Outpatient** | | | | | |
| Gross Outpatient Revenue | $20,005,569,335 | $17,572,433,747 | $14,608,268,942 | $13,088,918,718 | $11,360,904,338 |
| **Revenue and Expenses - Totals (Includes Inpatient and Outpatient)** | | | | | |
| Total Gross Revenue | $57,664,907,344 | $51,223,895,832 | $42,421,738,408 | $38,509,559,572 | $34,163,864,111 |
| Deductions from Revenue | 34,069,882,506 | 29,266,253,620 | 23,195,132,956 | 20,763,767,673 | 17,542,214,999 |
| Net Patient Revenue | 23,595,024,838 | 21,957,642,212 | 19,226,605,452 | 17,745,791,899 | 16,621,649,112 |
| Other Operating Revenue | 1,183,351,784 | 1,082,083,144 | 1,165,866,873 | 914,977,655 | 857,114,840 |
| Other Nonoperating Revenue | 279,791,570 | 247,116,847 | 355,603,623 | 350,531,542 | 333,030,721 |
| Total Net Revenue | 25,058,168,192 | 23,286,842,203 | 20,748,075,948 | 19,011,301,096 | 17,811,794,673 |
| Total Expenses | 23,296,281,246 | 21,439,442,983 | 19,222,843,051 | 17,634,866,621 | 16,728,824,652 |
| **HOSPITAL UNIT (Excludes Separate Nursing Home Units)** | | | | | |
| **Utilization - Inpatient** | | | | | |
| Beds | 38,192 | 38,104 | 37,453 | 36,716 | 35,984 |
| Admissions | 1,922,484 | 1,878,936 | 1,804,483 | 1,750,242 | 1,659,661 |
| Inpatient Days | 8,601,499 | 8,282,586 | 7,973,579 | 7,691,884 | 7,569,524 |
| Average Length of Stay | 4.5 | 4.4 | 4.4 | 4.4 | 4.6 |
| **Personnel** | | | | | |
| Total Full Time | 183,583 | 176,918 | 167,386 | 159,111 | 160,221 |
| Total Part Time | 65,741 | 63,778 | 58,435 | 63,895 | 57,735 |
| **Revenue and Expenses - Totals (Includes Inpatient and Outpatient)** | | | | | |
| Total Net Revenue | $24,854,081,925 | $23,087,760,662 | $20,511,142,311 | $18,801,244,040 | $17,573,081,317 |
| Total Expenses | 23,103,787,089 | 21,258,843,110 | 19,017,095,330 | 17,452,526,303 | 16,526,820,028 |
| **COMMUNITY HEALTH INDICATORS PER 1000 POPULATION** | | | | | |
| Total Population (in thousands) | 19,384 | 19,033 | 18,651 | 18,272 | 17,861 |
| **Inpatient** | | | | | |
| Beds | 2.2 | 2.2 | 2.3 | 2.3 | 2.3 |
| Admissions | 99.9 | 99.5 | 97.9 | 97.0 | 95.6 |
| Inpatient Days | 506.9 | 506.7 | 505.8 | 503.4 | 511.4 |
| Inpatient Surgeries | 29.4 | 30.2 | 29.6 | 30.2 | 31.1 |
| Births | 15.4 | 15.4 | 14.9 | 15.0 | 14.8 |
| **Outpatient** | | | | | |
| Emergency Outpatient Visits | 319.4 | 321.8 | 291.9 | 305.4 | 294.2 |
| Other Outpatient Visits | 1,300.6 | 1,230.7 | 1,211.7 | 1,197.4 | 1,194.9 |
| Total Outpatient Visits | 1,620.0 | 1,552.5 | 1,503.7 | 1,502.8 | 1,489.1 |
| Outpatient Surgeries | 42.5 | 45.7 | 43.6 | 45.9 | 47.6 |
| **Expense per Capita (per person)** | $1,201.8 | $1,126.4 | $1,030.7 | $965.1 | $936.6 |

# TABLE 5

## U.S. CENSUS DIVISION 9: PACIFIC

*U.S. Registered Community Hospitals*
*(Nonfederal, short-term general and other special hospitals)*

## Overview 1999–2003

| | 2003 | 2002 | 2001 | 2000 | 1999 |
|---|---|---|---|---|---|
| **Total Community Hospitals in Census Division 9, Pacific** | **556** | **573** | **570** | **571** | **579** |
| **Bed Size Category** | | | | | |
| 6-24 | 32 | 32 | 27 | 31 | 36 |
| 25-49 | 98 | 96 | 90 | 91 | 91 |
| 50-99 | 92 | 105 | 110 | 108 | 108 |
| 100-199 | 144 | 153 | 158 | 159 | 162 |
| 200-299 | 96 | 95 | 94 | 97 | 96 |
| 300-399 | 50 | 48 | 49 | 50 | 51 |
| 400-499 | 22 | 25 | 29 | 21 | 21 |
| 500 + | 22 | 19 | 13 | 14 | 14 |
| **Location** | | | | | |
| Hospitals Urban | 418 | 433 | 432 | 434 | 441 |
| Hospitals Rural | 138 | 140 | 138 | 137 | 138 |
| **Control** | | | | | |
| State and Local Government | 135 | 140 | 142 | 138 | 143 |
| Not for Profit | 319 | 332 | 329 | 330 | 328 |
| Investor owned | 102 | 101 | 99 | 103 | 108 |
| **Physician Models** | | | | | |
| Independent Practice Association | 123 | 142 | 142 | 140 | 146 |
| Group Practice without Walls | 18 | 27 | 28 | 25 | 24 |
| Open Physician-Hospital Organization | 28 | 33 | 33 | 37 | 39 |
| Closed Physician-Hospital Organization | 18 | 17 | 25 | 27 | 28 |
| Management Service Organization | 47 | 56 | 55 | 64 | 78 |
| Integrated Salary Model | 87 | 100 | 78 | 80 | 80 |
| Equity Model | — | 1 | 2 | 3 | 6 |
| Foundation | 32 | 33 | 29 | 43 | 42 |
| **Insurance Products** | | | | | |
| Health Maintenance Organization | 71 | 76 | 62 | 72 | 100 |
| Preferred Provider Organization | 56 | 58 | 44 | 52 | 72 |
| Indemnity Fee for Service | 26 | 23 | 16 | 15 | 20 |
| **Managed Care Contracts** | | | | | |
| Health Maintenance Organization | 247 | 275 | 243 | 260 | 285 |
| Preferred Provider Organization | 271 | 300 | 255 | 270 | 290 |
| **Affiliations** | | | | | |
| Hospitals in a System* | 336 | 342 | 339 | 337 | 345 |
| Hospitals in a Network | 76 | 80 | 80 | 65 | 68 |
| Hospitals in a Group Purchasing Organization | 327 | 359 | 333 | 295 | 301 |

* Please note that system affiliate information for hospitals is derived from AHA membership. In years prior to 2003 the affiliation was derived from a question on the AHA Annual Survey of hospitals; therefore, non-responding hospitals were not included in the system affiliation counts. Years prior to 2003 have been updated to reflect this change, which now include affiliation for non-reporting hospitals.

U.S. Census Divisions

# TABLE 5

## U.S. CENSUS DIVISION 9: PACIFIC

*U.S. Registered Community Hospitals*
*(Nonfederal, short-term general and other special hospitals)*

## Utilization, Personnel, Revenue and Expenses, Community Health Indicators 1999–2003

| | 2003 | 2002 | 2001 | 2000 | 1999 |
|---|---|---|---|---|---|
| **TOTAL FACILITY (Includes Hospital and Nursing Home Units)** | | | | | |
| **Utilization - Inpatient** | | | | | |
| Beds | 96,854 | 97,048 | 96,010 | 94,948 | 95,570 |
| Admissions | 4,489,795 | 4,453,054 | 4,347,642 | 4,296,908 | 4,192,529 |
| Inpatient Days | 23,850,078 | 23,756,101 | 22,968,771 | 22,490,293 | 21,953,126 |
| Average Length of Stay | 5.3 | 5.3 | 5.3 | 5.2 | 5.2 |
| Inpatient Surgeries | 1,254,159 | 1,309,119 | 1,200,316 | 1,197,879 | 1,153,469 |
| Births | 630,788 | 616,819 | 630,251 | 665,956 | 615,818 |
| **Utilization - Outpatient** | | | | | |
| Emergency Outpatient Visits | 12,947,101 | 13,731,605 | 13,916,852 | 13,085,734 | 12,507,125 |
| Other Outpatient Visits | 56,929,025 | 60,828,353 | 56,276,529 | 52,457,752 | 52,358,495 |
| Total Outpatient Visits | 69,876,126 | 74,559,958 | 70,193,381 | 65,543,486 | 64,865,620 |
| Outpatient Surgeries | 1,808,400 | 1,902,778 | 1,845,904 | 1,841,711 | 1,663,599 |
| **Personnel** | | | | | |
| Full Time RNs | 97,331 | 96,461 | 92,781 | 86,593 | 84,598 |
| Full Time LPNs | 11,134 | 11,299 | 11,012 | 10,753 | 10,705 |
| Part Time RNs | 63,567 | 53,794 | 51,294 | 64,202 | 59,976 |
| Part Time LPNs | 5,204 | 4,211 | 4,152 | 6,024 | 5,506 |
| Total Full Time | 419,189 | 426,704 | 411,166 | 387,216 | 380,054 |
| Total Part Time | 176,116 | 154,518 | 150,306 | 189,923 | 171,580 |
| **Revenue - Inpatient** | | | | | |
| Gross Inpatient Revenue | $131,147,209,263 | $104,936,331,959 | $89,170,723,161 | $75,477,661,383 | $69,198,015,940 |
| **Revenue - Outpatient** | | | | | |
| Gross Outpatient Revenue | $55,318,628,115 | $46,066,247,391 | $38,916,573,129 | $34,417,684,249 | $30,111,292,438 |
| **Revenue and Expenses - Totals (Includes Inpatient and Outpatient)** | | | | | |
| Total Gross Revenue | $186,465,837,378 | $151,002,579,350 | $128,087,296,290 | $109,895,345,632 | $99,309,308,378 |
| Deductions from Revenue | 125,667,694,248 | 95,502,859,945 | 77,374,399,517 | 62,997,781,765 | 55,746,141,428 |
| Net Patient Revenue | 60,798,143,130 | 55,499,719,405 | 50,712,896,773 | 46,897,563,867 | 43,563,166,950 |
| Other Operating Revenue | 3,547,025,742 | 3,077,494,277 | 2,797,221,202 | 2,794,056,480 | 2,556,475,389 |
| Other Nonoperating Revenue | 1,397,694,045 | 1,219,640,462 | 1,328,607,343 | 1,212,144,701 | 1,359,542,968 |
| Total Net Revenue | 65,742,862,917 | 59,796,854,144 | 54,838,725,318 | 50,903,765,048 | 47,479,185,307 |
| Total Expenses | 62,875,657,935 | 57,386,669,321 | 52,988,295,607 | 49,162,814,581 | 46,213,076,154 |
| **HOSPITAL UNIT (Excludes Separate Nursing Home Units)** | | | | | |
| **Utilization - Inpatient** | | | | | |
| Beds | 88,955 | 87,870 | 88,815 | 89,168 | 88,931 |
| Admissions | 4,437,867 | 4,385,440 | 4,286,501 | 4,248,674 | 4,133,064 |
| Inpatient Days | 21,468,884 | 21,145,589 | 20,858,375 | 20,803,528 | 20,024,988 |
| Average Length of Stay | 4.8 | 4.8 | 4.9 | 4.9 | 4.8 |
| **Personnel** | | | | | |
| Total Full Time | 413,600 | 420,265 | 406,127 | 383,153 | 375,756 |
| Total Part Time | 173,941 | 152,674 | 148,479 | 187,897 | 169,565 |
| **Revenue and Expenses - Totals (Includes Inpatient and Outpatient)** | | | | | |
| Total Net Revenue | $64,948,547,194 | $59,059,246,409 | $54,279,461,564 | $50,442,556,359 | $46,970,677,731 |
| Total Expenses | 62,298,298,365 | 56,802,766,053 | 52,589,699,252 | 48,846,089,081 | 45,852,689,635 |
| **COMMUNITY HEALTH INDICATORS PER 1000 POPULATION** | | | | | |
| Total Population (in thousands) | 47,082 | 46,472 | 45,856 | 45,182 | 44,571 |
| **Inpatient** | | | | | |
| Beds | 2.1 | 2.1 | 2.1 | 2.1 | 2.1 |
| Admissions | 95.4 | 95.8 | 94.8 | 95.1 | 94.1 |
| Inpatient Days | 506.6 | 511.2 | 500.9 | 497.8 | 492.5 |
| Inpatient Surgeries | 26.6 | 28.2 | 26.2 | 26.5 | 25.9 |
| Births | 13.4 | 13.3 | 13.7 | 14.7 | 13.8 |
| **Outpatient** | | | | | |
| Emergency Outpatient Visits | 275.0 | 295.5 | 303.5 | 289.6 | 280.6 |
| Other Outpatient Visits | 1,209.1 | 1,308.9 | 1,227.2 | 1,161.0 | 1,174.7 |
| Total Outpatient Visits | 1,484.1 | 1,604.4 | 1,530.7 | 1,450.7 | 1,455.3 |
| Outpatient Surgeries | 38.4 | 40.9 | 40.3 | 40.8 | 37.3 |
| **Expense per Capita (per person)** | $1,335.5 | $1,234.9 | $1,155.5 | $1,088.1 | $1,036.8 |

# TABLE 6

# ALABAMA

*U.S. Registered Community Hospitals*
*(Nonfederal, short-term general and other special hospitals)*

## Overview 1999–2003

| | 2003 | 2002 | 2001 | 2000 | 1999 |
|---|---|---|---|---|---|
| **Total Community Hospitals in Alabama** | **107** | **106** | **107** | **108** | **109** |
| **Bed Size Category** | | | | | |
| 6-24 | 7 | 6 | 4 | 4 | 4 |
| 25-49 | 19 | 15 | 18 | 17 | 17 |
| 50-99 | 24 | 30 | 26 | 28 | 29 |
| 100-199 | 34 | 30 | 34 | 34 | 33 |
| 200-299 | 11 | 13 | 11 | 13 | 14 |
| 300-399 | 6 | 7 | 7 | 7 | 6 |
| 400-499 | 2 | 1 | 4 | 3 | 3 |
| 500 + | 4 | 4 | 3 | 2 | 3 |
| **Location** | | | | | |
| Hospitals Urban | 57 | 57 | 57 | 57 | 57 |
| Hospitals Rural | 50 | 49 | 50 | 51 | 52 |
| **Control** | | | | | |
| State and Local Government | 37 | 36 | 40 | 40 | 43 |
| Not for Profit | 35 | 35 | 37 | 39 | 40 |
| Investor owned | 35 | 35 | 30 | 29 | 26 |
| **Physician Models** | | | | | |
| Independent Practice Association | 11 | 4 | 6 | 9 | 13 |
| Group Practice without Walls | 1 | 3 | 1 | 4 | 3 |
| Open Physician-Hospital Organization | 4 | 2 | 4 | 7 | 7 |
| Closed Physician-Hospital Organization | 0 | 0 | 1 | 1 | 2 |
| Management Service Organization | 8 | 8 | 8 | 9 | 15 |
| Integrated Salary Model | 13 | 9 | 8 | 11 | 10 |
| Equity Model | 0 | 0 | 2 | 3 | 1 |
| Foundation | 8 | 6 | 4 | 6 | 2 |
| **Insurance Products** | | | | | |
| Health Maintenance Organization | 5 | 2 | 3 | 14 | 19 |
| Preferred Provider Organization | 16 | 13 | 14 | 20 | 25 |
| Indemnity Fee for Service | 3 | 3 | 2 | 1 | 4 |
| **Managed Care Contracts** | | | | | |
| Health Maintenance Organization | 41 | 33 | 34 | 40 | 48 |
| Preferred Provider Organization | 56 | 42 | 46 | 56 | 60 |
| **Affiliations** | | | | | |
| Hospitals in a System* | 70 | 66 | 69 | 72 | 70 |
| Hospitals in a Network | 12 | 8 | 7 | 9 | 9 |
| Hospitals in a Group Purchasing Organization | 66 | 49 | 52 | 58 | 59 |

* Please note that system affiliate information for hospitals is derived from AHA membership. In years prior to 2003 the affiliation was derived from a question on the AHA Annual Survey of hospitals; therefore, non-responding hospitals were not included in the system affiliation counts. Years prior to 2003 have been updated to reflect this change, which now include affiliation for non-reporting hospitals.

# TABLE 6

## ALABAMA

*U.S. Registered Community Hospitals*
*(Nonfederal, short-term general and other special hospitals)*

## Utilization, Personnel, Revenue and Expenses, Community Health Indicators 1999–2003

| | 2003 | 2002 | 2001 | 2000 | 1999 |
|---|---|---|---|---|---|
| **TOTAL FACILITY (Includes Hospital and Nursing Home Units)** | | | | | |
| **Utilization - Inpatient** | | | | | |
| Beds | 15,666 | 15,935 | 16,627 | 16,370 | 16,306 |
| Admissions | 708,995 | 676,337 | 684,923 | 680,395 | 670,059 |
| Inpatient Days | 3,547,203 | 3,244,123 | 3,570,273 | 3,585,804 | 3,603,498 |
| Average Length of Stay | 5.0 | 4.8 | 5.2 | 5.3 | 5.4 |
| Inpatient Surgeries | 210,149 | 198,225 | 190,655 | 198,439 | 196,715 |
| Births | 57,580 | 55,677 | 55,794 | 57,501 | 57,787 |
| **Utilization - Outpatient** | | | | | |
| Emergency Outpatient Visits | 2,145,885 | 2,162,011 | 1,959,967 | 2,070,702 | 1,969,275 |
| Other Outpatient Visits | 6,753,290 | 7,883,504 | 5,826,096 | 5,893,511 | 5,866,213 |
| Total Outpatient Visits | 8,899,175 | 10,045,515 | 7,786,063 | 7,964,213 | 7,835,488 |
| Outpatient Surgeries | 323,743 | 319,658 | 293,428 | 287,725 | 279,495 |
| **Personnel** | | | | | |
| Full Time RNs | 16,063 | 15,328 | 14,825 | 14,551 | 14,642 |
| Full Time LPNs | 2,975 | 2,680 | 2,905 | 2,693 | 3,060 |
| Part Time RNs | 5,543 | 5,382 | 4,799 | 4,782 | 4,285 |
| Part Time LPNs | 784 | 750 | 695 | 745 | 709 |
| Total Full Time | 64,944 | 63,011 | 62,655 | 60,209 | 60,570 |
| Total Part Time | 16,435 | 14,924 | 13,575 | 13,408 | 12,302 |
| **Revenue - Inpatient** | | | | | |
| Gross Inpatient Revenue | $13,225,879,008 | $10,908,904,536 | $9,398,051,190 | $8,966,154,419 | $8,625,893,202 |
| **Revenue - Outpatient** | | | | | |
| Gross Outpatient Revenue | $6,504,097,756 | $5,203,241,240 | $4,564,975,896 | $4,271,722,359 | $3,898,882,021 |
| **Revenue and Expenses - Totals (Includes Inpatient and Outpatient)** | | | | | |
| Total Gross Revenue | $19,729,976,764 | $16,112,145,776 | $13,963,027,086 | $13,237,876,778 | $12,524,775,223 |
| Deductions from Revenue | 13,372,289,500 | 10,194,892,253 | 8,380,028,417 | 8,048,660,850 | 7,494,355,021 |
| Net Patient Revenue | 6,357,687,264 | 5,917,253,523 | 5,582,998,669 | 5,189,215,928 | 5,030,420,202 |
| Other Operating Revenue | 322,785,134 | 343,884,634 | 281,472,509 | 392,404,366 | 440,819,124 |
| Other Nonoperating Revenue | 165,592,463 | 66,577,418 | 112,779,032 | 138,535,799 | 137,896,417 |
| Total Net Revenue | 6,846,064,861 | 6,327,715,575 | 5,977,250,210 | 5,720,156,093 | 5,609,135,743 |
| Total Expenses | 6,507,392,947 | 5,767,179,494 | 5,664,284,252 | 5,461,919,463 | 5,222,381,900 |
| **HOSPITAL UNIT (Excludes Separate Nursing Home Units)** | | | | | |
| **Utilization - Inpatient** | | | | | |
| Beds | 14,823 | 15,678 | 15,704 | 15,382 | 15,052 |
| Admissions | 704,540 | 672,860 | 681,266 | 676,250 | 665,857 |
| Inpatient Days | 3,280,487 | 3,178,161 | 3,274,368 | 3,264,746 | 3,183,661 |
| Average Length of Stay | 4.7 | 4.7 | 4.8 | 4.8 | 4.8 |
| **Personnel** | | | | | |
| Total Full Time | 64,365 | 62,861 | 62,162 | 59,546 | 59,630 |
| Total Part Time | 16,309 | 14,895 | 13,518 | 13,272 | 12,117 |
| **Revenue and Expenses - Totals (Includes Inpatient and Outpatient)** | | | | | |
| Total Net Revenue | $6,778,019,599 | $6,315,357,773 | $5,942,050,549 | $5,695,856,842 | $5,567,541,618 |
| Total Expenses | 6,441,833,027 | 5,754,090,214 | 5,626,134,980 | 5,439,545,167 | 5,185,831,549 |
| **COMMUNITY HEALTH INDICATORS PER 1000 POPULATION** | | | | | |
| Total Population (in thousands) | 4,501 | 4,479 | 4,466 | 4,452 | 4,430 |
| **Inpatient** | | | | | |
| Beds | 3.5 | 3.6 | 3.7 | 3.7 | 3.7 |
| Admissions | 157.5 | 151.0 | 153.3 | 152.8 | 151.3 |
| Inpatient Days | 788.1 | 724.3 | 799.4 | 805.5 | 813.4 |
| Inpatient Surgeries | 46.7 | 44.3 | 42.7 | 44.6 | 44.4 |
| Births | 12.8 | 12.4 | 12.5 | 12.9 | 13.0 |
| **Outpatient** | | | | | |
| Emergency Outpatient Visits | 476.8 | 482.7 | 438.8 | 465.2 | 444.5 |
| Other Outpatient Visits | 1,500.5 | 1,760.1 | 1,304.4 | 1,323.9 | 1,324.2 |
| Total Outpatient Visits | 1,977.3 | 2,242.9 | 1,743.2 | 1,789.1 | 1,768.7 |
| Outpatient Surgeries | 71.9 | 71.4 | 65.7 | 64.6 | 63.1 |
| **Expense per Capita (per person)** | $1,445.8 | $1,287.6 | $1,268.2 | $1,227.0 | $1,178.8 |

# TABLE 6

## ALASKA

*U.S. Registered Community Hospitals*
*(Nonfederal, short-term general and other special hospitals)*

## Overview 1999–2003

| | 2003 | 2002 | 2001 | 2000 | 1999 |
|---|---|---|---|---|---|
| **Total Community Hospitals in Alaska** | **19** | **19** | **19** | **18** | **17** |
| **Bed Size Category** | | | | | |
| 6-24 | 5 | 5 | 5 | 4 | 5 |
| 25-49 | 7 | 6 | 6 | 7 | 6 |
| 50-99 | 3 | 4 | 4 | 3 | 3 |
| 100-199 | 2 | 3 | 2 | 2 | 1 |
| 200-299 | 1 | 0 | 1 | 1 | 1 |
| 300-399 | 1 | 1 | 1 | 1 | 1 |
| 400-499 | 0 | 0 | 0 | 0 | 0 |
| 500 + | 0 | 0 | 0 | 0 | 0 |
| **Location** | | | | | |
| Hospitals Urban | 3 | 3 | 3 | 3 | 2 |
| Hospitals Rural | 16 | 16 | 16 | 15 | 15 |
| **Control** | | | | | |
| State and Local Government | 7 | 7 | 8 | 7 | 7 |
| Not for Profit | 10 | 11 | 10 | 10 | 9 |
| Investor owned | 2 | 1 | 1 | 1 | 1 |
| **Physician Models** | | | | | |
| Independent Practice Association | 2 | 3 | 3 | 5 | 2 |
| Group Practice without Walls | 2 | 3 | 3 | 4 | 2 |
| Open Physician-Hospital Organization | 3 | 3 | 3 | 4 | 2 |
| Closed Physician-Hospital Organization | 0 | 0 | 0 | 1 | 0 |
| Management Service Organization | 0 | 0 | 1 | 2 | 2 |
| Integrated Salary Model | 6 | 5 | 3 | 3 | 2 |
| Equity Model | 0 | 0 | 0 | 1 | 0 |
| Foundation | 0 | 0 | 0 | 1 | 0 |
| **Insurance Products** | | | | | |
| Health Maintenance Organization | 0 | 0 | 0 | 0 | 0 |
| Preferred Provider Organization | 3 | 1 | 0 | 1 | 1 |
| Indemnity Fee for Service | 0 | 0 | 0 | 1 | 1 |
| **Managed Care Contracts** | | | | | |
| Health Maintenance Organization | 0 | 0 | 0 | 0 | 0 |
| Preferred Provider Organization | 7 | 6 | 3 | 7 | 5 |
| **Affiliations** | | | | | |
| Hospitals in a System* | 12 | 11 | 11 | 10 | 9 |
| Hospitals in a Network | 6 | 2 | 1 | 0 | 0 |
| Hospitals in a Group Purchasing Organization | 10 | 11 | 9 | 12 | 13 |

States

* Please note that system affiliate information for hospitals is derived from AHA membership. In years prior to 2003 the affiliation was derived from a question on the AHA Annual Survey of hospitals; therefore, non-responding hospitals were not included in the system affiliation counts. Years prior to 2003 have been updated to reflect this change, which now include affiliation for non-reporting hospitals.

# TABLE 6

## ALASKA

*U.S. Registered Community Hospitals*
*(Nonfederal, short-term general and other special hospitals)*

## Utilization, Personnel, Revenue and Expenses, Community Health Indicators 1999–2003

| | 2003 | 2002 | 2001 | 2000 | 1999 |
|---|---|---|---|---|---|
| **TOTAL FACILITY (Includes Hospital and Nursing Home Units)** | | | | | |
| **Utilization - Inpatient** | | | | | |
| Beds | 1,456 | 1,378 | 1,442 | 1,417 | 1,250 |
| Admissions | 45,982 | 47,560 | 49,065 | 46,887 | 40,785 |
| Inpatient Days | 287,351 | 300,060 | 303,092 | 293,707 | 246,872 |
| Average Length of Stay | 6.2 | 6.3 | 6.2 | 6.3 | 6.1 |
| Inpatient Surgeries | 15,879 | 22,359 | 15,888 | 15,196 | 12,762 |
| Births | 7,608 | 7,596 | 7,448 | 7,728 | 6,618 |
| **Utilization - Outpatient** | | | | | |
| Emergency Outpatient Visits | 213,380 | 254,592 | 205,595 | 187,226 | 164,113 |
| Other Outpatient Visits | 1,230,029 | 1,083,024 | 1,182,031 | 1,083,881 | 868,170 |
| Total Outpatient Visits | 1,443,409 | 1,337,616 | 1,387,626 | 1,271,107 | 1,032,283 |
| Outpatient Surgeries | 35,682 | 35,136 | 37,849 | 34,678 | 25,640 |
| **Personnel** | | | | | |
| Full Time RNs | 1,749 | 1,734 | 1,504 | 1,466 | 1,052 |
| Full Time LPNs | 155 | 144 | 189 | 200 | 86 |
| Part Time RNs | 758 | 752 | 956 | 768 | 832 |
| Part Time LPNs | 55 | 58 | 97 | 61 | 60 |
| Total Full Time | 6,990 | 7,447 | 6,544 | 5,763 | 4,154 |
| Total Part Time | 2,266 | 2,221 | 2,907 | 2,340 | 2,216 |
| **Revenue - Inpatient** | | | | | |
| Gross Inpatient Revenue | $1,034,651,499 | $960,861,590 | $875,560,013 | $741,246,222 | $625,651,216 |
| **Revenue - Outpatient** | | | | | |
| Gross Outpatient Revenue | $729,867,341 | $665,750,510 | $579,556,236 | $452,257,752 | $372,382,270 |
| **Revenue and Expenses - Totals (Includes Inpatient and Outpatient)** | | | | | |
| Total Gross Revenue | $1,764,518,840 | $1,626,612,100 | $1,455,116,249 | $1,193,503,974 | $998,033,486 |
| Deductions from Revenue | 864,446,975 | 755,063,643 | 624,227,686 | 460,734,350 | 383,654,287 |
| Net Patient Revenue | 900,071,865 | 871,548,457 | 830,888,563 | 732,769,624 | 614,379,199 |
| Other Operating Revenue | 45,996,074 | 40,119,994 | 72,758,253 | 34,360,208 | 29,498,177 |
| Other Nonoperating Revenue | 49,486,775 | 53,664,515 | 19,704,156 | 17,142,523 | 15,285,517 |
| Total Net Revenue | 995,554,714 | 965,332,966 | 923,350,972 | 784,272,355 | 659,162,893 |
| Total Expenses | 1,016,056,121 | 942,611,948 | 918,694,601 | 741,993,877 | 591,317,689 |
| **HOSPITAL UNIT (Excludes Separate Nursing Home Units)** | | | | | |
| **Utilization - Inpatient** | | | | | |
| Beds | 1,264 | 1,146 | 1,282 | 1,199 | 1,047 |
| Admissions | 45,690 | 47,038 | 48,661 | 46,246 | 40,167 |
| Inpatient Days | 229,735 | 228,355 | 252,692 | 227,379 | 182,521 |
| Average Length of Stay | 5.0 | 4.9 | 5.2 | 4.9 | 4.5 |
| **Personnel** | | | | | |
| Total Full Time | 6,896 | 7,261 | 6,404 | 5,619 | 4,021 |
| Total Part Time | 2,201 | 2,099 | 2,820 | 2,220 | 2,093 |
| **Revenue and Expenses - Totals (Includes Inpatient and Outpatient)** | | | | | |
| Total Net Revenue | $971,914,169 | $938,542,659 | $902,447,973 | $759,807,432 | $637,789,467 |
| Total Expenses | 997,720,331 | 923,049,072 | 902,546,954 | 727,117,622 | 577,708,366 |
| **COMMUNITY HEALTH INDICATORS PER 1000 POPULATION** | | | | | |
| Total Population (in thousands) | 649 | 641 | 633 | 628 | 625 |
| **Inpatient** | | | | | |
| Beds | 2.2 | 2.1 | 2.3 | 2.3 | 2.0 |
| Admissions | 70.9 | 74.1 | 77.6 | 74.7 | 65.3 |
| Inpatient Days | 442.9 | 467.8 | 479.1 | 468.0 | 395.1 |
| Inpatient Surgeries | 24.5 | 34.9 | 25.1 | 24.2 | 20.4 |
| Births | 11.7 | 11.8 | 11.8 | 12.3 | 10.6 |
| **Outpatient** | | | | | |
| Emergency Outpatient Visits | 328.9 | 396.9 | 325.0 | 298.3 | 262.7 |
| Other Outpatient Visits | 1,895.8 | 1,688.3 | 1,868.3 | 1,727.1 | 1,389.6 |
| Total Outpatient Visits | 2,224.7 | 2,085.2 | 2,193.3 | 2,025.4 | 1,652.2 |
| Outpatient Surgeries | 55.0 | 54.8 | 59.8 | 55.3 | 41.0 |
| **Expense per Capita (per person)** | $1,566.0 | $1,469.4 | $1,452.1 | $1,182.3 | $946.4 |

# TABLE 6

# ARIZONA

*U.S. Registered Community Hospitals*
*(Nonfederal, short-term general and other special hospitals)*

## Overview 1999–2003

| | 2003 | 2002 | 2001 | 2000 | 1999 |
|---|---|---|---|---|---|
| **Total Community Hospitals in Arizona** | **61** | **61** | **61** | **61** | **61** |
| **Bed Size Category** | | | | | |
| 6-24 | 4 | 3 | 1 | 2 | 3 |
| 25-49 | 8 | 10 | 10 | 9 | 8 |
| 50-99 | 12 | 11 | 12 | 13 | 14 |
| 100-199 | 14 | 14 | 16 | 17 | 16 |
| 200-299 | 12 | 13 | 12 | 10 | 12 |
| 300-399 | 5 | 4 | 5 | 5 | 3 |
| 400-499 | 2 | 3 | 2 | 2 | 2 |
| 500 + | 4 | 3 | 3 | 3 | 3 |
| **Location** | | | | | |
| Hospitals Urban | 46 | 46 | 46 | 46 | 45 |
| Hospitals Rural | 15 | 15 | 15 | 15 | 16 |
| **Control** | | | | | |
| State and Local Government | 5 | 5 | 4 | 5 | 6 |
| Not for Profit | 38 | 37 | 37 | 37 | 40 |
| Investor owned | 18 | 19 | 20 | 19 | 15 |
| **Physician Models** | | | | | |
| Independent Practice Association | 7 | 5 | 4 | 8 | 12 |
| Group Practice without Walls | 2 | 2 | 4 | 2 | 2 |
| Open Physician-Hospital Organization | 8 | 4 | 3 | 5 | 12 |
| Closed Physician-Hospital Organization | 2 | 3 | 4 | 6 | 8 |
| Management Service Organization | 3 | 1 | 3 | 5 | 10 |
| Integrated Salary Model | 13 | 7 | 10 | 8 | 12 |
| Equity Model | 1 | 0 | 0 | 0 | 1 |
| Foundation | 1 | 0 | 0 | 0 | 3 |
| **Insurance Products** | | | | | |
| Health Maintenance Organization | 7 | 7 | 6 | 6 | 8 |
| Preferred Provider Organization | 3 | 3 | 3 | 5 | 4 |
| Indemnity Fee for Service | 3 | 2 | 1 | 2 | 2 |
| **Managed Care Contracts** | | | | | |
| Health Maintenance Organization | 34 | 27 | 28 | 33 | 33 |
| Preferred Provider Organization | 36 | 29 | 30 | 34 | 31 |
| **Affiliations** | | | | | |
| Hospitals in a System* | 45 | 43 | 42 | 41 | 42 |
| Hospitals in a Network | 14 | 11 | 7 | 5 | 7 |
| Hospitals in a Group Purchasing Organization | 41 | 33 | 38 | 32 | 28 |

* Please note that system affiliate information for hospitals is derived from AHA membership. In years prior to 2003 the affiliation was derived from a question on the AHA Annual Survey of hospitals; therefore, non-responding hospitals were not included in the system affiliation counts. Years prior to 2003 have been updated to reflect this change, which now include affiliation for non-reporting hospitals.

# Table 6

## ARIZONA

*U.S. Registered Community Hospitals*
*(Nonfederal, short-term general and other special hospitals)*

## Utilization, Personnel, Revenue and Expenses, Community Health Indicators 1999–2003

| | 2003 | 2002 | 2001 | 2000 | 1999 |
|---|---|---|---|---|---|
| **TOTAL FACILITY (Includes Hospital and Nursing Home Units)** | | | | | |
| **Utilization - Inpatient** | | | | | |
| Beds | 10,801 | 10,930 | 10,732 | 10,864 | 10,576 |
| Admissions | 603,310 | 591,094 | 562,824 | 538,704 | 511,084 |
| Inpatient Days | 2,669,152 | 2,544,370 | 2,520,301 | 2,501,003 | 2,383,512 |
| Average Length of Stay | 4.4 | 4.3 | 4.5 | 4.6 | 4.7 |
| Inpatient Surgeries | 172,178 | 150,482 | 159,691 | 160,251 | 156,688 |
| Births | 87,912 | 85,418 | 80,408 | 77,851 | 74,255 |
| **Utilization - Outpatient** | | | | | |
| Emergency Outpatient Visits | 1,781,590 | 1,559,078 | 1,401,509 | 1,520,393 | 1,340,258 |
| Other Outpatient Visits | 4,925,127 | 3,577,803 | 3,670,119 | 3,779,713 | 3,602,695 |
| Total Outpatient Visits | 6,706,717 | 5,136,881 | 5,071,628 | 5,300,106 | 4,942,953 |
| Outpatient Surgeries | 210,079 | 208,797 | 197,227 | 212,829 | 200,933 |
| **Personnel** | | | | | |
| Full Time RNs | 12,411 | 11,156 | 10,027 | 10,777 | 10,564 |
| Full Time LPNs | 1,015 | 1,115 | 1,130 | 1,087 | 1,074 |
| Part Time RNs | 5,489 | 5,226 | 4,596 | 5,489 | 4,490 |
| Part Time LPNs | 348 | 388 | 339 | 483 | 342 |
| Total Full Time | 47,524 | 45,502 | 43,534 | 44,168 | 45,637 |
| Total Part Time | 14,299 | 15,229 | 13,146 | 16,142 | 12,958 |
| **Revenue - Inpatient** | | | | | |
| Gross Inpatient Revenue | $13,150,302,688 | $10,826,730,126 | $9,022,219,011 | $9,060,359,014 | $7,422,253,864 |
| **Revenue - Outpatient** | | | | | |
| Gross Outpatient Revenue | $5,741,277,192 | $4,770,650,607 | $3,772,046,879 | $3,805,828,209 | $2,988,190,051 |
| **Revenue and Expenses - Totals (Includes Inpatient and Outpatient)** | | | | | |
| Total Gross Revenue | $18,891,579,880 | $15,597,380,733 | $12,794,265,890 | $12,866,187,223 | $10,410,443,915 |
| Deductions from Revenue | 12,305,048,935 | 9,857,162,745 | 7,796,688,881 | 7,953,167,237 | 6,128,351,767 |
| Net Patient Revenue | 6,586,530,945 | 5,740,217,988 | 4,997,577,009 | 4,913,019,986 | 4,282,092,148 |
| Other Operating Revenue | 237,792,616 | 225,138,375 | 208,436,718 | 181,210,600 | 216,768,538 |
| Other Nonoperating Revenue | 41,239,855 | 34,008,928 | 50,890,354 | 82,678,089 | 92,131,062 |
| Total Net Revenue | 6,865,563,416 | 5,999,365,291 | 5,256,904,081 | 5,176,908,675 | 4,590,991,748 |
| Total Expenses | 6,256,631,400 | 5,647,682,344 | 4,986,268,299 | 4,797,810,319 | 4,496,686,959 |
| **HOSPITAL UNIT (Excludes Separate Nursing Home Units)** | | | | | |
| **Utilization - Inpatient** | | | | | |
| Beds | 10,584 | 10,653 | 10,325 | 10,205 | 9,687 |
| Admissions | 600,373 | 587,452 | 556,648 | 529,994 | 480,299 |
| Inpatient Days | 2,586,665 | 2,449,864 | 2,377,612 | 2,296,954 | 2,130,184 |
| Average Length of Stay | 4.3 | 4.2 | 4.3 | 4.3 | 4.4 |
| **Personnel** | | | | | |
| Total Full Time | 47,297 | 45,138 | 42,966 | 43,521 | 44,926 |
| Total Part Time | 14,247 | 15,130 | 13,025 | 15,952 | 12,773 |
| **Revenue and Expenses - Totals (Includes Inpatient and Outpatient)** | | | | | |
| Total Net Revenue | $6,835,799,648 | $5,976,493,274 | $5,225,561,891 | $5,127,715,363 | $4,525,282,814 |
| Total Expenses | 6,226,275,219 | 5,623,701,779 | 4,951,790,513 | 4,752,834,132 | 4,438,540,156 |
| **COMMUNITY HEALTH INDICATORS PER 1000 POPULATION** | | | | | |
| Total Population (in thousands) | 5,581 | 5,441 | 5,298 | 5,166 | 5,024 |
| **Inpatient** | | | | | |
| Beds | 1.9 | 2.0 | 2.0 | 2.1 | 2.1 |
| Admissions | 108.1 | 108.6 | 106.2 | 104.3 | 101.7 |
| Inpatient Days | 478.3 | 467.6 | 475.7 | 484.1 | 474.4 |
| Inpatient Surgeries | 30.9 | 27.7 | 30.1 | 31.0 | 31.2 |
| Births | 15.8 | 15.7 | 15.2 | 15.1 | 14.8 |
| **Outpatient** | | | | | |
| Emergency Outpatient Visits | 319.2 | 286.5 | 264.6 | 294.3 | 266.8 |
| Other Outpatient Visits | 882.5 | 657.5 | 692.8 | 731.7 | 717.1 |
| Total Outpatient Visits | 1,201.7 | 944.1 | 957.3 | 1,026.0 | 983.9 |
| Outpatient Surgeries | 37.6 | 38.4 | 37.2 | 41.2 | 40.0 |
| **Expense per Capita (per person)** | $1,121.1 | $1,038.0 | $941.2 | $928.8 | $895.1 |

# TABLE 6

## ARKANSAS

*U.S. Registered Community Hospitals*
*(Nonfederal, short-term general and other special hospitals)*

## Overview 1999–2003

| | 2003 | 2002 | 2001 | 2000 | 1999 |
|---|---|---|---|---|---|
| **Total Community Hospitals in Arkansas** | **88** | **87** | **83** | **83** | **83** |
| **Bed Size Category** | | | | | |
| 6-24 | 5 | 6 | 8 | 5 | 4 |
| 25-49 | 26 | 20 | 17 | 18 | 17 |
| 50-99 | 24 | 28 | 26 | 28 | 29 |
| 100-199 | 20 | 21 | 19 | 18 | 19 |
| 200-299 | 6 | 5 | 6 | 8 | 7 |
| 300-399 | 5 | 5 | 5 | 3 | 4 |
| 400-499 | 0 | 0 | 0 | 0 | 0 |
| 500 + | 2 | 2 | 2 | 3 | 3 |
| **Location** | | | | | |
| Hospitals Urban | 32 | 31 | 28 | 28 | 28 |
| Hospitals Rural | 56 | 56 | 55 | 55 | 55 |
| **Control** | | | | | |
| State and Local Government | 15 | 15 | 15 | 15 | 16 |
| Not for Profit | 52 | 51 | 49 | 49 | 48 |
| Investor owned | 21 | 21 | 19 | 19 | 19 |
| **Physician Models** | | | | | |
| Independent Practice Association | 22 | 18 | 12 | 11 | 7 |
| Group Practice without Walls | 6 | 6 | 4 | 4 | 4 |
| Open Physician-Hospital Organization | 32 | 29 | 24 | 30 | 24 |
| Closed Physician-Hospital Organization | 6 | 9 | 6 | 7 | 9 |
| Management Service Organization | 15 | 18 | 12 | 10 | 15 |
| Integrated Salary Model | 17 | 15 | 11 | 10 | 7 |
| Equity Model | 2 | 2 | 0 | 1 | 0 |
| Foundation | 9 | 10 | 11 | 13 | 14 |
| **Insurance Products** | | | | | |
| Health Maintenance Organization | 21 | 21 | 17 | 18 | 14 |
| Preferred Provider Organization | 31 | 30 | 22 | 24 | 19 |
| Indemnity Fee for Service | 6 | 8 | 3 | 7 | 6 |
| **Managed Care Contracts** | | | | | |
| Health Maintenance Organization | 48 | 48 | 47 | 48 | 36 |
| Preferred Provider Organization | 68 | 73 | 69 | 68 | 54 |
| **Affiliations** | | | | | |
| Hospitals in a System* | 48 | 47 | 42 | 45 | 46 |
| Hospitals in a Network | 27 | 28 | 24 | 25 | 18 |
| Hospitals in a Group Purchasing Organization | 82 | 79 | 74 | 70 | 51 |



* Please note that system affiliate information for hospitals is derived from AHA membership. In years prior to 2003 the affiliation was derived from a question on the AHA Annual Survey of hospitals; therefore, non-responding hospitals were not included in the system affiliation counts. Years prior to 2003 have been updated to reflect this change, which now include affiliation for non-reporting hospitals.

# ARKANSAS

*U.S. Registered Community Hospitals*
*(Nonfederal, short-term general and other special hospitals)*

## Utilization, Personnel, Revenue and Expenses, Community Health Indicators 1999–2003

| | 2003 | 2002 | 2001 | 2000 | 1999 |
|---|---|---|---|---|---|
| **TOTAL FACILITY (Includes Hospital and Nursing Home Units)** | | | | | |
| **Utilization - Inpatient** | | | | | |
| Beds | 9,909 | 9,942 | 9,535 | 9,784 | 10,051 |
| Admissions | 388,046 | 383,509 | 371,080 | 368,287 | 375,297 |
| Inpatient Days | 2,088,391 | 2,110,323 | 2,034,589 | 2,092,183 | 2,195,965 |
| Average Length of Stay | 5.4 | 5.5 | 5.5 | 5.7 | 5.9 |
| Inpatient Surgeries | 117,181 | 119,478 | 109,244 | 111,178 | 104,278 |
| Births | 38,892 | 38,191 | 36,863 | 37,723 | 36,561 |
| **Utilization - Outpatient** | | | | | |
| Emergency Outpatient Visits | 1,251,391 | 1,224,053 | 1,152,995 | 1,170,079 | 1,073,440 |
| Other Outpatient Visits | 3,330,961 | 3,614,451 | 3,340,779 | 3,237,000 | 2,882,432 |
| Total Outpatient Visits | 4,582,352 | 4,838,504 | 4,493,774 | 4,407,079 | 3,955,872 |
| Outpatient Surgeries | 151,653 | 159,314 | 151,651 | 154,713 | 154,726 |
| **Personnel** | | | | | |
| Full Time RNs | 9,019 | 8,417 | 8,359 | 8,817 | 9,235 |
| Full Time LPNs | 2,743 | 2,717 | 2,742 | 2,956 | 3,088 |
| Part Time RNs | 3,585 | 3,744 | 3,461 | 3,192 | 3,186 |
| Part Time LPNs | 1,045 | 969 | 976 | 879 | 888 |
| Total Full Time | 37,429 | 36,967 | 35,358 | 36,051 | 38,857 |
| Total Part Time | 12,127 | 11,843 | 11,629 | 11,110 | 10,349 |
| **Revenue - Inpatient** | | | | | |
| Gross Inpatient Revenue | $6,115,623,287 | $5,484,336,913 | $4,758,131,946 | $4,388,134,177 | $3,950,394,296 |
| **Revenue - Outpatient** | | | | | |
| Gross Outpatient Revenue | $3,592,960,043 | $3,139,609,992 | $2,687,321,039 | $2,451,987,458 | $2,145,741,679 |
| **Revenue and Expenses - Totals (Includes Inpatient and Outpatient)** | | | | | |
| Total Gross Revenue | $9,708,583,330 | $8,623,946,905 | $7,445,452,985 | $6,840,121,635 | $6,096,135,975 |
| Deductions from Revenue | 5,790,602,643 | 4,920,059,934 | 4,144,999,443 | 3,722,444,602 | 3,162,771,954 |
| Net Patient Revenue | 3,917,980,687 | 3,703,886,971 | 3,300,453,542 | 3,117,677,033 | 2,933,364,021 |
| Other Operating Revenue | 127,642,206 | 134,834,877 | 103,461,117 | 95,650,547 | 95,687,603 |
| Other Nonoperating Revenue | 49,276,715 | 34,677,549 | 42,618,122 | 48,896,908 | 42,627,476 |
| Total Net Revenue | 4,094,899,608 | 3,873,399,397 | 3,446,532,781 | 3,262,224,488 | 3,071,679,100 |
| Total Expenses | 3,947,107,676 | 3,612,279,530 | 3,249,943,830 | 3,176,562,841 | 2,972,492,256 |
| **HOSPITAL UNIT (Excludes Separate Nursing Home Units)** | | | | | |
| **Utilization - Inpatient** | | | | | |
| Beds | 9,341 | 9,388 | 9,041 | 9,018 | 9,372 |
| Admissions | 384,978 | 380,945 | 368,569 | 364,432 | 371,400 |
| Inpatient Days | 1,921,041 | 1,935,371 | 1,875,344 | 1,855,365 | 1,967,250 |
| Average Length of Stay | 5.0 | 5.1 | 5.1 | 5.1 | 5.3 |
| **Personnel** | | | | | |
| Total Full Time | 37,063 | 36,629 | 35,066 | 35,476 | 38,481 |
| Total Part Time | 11,998 | 11,717 | 11,549 | 10,979 | 10,282 |
| **Revenue and Expenses - Totals (Includes Inpatient and Outpatient)** | | | | | |
| Total Net Revenue | $4,072,785,097 | $3,850,828,585 | $3,427,559,010 | $3,241,028,997 | $3,048,845,221 |
| Total Expenses | 3,928,888,652 | 3,598,316,687 | 3,238,102,085 | 3,158,262,454 | 2,951,957,813 |
| **COMMUNITY HEALTH INDICATORS PER 1000 POPULATION** | | | | | |
| Total Population (in thousands) | 2,726 | 2,706 | 2,692 | 2,678 | 2,652 |
| **Inpatient** | | | | | |
| Beds | 3.6 | 3.7 | 3.5 | 3.7 | 3.8 |
| Admissions | 142.4 | 141.7 | 137.8 | 137.5 | 141.5 |
| Inpatient Days | 766.2 | 779.8 | 755.8 | 781.2 | 828.1 |
| Inpatient Surgeries | 43.0 | 44.1 | 40.6 | 41.5 | 39.3 |
| Births | 14.3 | 14.1 | 13.7 | 14.1 | 13.8 |
| **Outpatient** | | | | | |
| Emergency Outpatient Visits | 459.1 | 452.3 | 428.3 | 436.9 | 404.8 |
| Other Outpatient Visits | 1,222.1 | 1,335.6 | 1,241.0 | 1,208.6 | 1,086.9 |
| Total Outpatient Visits | 1,681.2 | 1,787.9 | 1,669.3 | 1,645.5 | 1,491.7 |
| Outpatient Surgeries | 55.6 | 58.9 | 56.3 | 57.8 | 58.3 |
| **Expense per Capita (per person)** | $1,448.1 | $1,334.8 | $1,207.2 | $1,186.0 | $1,120.9 |

# TABLE 6

# CALIFORNIA

*U.S. Registered Community Hospitals*
*(Nonfederal, short-term general and other special hospitals)*

## Overview 1999–2003

| | 2003 | 2002 | 2001 | 2000 | 1999 |
|---|---|---|---|---|---|
| **Total Community Hospitals in California** | **370** | **383** | **384** | **389** | **395** |
| **Bed Size Category** | | | | | |
| 6-24 | 9 | 10 | 10 | 14 | 16 |
| 25-49 | 42 | 47 | 39 | 38 | 38 |
| 50-99 | 63 | 63 | 67 | 72 | 74 |
| 100-199 | 105 | 114 | 121 | 123 | 121 |
| 200-299 | 74 | 74 | 74 | 73 | 76 |
| 300-399 | 41 | 38 | 38 | 40 | 40 |
| 400-499 | 16 | 20 | 24 | 17 | 18 |
| 500 + | 20 | 17 | 11 | 12 | 12 |
| **Location** | | | | | |
| Hospitals Urban | 330 | 343 | 344 | 348 | 354 |
| Hospitals Rural | 40 | 40 | 40 | 41 | 41 |
| **Control** | | | | | |
| State and Local Government | 71 | 74 | 75 | 71 | 73 |
| Not for Profit | 207 | 217 | 220 | 224 | 222 |
| Investor owned | 92 | 92 | 89 | 94 | 100 |
| **Physician Models** | | | | | |
| Independent Practice Association | 96 | 107 | 100 | 98 | 109 |
| Group Practice without Walls | 10 | 18 | 17 | 19 | 18 |
| Open Physician-Hospital Organization | 13 | 14 | 10 | 13 | 11 |
| Closed Physician-Hospital Organization | 9 | 11 | 17 | 20 | 18 |
| Management Service Organization | 37 | 43 | 39 | 48 | 60 |
| Integrated Salary Model | 24 | 35 | 27 | 30 | 35 |
| Equity Model | 0 | 1 | 1 | 0 | 3 |
| Foundation | 29 | 30 | 24 | 37 | 37 |
| **Insurance Products** | | | | | |
| Health Maintenance Organization | 51 | 50 | 40 | 50 | 64 |
| Preferred Provider Organization | 28 | 29 | 21 | 26 | 36 |
| Indemnity Fee for Service | 16 | 18 | 10 | 8 | 11 |
| **Managed Care Contracts** | | | | | |
| Health Maintenance Organization | 168 | 180 | 153 | 172 | 187 |
| Preferred Provider Organization | 174 | 184 | 155 | 170 | 185 |
| **Affiliations** | | | | | |
| Hospitals in a System* | 243 | 247 | 245 | 253 | 256 |
| Hospitals in a Network | 41 | 42 | 37 | 31 | 32 |
| Hospitals in a Group Purchasing Organization | 203 | 219 | 199 | 172 | 173 |

States

* Please note that system affiliate information for hospitals is derived from AHA membership. In years prior to 2003 the affiliation was derived from a question on the AHA Annual Survey of hospitals; therefore, non-responding hospitals were not included in the system affiliation counts. Years prior to 2003 have been updated to reflect this change, which now include affiliation for non-reporting hospitals.

# TABLE 6

# CALIFORNIA

*U.S. Registered Community Hospitals*
*(Nonfederal, short-term general and other special hospitals)*

## Utilization, Personnel, Revenue and Expenses, Community Health Indicators 1999–2003

| | 2003 | 2002 | 2001 | 2000 | 1999 |
|---|---|---|---|---|---|
| **TOTAL FACILITY (Includes Hospital and Nursing Home Units)** | | | | | |
| **Utilization - Inpatient** | | | | | |
| Beds | 74,330 | 74,343 | 73,291 | 72,707 | 73,672 |
| Admissions | 3,473,879 | 3,430,241 | 3,332,839 | 3,315,316 | 3,244,086 |
| Inpatient Days | 18,814,783 | 18,591,536 | 17,835,799 | 17,481,600 | 17,150,813 |
| Average Length of Stay | 5.4 | 5.4 | 5.4 | 5.3 | 5.3 |
| Inpatient Surgeries | 920,411 | 978,223 | 882,138 | 884,506 | 843,269 |
| Births | 492,547 | 475,383 | 493,383 | 528,444 | 480,910 |
| **Utilization - Outpatient** | | | | | |
| Emergency Outpatient Visits | 9,260,312 | 10,111,529 | 10,262,726 | 9,704,390 | 9,294,157 |
| Other Outpatient Visits | 38,775,827 | 43,221,919 | 38,284,808 | 35,240,037 | 35,484,904 |
| Total Outpatient Visits | 48,036,139 | 53,333,448 | 48,547,534 | 44,944,427 | 44,779,061 |
| Outpatient Surgeries | 1,252,323 | 1,342,641 | 1,270,674 | 1,331,626 | 1,181,547 |
| **Personnel** | | | | | |
| Full Time RNs | 73,628 | 74,071 | 69,584 | 63,988 | 65,955 |
| Full Time LPNs | 9,099 | 9,138 | 8,885 | 8,535 | 8,855 |
| Part Time RNs | 43,120 | 32,758 | 32,774 | 45,077 | 40,309 |
| Part Time LPNs | 3,811 | 2,607 | 3,008 | 4,430 | 3,840 |
| Total Full Time | 313,578 | 319,738 | 304,856 | 288,372 | 291,859 |
| Total Part Time | 117,232 | 92,674 | 97,102 | 133,503 | 115,347 |
| **Revenue - Inpatient** | | | | | |
| Gross Inpatient Revenue | $113,314,780,765 | $89,111,302,638 | $75,039,514,757 | $62,888,212,691 | $57,872,210,168 |
| **Revenue - Outpatient** | | | | | |
| Gross Outpatient Revenue | $42,148,908,089 | $34,457,820,473 | $29,444,438,788 | $26,342,290,083 | $22,979,554,909 |
| **Revenue and Expenses - Totals (Includes Inpatient and Outpatient)** | | | | | |
| Total Gross Revenue | $155,463,688,854 | $123,569,123,111 | $104,483,953,545 | $89,230,502,774 | $80,851,765,077 |
| Deductions from Revenue | 110,326,627,180 | 82,589,461,723 | 66,687,816,045 | 54,071,554,980 | 48,233,268,070 |
| Net Patient Revenue | 45,137,061,674 | 40,979,661,388 | 37,796,137,500 | 35,158,947,794 | 32,618,497,007 |
| Other Operating Revenue | 2,684,436,547 | 2,256,752,569 | 1,977,991,741 | 2,111,614,257 | 1,920,808,322 |
| Other Nonoperating Revenue | 1,172,015,105 | 1,114,663,017 | 1,133,993,257 | 931,691,027 | 1,113,488,295 |
| Total Net Revenue | 48,993,513,326 | 44,351,076,974 | 40,908,122,498 | 38,202,253,078 | 35,652,793,624 |
| Total Expenses | 46,910,735,231 | 42,504,560,362 | 39,559,376,603 | 37,075,150,430 | 34,970,489,094 |
| **HOSPITAL UNIT (Excludes Separate Nursing Home Units)** | | | | | |
| **Utilization - Inpatient** | | | | | |
| Beds | 68,069 | 67,012 | 67,949 | 69,021 | 69,254 |
| Admissions | 3,429,202 | 3,370,381 | 3,282,183 | 3,276,996 | 3,197,409 |
| Inpatient Days | 16,951,523 | 16,560,872 | 16,282,337 | 16,393,006 | 15,871,206 |
| Average Length of Stay | 4.9 | 4.9 | 5.0 | 5.0 | 5.0 |
| **Personnel** | | | | | |
| Total Full Time | 309,235 | 314,423 | 301,146 | 285,607 | 289,021 |
| Total Part Time | 115,650 | 91,515 | 95,942 | 132,111 | 114,039 |
| **Revenue and Expenses - Totals (Includes Inpatient and Outpatient)** | | | | | |
| Total Net Revenue | $48,316,168,890 | $43,726,173,992 | $40,457,487,441 | $37,843,321,779 | $35,260,844,072 |
| Total Expenses | 46,437,767,855 | 42,020,741,045 | 39,259,239,984 | 36,841,630,156 | 34,701,831,498 |
| **COMMUNITY HEALTH INDICATORS PER 1000 POPULATION** | | | | | |
| Total Population (in thousands) | 35,484 | 35,002 | 34,533 | 34,000 | 33,499 |
| **Inpatient** | | | | | |
| Beds | 2.1 | 2.1 | 2.1 | 2.1 | 2.2 |
| Admissions | 97.9 | 98.0 | 96.5 | 97.5 | 96.8 |
| Inpatient Days | 530.2 | 531.2 | 516.5 | 514.2 | 512.0 |
| Inpatient Surgeries | 25.9 | 27.9 | 25.5 | 26.0 | 25.2 |
| Births | 13.9 | 13.6 | 14.3 | 15.5 | 14.4 |
| **Outpatient** | | | | | |
| Emergency Outpatient Visits | 261.0 | 288.9 | 297.2 | 285.4 | 277.4 |
| Other Outpatient Visits | 1,092.8 | 1,234.8 | 1,108.6 | 1,036.5 | 1,059.3 |
| Total Outpatient Visits | 1,353.7 | 1,523.7 | 1,405.8 | 1,321.9 | 1,336.7 |
| Outpatient Surgeries | 35.3 | 38.4 | 36.8 | 39.2 | 35.3 |
| **Expense per Capita (per person)** | $1,322.0 | $1,214.3 | $1,145.6 | $1,090.4 | $1,043.9 |

# TABLE 6

# COLORADO

*U.S. Registered Community Hospitals*
*(Nonfederal, short-term general and other special hospitals)*

## Overview 1999–2003

| | 2003 | 2002 | 2001 | 2000 | 1999 |
|---|---|---|---|---|---|
| **Total Community Hospitals in Colorado** | **68** | **68** | **66** | **69** | **67** |
| **Bed Size Category** | | | | | |
| 6-24 | 7 | 7 | 7 | 9 | 8 |
| 25-49 | 17 | 17 | 16 | 17 | 16 |
| 50-99 | 17 | 16 | 16 | 16 | 16 |
| 100-199 | 7 | 8 | 8 | 8 | 9 |
| 200-299 | 8 | 9 | 7 | 8 | 6 |
| 300-399 | 7 | 8 | 8 | 6 | 8 |
| 400-499 | 5 | 3 | 3 | 5 | 4 |
| 500 + | 0 | 0 | 1 | 0 | 0 |
| **Location** | | | | | |
| Hospitals Urban | 32 | 32 | 31 | 32 | 32 |
| Hospitals Rural | 36 | 36 | 35 | 37 | 35 |
| **Control** | | | | | |
| State and Local Government | 27 | 27 | 26 | 28 | 27 |
| Not for Profit | 32 | 32 | 32 | 32 | 32 |
| Investor owned | 9 | 9 | 8 | 9 | 8 |
| **Physician Models** | | | | | |
| Independent Practice Association | 7 | 8 | 8 | 7 | 9 |
| Group Practice without Walls | 1 | 4 | 1 | 2 | 3 |
| Open Physician-Hospital Organization | 9 | 12 | 8 | 14 | 16 |
| Closed Physician-Hospital Organization | 3 | 5 | 3 | 8 | 4 |
| Management Service Organization | 5 | 7 | 6 | 7 | 7 |
| Integrated Salary Model | 20 | 22 | 18 | 16 | 17 |
| Equity Model | 0 | 2 | 0 | 1 | 1 |
| Foundation | 2 | 4 | 4 | 5 | 4 |
| **Insurance Products** | | | | | |
| Health Maintenance Organization | 7 | 7 | 8 | 11 | 11 |
| Preferred Provider Organization | 10 | 9 | 8 | 13 | 13 |
| Indemnity Fee for Service | 2 | 3 | 2 | 4 | 4 |
| **Managed Care Contracts** | | | | | |
| Health Maintenance Organization | 40 | 41 | 38 | 45 | 51 |
| Preferred Provider Organization | 40 | 41 | 39 | 46 | 48 |
| **Affiliations** | | | | | |
| Hospitals in a System* | 32 | 32 | 32 | 32 | 30 |
| Hospitals in a Network | 21 | 18 | 20 | 21 | 17 |
| Hospitals in a Group Purchasing Organization | 45 | 46 | 46 | 50 | 46 |

* Please note that system affiliate information for hospitals is derived from AHA membership. In years prior to 2003 the affiliation was derived from a question on the AHA Annual Survey of hospitals; therefore, non-responding hospitals were not included in the system affiliation counts. Years prior to 2003 have been updated to reflect this change, which now include affiliation for non-reporting hospitals.

# TABLE 6

## COLORADO

*U.S. Registered Community Hospitals*
*(Nonfederal, short-term general and other special hospitals)*

## Utilization, Personnel, Revenue and Expenses, Community Health Indicators 1999–2003

| | 2003 | 2002 | 2001 | 2000 | 1999 |
|---|---|---|---|---|---|
| **TOTAL FACILITY (Includes Hospital and Nursing Home Units)** | | | | | |
| **Utilization - Inpatient** | | | | | |
| Beds | 9,479 | 9,575 | 9,442 | 9,391 | 9,349 |
| Admissions | 443,773 | 426,560 | 413,605 | 397,026 | 383,283 |
| Inpatient Days | 2,252,174 | 2,172,074 | 2,111,549 | 1,986,526 | 1,947,693 |
| Average Length of Stay | 5.1 | 5.1 | 5.1 | 5.0 | 5.1 |
| Inpatient Surgeries | 128,846 | 129,569 | 124,570 | 125,630 | 121,742 |
| Births | 65,907 | 65,284 | 61,708 | 61,859 | 54,800 |
| **Utilization - Outpatient** | | | | | |
| Emergency Outpatient Visits | 1,384,544 | 1,501,013 | 1,380,740 | 1,377,130 | 1,324,504 |
| Other Outpatient Visits | 5,602,749 | 5,511,485 | 5,531,785 | 5,335,591 | 5,115,007 |
| Total Outpatient Visits | 6,987,293 | 7,012,498 | 6,912,525 | 6,712,721 | 6,439,511 |
| Outpatient Surgeries | 177,347 | 185,162 | 201,029 | 219,396 | 207,411 |
| **Personnel** | | | | | |
| Full Time RNs | 11,462 | 10,881 | 10,136 | 9,656 | 9,417 |
| Full Time LPNs | 865 | 960 | 824 | 694 | 820 |
| Part Time RNs | 4,694 | 4,522 | 4,179 | 4,346 | 4,221 |
| Part Time LPNs | 285 | 298 | 280 | 283 | 317 |
| Total Full Time | 46,172 | 44,913 | 43,027 | 39,556 | 39,830 |
| Total Part Time | 13,657 | 13,444 | 12,781 | 13,204 | 12,649 |
| **Revenue - Inpatient** | | | | | |
| Gross Inpatient Revenue | $9,509,561,663 | $8,494,295,044 | $7,227,257,609 | $5,902,881,921 | $5,465,908,323 |
| **Revenue - Outpatient** | | | | | |
| Gross Outpatient Revenue | $5,531,332,071 | $4,938,808,685 | $4,189,489,714 | $3,614,340,221 | $3,052,304,763 |
| **Revenue and Expenses - Totals (Includes Inpatient and Outpatient)** | | | | | |
| Total Gross Revenue | $15,040,893,734 | $13,433,103,729 | $11,416,747,323 | $9,517,222,142 | $8,518,213,086 |
| Deductions from Revenue | 8,988,839,107 | 7,638,320,935 | 6,439,372,017 | 4,994,563,358 | 4,429,949,594 |
| Net Patient Revenue | 6,052,054,627 | 5,794,782,794 | 4,977,375,306 | 4,522,658,784 | 4,088,263,492 |
| Other Operating Revenue | 379,770,612 | 250,396,757 | 479,100,659 | 321,544,924 | 244,779,945 |
| Other Nonoperating Revenue | 112,452,988 | 97,026,733 | 141,537,462 | 106,349,090 | 99,153,654 |
| Total Net Revenue | 6,544,278,227 | 6,142,206,284 | 5,598,013,427 | 4,950,552,798 | 4,432,197,091 |
| Total Expenses | 5,886,657,882 | 5,472,452,136 | 4,948,616,302 | 4,453,861,107 | 4,188,116,091 |
| **HOSPITAL UNIT (Excludes Separate Nursing Home Units)** | | | | | |
| **Utilization - Inpatient** | | | | | |
| Beds | 8,845 | 8,890 | 8,661 | 8,715 | 8,695 |
| Admissions | 441,220 | 423,839 | 410,743 | 394,223 | 379,249 |
| Inpatient Days | 2,063,902 | 1,966,328 | 1,867,438 | 1,767,350 | 1,749,055 |
| Average Length of Stay | 4.7 | 4.6 | 4.5 | 4.5 | 4.6 |
| **Personnel** | | | | | |
| Total Full Time | 45,730 | 44,448 | 42,445 | 39,056 | 39,356 |
| Total Part Time | 13,498 | 13,270 | 12,595 | 12,997 | 12,429 |
| **Revenue and Expenses - Totals (Includes Inpatient and Outpatient)** | | | | | |
| Total Net Revenue | $6,511,160,076 | $6,107,394,817 | $5,547,464,684 | $4,922,342,002 | $4,401,477,273 |
| Total Expenses | 5,854,637,695 | 5,440,791,541 | 4,910,277,563 | 4,425,039,103 | 4,161,145,943 |
| **COMMUNITY HEALTH INDICATORS PER 1000 POPULATION** | | | | | |
| Total Population (in thousands) | 4,551 | 4,501 | 4,429 | 4,327 | 4,226 |
| **Inpatient** | | | | | |
| Beds | 2.1 | 2.1 | 2.1 | 2.2 | 2.2 |
| Admissions | 97.5 | 94.8 | 93.4 | 91.8 | 90.7 |
| Inpatient Days | 494.9 | 482.6 | 476.8 | 459.1 | 460.9 |
| Inpatient Surgeries | 28.3 | 28.8 | 28.1 | 29.0 | 28.8 |
| Births | 14.5 | 14.5 | 13.9 | 14.3 | 13.0 |
| **Outpatient** | | | | | |
| Emergency Outpatient Visits | 304.2 | 333.5 | 311.8 | 318.3 | 313.4 |
| Other Outpatient Visits | 1,231.2 | 1,224.5 | 1,249.1 | 1,233.1 | 1,210.4 |
| Total Outpatient Visits | 1,535.4 | 1,558.0 | 1,560.8 | 1,551.4 | 1,523.8 |
| Outpatient Surgeries | 39.0 | 41.1 | 45.4 | 50.7 | 49.1 |
| **Expense per Capita (per person)** | $1,293.6 | $1,215.8 | $1,117.4 | $1,029.3 | $991.0 |

# TABLE 6

## CONNECTICUT

*U.S. Registered Community Hospitals*
*(Nonfederal, short-term general and other special hospitals)*

## Overview 1999–2003

| | 2003 | 2002 | 2001 | 2000 | 1999 |
|---|---|---|---|---|---|
| **Total Community Hospitals in Connecticut** | **34** | **35** | **35** | **35** | **35** |
| **Bed Size Category** | | | | | |
| 6-24 | 0 | 0 | 0 | 0 | 0 |
| 25-49 | 0 | 0 | 1 | 1 | 0 |
| 50-99 | 10 | 10 | 10 | 10 | 10 |
| 100-199 | 11 | 11 | 9 | 11 | 11 |
| 200-299 | 6 | 5 | 6 | 4 | 7 |
| 300-399 | 3 | 5 | 4 | 4 | 2 |
| 400-499 | 1 | 0 | 1 | 1 | 1 |
| 500 + | 3 | 4 | 4 | 4 | 4 |
| **Location** | | | | | |
| Hospitals Urban | 28 | 29 | 29 | 29 | 29 |
| Hospitals Rural | 6 | 6 | 6 | 6 | 6 |
| **Control** | | | | | |
| State and Local Government | 1 | 1 | 1 | 1 | 2 |
| Not for Profit | 32 | 34 | 34 | 33 | 33 |
| Investor owned | 1 | 0 | 0 | 1 | 0 |
| **Physician Models** | | | | | |
| Independent Practice Association | 10 | 10 | 12 | 12 | 15 |
| Group Practice without Walls | 1 | 1 | 2 | 3 | 5 |
| Open Physician-Hospital Organization | 12 | 13 | 13 | 14 | 17 |
| Closed Physician-Hospital Organization | 0 | 0 | 2 | 2 | 4 |
| Management Service Organization | 5 | 6 | 7 | 8 | 10 |
| Integrated Salary Model | 7 | 6 | 5 | 5 | 8 |
| Equity Model | 0 | 0 | 0 | 0 | 0 |
| Foundation | 1 | 0 | 2 | 2 | 1 |
| **Insurance Products** | | | | | |
| Health Maintenance Organization | 0 | 2 | 9 | 12 | 15 |
| Preferred Provider Organization | 6 | 5 | 7 | 7 | 7 |
| Indemnity Fee for Service | 0 | 0 | 0 | 0 | 0 |
| **Managed Care Contracts** | | | | | |
| Health Maintenance Organization | 26 | 25 | 28 | 32 | 32 |
| Preferred Provider Organization | 26 | 24 | 27 | 30 | 29 |
| **Affiliations** | | | | | |
| Hospitals in a System* | 7 | 7 | 7 | 4 | 4 |
| Hospitals in a Network | 10 | 10 | 11 | 15 | 12 |
| Hospitals in a Group Purchasing Organization | 29 | 27 | 29 | 32 | 31 |

States

* Please note that system affiliate information for hospitals is derived from AHA membership. In years prior to 2003 the affiliation was derived from a question on the AHA Annual Survey of hospitals; therefore, non-responding hospitals were not included in the system affiliation counts. Years prior to 2003 have been updated to reflect this change, which now include affiliation for non-reporting hospitals.

# TABLE 6

## CONNECTICUT

*U.S. Registered Community Hospitals*
*(Nonfederal, short-term general and other special hospitals)*

## Utilization, Personnel, Revenue and Expenses, Community Health Indicators 1999–2003

| | 2003 | 2002 | 2001 | 2000 | 1999 |
|---|---|---|---|---|---|
| **TOTAL FACILITY (Includes Hospital and Nursing Home Units)** | | | | | |
| **Utilization - Inpatient** | | | | | |
| Beds | 7,185 | 7,714 | 8,041 | 7,719 | 7,872 |
| Admissions | 372,630 | 375,686 | 360,007 | 348,780 | 337,821 |
| Inpatient Days | 2,029,059 | 2,239,055 | 2,184,918 | 2,114,362 | 2,070,480 |
| Average Length of Stay | 5.4 | 6.0 | 6.1 | 6.1 | 6.1 |
| Inpatient Surgeries | 110,964 | 108,975 | 102,924 | 101,548 | 105,211 |
| Births | 43,131 | 42,607 | 42,694 | 42,839 | 43,063 |
| **Utilization - Outpatient** | | | | | |
| Emergency Outpatient Visits | 1,372,015 | 1,392,274 | 1,328,651 | 1,323,999 | 1,344,816 |
| Other Outpatient Visits | 5,490,783 | 5,249,471 | 5,160,775 | 5,409,523 | 5,473,361 |
| Total Outpatient Visits | 6,862,798 | 6,641,745 | 6,489,426 | 6,733,522 | 6,818,177 |
| Outpatient Surgeries | 194,907 | 190,334 | 192,473 | 192,522 | 185,381 |
| **Personnel** | | | | | |
| Full Time RNs | 8,322 | 7,275 | 6,817 | 6,784 | 6,597 |
| Full Time LPNs | 375 | 403 | 323 | 360 | 331 |
| Part Time RNs | 6,679 | 6,952 | 6,866 | 5,413 | 5,727 |
| Part Time LPNs | 357 | 431 | 397 | 321 | 363 |
| Total Full Time | 37,725 | 36,424 | 35,996 | 34,079 | 33,264 |
| Total Part Time | 21,207 | 22,010 | 22,275 | 19,311 | 19,557 |
| **Revenue - Inpatient** | | | | | |
| Gross Inpatient Revenue | $6,887,232,102 | $6,057,484,644 | $5,235,105,389 | $4,793,838,712 | $4,607,260,826 |
| **Revenue - Outpatient** | | | | | |
| Gross Outpatient Revenue | $4,321,108,239 | $3,680,120,901 | $3,092,163,110 | $2,787,895,246 | $2,554,529,729 |
| **Revenue and Expenses - Totals (Includes Inpatient and Outpatient)** | | | | | |
| Total Gross Revenue | $11,208,340,341 | $9,737,605,545 | $8,327,268,499 | $7,581,733,958 | $7,161,790,555 |
| Deductions from Revenue | 5,855,457,310 | 4,688,468,374 | 3,787,142,271 | 3,417,644,028 | 3,082,461,893 |
| Net Patient Revenue | 5,352,883,031 | 5,049,137,171 | 4,540,126,228 | 4,164,089,930 | 4,079,328,662 |
| Other Operating Revenue | 206,489,799 | 190,947,384 | 187,046,158 | 180,038,222 | 235,827,532 |
| Other Nonoperating Revenue | 37,820,924 | 37,644,997 | 89,196,050 | 139,597,475 | 130,391,249 |
| Total Net Revenue | 5,597,193,754 | 5,277,729,552 | 4,816,368,436 | 4,483,725,627 | 4,445,547,443 |
| Total Expenses | 5,543,271,562 | 5,243,316,266 | 4,718,315,413 | 4,396,429,072 | 4,339,548,425 |
| **HOSPITAL UNIT (Excludes Separate Nursing Home Units)** | | | | | |
| **Utilization - Inpatient** | | | | | |
| Beds | 6,892 | 7,228 | 7,262 | 6,854 | 7,007 |
| Admissions | 371,894 | 374,638 | 358,242 | 347,414 | 336,878 |
| Inpatient Days | 1,909,689 | 2,036,015 | 1,863,319 | 1,795,186 | 1,781,174 |
| Average Length of Stay | 5.1 | 5.4 | 5.2 | 5.2 | 5.3 |
| **Personnel** | | | | | |
| Total Full Time | 37,176 | 36,321 | 35,093 | 33,092 | 32,782 |
| Total Part Time | 20,946 | 21,930 | 21,647 | 18,570 | 19,062 |
| **Revenue and Expenses - Totals (Includes Inpatient and Outpatient)** | | | | | |
| Total Net Revenue | $5,570,234,174 | $5,229,759,070 | $4,750,389,473 | $4,425,572,619 | $4,401,579,596 |
| Total Expenses | 5,518,804,682 | 5,183,998,846 | 4,644,731,988 | 4,334,999,636 | 4,295,663,582 |
| **COMMUNITY HEALTH INDICATORS PER 1000 POPULATION** | | | | | |
| Total Population (in thousands) | 3,483 | 3,459 | 3,433 | 3,412 | 3,386 |
| **Inpatient** | | | | | |
| Beds | 2.1 | 2.2 | 2.3 | 2.3 | 2.3 |
| Admissions | 107.0 | 108.6 | 104.9 | 102.2 | 99.8 |
| Inpatient Days | 582.5 | 647.4 | 636.5 | 619.7 | 611.4 |
| Inpatient Surgeries | 31.9 | 31.5 | 30.0 | 29.8 | 31.1 |
| Births | 12.4 | 12.3 | 12.4 | 12.6 | 12.7 |
| **Outpatient** | | | | | |
| Emergency Outpatient Visits | 393.9 | 402.6 | 387.1 | 388.1 | 397.1 |
| Other Outpatient Visits | 1,576.3 | 1,517.8 | 1,503.5 | 1,585.6 | 1,616.3 |
| Total Outpatient Visits | 1,970.2 | 1,920.4 | 1,890.6 | 1,973.6 | 2,013.4 |
| Outpatient Surgeries | 56.0 | 55.0 | 56.1 | 56.4 | 54.7 |
| **Expense per Capita (per person)** | $1,591.4 | $1,516.0 | $1,374.6 | $1,288.6 | $1,281.5 |

# TABLE 6

## DELAWARE

*U.S. Registered Community Hospitals*
*(Nonfederal, short-term general and other special hospitals)*

## Overview 1999–2003

| | 2003 | 2002 | 2001 | 2000 | 1999 |
|---|---|---|---|---|---|
| **Total Community Hospitals in Delaware** | **6** | **6** | **5** | **5** | **6** |
| **Bed Size Category** | | | | | |
| 6-24 | 0 | 0 | 0 | 0 | 0 |
| 25-49 | 0 | 0 | 0 | 0 | 0 |
| 50-99 | 0 | 0 | 0 | 0 | 0 |
| 100-199 | 2 | 2 | 1 | 0 | 1 |
| 200-299 | 2 | 2 | 2 | 3 | 3 |
| 300-399 | 1 | 1 | 1 | 1 | 1 |
| 400-499 | 0 | 0 | 0 | 0 | 0 |
| 500 + | 1 | 1 | 1 | 1 | 1 |
| **Location** | | | | | |
| Hospitals Urban | 4 | 4 | 3 | 3 | 4 |
| Hospitals Rural | 2 | 2 | 2 | 2 | 2 |
| **Control** | | | | | |
| State and Local Government | 0 | 0 | 0 | 0 | 0 |
| Not for Profit | 6 | 6 | 5 | 5 | 6 |
| Investor owned | 0 | 0 | 0 | 0 | 0 |
| **Physician Models** | | | | | |
| Independent Practice Association | 0 | 0 | 0 | 1 | 1 |
| Group Practice without Walls | 0 | 0 | 0 | 0 | 0 |
| Open Physician-Hospital Organization | 1 | 1 | 1 | 1 | 2 |
| Closed Physician-Hospital Organization | 0 | 0 | 0 | 1 | 1 |
| Management Service Organization | 0 | 0 | 0 | 0 | 0 |
| Integrated Salary Model | 4 | 4 | 2 | 3 | 2 |
| Equity Model | 0 | 0 | 0 | 0 | 0 |
| Foundation | 0 | 0 | 0 | 0 | 1 |
| **Insurance Products** | | | | | |
| Health Maintenance Organization | 2 | 1 | 1 | 1 | 1 |
| Preferred Provider Organization | 1 | 1 | 0 | 0 | 0 |
| Indemnity Fee for Service | 1 | 1 | 0 | 0 | 0 |
| **Managed Care Contracts** | | | | | |
| Health Maintenance Organization | 5 | 5 | 4 | 3 | 6 |
| Preferred Provider Organization | 5 | 5 | 4 | 3 | 6 |
| **Affiliations** | | | | | |
| Hospitals in a System* | 2 | 2 | 2 | 2 | 2 |
| Hospitals in a Network | 0 | 0 | 0 | 0 | 0 |
| Hospitals in a Group Purchasing Organization | 6 | 6 | 5 | 4 | 6 |

States

* Please note that system affiliate information for hospitals is derived from AHA membership. In years prior to 2003 the affiliation was derived from a question on the AHA Annual Survey of hospitals; therefore, non-responding hospitals were not included in the system affiliation counts. Years prior to 2003 have been updated to reflect this change, which now include affiliation for non-reporting hospitals.

# TABLE 6

# DELAWARE

*U.S. Registered Community Hospitals*
*(Nonfederal, short-term general and other special hospitals)*

## Utilization, Personnel, Revenue and Expenses, Community Health Indicators 1999–2003

| | 2003 | 2002 | 2001 | 2000 | 1999 |
|---|---|---|---|---|---|
| **TOTAL FACILITY (Includes Hospital and Nursing Home Units)** | | | | | |
| **Utilization - Inpatient** | | | | | |
| Beds | 2,051 | 2,014 | 1,853 | 1,839 | 2,000 |
| Admissions | 97,074 | 93,275 | 83,047 | 83,318 | 87,200 |
| Inpatient Days | 606,183 | 546,058 | 502,238 | 505,422 | 492,551 |
| Average Length of Stay | 6.2 | 5.9 | 6.0 | 6.1 | 5.6 |
| Inpatient Surgeries | 31,611 | 29,696 | 24,321 | 25,878 | 27,295 |
| Births | 11,837 | 11,350 | 11,286 | 11,375 | 10,896 |
| **Utilization - Outpatient** | | | | | |
| Emergency Outpatient Visits | 300,450 | 305,634 | 268,517 | 286,231 | 285,276 |
| Other Outpatient Visits | 1,721,410 | 1,642,184 | 1,216,401 | 1,175,657 | 1,062,037 |
| Total Outpatient Visits | 2,021,860 | 1,947,818 | 1,484,918 | 1,461,888 | 1,347,313 |
| Outpatient Surgeries | 62,989 | 66,987 | 57,342 | 52,972 | 66,234 |
| **Personnel** | | | | | |
| Full Time RNs | 2,170 | 2,609 | 2,058 | 2,179 | 2,455 |
| Full Time LPNs | 202 | 198 | 171 | 174 | 173 |
| Part Time RNs | 1,865 | 1,671 | 1,522 | 1,433 | 1,347 |
| Part Time LPNs | 145 | 86 | 77 | 74 | 84 |
| Total Full Time | 11,585 | 12,044 | 9,465 | 9,412 | 8,772 |
| Total Part Time | 5,771 | 4,759 | 3,936 | 3,798 | 3,933 |
| **Revenue - Inpatient** | | | | | |
| Gross Inpatient Revenue | $1,483,137,026 | $1,257,109,446 | $934,270,274 | $899,982,681 | $931,058,817 |
| **Revenue - Outpatient** | | | | | |
| Gross Outpatient Revenue | $840,915,945 | $697,074,088 | $543,554,090 | $465,864,889 | $474,399,061 |
| **Revenue and Expenses - Totals (Includes Inpatient and Outpatient)** | | | | | |
| Total Gross Revenue | $2,324,052,971 | $1,954,183,534 | $1,477,824,364 | $1,365,847,570 | $1,405,457,878 |
| Deductions from Revenue | 984,738,879 | 821,168,346 | 535,555,319 | 484,935,362 | 489,660,170 |
| Net Patient Revenue | 1,339,314,092 | 1,133,015,188 | 942,269,045 | 880,912,208 | 915,797,708 |
| Other Operating Revenue | 109,287,307 | 81,264,100 | 64,471,002 | 120,518,768 | 102,355,170 |
| Other Nonoperating Revenue | -21,627,318 | -14,105,872 | -6,015,492 | 39,475,261 | 43,155,449 |
| Total Net Revenue | 1,426,974,081 | 1,200,173,416 | 1,000,724,555 | 1,040,906,237 | 1,061,308,327 |
| Total Expenses | 1,444,199,303 | 1,201,883,266 | 1,049,014,326 | 1,020,468,822 | 990,513,404 |
| **HOSPITAL UNIT (Excludes Separate Nursing Home Units)** | | | | | |
| **Utilization - Inpatient** | | | | | |
| Beds | 1,723 | 1,686 | 1,561 | 1,561 | 1,786 |
| Admissions | 95,493 | 91,880 | 81,719 | 82,238 | 85,787 |
| Inpatient Days | 493,165 | 440,860 | 395,736 | 405,399 | 421,774 |
| Average Length of Stay | 5.2 | 4.8 | 4.8 | 4.9 | 4.9 |
| **Personnel** | | | | | |
| Total Full Time | 11,300 | 11,753 | 9,181 | 9,194 | 8,625 |
| Total Part Time | 5,676 | 4,630 | 3,806 | 3,736 | 3,846 |
| **Revenue and Expenses - Totals (Includes Inpatient and Outpatient)** | | | | | |
| Total Net Revenue | $1,406,722,580 | $1,174,652,121 | $978,200,536 | $1,003,754,485 | $1,042,456,545 |
| Total Expenses | 1,421,578,543 | 1,174,014,509 | 1,023,947,668 | 1,004,383,808 | 968,889,580 |
| **COMMUNITY HEALTH INDICATORS PER 1000 POPULATION** | | | | | |
| Total Population (in thousands) | 817 | 806 | 796 | 786 | 775 |
| **Inpatient** | | | | | |
| Beds | 2.5 | 2.5 | 2.3 | 2.3 | 2.6 |
| Admissions | 118.7 | 115.7 | 104.4 | 105.9 | 112.5 |
| Inpatient Days | 741.5 | 677.5 | 631.3 | 642.7 | 635.6 |
| Inpatient Surgeries | 38.7 | 36.8 | 30.6 | 32.9 | 35.2 |
| Births | 14.5 | 14.1 | 14.2 | 14.5 | 14.1 |
| **Outpatient** | | | | | |
| Emergency Outpatient Visits | 367.5 | 379.2 | 337.5 | 364.0 | 368.1 |
| Other Outpatient Visits | 2,105.7 | 2,037.6 | 1,529.0 | 1,495.0 | 1,370.4 |
| Total Outpatient Visits | 2,473.3 | 2,416.8 | 1,866.5 | 1,859.0 | 1,738.5 |
| Outpatient Surgeries | 77.1 | 83.1 | 72.1 | 67.4 | 85.5 |
| **Expense per Capita (per person)** | $1,766.6 | $1,491.3 | $1,318.6 | $1,297.7 | $1,278.1 |

# TABLE 6

# DISTRICT OF COLUMBIA

*U.S. Registered Community Hospitals*
*(Nonfederal, short-term general and other special hospitals)*

## Overview 1999–2003

| | 2003 | 2002 | 2001 | 2000 | 1999 |
|---|---|---|---|---|---|
| **Total Community Hospitals in District of Columbia** | **10** | **10** | **10** | **11** | **12** |
| **Bed Size Category** | | | | | |
| 6-24 | 0 | 0 | 0 | 0 | 0 |
| 25-49 | 0 | 0 | 0 | 0 | 0 |
| 50-99 | 0 | 0 | 0 | 1 | 1 |
| 100-199 | 3 | 3 | 3 | 3 | 3 |
| 200-299 | 2 | 1 | 2 | 3 | 4 |
| 300-399 | 3 | 4 | 3 | 2 | 2 |
| 400-499 | 0 | 0 | 0 | 0 | 0 |
| 500 + | 2 | 2 | 2 | 2 | 2 |
| **Location** | | | | | |
| Hospitals Urban | 10 | 10 | 10 | 11 | 12 |
| Hospitals Rural | 0 | 0 | 0 | 0 | 0 |
| **Control** | | | | | |
| State and Local Government | 0 | 0 | 0 | 0 | 1 |
| Not for Profit | 7 | 7 | 7 | 8 | 8 |
| Investor owned | 3 | 3 | 3 | 3 | 3 |
| **Physician Models** | | | | | |
| Independent Practice Association | 1 | 1 | 0 | 0 | 2 |
| Group Practice without Walls | 0 | 0 | 1 | 1 | 0 |
| Open Physician-Hospital Organization | 1 | 1 | 1 | 2 | 1 |
| Closed Physician-Hospital Organization | 1 | 2 | 2 | 2 | 3 |
| Management Service Organization | 1 | 1 | 1 | 2 | 3 |
| Integrated Salary Model | 4 | 4 | 5 | 4 | 5 |
| Equity Model | 0 | 0 | 0 | 0 | 0 |
| Foundation | 0 | 0 | 0 | 0 | 0 |
| **Insurance Products** | | | | | |
| Health Maintenance Organization | 5 | 3 | 4 | 4 | 5 |
| Preferred Provider Organization | 2 | 1 | 1 | 2 | 0 |
| Indemnity Fee for Service | 2 | 0 | 0 | 1 | 0 |
| **Managed Care Contracts** | | | | | |
| Health Maintenance Organization | 7 | 8 | 8 | 7 | 9 |
| Preferred Provider Organization | 7 | 6 | 7 | 7 | 6 |
| **Affiliations** | | | | | |
| Hospitals in a System* | 4 | 7 | 7 | 7 | 7 |
| Hospitals in a Network | 0 | 0 | 2 | 2 | 1 |
| Hospitals in a Group Purchasing Organization | 8 | 7 | 7 | 7 | 8 |

* Please note that system affiliate information for hospitals is derived from AHA membership. In years prior to 2003 the affiliation was derived from a question on the AHA Annual Survey of hospitals; therefore, non-responding hospitals were not included in the system affiliation counts. Years prior to 2003 have been updated to reflect this change, which now include affiliation for non-reporting hospitals.

## TABLE 6

# DISTRICT OF COLUMBIA

*U.S. Registered Community Hospitals*
*(Nonfederal, short-term general and other special hospitals)*

## Utilization, Personnel, Revenue and Expenses, Community Health Indicators 1999–2003

| | 2003 | 2002 | 2001 | 2000 | 1999 |
|---|---|---|---|---|---|
| **TOTAL FACILITY (Includes Hospital and Nursing Home Units)** | | | | | |
| **Utilization - Inpatient** | | | | | |
| Beds | 3,375 | 3,352 | 3,372 | 3,339 | 3,541 |
| Admissions | 134,685 | 137,172 | 131,906 | 129,056 | 138,408 |
| Inpatient Days | 905,107 | 936,124 | 903,469 | 901,167 | 984,094 |
| Average Length of Stay | 6.7 | 6.8 | 6.8 | 7.0 | 7.1 |
| Inpatient Surgeries | 44,062 | 43,815 | 42,789 | 58,333 | 61,982 |
| Births | 14,137 | 13,843 | 12,583 | 11,439 | 11,824 |
| **Utilization - Outpatient** | | | | | |
| Emergency Outpatient Visits | 359,624 | 352,942 | 337,851 | 284,075 | 330,143 |
| Other Outpatient Visits | 1,228,652 | 1,173,119 | 1,081,197 | 1,047,332 | 1,053,206 |
| Total Outpatient Visits | 1,588,276 | 1,526,061 | 1,419,048 | 1,331,407 | 1,383,349 |
| Outpatient Surgeries | 61,488 | 62,102 | 55,491 | 74,848 | 95,860 |
| **Personnel** | | | | | |
| Full Time RNs | 3,884 | 3,700 | 3,731 | 4,041 | 4,249 |
| Full Time LPNs | 242 | 285 | 261 | 286 | 324 |
| Part Time RNs | 1,620 | 1,835 | 1,695 | 1,908 | 1,328 |
| Part Time LPNs | 39 | 75 | 64 | 93 | 99 |
| Total Full Time | 18,110 | 18,939 | 18,187 | 18,519 | 17,209 |
| Total Part Time | 3,964 | 5,321 | 4,877 | 5,266 | 4,514 |
| **Revenue - Inpatient** | | | | | |
| Gross Inpatient Revenue | $3,523,798,623 | $3,403,763,454 | $3,109,126,002 | $2,730,685,206 | $2,761,995,772 |
| **Revenue - Outpatient** | | | | | |
| Gross Outpatient Revenue | $1,619,646,872 | $1,443,430,513 | $1,192,439,734 | $963,364,001 | $972,983,386 |
| **Revenue and Expenses - Totals (Includes Inpatient and Outpatient)** | | | | | |
| Total Gross Revenue | $5,143,445,495 | $4,847,193,967 | $4,301,565,736 | $3,694,049,207 | $3,734,979,158 |
| Deductions from Revenue | 2,928,873,497 | 2,709,835,364 | 2,344,359,123 | 1,987,583,335 | 2,036,092,141 |
| Net Patient Revenue | 2,214,571,998 | 2,137,358,603 | 1,957,206,613 | 1,706,465,872 | 1,698,887,017 |
| Other Operating Revenue | 170,762,223 | 153,122,453 | 151,214,377 | 111,158,200 | 144,298,148 |
| Other Nonoperating Revenue | 61,380,891 | -14,807,356 | 42,742,302 | 53,069,156 | 97,579,393 |
| Total Net Revenue | 2,446,715,112 | 2,275,673,700 | 2,151,163,292 | 1,870,693,228 | 1,940,764,558 |
| Total Expenses | 2,415,900,022 | 2,313,103,242 | 2,157,226,423 | 1,845,801,885 | 1,971,499,970 |
| **HOSPITAL UNIT (Excludes Separate Nursing Home Units)** | | | | | |
| **Utilization - Inpatient** | | | | | |
| Beds | 3,307 | 3,052 | 3,080 | 3,056 | 3,256 |
| Admissions | 133,262 | 135,377 | 130,307 | 127,615 | 136,998 |
| Inpatient Days | 886,341 | 833,747 | 804,586 | 803,418 | 880,583 |
| Average Length of Stay | 6.7 | 6.2 | 6.2 | 6.3 | 6.4 |
| **Personnel** | | | | | |
| Total Full Time | 18,054 | 18,654 | 17,880 | 18,235 | 16,977 |
| Total Part Time | 3,951 | 5,234 | 4,755 | 5,163 | 4,409 |
| **Revenue and Expenses - Totals (Includes Inpatient and Outpatient)** | | | | | |
| Total Net Revenue | $2,433,743,522 | $2,244,040,209 | $2,119,026,870 | $1,846,118,330 | $1,910,666,848 |
| Total Expenses | 2,405,630,003 | 2,282,999,519 | 2,130,816,375 | 1,824,373,545 | 1,946,444,149 |
| **COMMUNITY HEALTH INDICATORS PER 1000 POPULATION** | | | | | |
| Total Population (in thousands) | 563 | 569 | 573 | 571 | 570 |
| **Inpatient** | | | | | |
| Beds | 6.0 | 5.9 | 5.9 | 5.8 | 6.2 |
| Admissions | 239.1 | 241.0 | 230.3 | 225.8 | 242.7 |
| Inpatient Days | 1,606.6 | 1,644.8 | 1,577.5 | 1,577.0 | 1,725.8 |
| Inpatient Surgeries | 78.2 | 77.0 | 74.7 | 102.1 | 108.7 |
| Births | 25.1 | 24.3 | 22.0 | 20.0 | 20.7 |
| **Outpatient** | | | | | |
| Emergency Outpatient Visits | 638.3 | 620.1 | 589.9 | 497.1 | 579.0 |
| Other Outpatient Visits | 2,180.8 | 2,061.2 | 1,887.8 | 1,832.8 | 1,847.0 |
| Total Outpatient Visits | 2,819.2 | 2,681.3 | 2,477.8 | 2,329.9 | 2,426.0 |
| Outpatient Surgeries | 109.1 | 109.1 | 96.9 | 131.0 | 168.1 |
| **Expense per Capita (per person)** | $4,288.2 | $4,064.1 | $3,766.7 | $3,230.1 | $3,457.5 |

# TABLE 6

## FLORIDA

*U.S. Registered Community Hospitals*
*(Nonfederal, short-term general and other special hospitals)*

## Overview 1999–2003

| | 2003 | 2002 | 2001 | 2000 | 1999 |
|---|---|---|---|---|---|
| **Total Community Hospitals in Florida** | **203** | **202** | **202** | **202** | **203** |
| **Bed Size Category** | | | | | |
| 6-24 | 6 | 3 | 2 | 2 | 3 |
| 25-49 | 20 | 21 | 21 | 22 | 20 |
| 50-99 | 33 | 29 | 30 | 27 | 32 |
| 100-199 | 52 | 50 | 51 | 53 | 52 |
| 200-299 | 34 | 38 | 37 | 38 | 37 |
| 300-399 | 25 | 27 | 24 | 24 | 24 |
| 400-499 | 9 | 11 | 14 | 14 | 13 |
| 500 + | 24 | 23 | 23 | 22 | 22 |
| **Location** | | | | | |
| Hospitals Urban | 170 | 170 | 170 | 171 | 172 |
| Hospitals Rural | 33 | 32 | 32 | 31 | 31 |
| **Control** | | | | | |
| State and Local Government | 20 | 20 | 20 | 19 | 24 |
| Not for Profit | 88 | 86 | 87 | 88 | 86 |
| Investor owned | 95 | 96 | 95 | 95 | 93 |
| **Physician Models** | | | | | |
| Independent Practice Association | 13 | 9 | 22 | 22 | 21 |
| Group Practice without Walls | 3 | 2 | 6 | 7 | 7 |
| Open Physician-Hospital Organization | 15 | 16 | 20 | 24 | 23 |
| Closed Physician-Hospital Organization | 10 | 7 | 7 | 13 | 18 |
| Management Service Organization | 13 | 13 | 16 | 27 | 30 |
| Integrated Salary Model | 28 | 27 | 30 | 29 | 31 |
| Equity Model | 1 | 1 | 1 | 2 | 3 |
| Foundation | 1 | 1 | 1 | 2 | 4 |
| **Insurance Products** | | | | | |
| Health Maintenance Organization | 17 | 16 | 20 | 25 | 30 |
| Preferred Provider Organization | 18 | 17 | 19 | 22 | 34 |
| Indemnity Fee for Service | 9 | 8 | 8 | 10 | 3 |
| **Managed Care Contracts** | | | | | |
| Health Maintenance Organization | 100 | 93 | 90 | 94 | 97 |
| Preferred Provider Organization | 104 | 98 | 97 | 96 | 96 |
| **Affiliations** | | | | | |
| Hospitals in a System* | 153 | 153 | 147 | 148 | 149 |
| Hospitals in a Network | 36 | 36 | 31 | 31 | 38 |
| Hospitals in a Group Purchasing Organization | 116 | 110 | 98 | 93 | 89 |

States

* Please note that system affiliate information for hospitals is derived from AHA membership. In years prior to 2003 the affiliation was derived from a question on the AHA Annual Survey of hospitals; therefore, non-responding hospitals were not included in the system affiliation counts. Years prior to 2003 have been updated to reflect this change, which now include affiliation for non-reporting hospitals.

# Table 6 FLORIDA

*U.S. Registered Community Hospitals*
*(Nonfederal, short-term general and other special hospitals)*

## Utilization, Personnel, Revenue and Expenses, Community Health Indicators 1999–2003

| | 2003 | 2002 | 2001 | 2000 | 1999 |
|---|---|---|---|---|---|
| **TOTAL FACILITY (Includes Hospital and Nursing Home Units)** | | | | | |
| **Utilization - Inpatient** | | | | | |
| Beds | 50,687 | 51,201 | 51,762 | 51,170 | 49,434 |
| Admissions | 2,296,184 | 2,315,230 | 2,207,147 | 2,119,052 | 2,020,073 |
| Inpatient Days | 11,966,726 | 12,303,559 | 11,521,025 | 11,345,469 | 11,135,544 |
| Average Length of Stay | 5.2 | 5.3 | 5.2 | 5.4 | 5.5 |
| Inpatient Surgeries | 642,112 | 688,383 | 660,330 | 614,345 | 570,283 |
| Births | 197,538 | 208,996 | 204,753 | 193,344 | 180,857 |
| **Utilization - Outpatient** | | | | | |
| Emergency Outpatient Visits | 6,668,184 | 6,623,448 | 5,879,596 | 6,041,546 | 5,488,609 |
| Other Outpatient Visits | 15,355,370 | 15,866,843 | 14,891,198 | 15,752,042 | 14,210,881 |
| Total Outpatient Visits | 22,023,554 | 22,490,291 | 20,770,794 | 21,793,588 | 19,699,490 |
| Outpatient Surgeries | 833,259 | 912,233 | 857,272 | 816,677 | 803,554 |
| **Personnel** | | | | | |
| Full Time RNs | 51,591 | 49,218 | 48,277 | 47,635 | 45,140 |
| Full Time LPNs | 5,881 | 6,111 | 6,224 | 6,258 | 6,898 |
| Part Time RNs | 16,601 | 16,534 | 14,235 | 17,432 | 15,741 |
| Part Time LPNs | 1,622 | 1,615 | 1,550 | 1,799 | 1,894 |
| Total Full Time | 200,516 | 203,256 | 198,925 | 193,653 | 186,175 |
| Total Part Time | 51,128 | 49,095 | 40,983 | 52,267 | 48,474 |
| **Revenue - Inpatient** | | | | | |
| Gross Inpatient Revenue | $51,343,112,371 | $46,105,920,999 | $38,526,016,053 | $36,166,618,934 | $30,772,909,076 |
| **Revenue - Outpatient** | | | | | |
| Gross Outpatient Revenue | $24,147,744,686 | $21,541,764,183 | $17,579,375,385 | $16,339,412,601 | $14,207,698,162 |
| **Revenue and Expenses - Totals (Includes Inpatient and Outpatient)** | | | | | |
| Total Gross Revenue | $75,490,857,057 | $67,647,685,182 | $56,105,391,438 | $52,506,031,535 | $44,980,607,238 |
| Deductions from Revenue | 50,847,577,350 | 44,385,926,589 | 35,545,733,610 | 33,270,201,252 | 27,234,827,859 |
| Net Patient Revenue | 24,643,279,707 | 23,261,758,593 | 20,559,657,828 | 19,235,830,283 | 17,745,779,379 |
| Other Operating Revenue | 1,325,328,179 | 1,443,094,405 | 1,232,856,710 | 1,060,248,158 | 993,711,653 |
| Other Nonoperating Revenue | 324,632,193 | 113,856,010 | 287,972,889 | 516,162,789 | 438,224,356 |
| Total Net Revenue | 26,293,240,079 | 24,818,709,008 | 22,080,487,427 | 20,812,241,230 | 19,177,715,388 |
| Total Expenses | 24,774,272,657 | 23,194,124,932 | 20,475,866,330 | 19,289,627,098 | 17,522,447,345 |
| **HOSPITAL UNIT (Excludes Separate Nursing Home Units)** | | | | | |
| **Utilization - Inpatient** | | | | | |
| Beds | 49,515 | 49,786 | 49,865 | 48,979 | 47,342 |
| Admissions | 2,289,785 | 2,304,044 | 2,193,104 | 2,098,216 | 1,999,574 |
| Inpatient Days | 11,583,859 | 11,864,811 | 10,918,750 | 10,688,767 | 10,464,347 |
| Average Length of Stay | 5.1 | 5.1 | 5.0 | 5.1 | 5.2 |
| **Personnel** | | | | | |
| Total Full Time | 199,135 | 201,890 | 197,587 | 191,191 | 183,992 |
| Total Part Time | 50,822 | 48,872 | 40,716 | 51,396 | 47,889 |
| **Revenue and Expenses - Totals (Includes Inpatient and Outpatient)** | | | | | |
| Total Net Revenue | $25,984,400,882 | $24,696,657,727 | $21,928,434,635 | $20,649,613,293 | $18,999,058,161 |
| Total Expenses | 24,455,800,098 | 23,082,690,334 | 20,345,809,450 | 19,160,212,008 | 17,374,197,783 |
| **COMMUNITY HEALTH INDICATORS PER 1000 POPULATION** | | | | | |
| Total Population (in thousands) | 17,019 | 16,692 | 16,355 | 16,048 | 15,759 |
| **Inpatient** | | | | | |
| Beds | 3.0 | 3.1 | 3.2 | 3.2 | 3.1 |
| Admissions | 134.9 | 138.7 | 135.0 | 132.0 | 128.2 |
| Inpatient Days | 703.1 | 737.1 | 704.4 | 707.0 | 706.6 |
| Inpatient Surgeries | 37.7 | 41.2 | 40.4 | 38.3 | 36.2 |
| Births | 11.6 | 12.5 | 12.5 | 12.0 | 11.5 |
| **Outpatient** | | | | | |
| Emergency Outpatient Visits | 391.8 | 396.8 | 359.5 | 376.5 | 348.3 |
| Other Outpatient Visits | 902.2 | 950.6 | 910.5 | 981.6 | 901.7 |
| Total Outpatient Visits | 1,294.1 | 1,347.4 | 1,270.0 | 1,358.0 | 1,250.0 |
| Outpatient Surgeries | 49.0 | 54.7 | 52.4 | 50.9 | 51.0 |
| **Expense per Capita (per person)** | $1,455.7 | $1,389.6 | $1,251.9 | $1,202.0 | $1,111.9 |

# TABLE 6

# GEORGIA

*U.S. Registered Community Hospitals*
*(Nonfederal, short-term general and other special hospitals)*

## Overview 1999–2003

| | 2003 | 2002 | 2001 | 2000 | 1999 |
|---|---|---|---|---|---|
| **Total Community Hospitals in Georgia** | **146** | **146** | **147** | **151** | **154** |
| **Bed Size Category** | | | | | |
| 6-24 | 6 | 7 | 4 | 5 | 4 |
| 25-49 | 30 | 30 | 34 | 36 | 36 |
| 50-99 | 25 | 25 | 28 | 28 | 23 |
| 100-199 | 43 | 42 | 42 | 43 | 51 |
| 200-299 | 15 | 15 | 13 | 14 | 14 |
| 300-399 | 11 | 12 | 10 | 11 | 14 |
| 400-499 | 11 | 10 | 9 | 9 | 9 |
| 500 + | 5 | 5 | 7 | 5 | 3 |
| **Location** | | | | | |
| Hospitals Urban | 63 | 63 | 64 | 67 | 68 |
| Hospitals Rural | 83 | 83 | 83 | 84 | 86 |
| **Control** | | | | | |
| State and Local Government | 54 | 52 | 53 | 56 | 55 |
| Not for Profit | 62 | 64 | 62 | 62 | 63 |
| Investor owned | 30 | 30 | 32 | 33 | 36 |
| **Physician Models** | | | | | |
| Independent Practice Association | 14 | 15 | 16 | 18 | 16 |
| Group Practice without Walls | 3 | 1 | 2 | 4 | 2 |
| Open Physician-Hospital Organization | 26 | 22 | 22 | 21 | 21 |
| Closed Physician-Hospital Organization | 15 | 18 | 24 | 25 | 16 |
| Management Service Organization | 11 | 14 | 17 | 17 | 15 |
| Integrated Salary Model | 25 | 25 | 18 | 26 | 14 |
| Equity Model | 1 | 2 | 2 | 2 | 1 |
| Foundation | 4 | 5 | 4 | 4 | 3 |
| **Insurance Products** | | | | | |
| Health Maintenance Organization | 11 | 9 | 14 | 16 | 20 |
| Preferred Provider Organization | 38 | 39 | 41 | 36 | 43 |
| Indemnity Fee for Service | 6 | 9 | 10 | 9 | 8 |
| **Managed Care Contracts** | | | | | |
| Health Maintenance Organization | 63 | 56 | 58 | 65 | 60 |
| Preferred Provider Organization | 105 | 99 | 98 | 103 | 111 |
| **Affiliations** | | | | | |
| Hospitals in a System* | 61 | 65 | 66 | 69 | 72 |
| Hospitals in a Network | 57 | 62 | 69 | 61 | 58 |
| Hospitals in a Group Purchasing Organization | 111 | 103 | 109 | 103 | 98 |

* Please note that system affiliate information for hospitals is derived from AHA membership. In years prior to 2003 the affiliation was derived from a question on the AHA Annual Survey of hospitals; therefore, non-responding hospitals were not included in the system affiliation counts. Years prior to 2003 have been updated to reflect this change, which now include affiliation for non-reporting hospitals.

# TABLE 6

# GEORGIA

*U.S. Registered Community Hospitals*
*(Nonfederal, short-term general and other special hospitals)*

## Utilization, Personnel, Revenue and Expenses, Community Health Indicators 1999–2003

| | 2003 | 2002 | 2001 | 2000 | 1999 |
|---|---|---|---|---|---|
| **TOTAL FACILITY (Includes Hospital and Nursing Home Units)** | | | | | |
| **Utilization - Inpatient** | | | | | |
| Beds | 24,624 | 24,500 | 24,113 | 23,875 | 24,784 |
| Admissions | 925,681 | 885,142 | 903,663 | 862,797 | 824,376 |
| Inpatient Days | 6,024,083 | 5,774,911 | 5,484,805 | 5,479,389 | 5,625,261 |
| Average Length of Stay | 6.5 | 6.5 | 6.1 | 6.4 | 6.8 |
| Inpatient Surgeries | 276,917 | 288,573 | 284,283 | 257,624 | 257,164 |
| Births | 133,692 | 128,981 | 130,673 | 129,084 | 113,784 |
| **Utilization - Outpatient** | | | | | |
| Emergency Outpatient Visits | 3,542,261 | 3,227,698 | 3,149,115 | 3,128,275 | 2,854,136 |
| Other Outpatient Visits | 9,307,084 | 9,256,245 | 8,865,939 | 8,113,649 | 7,984,774 |
| Total Outpatient Visits | 12,849,345 | 12,483,943 | 12,015,054 | 11,241,924 | 10,838,910 |
| Outpatient Surgeries | 507,592 | 511,906 | 497,614 | 459,852 | 429,526 |
| **Personnel** | | | | | |
| Full Time RNs | 23,431 | 22,730 | 21,881 | 22,259 | 20,681 |
| Full Time LPNs | 4,053 | 4,063 | 3,888 | 3,466 | 3,854 |
| Part Time RNs | 11,974 | 12,269 | 12,896 | 11,977 | 8,977 |
| Part Time LPNs | 1,277 | 1,189 | 1,224 | 1,147 | 1,147 |
| Total Full Time | 100,288 | 98,246 | 95,397 | 92,094 | 90,711 |
| Total Part Time | 31,452 | 32,518 | 34,238 | 32,304 | 27,457 |
| **Revenue - Inpatient** | | | | | |
| Gross Inpatient Revenue | $16,113,698,381 | $14,445,750,952 | $12,699,629,255 | $11,757,965,146 | $10,148,108,959 |
| **Revenue - Outpatient** | | | | | |
| Gross Outpatient Revenue | $10,259,708,558 | $9,240,551,617 | $7,748,463,309 | $7,353,248,681 | $5,911,411,142 |
| **Revenue and Expenses - Totals (Includes Inpatient and Outpatient)** | | | | | |
| Total Gross Revenue | $26,373,406,939 | $23,686,302,569 | $20,448,092,564 | $19,111,213,827 | $16,059,520,101 |
| Deductions from Revenue | 15,113,531,785 | 13,112,710,432 | 10,910,867,874 | 9,922,910,066 | 7,822,591,409 |
| Net Patient Revenue | 11,259,875,154 | 10,573,592,137 | 9,537,224,690 | 9,188,303,761 | 8,236,928,692 |
| Other Operating Revenue | 634,628,403 | 553,755,731 | 582,210,731 | 496,378,760 | 632,168,142 |
| Other Nonoperating Revenue | 227,288,500 | 29,263,979 | 247,374,354 | 242,231,703 | 227,205,059 |
| Total Net Revenue | 12,121,792,057 | 11,156,611,847 | 10,366,809,775 | 9,926,914,224 | 9,096,301,893 |
| Total Expenses | 11,386,865,460 | 10,576,054,877 | 9,839,984,105 | 9,217,250,307 | 8,225,718,150 |
| **HOSPITAL UNIT (Excludes Separate Nursing Home Units)** | | | | | |
| **Utilization - Inpatient** | | | | | |
| Beds | 19,969 | 20,655 | 20,813 | 20,138 | 20,540 |
| Admissions | 918,417 | 880,499 | 898,539 | 856,482 | 816,709 |
| Inpatient Days | 4,426,838 | 4,466,878 | 4,396,989 | 4,184,817 | 4,200,321 |
| Average Length of Stay | 4.8 | 5.1 | 4.9 | 4.9 | 5.1 |
| **Personnel** | | | | | |
| Total Full Time | 96,825 | 95,471 | 93,155 | 89,656 | 88,053 |
| Total Part Time | 30,446 | 31,711 | 33,610 | 31,527 | 26,714 |
| **Revenue and Expenses - Totals (Includes Inpatient and Outpatient)** | | | | | |
| Total Net Revenue | $11,896,757,187 | $11,012,776,470 | $10,228,892,959 | $9,802,309,486 | $8,956,729,154 |
| Total Expenses | 11,201,806,143 | 10,446,159,150 | 9,716,646,918 | 9,104,562,407 | 8,091,415,980 |
| **COMMUNITY HEALTH INDICATORS PER 1000 POPULATION** | | | | | |
| Total Population (in thousands) | 8,685 | 8,544 | 8,395 | 8,230 | 8,046 |
| **Inpatient** | | | | | |
| Beds | 2.8 | 2.9 | 2.9 | 2.9 | 3.1 |
| Admissions | 106.6 | 103.6 | 107.6 | 104.8 | 102.5 |
| Inpatient Days | 693.6 | 675.9 | 653.4 | 665.8 | 699.1 |
| Inpatient Surgeries | 31.9 | 33.8 | 33.9 | 31.3 | 32.0 |
| Births | 15.4 | 15.1 | 15.6 | 15.7 | 14.1 |
| **Outpatient** | | | | | |
| Emergency Outpatient Visits | 407.9 | 377.8 | 375.1 | 380.1 | 354.7 |
| Other Outpatient Visits | 1,071.7 | 1,083.4 | 1,056.1 | 985.9 | 992.4 |
| Total Outpatient Visits | 1,479.5 | 1,461.1 | 1,431.3 | 1,366.0 | 1,347.1 |
| Outpatient Surgeries | 58.4 | 59.9 | 59.3 | 55.9 | 53.4 |
| **Expense per Capita (per person)** | $1,311.1 | $1,237.8 | $1,172.2 | $1,119.9 | $1,022.3 |

# TABLE 6

## HAWAII

*U.S. Registered Community Hospitals*
*(Nonfederal, short-term general and other special hospitals)*

## Overview 1999–2003

| | 2003 | 2002 | 2001 | 2000 | 1999 |
|---|---|---|---|---|---|
| **Total Community Hospitals in Hawaii** | **24** | **25** | **23** | **21** | **22** |
| **Bed Size Category** | | | | | |
| 6-24 | 3 | 3 | 2 | 2 | 2 |
| 25-49 | 5 | 5 | 4 | 3 | 4 |
| 50-99 | 2 | 3 | 4 | 3 | 3 |
| 100-199 | 9 | 9 | 8 | 8 | 10 |
| 200-299 | 4 | 4 | 4 | 4 | 2 |
| 300-399 | 0 | 0 | 0 | 0 | 0 |
| 400-499 | 1 | 1 | 1 | 1 | 1 |
| 500 + | 0 | 0 | 0 | 0 | 0 |
| **Location** | | | | | |
| Hospitals Urban | 13 | 13 | 13 | 12 | 12 |
| Hospitals Rural | 11 | 12 | 10 | 9 | 10 |
| **Control** | | | | | |
| State and Local Government | 6 | 7 | 8 | 7 | 8 |
| Not for Profit | 18 | 18 | 14 | 13 | 13 |
| Investor owned | 0 | 0 | 1 | 1 | 1 |
| **Physician Models** | | | | | |
| Independent Practice Association | 4 | 3 | 4 | 6 | 5 |
| Group Practice without Walls | 0 | 0 | 0 | 0 | 1 |
| Open Physician-Hospital Organization | 1 | 1 | 3 | 4 | 5 |
| Closed Physician-Hospital Organization | 1 | 1 | 0 | 0 | 0 |
| Management Service Organization | 0 | 0 | 0 | 0 | 1 |
| Integrated Salary Model | 3 | 3 | 2 | 2 | 2 |
| Equity Model | 0 | 0 | 0 | 0 | 1 |
| Foundation | 1 | 1 | 1 | 1 | 1 |
| **Insurance Products** | | | | | |
| Health Maintenance Organization | 3 | 3 | 3 | 3 | 6 |
| Preferred Provider Organization | 2 | 1 | 2 | 2 | 5 |
| Indemnity Fee for Service | 1 | 0 | 1 | 1 | 1 |
| **Managed Care Contracts** | | | | | |
| Health Maintenance Organization | 9 | 13 | 11 | 11 | 14 |
| Preferred Provider Organization | 6 | 9 | 9 | 7 | 10 |
| **Affiliations** | | | | | |
| Hospitals in a System* | 19 | 21 | 19 | 15 | 16 |
| Hospitals in a Network | 1 | 1 | 2 | 3 | 2 |
| Hospitals in a Group Purchasing Organization | 11 | 14 | 16 | 14 | 14 |

States

* Please note that system affiliate information for hospitals is derived from AHA membership. In years prior to 2003 the affiliation was derived from a question on the AHA Annual Survey of hospitals; therefore, non-responding hospitals were not included in the system affiliation counts. Years prior to 2003 have been updated to reflect this change, which now include affiliation for non-reporting hospitals.

# HAWAII

*U.S. Registered Community Hospitals*
*(Nonfederal, short-term general and other special hospitals)*

## Utilization, Personnel, Revenue and Expenses, Community Health Indicators 1999–2003

| | 2003 | 2002 | 2001 | 2000 | 1999 |
|---|---|---|---|---|---|
| **TOTAL FACILITY (Includes Hospital and Nursing Home Units)** | | | | | |
| **Utilization - Inpatient** | | | | | |
| Beds | 3,121 | 3,191 | 3,235 | 3,057 | 2,913 |
| Admissions | 111,713 | 111,498 | 108,252 | 99,937 | 99,191 |
| Inpatient Days | 815,796 | 866,160 | 879,258 | 847,352 | 769,824 |
| Average Length of Stay | 7.3 | 7.8 | 8.1 | 8.5 | 7.8 |
| Inpatient Surgeries | 31,628 | 32,059 | 31,003 | 28,912 | 30,001 |
| Births | 12,476 | 15,845 | 10,007 | 9,903 | 10,148 |
| **Utilization - Outpatient** | | | | | |
| Emergency Outpatient Visits | 330,034 | 311,713 | 287,017 | 253,452 | 239,560 |
| Other Outpatient Visits | 1,587,707 | 1,652,619 | 2,880,570 | 2,212,552 | 2,197,092 |
| Total Outpatient Visits | 1,917,741 | 1,964,332 | 3,167,587 | 2,466,004 | 2,436,652 |
| Outpatient Surgeries | 55,107 | 52,498 | 52,624 | 46,250 | 45,328 |
| **Personnel** | | | | | |
| Full Time RNs | 3,405 | 3,328 | 2,727 | 3,002 | 2,738 |
| Full Time LPNs | 435 | 410 | 420 | 395 | 423 |
| Part Time RNs | 1,066 | 1,353 | 1,409 | 968 | 1,053 |
| Part Time LPNs | 101 | 112 | 138 | 93 | 81 |
| Total Full Time | 13,866 | 13,264 | 12,621 | 11,854 | 11,697 |
| Total Part Time | 3,092 | 3,791 | 3,953 | 3,051 | 2,978 |
| **Revenue - Inpatient** | | | | | |
| Gross Inpatient Revenue | $2,234,373,694 | $2,089,877,140 | $1,932,544,979 | $1,803,657,551 | $1,649,885,281 |
| **Revenue - Outpatient** | | | | | |
| Gross Outpatient Revenue | $1,428,134,717 | $1,175,498,990 | $1,063,359,978 | $826,991,000 | $730,624,505 |
| **Revenue and Expenses - Totals (Includes Inpatient and Outpatient)** | | | | | |
| Total Gross Revenue | $3,662,508,411 | $3,265,376,130 | $2,995,904,957 | $2,630,648,551 | $2,380,509,786 |
| Deductions from Revenue | 2,047,040,507 | 1,773,759,884 | 1,574,104,007 | 1,382,408,955 | 1,199,936,747 |
| Net Patient Revenue | 1,615,467,904 | 1,491,616,246 | 1,421,800,950 | 1,248,239,596 | 1,180,573,039 |
| Other Operating Revenue | 100,988,680 | 87,285,962 | 82,464,076 | 70,164,871 | 74,945,697 |
| Other Nonoperating Revenue | 24,424,255 | -1,274,071 | 30,318,193 | 33,274,738 | 28,166,307 |
| Total Net Revenue | 1,740,880,839 | 1,577,628,137 | 1,534,583,219 | 1,351,679,205 | 1,283,685,043 |
| Total Expenses | 1,783,815,570 | 1,640,541,613 | 1,587,146,492 | 1,360,759,208 | 1,273,162,963 |
| **HOSPITAL UNIT (Excludes Separate Nursing Home Units)** | | | | | |
| **Utilization - Inpatient** | | | | | |
| Beds | 2,687 | 2,766 | 2,704 | 2,511 | 2,386 |
| Admissions | 109,814 | 109,535 | 106,717 | 97,822 | 96,915 |
| Inpatient Days | 670,099 | 730,123 | 704,963 | 676,735 | 594,519 |
| Average Length of Stay | 6.1 | 6.7 | 6.6 | 6.9 | 6.1 |
| **Personnel** | | | | | |
| Total Full Time | 13,455 | 13,053 | 12,228 | 11,517 | 11,299 |
| Total Part Time | 3,033 | 3,758 | 3,889 | 2,992 | 2,885 |
| **Revenue and Expenses - Totals (Includes Inpatient and Outpatient)** | | | | | |
| Total Net Revenue | $1,709,471,083 | $1,555,292,196 | $1,513,078,577 | $1,331,297,637 | $1,255,628,493 |
| Total Expenses | 1,750,929,948 | 1,615,200,267 | 1,567,775,123 | 1,342,654,703 | 1,246,855,789 |
| **COMMUNITY HEALTH INDICATORS PER 1000 POPULATION** | | | | | |
| Total Population (in thousands) | 1,258 | 1,241 | 1,225 | 1,212 | 1,210 |
| **Inpatient** | | | | | |
| Beds | 2.5 | 2.6 | 2.6 | 2.5 | 2.4 |
| Admissions | 88.8 | 89.9 | 88.4 | 82.4 | 82.0 |
| Inpatient Days | 648.7 | 698.1 | 717.7 | 698.9 | 636.1 |
| Inpatient Surgeries | 25.1 | 25.8 | 25.3 | 23.8 | 24.8 |
| Births | 9.9 | 12.8 | 8.2 | 8.2 | 8.4 |
| **Outpatient** | | | | | |
| Emergency Outpatient Visits | 262.4 | 251.2 | 234.3 | 209.1 | 197.9 |
| Other Outpatient Visits | 1,262.5 | 1,332.0 | 2,351.4 | 1,825.0 | 1,815.3 |
| Total Outpatient Visits | 1,524.9 | 1,583.3 | 2,585.7 | 2,034.1 | 2,013.3 |
| Outpatient Surgeries | 43.8 | 42.3 | 43.0 | 38.1 | 37.5 |
| **Expense per Capita (per person)** | $1,418.4 | $1,322.3 | $1,295.6 | $1,122.4 | $1,051.9 |

## TABLE 6

# IDAHO

*U.S. Registered Community Hospitals*
*(Nonfederal, short-term general and other special hospitals)*

## Overview 1999–2003

| | 2003 | 2002 | 2001 | 2000 | 1999 |
|---|---|---|---|---|---|
| **Total Community Hospitals in Idaho** | **39** | **39** | **40** | **42** | **42** |
| **Bed Size Category** | | | | | |
| 6-24 | 11 | 11 | 9 | 8 | 8 |
| 25-49 | 8 | 8 | 8 | 11 | 10 |
| 50-99 | 10 | 9 | 12 | 12 | 13 |
| 100-199 | 4 | 6 | 6 | 6 | 6 |
| 200-299 | 3 | 3 | 3 | 3 | 4 |
| 300-399 | 2 | 1 | 2 | 2 | 1 |
| 400-499 | 1 | 1 | 0 | 0 | 0 |
| 500 + | 0 | 0 | 0 | 0 | 0 |
| **Location** | | | | | |
| Hospitals Urban | 6 | 6 | 7 | 7 | 7 |
| Hospitals Rural | 33 | 33 | 33 | 35 | 35 |
| **Control** | | | | | |
| State and Local Government | 24 | 24 | 27 | 28 | 28 |
| Not for Profit | 13 | 13 | 11 | 11 | 11 |
| Investor owned | 2 | 2 | 2 | 3 | 3 |
| **Physician Models** | | | | | |
| Independent Practice Association | 7 | 6 | 6 | 5 | 7 |
| Group Practice without Walls | 1 | 1 | 1 | 0 | 2 |
| Open Physician-Hospital Organization | 5 | 6 | 6 | 8 | 10 |
| Closed Physician-Hospital Organization | 4 | 5 | 5 | 4 | 2 |
| Management Service Organization | 2 | 1 | 1 | 1 | 2 |
| Integrated Salary Model | 5 | 4 | 7 | 5 | 5 |
| Equity Model | 2 | 1 | 1 | 0 | 1 |
| Foundation | 0 | 0 | 0 | 0 | 3 |
| **Insurance Products** | | | | | |
| Health Maintenance Organization | 4 | 6 | 7 | 6 | 5 |
| Preferred Provider Organization | 6 | 6 | 8 | 9 | 6 |
| Indemnity Fee for Service | 2 | 3 | 4 | 5 | 5 |
| **Managed Care Contracts** | | | | | |
| Health Maintenance Organization | 12 | 10 | 12 | 11 | 13 |
| Preferred Provider Organization | 18 | 17 | 22 | 19 | 19 |
| **Affiliations** | | | | | |
| Hospitals in a System* | 15 | 13 | 14 | 15 | 16 |
| Hospitals in a Network | 14 | 13 | 17 | 13 | 14 |
| Hospitals in a Group Purchasing Organization | 27 | 25 | 28 | 29 | 27 |

States

* Please note that system affiliate information for hospitals is derived from AHA membership. In years prior to 2003 the affiliation was derived from a question on the AHA Annual Survey of hospitals; therefore, non-responding hospitals were not included in the system affiliation counts. Years prior to 2003 have been updated to reflect this change, which now include affiliation for non-reporting hospitals.

# TABLE 6

## IDAHO

*U.S. Registered Community Hospitals*
*(Nonfederal, short-term general and other special hospitals)*

## Utilization, Personnel, Revenue and Expenses, Community Health Indicators 1999–2003

| | 2003 | 2002 | 2001 | 2000 | 1999 |
|---|---|---|---|---|---|
| **TOTAL FACILITY (Includes Hospital and Nursing Home Units)** | | | | | |
| **Utilization - Inpatient** | | | | | |
| Beds | 3,412 | 3,349 | 3,439 | 3,485 | 3,499 |
| Admissions | 135,920 | 123,046 | 122,510 | 123,187 | 119,928 |
| Inpatient Days | 698,748 | 648,640 | 682,010 | 669,186 | 694,361 |
| Average Length of Stay | 5.1 | 5.3 | 5.6 | 5.4 | 5.8 |
| Inpatient Surgeries | 44,640 | 40,816 | 41,062 | 38,270 | 38,624 |
| Births | 19,796 | 19,601 | 19,672 | 17,738 | 17,990 |
| **Utilization - Outpatient** | | | | | |
| Emergency Outpatient Visits | 468,818 | 445,100 | 411,533 | 409,030 | 414,388 |
| Other Outpatient Visits | 2,300,786 | 1,942,986 | 2,228,545 | 1,748,372 | 1,767,925 |
| Total Outpatient Visits | 2,769,604 | 2,388,086 | 2,640,078 | 2,157,402 | 2,182,313 |
| Outpatient Surgeries | 59,016 | 60,626 | 57,886 | 53,171 | 60,607 |
| **Personnel** | | | | | |
| Full Time RNs | 2,877 | 3,045 | 2,411 | 2,370 | 2,556 |
| Full Time LPNs | 481 | 533 | 489 | 502 | 525 |
| Part Time RNs | 2,234 | 2,034 | 1,918 | 1,759 | 1,676 |
| Part Time LPNs | 307 | 309 | 275 | 310 | 324 |
| Total Full Time | 12,935 | 13,827 | 11,650 | 11,074 | 11,354 |
| Total Part Time | 7,083 | 6,716 | 6,681 | 5,678 | 5,373 |
| **Revenue - Inpatient** | | | | | |
| Gross Inpatient Revenue | $1,531,029,736 | $1,689,244,058 | $1,311,305,096 | $1,243,357,709 | $1,132,120,798 |
| **Revenue - Outpatient** | | | | | |
| Gross Outpatient Revenue | $1,153,678,786 | $875,193,822 | $841,069,903 | $785,301,536 | $682,496,769 |
| **Revenue and Expenses - Totals (Includes Inpatient and Outpatient)** | | | | | |
| Total Gross Revenue | $2,684,708,522 | $2,564,437,880 | $2,152,374,999 | $2,028,659,245 | $1,814,617,567 |
| Deductions from Revenue | 1,042,369,113 | 1,085,024,888 | 817,619,918 | 826,933,247 | 675,699,809 |
| Net Patient Revenue | 1,642,339,409 | 1,479,412,992 | 1,334,755,081 | 1,201,725,998 | 1,138,917,758 |
| Other Operating Revenue | 70,613,156 | 62,644,590 | 43,219,742 | 42,583,119 | 55,873,470 |
| Other Nonoperating Revenue | 22,929,734 | 17,699,166 | 38,074,932 | 28,837,697 | 31,708,471 |
| Total Net Revenue | 1,735,882,299 | 1,559,756,748 | 1,416,049,755 | 1,273,146,814 | 1,226,499,699 |
| Total Expenses | 1,636,080,398 | 1,488,003,696 | 1,313,949,886 | 1,167,101,520 | 1,116,899,654 |
| **HOSPITAL UNIT (Excludes Separate Nursing Home Units)** | | | | | |
| **Utilization - Inpatient** | | | | | |
| Beds | 2,966 | 2,744 | 2,828 | 2,874 | 2,816 |
| Admissions | 133,599 | 120,656 | 119,945 | 120,655 | 115,670 |
| Inpatient Days | 572,243 | 478,779 | 504,028 | 497,049 | 503,844 |
| Average Length of Stay | 4.3 | 4.0 | 4.2 | 4.1 | 4.4 |
| **Personnel** | | | | | |
| Total Full Time | 12,666 | 13,513 | 11,265 | 10,801 | 10,839 |
| Total Part Time | 6,806 | 6,443 | 6,431 | 5,396 | 5,097 |
| **Revenue and Expenses - Totals (Includes Inpatient and Outpatient)** | | | | | |
| Total Net Revenue | $1,707,677,232 | $1,529,409,854 | $1,390,073,406 | $1,249,236,753 | $1,191,632,434 |
| Total Expenses | 1,611,236,547 | 1,465,901,906 | 1,292,299,636 | 1,151,521,698 | 1,093,475,829 |
| **COMMUNITY HEALTH INDICATORS PER 1000 POPULATION** | | | | | |
| Total Population (in thousands) | 1,366 | 1,343 | 1,321 | 1,300 | 1,276 |
| **Inpatient** | | | | | |
| Beds | 2.5 | 2.5 | 2.6 | 2.7 | 2.7 |
| Admissions | 99.5 | 91.6 | 92.7 | 94.8 | 94.0 |
| Inpatient Days | 511.4 | 482.9 | 516.2 | 514.9 | 544.3 |
| Inpatient Surgeries | 32.7 | 30.4 | 31.1 | 29.4 | 30.3 |
| Births | 14.5 | 14.6 | 14.9 | 13.6 | 14.1 |
| **Outpatient** | | | | | |
| Emergency Outpatient Visits | 343.1 | 331.4 | 311.5 | 314.7 | 324.8 |
| Other Outpatient Visits | 1,683.9 | 1,446.6 | 1,686.6 | 1,345.3 | 1,385.9 |
| Total Outpatient Visits | 2,027.0 | 1,778.0 | 1,998.1 | 1,660.0 | 1,710.7 |
| Outpatient Surgeries | 43.2 | 45.1 | 43.8 | 40.9 | 47.5 |
| **Expense per Capita (per person)** | $1,197.4 | $1,107.9 | $994.4 | $898.0 | $875.5 |

# TABLE 6

## ILLINOIS

*U.S. Registered Community Hospitals*
*(Nonfederal, short-term general and other special hospitals)*

## Overview 1999–2003

| | 2003 | 2002 | 2001 | 2000 | 1999 |
|---|---|---|---|---|---|
| **Total Community Hospitals in Illinois** | **192** | **192** | **192** | **196** | **198** |
| **Bed Size Category** | | | | | |
| 6-24 | 5 | 6 | 3 | 4 | 3 |
| 25-49 | 23 | 18 | 18 | 18 | 20 |
| 50-99 | 39 | 39 | 36 | 34 | 37 |
| 100-199 | 60 | 63 | 67 | 68 | 66 |
| 200-299 | 30 | 31 | 29 | 33 | 34 |
| 300-399 | 18 | 17 | 21 | 21 | 19 |
| 400-499 | 8 | 6 | 7 | 7 | 6 |
| 500 + | 9 | 12 | 11 | 11 | 13 |
| **Location** | | | | | |
| Hospitals Urban | 120 | 120 | 120 | 124 | 125 |
| Hospitals Rural | 72 | 72 | 72 | 72 | 73 |
| **Control** | | | | | |
| State and Local Government | 28 | 29 | 28 | 28 | 30 |
| Not for Profit | 154 | 154 | 156 | 159 | 161 |
| Investor owned | 10 | 9 | 8 | 9 | 7 |
| **Physician Models** | | | | | |
| Independent Practice Association | 40 | 36 | 36 | 42 | 42 |
| Group Practice without Walls | 5 | 7 | 8 | 9 | 7 |
| Open Physician-Hospital Organization | 51 | 50 | 53 | 51 | 51 |
| Closed Physician-Hospital Organization | 17 | 16 | 14 | 19 | 26 |
| Management Service Organization | 29 | 28 | 37 | 42 | 48 |
| Integrated Salary Model | 54 | 52 | 50 | 65 | 65 |
| Equity Model | 0 | 3 | 2 | 2 | 4 |
| Foundation | 11 | 9 | 9 | 11 | 10 |
| **Insurance Products** | | | | | |
| Health Maintenance Organization | 25 | 26 | 27 | 35 | 48 |
| Preferred Provider Organization | 30 | 28 | 29 | 35 | 44 |
| Indemnity Fee for Service | 8 | 7 | 10 | 15 | 11 |
| **Managed Care Contracts** | | | | | |
| Health Maintenance Organization | 133 | 121 | 122 | 140 | 143 |
| Preferred Provider Organization | 154 | 140 | 141 | 153 | 161 |
| **Affiliations** | | | | | |
| Hospitals in a System* | 94 | 90 | 92 | 91 | 97 |
| Hospitals in a Network | 42 | 31 | 32 | 32 | 38 |
| Hospitals in a Group Purchasing Organization | 163 | 146 | 150 | 158 | 153 |

* Please note that system affiliate information for hospitals is derived from AHA membership. In years prior to 2003 the affiliation was derived from a question on the AHA Annual Survey of hospitals; therefore, non-responding hospitals were not included in the system affiliation counts. Years prior to 2003 have been updated to reflect this change, which now include affiliation for non-reporting hospitals.

# TABLE 6 — ILLINOIS

*U.S. Registered Community Hospitals*
*(Nonfederal, short-term general and other special hospitals)*

## Utilization, Personnel, Revenue and Expenses, Community Health Indicators 1999–2003

| | 2003 | 2002 | 2001 | 2000 | 1999 |
|---|---|---|---|---|---|
| **TOTAL FACILITY (Includes Hospital and Nursing Home Units)** | | | | | |
| **Utilization - Inpatient** | | | | | |
| Beds | 35,048 | 36,309 | 36,834 | 37,310 | 37,658 |
| Admissions | 1,594,007 | 1,615,269 | 1,559,357 | 1,530,800 | 1,508,816 |
| Inpatient Days | 8,174,779 | 8,326,561 | 8,215,380 | 8,189,818 | 8,267,158 |
| Average Length of Stay | 5.1 | 5.2 | 5.3 | 5.4 | 5.5 |
| Inpatient Surgeries | 419,711 | 429,366 | 414,121 | 404,231 | 387,355 |
| Births | 177,192 | 172,338 | 173,967 | 179,057 | 176,435 |
| **Utilization - Outpatient** | | | | | |
| Emergency Outpatient Visits | 4,867,066 | 4,699,328 | 4,582,408 | 4,497,815 | 4,420,908 |
| Other Outpatient Visits | 22,358,135 | 21,811,988 | 20,687,505 | 20,601,748 | 19,495,093 |
| Total Outpatient Visits | 27,225,201 | 26,511,316 | 25,269,913 | 25,099,563 | 23,916,001 |
| Outpatient Surgeries | 710,827 | 745,579 | 710,346 | 691,824 | 654,078 |
| **Personnel** | | | | | |
| Full Time RNs | 34,297 | 32,720 | 33,093 | 33,905 | 34,481 |
| Full Time LPNs | 2,590 | 2,608 | 2,781 | 2,789 | 3,042 |
| Part Time RNs | 25,372 | 25,875 | 23,596 | 21,807 | 21,044 |
| Part Time LPNs | 1,376 | 1,361 | 1,116 | 1,239 | 1,186 |
| Total Full Time | 157,106 | 156,627 | 160,545 | 161,303 | 157,818 |
| Total Part Time | 76,983 | 80,497 | 71,502 | 69,069 | 65,200 |
| **Revenue - Inpatient** | | | | | |
| Gross Inpatient Revenue | $30,474,701,629 | $27,722,800,143 | $24,926,910,293 | $22,597,529,237 | $20,652,014,700 |
| **Revenue - Outpatient** | | | | | |
| Gross Outpatient Revenue | $18,096,235,944 | $15,980,470,692 | $14,044,549,597 | $12,699,517,400 | $11,241,559,394 |
| **Revenue and Expenses - Totals (Includes Inpatient and Outpatient)** | | | | | |
| Total Gross Revenue | $48,570,937,573 | $43,703,270,835 | $38,971,459,890 | $35,297,046,637 | $31,893,574,094 |
| Deductions from Revenue | 28,856,859,436 | 25,017,360,640 | 21,796,610,516 | 19,210,165,443 | 17,010,439,012 |
| Net Patient Revenue | 19,714,078,137 | 18,685,910,195 | 17,174,849,374 | 16,086,881,194 | 14,883,135,082 |
| Other Operating Revenue | 1,137,597,475 | 1,174,384,266 | 1,057,250,792 | 984,694,243 | 846,212,294 |
| Other Nonoperating Revenue | 320,997,567 | 56,898,594 | 384,325,832 | 937,308,890 | 975,103,585 |
| Total Net Revenue | 21,172,673,179 | 19,917,193,055 | 18,616,425,998 | 18,008,884,327 | 16,704,450,961 |
| Total Expenses | 20,458,310,850 | 19,597,944,423 | 18,304,829,361 | 17,215,623,885 | 16,050,659,864 |
| **HOSPITAL UNIT (Excludes Separate Nursing Home Units)** | | | | | |
| **Utilization - Inpatient** | | | | | |
| Beds | 32,267 | 33,876 | 33,998 | 33,695 | 33,806 |
| Admissions | 1,568,413 | 1,588,707 | 1,526,030 | 1,495,873 | 1,469,587 |
| Inpatient Days | 7,382,487 | 7,652,143 | 7,417,273 | 7,180,518 | 7,202,654 |
| Average Length of Stay | 4.7 | 4.8 | 4.9 | 4.8 | 4.9 |
| **Personnel** | | | | | |
| Total Full Time | 155,219 | 154,973 | 158,634 | 158,538 | 154,891 |
| Total Part Time | 75,920 | 79,653 | 70,507 | 67,735 | 63,943 |
| **Revenue and Expenses - Totals (Includes Inpatient and Outpatient)** | | | | | |
| Total Net Revenue | $21,024,338,670 | $19,771,409,995 | $18,410,732,829 | $17,824,208,519 | $16,449,642,798 |
| Total Expenses | 20,332,186,270 | 19,476,432,848 | 18,152,199,024 | 17,076,598,221 | 15,858,782,696 |
| **COMMUNITY HEALTH INDICATORS PER 1000 POPULATION** | | | | | |
| Total Population (in thousands) | 12,654 | 12,586 | 12,517 | 12,439 | 12,359 |
| **Inpatient** | | | | | |
| Beds | 2.8 | 2.9 | 2.9 | 3.0 | 3.0 |
| Admissions | 126.0 | 128.3 | 124.6 | 123.1 | 122.1 |
| Inpatient Days | 646.0 | 661.5 | 656.3 | 658.4 | 668.9 |
| Inpatient Surgeries | 33.2 | 34.1 | 33.1 | 32.5 | 31.3 |
| Births | 14.0 | 13.7 | 13.9 | 14.4 | 14.3 |
| **Outpatient** | | | | | |
| Emergency Outpatient Visits | 384.6 | 373.4 | 366.1 | 361.6 | 357.7 |
| Other Outpatient Visits | 1,766.9 | 1,733.0 | 1,652.7 | 1,656.2 | 1,577.4 |
| Total Outpatient Visits | 2,151.6 | 2,106.3 | 2,018.8 | 2,017.8 | 1,935.1 |
| Outpatient Surgeries | 56.2 | 59.2 | 56.7 | 55.6 | 52.9 |
| **Expense per Capita (per person)** | $1,616.8 | $1,557.1 | $1,462.4 | $1,384.0 | $1,298.7 |

# TABLE 6

## INDIANA

*U.S. Registered Community Hospitals*
*(Nonfederal, short-term general and other special hospitals)*

## Overview 1999–2003

| | 2003 | 2002 | 2001 | 2000 | 1999 |
|---|---|---|---|---|---|
| **Total Community Hospitals in Indiana** | **112** | **112** | **110** | **109** | **111** |
| **Bed Size Category** | | | | | |
| 6-24 | 4 | 5 | 5 | 4 | 5 |
| 25-49 | 28 | 23 | 21 | 22 | 23 |
| 50-99 | 28 | 33 | 30 | 29 | 30 |
| 100-199 | 20 | 21 | 24 | 24 | 23 |
| 200-299 | 15 | 13 | 13 | 13 | 13 |
| 300-399 | 6 | 6 | 5 | 5 | 5 |
| 400-499 | 2 | 3 | 4 | 3 | 4 |
| 500 + | 9 | 8 | 8 | 9 | 8 |
| **Location** | | | | | |
| Hospitals Urban | 67 | 67 | 64 | 64 | 65 |
| Hospitals Rural | 45 | 45 | 46 | 45 | 46 |
| **Control** | | | | | |
| State and Local Government | 38 | 40 | 41 | 41 | 45 |
| Not for Profit | 59 | 58 | 57 | 56 | 54 |
| Investor owned | 15 | 14 | 12 | 12 | 12 |
| **Physician Models** | | | | | |
| Independent Practice Association | 11 | 14 | 15 | 15 | 10 |
| Group Practice without Walls | 5 | 4 | 4 | 1 | 0 |
| Open Physician-Hospital Organization | 27 | 29 | 26 | 32 | 31 |
| Closed Physician-Hospital Organization | 11 | 13 | 14 | 16 | 14 |
| Management Service Organization | 15 | 16 | 17 | 20 | 19 |
| Integrated Salary Model | 33 | 37 | 31 | 32 | 36 |
| Equity Model | 0 | 0 | 1 | 1 | 1 |
| Foundation | 3 | 3 | 2 | 1 | 4 |
| **Insurance Products** | | | | | |
| Health Maintenance Organization | 25 | 17 | 20 | 32 | 34 |
| Preferred Provider Organization | 35 | 31 | 28 | 42 | 42 |
| Indemnity Fee for Service | 10 | 6 | 8 | 11 | 11 |
| **Managed Care Contracts** | | | | | |
| Health Maintenance Organization | 66 | 65 | 60 | 73 | 72 |
| Preferred Provider Organization | 82 | 78 | 71 | 82 | 86 |
| **Affiliations** | | | | | |
| Hospitals in a System* | 56 | 57 | 56 | 57 | 51 |
| Hospitals in a Network | 37 | 41 | 36 | 40 | 32 |
| Hospitals in a Group Purchasing Organization | 87 | 87 | 78 | 87 | 84 |

States

* Please note that system affiliate information for hospitals is derived from AHA membership. In years prior to 2003 the affiliation was derived from a question on the AHA Annual Survey of hospitals; therefore, non-responding hospitals were not included in the system affiliation counts. Years prior to 2003 have been updated to reflect this change, which now include affiliation for non-reporting hospitals.

# TABLE 6

## INDIANA

*U.S. Registered Community Hospitals*
*(Nonfederal, short-term general and other special hospitals)*

## Utilization, Personnel, Revenue and Expenses, Community Health Indicators 1999–2003

| | 2003 | 2002 | 2001 | 2000 | 1999 |
|---|---|---|---|---|---|
| **TOTAL FACILITY (Includes Hospital and Nursing Home Units)** | | | | | |
| **Utilization - Inpatient** | | | | | |
| Beds | 18,932 | 18,961 | 19,036 | 19,160 | 19,225 |
| Admissions | 712,151 | 715,936 | 718,369 | 699,511 | 683,264 |
| Inpatient Days | 3,997,353 | 4,077,032 | 3,944,457 | 3,943,695 | 3,998,799 |
| Average Length of Stay | 5.6 | 5.7 | 5.5 | 5.6 | 5.9 |
| Inpatient Surgeries | 201,344 | 199,279 | 195,206 | 216,204 | 189,678 |
| Births | 81,200 | 78,921 | 80,485 | 81,052 | 75,076 |
| **Utilization - Outpatient** | | | | | |
| Emergency Outpatient Visits | 2,492,597 | 2,437,268 | 2,385,242 | 2,187,447 | 2,120,329 |
| Other Outpatient Visits | 12,505,299 | 11,650,167 | 12,008,043 | 11,946,547 | 10,993,509 |
| Total Outpatient Visits | 14,997,896 | 14,087,435 | 14,393,285 | 14,133,994 | 13,113,838 |
| Outpatient Surgeries | 452,206 | 416,641 | 386,704 | 388,192 | 408,893 |
| **Personnel** | | | | | |
| Full Time RNs | 16,836 | 17,176 | 15,997 | 17,308 | 17,831 |
| Full Time LPNs | 2,292 | 2,408 | 2,486 | 2,430 | 2,373 |
| Part Time RNs | 12,701 | 11,544 | 10,944 | 11,696 | 10,222 |
| Part Time LPNs | 1,456 | 1,399 | 1,344 | 1,403 | 1,207 |
| Total Full Time | 76,985 | 79,408 | 77,258 | 76,219 | 75,902 |
| Total Part Time | 37,643 | 35,876 | 35,540 | 35,901 | 32,134 |
| **Revenue - Inpatient** | | | | | |
| Gross Inpatient Revenue | $11,665,904,141 | $10,700,904,487 | $9,449,404,551 | $8,288,484,221 | $7,574,440,688 |
| **Revenue - Outpatient** | | | | | |
| Gross Outpatient Revenue | $8,771,505,233 | $7,508,632,761 | $6,380,741,910 | $5,799,391,724 | $5,058,777,890 |
| **Revenue and Expenses - Totals (Includes Inpatient and Outpatient)** | | | | | |
| Total Gross Revenue | $20,437,409,374 | $18,209,537,248 | $15,830,146,461 | $14,087,875,945 | $12,633,218,578 |
| Deductions from Revenue | 10,322,060,345 | 8,632,745,626 | 7,243,961,000 | 6,058,831,246 | 5,130,679,610 |
| Net Patient Revenue | 10,115,349,029 | 9,576,791,622 | 8,586,185,461 | 8,029,044,699 | 7,502,538,968 |
| Other Operating Revenue | 584,230,112 | 433,611,706 | 501,261,342 | 496,781,927 | 439,652,541 |
| Other Nonoperating Revenue | 196,893,476 | 63,204,269 | 145,445,011 | 282,308,259 | 262,145,842 |
| Total Net Revenue | 10,896,472,617 | 10,073,607,597 | 9,232,891,814 | 8,808,134,885 | 8,204,337,351 |
| Total Expenses | 9,985,287,171 | 9,272,854,799 | 8,446,387,337 | 7,865,789,801 | 7,490,717,665 |
| **HOSPITAL UNIT (Excludes Separate Nursing Home Units)** | | | | | |
| **Utilization - Inpatient** | | | | | |
| Beds | 17,907 | 17,867 | 17,157 | 16,957 | 16,801 |
| Admissions | 701,648 | 704,094 | 705,746 | 684,461 | 664,977 |
| Inpatient Days | 3,690,772 | 3,751,265 | 3,404,916 | 3,337,863 | 3,341,593 |
| Average Length of Stay | 5.3 | 5.3 | 4.8 | 4.9 | 5.0 |
| **Personnel** | | | | | |
| Total Full Time | 76,249 | 78,630 | 75,807 | 74,693 | 74,041 |
| Total Part Time | 36,759 | 35,272 | 34,952 | 35,169 | 31,265 |
| **Revenue and Expenses - Totals (Includes Inpatient and Outpatient)** | | | | | |
| Total Net Revenue | $10,836,544,994 | $9,996,393,418 | $9,142,546,269 | $8,721,330,380 | $8,064,204,896 |
| Total Expenses | 9,927,768,129 | 9,204,932,252 | 8,353,731,881 | 7,780,952,771 | 7,368,487,400 |
| **COMMUNITY HEALTH INDICATORS PER 1000 POPULATION** | | | | | |
| Total Population (in thousands) | 6,196 | 6,157 | 6,126 | 6,092 | 6,045 |
| **Inpatient** | | | | | |
| Beds | 3.1 | 3.1 | 3.1 | 3.1 | 3.2 |
| Admissions | 114.9 | 116.3 | 117.3 | 114.8 | 113.0 |
| Inpatient Days | 645.2 | 662.2 | 643.8 | 647.4 | 661.5 |
| Inpatient Surgeries | 32.5 | 32.4 | 31.9 | 35.5 | 31.4 |
| Births | 13.1 | 12.8 | 13.1 | 13.3 | 12.4 |
| **Outpatient** | | | | | |
| Emergency Outpatient Visits | 402.3 | 395.9 | 389.3 | 359.1 | 350.8 |
| Other Outpatient Visits | 2,018.4 | 1,892.2 | 1,960.0 | 1,961.2 | 1,818.6 |
| Total Outpatient Visits | 2,420.7 | 2,288.1 | 2,349.4 | 2,320.3 | 2,169.4 |
| Outpatient Surgeries | 73.0 | 67.7 | 63.1 | 63.7 | 67.6 |
| **Expense per Capita (per person)** | $1,611.7 | $1,506.1 | $1,378.7 | $1,291.3 | $1,239.2 |

# Table 6

## IOWA

*U.S. Registered Community Hospitals*
*(Nonfederal, short-term general and other special hospitals)*

## Overview 1999–2003

| | 2003 | 2002 | 2001 | 2000 | 1999 |
|---|---|---|---|---|---|
| **Total Community Hospitals in Iowa** | **116** | **116** | **116** | **115** | **115** |
| **Bed Size Category** | | | | | |
| 6-24 | 11 | 12 | 12 | 11 | 11 |
| 25-49 | 47 | 45 | 42 | 41 | 40 |
| 50-99 | 30 | 29 | 31 | 29 | 31 |
| 100-199 | 13 | 14 | 15 | 17 | 18 |
| 200-299 | 6 | 7 | 7 | 8 | 6 |
| 300-399 | 5 | 5 | 5 | 5 | 5 |
| 400-499 | 2 | 2 | 2 | 2 | 2 |
| 500 + | 2 | 2 | 2 | 2 | 2 |
| **Location** | | | | | |
| Hospitals Urban | 21 | 21 | 21 | 21 | 21 |
| Hospitals Rural | 95 | 95 | 95 | 94 | 94 |
| **Control** | | | | | |
| State and Local Government | 59 | 59 | 59 | 58 | 59 |
| Not for Profit | 57 | 57 | 56 | 57 | 56 |
| Investor owned | 0 | 0 | 1 | 0 | 0 |
| **Physician Models** | | | | | |
| Independent Practice Association | 18 | 21 | 14 | 15 | 17 |
| Group Practice without Walls | 4 | 3 | 4 | 3 | 3 |
| Open Physician-Hospital Organization | 19 | 18 | 21 | 21 | 20 |
| Closed Physician-Hospital Organization | 16 | 17 | 17 | 19 | 20 |
| Management Service Organization | 13 | 12 | 14 | 13 | 15 |
| Integrated Salary Model | 58 | 51 | 44 | 41 | 39 |
| Equity Model | 2 | 3 | 1 | 1 | 0 |
| Foundation | 3 | 3 | 4 | 6 | 7 |
| **Insurance Products** | | | | | |
| Health Maintenance Organization | 16 | 18 | 17 | 18 | 21 |
| Preferred Provider Organization | 37 | 35 | 34 | 40 | 40 |
| Indemnity Fee for Service | 9 | 8 | 7 | 6 | 6 |
| **Managed Care Contracts** | | | | | |
| Health Maintenance Organization | 66 | 66 | 69 | 69 | 70 |
| Preferred Provider Organization | 97 | 96 | 98 | 100 | 104 |
| **Affiliations** | | | | | |
| Hospitals in a System* | 59 | 61 | 58 | 56 | 57 |
| Hospitals in a Network | 59 | 59 | 55 | 52 | 46 |
| Hospitals in a Group Purchasing Organization | 105 | 105 | 109 | 108 | 104 |

* Please note that system affiliate information for hospitals is derived from AHA membership. In years prior to 2003 the affiliation was derived from a question on the AHA Annual Survey of hospitals; therefore, non-responding hospitals were not included in the system affiliation counts. Years prior to 2003 have been updated to reflect this change, which now include affiliation for non-reporting hospitals.

# TABLE 6

# IOWA

*U.S. Registered Community Hospitals*
*(Nonfederal, short-term general and other special hospitals)*

## Utilization, Personnel, Revenue and Expenses, Community Health Indicators 1999–2003

| | 2003 | 2002 | 2001 | 2000 | 1999 |
|---|---|---|---|---|---|
| **TOTAL FACILITY (Includes Hospital and Nursing Home Units)** | | | | | |
| **Utilization - Inpatient** | | | | | |
| Beds | 11,002 | 11,267 | 11,538 | 11,811 | 11,838 |
| Admissions | 363,008 | 370,968 | 370,885 | 359,682 | 359,142 |
| Inpatient Days | 2,369,769 | 2,447,672 | 2,491,172 | 2,493,185 | 2,498,984 |
| Average Length of Stay | 6.5 | 6.6 | 6.7 | 6.9 | 7.0 |
| Inpatient Surgeries | 100,020 | 106,987 | 107,252 | 105,897 | 105,951 |
| Births | 37,936 | 37,342 | 37,628 | 37,692 | 37,162 |
| **Utilization - Outpatient** | | | | | |
| Emergency Outpatient Visits | 1,066,268 | 1,072,319 | 1,063,304 | 1,050,606 | 1,051,682 |
| Other Outpatient Visits | 8,669,111 | 8,258,357 | 8,336,049 | 8,106,385 | 7,511,574 |
| Total Outpatient Visits | 9,735,379 | 9,330,676 | 9,399,353 | 9,156,991 | 8,563,256 |
| Outpatient Surgeries | 273,026 | 302,995 | 289,647 | 289,715 | 280,264 |
| **Personnel** | | | | | |
| Full Time RNs | 8,926 | 8,967 | 8,519 | 8,855 | 8,581 |
| Full Time LPNs | 922 | 996 | 904 | 897 | 826 |
| Part Time RNs | 7,045 | 7,391 | 7,027 | 6,698 | 6,988 |
| Part Time LPNs | 832 | 836 | 818 | 757 | 781 |
| Total Full Time | 40,849 | 41,179 | 40,716 | 40,602 | 39,836 |
| Total Part Time | 24,861 | 25,648 | 25,215 | 23,512 | 23,967 |
| **Revenue - Inpatient** | | | | | |
| Gross Inpatient Revenue | $4,676,641,630 | $4,245,474,792 | $3,868,944,808 | $3,523,992,700 | $3,291,048,997 |
| **Revenue - Outpatient** | | | | | |
| Gross Outpatient Revenue | $3,946,331,686 | $3,390,410,867 | $2,990,618,965 | $2,693,739,475 | $2,389,853,804 |
| **Revenue and Expenses - Totals (Includes Inpatient and Outpatient)** | | | | | |
| Total Gross Revenue | $8,622,973,316 | $7,635,885,659 | $6,859,563,773 | $6,217,732,175 | $5,680,902,801 |
| Deductions from Revenue | 3,993,879,715 | 3,333,435,082 | 2,824,125,097 | 2,466,317,174 | 2,114,838,477 |
| Net Patient Revenue | 4,629,093,601 | 4,302,450,577 | 4,035,438,676 | 3,751,415,001 | 3,566,064,324 |
| Other Operating Revenue | 352,052,586 | 328,828,491 | 319,656,799 | 308,982,657 | 265,943,571 |
| Other Nonoperating Revenue | 52,808,563 | 51,699,288 | 93,484,169 | 83,255,612 | 90,128,303 |
| Total Net Revenue | 5,033,954,750 | 4,682,978,356 | 4,448,579,644 | 4,143,653,270 | 3,922,136,198 |
| Total Expenses | 4,779,866,027 | 4,483,595,177 | 4,202,394,287 | 3,932,103,219 | 3,669,806,143 |
| **HOSPITAL UNIT (Excludes Separate Nursing Home Units)** | | | | | |
| **Utilization - Inpatient** | | | | | |
| Beds | 8,777 | 9,038 | 9,251 | 9,481 | 9,440 |
| Admissions | 352,526 | 360,065 | 359,577 | 347,688 | 345,654 |
| Inpatient Days | 1,643,007 | 1,723,431 | 1,748,201 | 1,739,816 | 1,733,617 |
| Average Length of Stay | 4.7 | 4.8 | 4.9 | 5.0 | 5.0 |
| **Personnel** | | | | | |
| Total Full Time | 39,856 | 40,108 | 39,690 | 39,540 | 38,830 |
| Total Part Time | 23,844 | 24,625 | 24,220 | 22,599 | 23,099 |
| **Revenue and Expenses - Totals (Includes Inpatient and Outpatient)** | | | | | |
| Total Net Revenue | $4,927,832,564 | $4,581,452,200 | $4,348,039,384 | $4,048,875,825 | $3,830,086,493 |
| Total Expenses | 4,695,594,251 | 4,406,423,753 | 4,123,430,546 | 3,857,836,935 | 3,590,355,032 |
| **COMMUNITY HEALTH INDICATORS PER 1000 POPULATION** | | | | | |
| Total Population (in thousands) | 2,944 | 2,936 | 2,932 | 2,929 | 2,918 |
| **Inpatient** | | | | | |
| Beds | 3.7 | 3.8 | 3.9 | 4.0 | 4.1 |
| Admissions | 123.3 | 126.4 | 126.5 | 122.8 | 123.1 |
| Inpatient Days | 804.9 | 833.7 | 849.6 | 851.3 | 856.5 |
| Inpatient Surgeries | 34.0 | 36.4 | 36.6 | 36.2 | 36.3 |
| Births | 12.9 | 12.7 | 12.8 | 12.9 | 12.7 |
| **Outpatient** | | | | | |
| Emergency Outpatient Visits | 362.2 | 365.3 | 362.6 | 358.8 | 360.5 |
| Other Outpatient Visits | 2,944.6 | 2,812.9 | 2,842.9 | 2,768.1 | 2,574.5 |
| Total Outpatient Visits | 3,306.8 | 3,178.2 | 3,205.5 | 3,126.8 | 2,935.0 |
| Outpatient Surgeries | 92.7 | 103.2 | 98.8 | 98.9 | 96.1 |
| **Expense per Capita (per person)** | $1,623.6 | $1,527.2 | $1,433.2 | $1,342.7 | $1,257.8 |

# TABLE 6

## KANSAS

*U.S. Registered Community Hospitals*
*(Nonfederal, short-term general and other special hospitals)*

## Overview 1999–2003

| | 2003 | 2002 | 2001 | 2000 | 1999 |
|---|---|---|---|---|---|
| **Total Community Hospitals in Kansas** | **134** | **132** | **133** | **129** | **131** |
| **Bed Size Category** | | | | | |
| 6-24 | 17 | 15 | 15 | 18 | 17 |
| 25-49 | 45 | 42 | 44 | 39 | 41 |
| 50-99 | 48 | 50 | 46 | 46 | 44 |
| 100-199 | 14 | 14 | 18 | 16 | 17 |
| 200-299 | 5 | 6 | 5 | 5 | 7 |
| 300-399 | 2 | 2 | 2 | 3 | 3 |
| 400-499 | 1 | 2 | 2 | 1 | 0 |
| 500 + | 2 | 1 | 1 | 1 | 2 |
| **Location** | | | | | |
| Hospitals Urban | 27 | 25 | 28 | 25 | 26 |
| Hospitals Rural | 107 | 107 | 105 | 104 | 105 |
| **Control** | | | | | |
| State and Local Government | 61 | 61 | 62 | 63 | 63 |
| Not for Profit | 60 | 62 | 62 | 60 | 61 |
| Investor owned | 13 | 9 | 9 | 6 | 7 |
| **Physician Models** | | | | | |
| Independent Practice Association | 18 | 16 | 19 | 15 | 12 |
| Group Practice without Walls | 6 | 5 | 9 | 7 | 7 |
| Open Physician-Hospital Organization | 16 | 18 | 19 | 19 | 21 |
| Closed Physician-Hospital Organization | 2 | 4 | 3 | 4 | 3 |
| Management Service Organization | 2 | 5 | 5 | 6 | 12 |
| Integrated Salary Model | 52 | 45 | 45 | 42 | 43 |
| Equity Model | 0 | 0 | 0 | 0 | 0 |
| Foundation | 2 | 3 | 2 | 5 | 10 |
| **Insurance Products** | | | | | |
| Health Maintenance Organization | 8 | 7 | 9 | 15 | 16 |
| Preferred Provider Organization | 34 | 22 | 21 | 23 | 27 |
| Indemnity Fee for Service | 6 | 6 | 6 | 7 | 6 |
| **Managed Care Contracts** | | | | | |
| Health Maintenance Organization | 42 | 41 | 48 | 41 | 45 |
| Preferred Provider Organization | 103 | 105 | 108 | 106 | 103 |
| **Affiliations** | | | | | |
| Hospitals in a System* | 54 | 52 | 50 | 48 | 50 |
| Hospitals in a Network | 78 | 73 | 76 | 79 | 76 |
| Hospitals in a Group Purchasing Organization | 124 | 121 | 124 | 119 | 115 |

States

* Please note that system affiliate information for hospitals is derived from AHA membership. In years prior to 2003 the affiliation was derived from a question on the AHA Annual Survey of hospitals; therefore, non-responding hospitals were not included in the system affiliation counts. Years prior to 2003 have been updated to reflect this change, which now include affiliation for non-reporting hospitals.

# TABLE 6

# KANSAS

*U.S. Registered Community Hospitals*
*(Nonfederal, short-term general and other special hospitals)*

## Utilization, Personnel, Revenue and Expenses, Community Health Indicators 1999–2003

| | 2003 | 2002 | 2001 | 2000 | 1999 |
|---|---|---|---|---|---|
| **TOTAL FACILITY (Includes Hospital and Nursing Home Units)** | | | | | |
| **Utilization - Inpatient** | | | | | |
| Beds | 10,554 | 10,850 | 11,211 | 10,821 | 11,615 |
| Admissions | 331,244 | 328,987 | 322,067 | 310,256 | 326,352 |
| Inpatient Days | 2,148,111 | 2,165,195 | 2,175,989 | 2,081,932 | 2,232,737 |
| Average Length of Stay | 6.5 | 6.6 | 6.8 | 6.7 | 6.8 |
| Inpatient Surgeries | 89,889 | 88,704 | 86,949 | 84,051 | 91,259 |
| Births | 39,341 | 38,591 | 37,847 | 37,599 | 38,971 |
| **Utilization - Outpatient** | | | | | |
| Emergency Outpatient Visits | 945,208 | 940,408 | 907,083 | 889,390 | 921,066 |
| Other Outpatient Visits | 5,004,830 | 4,734,607 | 4,486,945 | 4,365,883 | 4,103,314 |
| Total Outpatient Visits | 5,950,038 | 5,675,015 | 5,394,028 | 5,255,273 | 5,024,380 |
| Outpatient Surgeries | 162,583 | 155,965 | 161,789 | 162,669 | 176,375 |
| **Personnel** | | | | | |
| Full Time RNs | 7,839 | 7,600 | 6,906 | 7,158 | 7,601 |
| Full Time LPNs | 1,169 | 1,138 | 1,079 | 1,038 | 1,075 |
| Part Time RNs | 4,217 | 4,088 | 4,041 | 4,072 | 4,415 |
| Part Time LPNs | 490 | 558 | 549 | 523 | 590 |
| Total Full Time | 34,022 | 33,790 | 32,609 | 31,548 | 33,931 |
| Total Part Time | 14,736 | 14,290 | 14,668 | 13,944 | 12,984 |
| **Revenue - Inpatient** | | | | | |
| Gross Inpatient Revenue | $5,466,344,640 | $4,837,931,215 | $4,299,715,760 | $3,829,510,816 | $3,772,245,204 |
| **Revenue - Outpatient** | | | | | |
| Gross Outpatient Revenue | $3,554,053,357 | $3,020,822,797 | $2,632,758,324 | $2,374,823,658 | $2,198,345,422 |
| **Revenue and Expenses - Totals (Includes Inpatient and Outpatient)** | | | | | |
| Total Gross Revenue | $9,020,397,997 | $7,858,754,012 | $6,932,474,084 | $6,204,334,474 | $5,970,590,626 |
| Deductions from Revenue | 5,192,082,605 | 4,306,839,200 | 3,693,649,527 | 3,189,390,696 | 2,949,255,620 |
| Net Patient Revenue | 3,828,315,392 | 3,551,914,812 | 3,238,824,557 | 3,014,943,778 | 3,021,335,006 |
| Other Operating Revenue | 145,873,173 | 150,197,636 | 162,388,962 | 147,629,759 | 144,033,337 |
| Other Nonoperating Revenue | 27,634,261 | 18,174,135 | 42,943,502 | 71,565,700 | 65,565,230 |
| Total Net Revenue | 4,001,822,826 | 3,720,286,583 | 3,444,157,021 | 3,234,139,237 | 3,230,933,573 |
| Total Expenses | 3,816,798,953 | 3,576,366,207 | 3,285,567,037 | 3,065,466,141 | 3,036,739,861 |
| **HOSPITAL UNIT (Excludes Separate Nursing Home Units)** | | | | | |
| **Utilization - Inpatient** | | | | | |
| Beds | 8,785 | 9,004 | 9,171 | 8,658 | 9,380 |
| Admissions | 326,144 | 322,983 | 314,556 | 301,101 | 316,200 |
| Inpatient Days | 1,600,483 | 1,630,230 | 1,576,671 | 1,489,124 | 1,615,520 |
| Average Length of Stay | 4.9 | 5.0 | 5.0 | 4.9 | 5.1 |
| **Personnel** | | | | | |
| Total Full Time | 32,915 | 32,669 | 31,407 | 30,303 | 32,649 |
| Total Part Time | 14,149 | 13,618 | 13,885 | 13,199 | 12,225 |
| **Revenue and Expenses - Totals (Includes Inpatient and Outpatient)** | | | | | |
| Total Net Revenue | $3,940,784,536 | $3,656,845,788 | $3,372,688,086 | $3,169,162,014 | $3,160,271,291 |
| Total Expenses | 3,760,914,701 | 3,520,829,715 | 3,229,152,871 | 3,011,711,334 | 2,981,430,308 |
| **COMMUNITY HEALTH INDICATORS PER 1000 POPULATION** | | | | | |
| Total Population (in thousands) | 2,724 | 2,712 | 2,700 | 2,693 | 2,678 |
| **Inpatient** | | | | | |
| Beds | 3.9 | 4.0 | 4.2 | 4.0 | 4.3 |
| Admissions | 121.6 | 121.3 | 119.3 | 115.2 | 121.8 |
| Inpatient Days | 788.7 | 798.4 | 805.8 | 773.2 | 833.6 |
| Inpatient Surgeries | 33.0 | 32.7 | 32.2 | 31.2 | 34.1 |
| Births | 14.4 | 14.2 | 14.0 | 14.0 | 14.6 |
| **Outpatient** | | | | | |
| Emergency Outpatient Visits | 347.1 | 346.8 | 335.9 | 330.3 | 343.9 |
| Other Outpatient Visits | 1,837.6 | 1,745.9 | 1,661.6 | 1,621.4 | 1,532.0 |
| Total Outpatient Visits | 2,184.7 | 2,092.7 | 1,997.5 | 1,951.7 | 1,875.9 |
| Outpatient Surgeries | 59.7 | 57.5 | 59.9 | 60.4 | 65.9 |
| **Expense per Capita (per person)** | $1,401.4 | $1,318.8 | $1,216.7 | $1,138.5 | $1,133.8 |

# TABLE 6

# KENTUCKY

*U.S. Registered Community Hospitals*
*(Nonfederal, short-term general and other special hospitals)*

## Overview 1999–2003

| | 2003 | 2002 | 2001 | 2000 | 1999 |
|---|---|---|---|---|---|
| **Total Community Hospitals in Kentucky** | **103** | **104** | **103** | **105** | **105** |
| **Bed Size Category** | | | | | |
| 6-24 | 1 | 2 | 1 | 3 | 2 |
| 25-49 | 27 | 21 | 20 | 19 | 22 |
| 50-99 | 26 | 33 | 33 | 30 | 29 |
| 100-199 | 21 | 21 | 22 | 27 | 27 |
| 200-299 | 13 | 13 | 14 | 14 | 12 |
| 300-399 | 7 | 6 | 6 | 6 | 9 |
| 400-499 | 5 | 5 | 5 | 4 | 2 |
| 500 + | 3 | 3 | 2 | 2 | 2 |
| **Location** | | | | | |
| Hospitals Urban | 32 | 32 | 32 | 33 | 33 |
| Hospitals Rural | 71 | 72 | 71 | 72 | 72 |
| **Control** | | | | | |
| State and Local Government | 13 | 14 | 14 | 15 | 14 |
| Not for Profit | 73 | 73 | 71 | 72 | 73 |
| Investor owned | 17 | 17 | 18 | 18 | 18 |
| **Physician Models** | | | | | |
| Independent Practice Association | 9 | 8 | 7 | 6 | 8 |
| Group Practice without Walls | 2 | 2 | 2 | 3 | 1 |
| Open Physician-Hospital Organization | 14 | 11 | 11 | 12 | 15 |
| Closed Physician-Hospital Organization | 1 | 1 | 1 | 1 | 6 |
| Management Service Organization | 4 | 3 | 3 | 12 | 14 |
| Integrated Salary Model | 29 | 31 | 29 | 24 | 21 |
| Equity Model | 0 | 0 | 0 | 0 | 1 |
| Foundation | 2 | 9 | 10 | 11 | 10 |
| **Insurance Products** | | | | | |
| Health Maintenance Organization | 25 | 23 | 22 | 17 | 20 |
| Preferred Provider Organization | 20 | 23 | 17 | 8 | 18 |
| Indemnity Fee for Service | 3 | 1 | 2 | 0 | 3 |
| **Managed Care Contracts** | | | | | |
| Health Maintenance Organization | 61 | 59 | 53 | 48 | 52 |
| Preferred Provider Organization | 73 | 70 | 68 | 54 | 69 |
| **Affiliations** | | | | | |
| Hospitals in a System* | 64 | 63 | 64 | 70 | 69 |
| Hospitals in a Network | 18 | 15 | 13 | 13 | 15 |
| Hospitals in a Group Purchasing Organization | 91 | 82 | 76 | 63 | 62 |

States

* Please note that system affiliate information for hospitals is derived from AHA membership. In years prior to 2003 the affiliation was derived from a question on the AHA Annual Survey of hospitals; therefore, non-responding hospitals were not included in the system affiliation counts. Years prior to 2003 have been updated to reflect this change, which now include affiliation for non-reporting hospitals.

# TABLE 6

# KENTUCKY

*U.S. Registered Community Hospitals*
*(Nonfederal, short-term general and other special hospitals)*

## Utilization, Personnel, Revenue and Expenses, Community Health Indicators 1999–2003

| | 2003 | 2002 | 2001 | 2000 | 1999 |
|---|---|---|---|---|---|
| **TOTAL FACILITY (Includes Hospital and Nursing Home Units)** | | | | | |
| **Utilization - Inpatient** | | | | | |
| Beds | 14,940 | 15,066 | 15,001 | 14,827 | 14,956 |
| Admissions | 600,454 | 601,644 | 594,899 | 581,620 | 569,792 |
| Inpatient Days | 3,394,239 | 3,393,525 | 3,315,218 | 3,333,314 | 3,296,591 |
| Average Length of Stay | 5.7 | 5.6 | 5.6 | 5.7 | 5.8 |
| Inpatient Surgeries | 169,619 | 180,073 | 167,283 | 170,029 | 164,304 |
| Births | 52,813 | 52,098 | 52,818 | 53,547 | 51,637 |
| **Utilization - Outpatient** | | | | | |
| Emergency Outpatient Visits | 2,137,500 | 2,109,556 | 1,985,284 | 1,953,727 | 1,990,266 |
| Other Outpatient Visits | 6,405,609 | 6,536,556 | 6,692,104 | 6,742,993 | 5,991,574 |
| Total Outpatient Visits | 8,543,109 | 8,646,112 | 8,677,388 | 8,696,720 | 7,981,840 |
| Outpatient Surgeries | 370,684 | 363,052 | 359,153 | 349,830 | 333,683 |
| **Personnel** | | | | | |
| Full Time RNs | 13,620 | 13,224 | 12,892 | 13,138 | 13,532 |
| Full Time LPNs | 2,749 | 2,361 | 2,427 | 2,206 | 2,362 |
| Part Time RNs | 6,706 | 6,354 | 5,229 | 5,041 | 5,217 |
| Part Time LPNs | 655 | 714 | 540 | 544 | 648 |
| Total Full Time | 56,016 | 56,104 | 57,175 | 55,775 | 54,147 |
| Total Part Time | 19,332 | 20,611 | 17,162 | 17,452 | 16,457 |
| **Revenue - Inpatient** | | | | | |
| Gross Inpatient Revenue | $9,477,812,427 | $8,677,558,625 | $7,787,598,143 | $6,926,847,867 | $6,349,440,581 |
| **Revenue - Outpatient** | | | | | |
| Gross Outpatient Revenue | $6,435,990,027 | $5,544,182,284 | $4,733,719,223 | $4,237,568,311 | $3,654,809,995 |
| **Revenue and Expenses - Totals (Includes Inpatient and Outpatient)** | | | | | |
| Total Gross Revenue | $15,913,802,454 | $14,221,740,909 | $12,521,317,366 | $11,164,416,178 | $10,004,250,576 |
| Deductions from Revenue | 9,289,949,832 | 7,943,529,393 | 6,819,797,436 | 5,892,730,890 | 5,113,919,722 |
| Net Patient Revenue | 6,623,852,622 | 6,278,211,516 | 5,701,519,930 | 5,271,685,288 | 4,890,330,854 |
| Other Operating Revenue | 286,235,427 | 264,424,862 | 264,715,481 | 250,730,317 | 237,393,468 |
| Other Nonoperating Revenue | 38,680,240 | 55,509,283 | 61,362,641 | 91,895,438 | 108,001,346 |
| Total Net Revenue | 6,948,768,289 | 6,598,145,661 | 6,027,598,052 | 5,614,311,043 | 5,235,725,668 |
| Total Expenses | 6,606,931,221 | 6,201,408,483 | 5,731,885,674 | 5,262,215,893 | 4,962,196,037 |
| **HOSPITAL UNIT (Excludes Separate Nursing Home Units)** | | | | | |
| **Utilization - Inpatient** | | | | | |
| Beds | 13,408 | 13,640 | 13,587 | 13,295 | 13,125 |
| Admissions | 590,914 | 591,970 | 584,628 | 570,135 | 555,394 |
| Inpatient Days | 2,932,767 | 2,999,495 | 2,863,991 | 2,844,864 | 2,716,093 |
| Average Length of Stay | 5.0 | 5.1 | 4.9 | 5.0 | 4.9 |
| **Personnel** | | | | | |
| Total Full Time | 54,630 | 54,958 | 55,916 | 54,545 | 52,598 |
| Total Part Time | 18,897 | 20,115 | 16,843 | 17,049 | 15,919 |
| **Revenue and Expenses - Totals (Includes Inpatient and Outpatient)** | | | | | |
| Total Net Revenue | $6,840,739,073 | $6,505,926,611 | $5,922,961,820 | $5,467,691,050 | $5,083,079,627 |
| Total Expenses | 6,523,073,019 | 6,126,969,102 | 5,659,683,174 | 5,142,390,665 | 4,876,938,853 |
| **COMMUNITY HEALTH INDICATORS PER 1000 POPULATION** | | | | | |
| Total Population (in thousands) | 4,118 | 4,090 | 4,067 | 4,049 | 4,018 |
| **Inpatient** | | | | | |
| Beds | 3.6 | 3.7 | 3.7 | 3.7 | 3.7 |
| Admissions | 145.8 | 147.1 | 146.3 | 143.7 | 141.8 |
| Inpatient Days | 824.3 | 829.7 | 815.1 | 823.3 | 820.4 |
| Inpatient Surgeries | 41.2 | 44.0 | 41.1 | 42.0 | 40.9 |
| Births | 12.8 | 12.7 | 13.0 | 13.2 | 12.9 |
| **Outpatient** | | | | | |
| Emergency Outpatient Visits | 519.1 | 515.8 | 488.1 | 482.6 | 495.3 |
| Other Outpatient Visits | 1,555.6 | 1,598.2 | 1,645.3 | 1,665.5 | 1,491.2 |
| Total Outpatient Visits | 2,074.7 | 2,114.1 | 2,133.4 | 2,148.1 | 1,986.5 |
| Outpatient Surgeries | 90.0 | 88.8 | 88.3 | 86.4 | 83.0 |
| **Expense per Capita (per person)** | $1,604.5 | $1,516.3 | $1,409.2 | $1,299.8 | $1,235.0 |

# TABLE 6

## LOUISIANA

*U.S. Registered Community Hospitals*
*(Nonfederal, short-term general and other special hospitals)*

## Overview 1999–2003

| | 2003 | 2002 | 2001 | 2000 | 1999 |
|---|---|---|---|---|---|
| **Total Community Hospitals in Louisiana** | **127** | **128** | **125** | **123** | **122** |
| **Bed Size Category** | | | | | |
| 6-24 | 11 | 10 | 9 | 6 | 5 |
| 25-49 | 32 | 33 | 29 | 29 | 29 |
| 50-99 | 29 | 30 | 30 | 33 | 31 |
| 100-199 | 25 | 28 | 30 | 27 | 32 |
| 200-299 | 12 | 8 | 11 | 11 | 8 |
| 300-399 | 8 | 9 | 6 | 8 | 11 |
| 400-499 | 5 | 5 | 4 | 4 | 4 |
| 500 + | 5 | 5 | 6 | 5 | 2 |
| **Location** | | | | | |
| Hospitals Urban | 78 | 77 | 76 | 75 | 74 |
| Hospitals Rural | 49 | 51 | 49 | 48 | 48 |
| **Control** | | | | | |
| State and Local Government | 50 | 52 | 55 | 55 | 55 |
| Not for Profit | 34 | 35 | 33 | 31 | 30 |
| Investor owned | 43 | 41 | 37 | 37 | 37 |
| **Physician Models** | | | | | |
| Independent Practice Association | 13 | 13 | 17 | 15 | 11 |
| Group Practice without Walls | 4 | 5 | 2 | 3 | 1 |
| Open Physician-Hospital Organization | 14 | 17 | 17 | 25 | 20 |
| Closed Physician-Hospital Organization | 4 | 8 | 15 | 14 | 13 |
| Management Service Organization | 7 | 8 | 10 | 15 | 18 |
| Integrated Salary Model | 18 | 19 | 16 | 19 | 14 |
| Equity Model | 1 | 1 | 0 | 0 | 1 |
| Foundation | 1 | 3 | 2 | 2 | 1 |
| **Insurance Products** | | | | | |
| Health Maintenance Organization | 8 | 8 | 9 | 12 | 18 |
| Preferred Provider Organization | 10 | 14 | 15 | 19 | 27 |
| Indemnity Fee for Service | 1 | 3 | 2 | 3 | 5 |
| **Managed Care Contracts** | | | | | |
| Health Maintenance Organization | 55 | 51 | 54 | 55 | 57 |
| Preferred Provider Organization | 65 | 62 | 69 | 70 | 72 |
| **Affiliations** | | | | | |
| Hospitals in a System* | 68 | 68 | 69 | 67 | 63 |
| Hospitals in a Network | 20 | 18 | 18 | 22 | 17 |
| Hospitals in a Group Purchasing Organization | 70 | 64 | 71 | 62 | 60 |

States

* Please note that system affiliate information for hospitals is derived from AHA membership. In years prior to 2003 the affiliation was derived from a question on the AHA Annual Survey of hospitals; therefore, non-responding hospitals were not included in the system affiliation counts. Years prior to 2003 have been updated to reflect this change, which now include affiliation for non-reporting hospitals.

# TABLE 6

# LOUISIANA

*U.S. Registered Community Hospitals*
*(Nonfederal, short-term general and other special hospitals)*

## Utilization, Personnel, Revenue and Expenses, Community Health Indicators 1999–2003

| | 2003 | 2002 | 2001 | 2000 | 1999 |
|---|---|---|---|---|---|
| **TOTAL FACILITY (Includes Hospital and Nursing Home Units)** | | | | | |
| **Utilization - Inpatient** | | | | | |
| Beds | 17,829 | 17,867 | 17,975 | 17,544 | 16,782 |
| Admissions | 690,246 | 692,011 | 682,586 | 654,323 | 626,801 |
| Inpatient Days | 3,872,912 | 3,873,634 | 3,736,536 | 3,569,621 | 3,472,409 |
| Average Length of Stay | 5.6 | 5.6 | 5.5 | 5.5 | 5.5 |
| Inpatient Surgeries | 171,599 | 179,986 | 172,824 | 179,651 | 174,051 |
| Births | 63,923 | 57,564 | 63,248 | 64,904 | 63,553 |
| **Utilization - Outpatient** | | | | | |
| Emergency Outpatient Visits | 2,498,935 | 2,468,832 | 2,267,490 | 2,143,846 | 2,182,109 |
| Other Outpatient Visits | 8,325,075 | 8,262,795 | 7,792,891 | 7,882,211 | 7,331,885 |
| Total Outpatient Visits | 10,824,010 | 10,731,627 | 10,060,381 | 10,026,057 | 9,513,994 |
| Outpatient Surgeries | 254,242 | 287,954 | 285,927 | 278,438 | 272,852 |
| **Personnel** | | | | | |
| Full Time RNs | 15,350 | 15,320 | 14,845 | 15,634 | 15,460 |
| Full Time LPNs | 3,296 | 3,186 | 3,202 | 3,711 | 3,849 |
| Part Time RNs | 5,413 | 5,973 | 5,472 | 5,630 | 4,586 |
| Part Time LPNs | 853 | 921 | 1,046 | 1,073 | 1,018 |
| Total Full Time | 69,524 | 69,541 | 68,540 | 70,010 | 68,263 |
| Total Part Time | 17,344 | 19,700 | 18,200 | 18,093 | 16,056 |
| **Revenue - Inpatient** | | | | | |
| Gross Inpatient Revenue | $12,094,846,990 | $10,679,535,909 | $9,096,048,174 | $8,243,500,319 | $7,543,819,679 |
| **Revenue - Outpatient** | | | | | |
| Gross Outpatient Revenue | $6,409,128,381 | $5,523,762,540 | $4,760,161,472 | $4,251,539,053 | $3,934,910,084 |
| **Revenue and Expenses - Totals (Includes Inpatient and Outpatient)** | | | | | |
| Total Gross Revenue | $18,503,975,371 | $16,203,298,449 | $13,856,209,646 | $12,495,039,372 | $11,478,729,763 |
| Deductions from Revenue | 11,323,461,934 | 9,401,154,343 | 7,622,952,381 | 6,598,655,986 | 5,462,495,406 |
| Net Patient Revenue | 7,180,513,437 | 6,802,144,106 | 6,233,257,265 | 5,896,383,386 | 6,016,234,357 |
| Other Operating Revenue | 342,156,916 | 271,896,066 | 267,094,438 | 242,589,117 | 431,151,639 |
| Other Nonoperating Revenue | 124,878,279 | 49,925,463 | 118,755,497 | 132,937,013 | 123,928,310 |
| Total Net Revenue | 7,647,548,632 | 7,123,965,635 | 6,619,107,200 | 6,271,909,516 | 6,571,314,306 |
| Total Expenses | 7,170,688,383 | 6,751,804,011 | 6,231,829,149 | 5,944,697,229 | 5,552,067,184 |
| **HOSPITAL UNIT (Excludes Separate Nursing Home Units)** | | | | | |
| **Utilization - Inpatient** | | | | | |
| Beds | 17,430 | 17,026 | 16,772 | 16,724 | 16,031 |
| Admissions | 687,450 | 687,478 | 676,446 | 645,795 | 617,298 |
| Inpatient Days | 3,747,426 | 3,657,799 | 3,433,204 | 3,333,668 | 3,256,709 |
| Average Length of Stay | 5.5 | 5.3 | 5.1 | 5.2 | 5.3 |
| **Personnel** | | | | | |
| Total Full Time | 68,913 | 68,904 | 67,852 | 68,743 | 67,579 |
| Total Part Time | 17,029 | 19,388 | 17,972 | 17,855 | 15,884 |
| **Revenue and Expenses - Totals (Includes Inpatient and Outpatient)** | | | | | |
| Total Net Revenue | $7,623,909,158 | $7,079,640,911 | $6,575,698,935 | $6,196,038,147 | $6,306,351,941 |
| Total Expenses | 7,147,825,517 | 6,714,901,922 | 6,196,893,942 | 5,901,358,320 | 5,509,175,610 |
| **COMMUNITY HEALTH INDICATORS PER 1000 POPULATION** | | | | | |
| Total Population (in thousands) | 4,496 | 4,476 | 4,466 | 4,469 | 4,461 |
| **Inpatient** | | | | | |
| Beds | 4.0 | 4.0 | 4.0 | 3.9 | 3.8 |
| Admissions | 153.5 | 154.6 | 152.8 | 146.4 | 140.5 |
| Inpatient Days | 861.3 | 865.4 | 836.7 | 798.7 | 778.4 |
| Inpatient Surgeries | 38.2 | 40.2 | 38.7 | 40.2 | 39.0 |
| Births | 14.2 | 12.9 | 14.2 | 14.5 | 14.2 |
| **Outpatient** | | | | | |
| Emergency Outpatient Visits | 555.8 | 551.5 | 507.7 | 479.7 | 489.2 |
| Other Outpatient Visits | 1,851.5 | 1,845.9 | 1,744.9 | 1,763.7 | 1,643.6 |
| Total Outpatient Visits | 2,407.3 | 2,397.5 | 2,252.7 | 2,243.4 | 2,132.8 |
| Outpatient Surgeries | 56.5 | 64.3 | 64.0 | 62.3 | 61.2 |
| **Expense per Capita (per person)** | $1,594.8 | $1,508.4 | $1,395.4 | $1,330.1 | $1,244.6 |

# TABLE 6

# MAINE

*U.S. Registered Community Hospitals*
*(Nonfederal, short-term general and other special hospitals)*

## Overview 1999–2003

| | 2003 | 2002 | 2001 | 2000 | 1999 |
|---|---|---|---|---|---|
| **Total Community Hospitals in Maine** | **37** | **37** | **37** | **37** | **37** |
| **Bed Size Category** | | | | | |
| 6-24 | 2 | 3 | 0 | 1 | 2 |
| 25-49 | 12 | 11 | 14 | 13 | 12 |
| 50-99 | 12 | 12 | 11 | 12 | 12 |
| 100-199 | 8 | 8 | 9 | 8 | 8 |
| 200-299 | 0 | 0 | 0 | 0 | 0 |
| 300-399 | 2 | 2 | 2 | 2 | 2 |
| 400-499 | 0 | 0 | 0 | 0 | 0 |
| 500 + | 1 | 1 | 1 | 1 | 1 |
| **Location** | | | | | |
| Hospitals Urban | 8 | 8 | 8 | 8 | 8 |
| Hospitals Rural | 29 | 29 | 29 | 29 | 29 |
| **Control** | | | | | |
| State and Local Government | 2 | 2 | 3 | 3 | 3 |
| Not for Profit | 34 | 34 | 33 | 33 | 33 |
| Investor owned | 1 | 1 | 1 | 1 | 1 |
| **Physician Models** | | | | | |
| Independent Practice Association | 5 | 4 | 4 | 3 | 3 |
| Group Practice without Walls | 2 | 2 | 1 | 1 | 2 |
| Open Physician-Hospital Organization | 14 | 15 | 16 | 12 | 13 |
| Closed Physician-Hospital Organization | 0 | 0 | 0 | 2 | 2 |
| Management Service Organization | 3 | 4 | 4 | 4 | 5 |
| Integrated Salary Model | 15 | 14 | 13 | 14 | 16 |
| Equity Model | 1 | 2 | 2 | 2 | 2 |
| Foundation | 1 | 2 | 2 | 0 | 0 |
| **Insurance Products** | | | | | |
| Health Maintenance Organization | 2 | 3 | 2 | 3 | 6 |
| Preferred Provider Organization | 5 | 4 | 3 | 4 | 7 |
| Indemnity Fee for Service | 1 | 2 | 2 | 2 | 2 |
| **Managed Care Contracts** | | | | | |
| Health Maintenance Organization | 22 | 24 | 28 | 28 | 27 |
| Preferred Provider Organization | 19 | 21 | 24 | 25 | 22 |
| **Affiliations** | | | | | |
| Hospitals in a System* | 14 | 15 | 16 | 15 | 15 |
| Hospitals in a Network | 18 | 18 | 16 | 15 | 13 |
| Hospitals in a Group Purchasing Organization | 33 | 34 | 31 | 31 | 30 |

States

* Please note that system affiliate information for hospitals is derived from AHA membership. In years prior to 2003 the affiliation was derived from a question on the AHA Annual Survey of hospitals; therefore, non-responding hospitals were not included in the system affiliation counts. Years prior to 2003 have been updated to reflect this change, which now include affiliation for non-reporting hospitals.

# TABLE 6

## MAINE

*U.S. Registered Community Hospitals*
*(Nonfederal, short-term general and other special hospitals)*

## Utilization, Personnel, Revenue and Expenses, Community Health Indicators 1999–2003

| | 2003 | 2002 | 2001 | 2000 | 1999 |
|---|---|---|---|---|---|
| **TOTAL FACILITY (Includes Hospital and Nursing Home Units)** | | | | | |
| **Utilization - Inpatient** | | | | | |
| Beds | 3,702 | 3,694 | 3,844 | 3,700 | 3,691 |
| Admissions | 148,517 | 145,917 | 148,612 | 147,236 | 146,378 |
| Inpatient Days | 816,332 | 889,005 | 898,059 | 867,352 | 872,635 |
| Average Length of Stay | 5.5 | 6.1 | 6.0 | 5.9 | 6.0 |
| Inpatient Surgeries | 45,340 | 60,022 | 45,682 | 45,114 | 44,045 |
| Births | 13,263 | 13,072 | 13,320 | 13,294 | 13,284 |
| **Utilization - Outpatient** | | | | | |
| Emergency Outpatient Visits | 710,201 | 709,091 | 700,510 | 673,853 | 579,803 |
| Other Outpatient Visits | 3,215,263 | 3,022,170 | 2,812,088 | 2,573,641 | 2,197,596 |
| Total Outpatient Visits | 3,925,464 | 3,731,261 | 3,512,598 | 3,247,494 | 2,777,399 |
| Outpatient Surgeries | 115,386 | 97,665 | 114,146 | 108,086 | 96,653 |
| **Personnel** | | | | | |
| Full Time RNs | 4,035 | 3,754 | 3,573 | 3,628 | 3,517 |
| Full Time LPNs | 283 | 241 | 270 | 302 | 352 |
| Part Time RNs | 3,428 | 3,449 | 3,005 | 2,964 | 2,725 |
| Part Time LPNs | 185 | 193 | 183 | 212 | 199 |
| Total Full Time | 17,983 | 17,038 | 16,599 | 16,403 | 15,485 |
| Total Part Time | 10,496 | 10,681 | 9,641 | 9,180 | 7,239 |
| **Revenue - Inpatient** | | | | | |
| Gross Inpatient Revenue | $2,191,849,628 | $2,019,706,879 | $1,812,197,212 | $1,698,718,945 | $1,520,624,429 |
| **Revenue - Outpatient** | | | | | |
| Gross Outpatient Revenue | $1,869,295,933 | $1,567,817,352 | $1,304,548,466 | $1,154,754,197 | $999,290,257 |
| **Revenue and Expenses - Totals (Includes Inpatient and Outpatient)** | | | | | |
| Total Gross Revenue | $4,061,145,561 | $3,587,524,231 | $3,116,745,678 | $2,853,473,142 | $2,519,914,686 |
| Deductions from Revenue | 1,774,902,165 | 1,488,086,115 | 1,217,966,635 | 1,115,439,062 | 915,152,948 |
| Net Patient Revenue | 2,286,243,396 | 2,099,438,116 | 1,898,779,043 | 1,738,034,080 | 1,604,761,738 |
| Other Operating Revenue | 76,610,152 | 72,149,218 | 65,237,618 | 57,843,349 | 55,504,484 |
| Other Nonoperating Revenue | 29,473,853 | 19,653,975 | 44,611,020 | 65,070,578 | 60,959,561 |
| Total Net Revenue | 2,392,327,401 | 2,191,241,309 | 2,008,627,681 | 1,860,948,007 | 1,721,225,783 |
| Total Expenses | 2,291,786,577 | 2,105,062,300 | 1,895,302,775 | 1,728,203,811 | 1,590,697,508 |
| **HOSPITAL UNIT (Excludes Separate Nursing Home Units)** | | | | | |
| **Utilization - Inpatient** | | | | | |
| Beds | 3,351 | 3,151 | 3,266 | 3,308 | 3,146 |
| Admissions | 146,917 | 144,016 | 146,398 | 145,274 | 144,095 |
| Inpatient Days | 704,903 | 714,141 | 715,018 | 744,933 | 702,828 |
| Average Length of Stay | 4.8 | 5.0 | 4.9 | 5.1 | 4.9 |
| **Personnel** | | | | | |
| Total Full Time | 17,502 | 16,584 | 16,166 | 16,052 | 15,042 |
| Total Part Time | 9,843 | 10,351 | 9,376 | 8,910 | 6,920 |
| **Revenue and Expenses - Totals (Includes Inpatient and Outpatient)** | | | | | |
| Total Net Revenue | $2,369,627,414 | $2,161,952,361 | $1,978,598,927 | $1,840,086,132 | $1,689,929,697 |
| Total Expenses | 2,269,425,051 | 2,081,511,605 | 1,864,078,445 | 1,710,294,770 | 1,569,334,589 |
| **COMMUNITY HEALTH INDICATORS PER 1000 POPULATION** | | | | | |
| Total Population (in thousands) | 1,306 | 1,295 | 1,285 | 1,277 | 1,267 |
| **Inpatient** | | | | | |
| Beds | 2.8 | 2.9 | 3.0 | 2.9 | 2.9 |
| Admissions | 113.7 | 112.7 | 115.7 | 115.3 | 115.5 |
| Inpatient Days | 625.2 | 686.5 | 699.0 | 679.1 | 688.8 |
| Inpatient Surgeries | 34.7 | 46.4 | 35.6 | 35.3 | 34.8 |
| Births | 10.2 | 10.1 | 10.4 | 10.4 | 10.5 |
| **Outpatient** | | | | | |
| Emergency Outpatient Visits | 543.9 | 547.6 | 545.3 | 527.6 | 457.7 |
| Other Outpatient Visits | 2,462.4 | 2,333.9 | 2,188.9 | 2,014.9 | 1,734.8 |
| Total Outpatient Visits | 3,006.3 | 2,881.5 | 2,734.2 | 2,542.5 | 2,192.4 |
| Outpatient Surgeries | 88.4 | 75.4 | 88.9 | 84.6 | 76.3 |
| **Expense per Capita (per person)** | $1,755.2 | $1,625.7 | $1,475.3 | $1,353.0 | $1,255.7 |

# Table 6

## MARYLAND

*U.S. Registered Community Hospitals*
*(Nonfederal, short-term general and other special hospitals)*

## Overview 1999–2003

| | 2003 | 2002 | 2001 | 2000 | 1999 |
|---|---|---|---|---|---|
| **Total Community Hospitals in Maryland** | **51** | **49** | **49** | **49** | **49** |
| **Bed Size Category** | | | | | |
| 6-24 | 0 | 0 | 0 | 0 | 0 |
| 25-49 | 3 | 4 | 3 | 3 | 3 |
| 50-99 | 7 | 5 | 6 | 5 | 4 |
| 100-199 | 16 | 15 | 15 | 18 | 19 |
| 200-299 | 12 | 11 | 12 | 11 | 9 |
| 300-399 | 8 | 9 | 8 | 6 | 9 |
| 400-499 | 2 | 2 | 2 | 3 | 1 |
| 500 + | 3 | 3 | 3 | 3 | 4 |
| **Location** | | | | | |
| Hospitals Urban | 41 | 40 | 40 | 40 | 40 |
| Hospitals Rural | 10 | 9 | 9 | 9 | 9 |
| **Control** | | | | | |
| State and Local Government | 1 | 0 | 0 | 0 | 0 |
| Not for Profit | 47 | 46 | 47 | 47 | 47 |
| Investor owned | 3 | 3 | 2 | 2 | 2 |
| **Physician Models** | | | | | |
| Independent Practice Association | 7 | 5 | 6 | 7 | 11 |
| Group Practice without Walls | 2 | 2 | 1 | 1 | 2 |
| Open Physician-Hospital Organization | 8 | 7 | 7 | 9 | 11 |
| Closed Physician-Hospital Organization | 2 | 3 | 5 | 4 | 7 |
| Management Service Organization | 3 | 2 | 3 | 5 | 15 |
| Integrated Salary Model | 25 | 23 | 23 | 19 | 20 |
| Equity Model | 3 | 3 | 3 | 4 | 5 |
| Foundation | 2 | 2 | 2 | 2 | 4 |
| **Insurance Products** | | | | | |
| Health Maintenance Organization | 12 | 10 | 16 | 14 | 10 |
| Preferred Provider Organization | 7 | 4 | 8 | 10 | 10 |
| Indemnity Fee for Service | 3 | 1 | 3 | 3 | 4 |
| **Managed Care Contracts** | | | | | |
| Health Maintenance Organization | 39 | 36 | 38 | 37 | 33 |
| Preferred Provider Organization | 36 | 32 | 34 | 32 | 29 |
| **Affiliations** | | | | | |
| Hospitals in a System* | 30 | 26 | 27 | 28 | 26 |
| Hospitals in a Network | 11 | 9 | 8 | 6 | 5 |
| Hospitals in a Group Purchasing Organization | 48 | 41 | 43 | 41 | 34 |

States

* Please note that system affiliate information for hospitals is derived from AHA membership. In years prior to 2003 the affiliation was derived from a question on the AHA Annual Survey of hospitals; therefore, non-responding hospitals were not included in the system affiliation counts. Years prior to 2003 have been updated to reflect this change, which now include affiliation for non-reporting hospitals.

# MARYLAND

*U.S. Registered Community Hospitals*
*(Nonfederal, short-term general and other special hospitals)*

## Utilization, Personnel, Revenue and Expenses, Community Health Indicators 1999–2003

| | 2003 | 2002 | 2001 | 2000 | 1999 |
|---|---|---|---|---|---|
| **TOTAL FACILITY (Includes Hospital and Nursing Home Units)** | | | | | |
| **Utilization - Inpatient** | | | | | |
| Beds | 11,613 | 11,417 | 11,234 | 11,192 | 11,629 |
| Admissions | 645,158 | 634,914 | 608,165 | 586,809 | 576,551 |
| Inpatient Days | 3,167,111 | 3,049,647 | 2,981,003 | 2,993,513 | 3,023,508 |
| Average Length of Stay | 4.9 | 4.8 | 4.9 | 5.1 | 5.2 |
| Inpatient Surgeries | 185,674 | 186,084 | 183,287 | 178,327 | 175,733 |
| Births | 65,861 | 63,744 | 63,843 | 64,030 | 62,251 |
| **Utilization - Outpatient** | | | | | |
| Emergency Outpatient Visits | 2,079,674 | 1,943,614 | 1,854,562 | 1,765,739 | 1,667,655 |
| Other Outpatient Visits | 4,442,692 | 4,520,569 | 4,411,827 | 4,251,883 | 4,275,428 |
| Total Outpatient Visits | 6,522,366 | 6,464,183 | 6,266,389 | 6,017,622 | 5,943,083 |
| Outpatient Surgeries | 347,734 | 347,715 | 330,571 | 335,445 | 320,799 |
| **Personnel** | | | | | |
| Full Time RNs | 13,209 | 11,975 | 11,196 | 11,629 | 12,145 |
| Full Time LPNs | 583 | 705 | 593 | 629 | 702 |
| Part Time RNs | 8,825 | 8,418 | 8,804 | 8,458 | 7,152 |
| Part Time LPNs | 300 | 357 | 338 | 365 | 515 |
| Total Full Time | 58,458 | 56,379 | 54,035 | 52,045 | 51,194 |
| Total Part Time | 25,552 | 24,293 | 25,913 | 25,896 | 23,098 |
| **Revenue - Inpatient** | | | | | |
| Gross Inpatient Revenue | $6,419,579,015 | $6,314,536,604 | $5,524,686,729 | $4,869,935,847 | $4,872,474,817 |
| **Revenue - Outpatient** | | | | | |
| Gross Outpatient Revenue | $3,161,027,418 | $3,110,642,148 | $2,614,614,189 | $2,239,872,994 | $2,014,087,252 |
| **Revenue and Expenses - Totals (Includes Inpatient and Outpatient)** | | | | | |
| Total Gross Revenue | $9,580,606,433 | $9,425,178,752 | $8,139,300,918 | $7,109,808,841 | $6,886,562,069 |
| Deductions from Revenue | 2,111,602,747 | 2,597,808,764 | 1,898,515,253 | 1,433,510,257 | 1,603,233,392 |
| Net Patient Revenue | 7,469,003,686 | 6,827,369,988 | 6,240,785,665 | 5,676,298,584 | 5,283,328,677 |
| Other Operating Revenue | 293,576,216 | 303,127,043 | 266,638,563 | 255,723,354 | 217,607,190 |
| Other Nonoperating Revenue | 58,685,721 | 25,174,124 | 43,785,690 | 91,201,507 | 82,290,784 |
| Total Net Revenue | 7,821,265,623 | 7,155,671,155 | 6,551,209,918 | 6,023,223,445 | 5,583,226,651 |
| Total Expenses | 7,601,418,187 | 6,971,693,586 | 6,345,348,924 | 5,872,418,845 | 5,457,297,063 |
| **HOSPITAL UNIT (Excludes Separate Nursing Home Units)** | | | | | |
| **Utilization - Inpatient** | | | | | |
| Beds | 10,796 | 10,726 | 10,575 | 10,297 | 10,699 |
| Admissions | 634,981 | 624,477 | 598,350 | 574,952 | 564,358 |
| Inpatient Days | 2,899,226 | 2,832,577 | 2,773,678 | 2,708,689 | 2,753,302 |
| Average Length of Stay | 4.6 | 4.5 | 4.6 | 4.7 | 4.9 |
| **Personnel** | | | | | |
| Total Full Time | 57,729 | 55,681 | 53,463 | 51,409 | 50,461 |
| Total Part Time | 25,201 | 23,927 | 25,579 | 25,392 | 22,627 |
| **Revenue and Expenses - Totals (Includes Inpatient and Outpatient)** | | | | | |
| Total Net Revenue | $7,736,373,266 | $7,070,224,974 | $6,462,828,420 | $5,938,396,900 | $5,486,858,411 |
| Total Expenses | 7,516,936,241 | 6,892,430,543 | 6,281,919,803 | 5,796,277,170 | 5,372,382,741 |
| **COMMUNITY HEALTH INDICATORS PER 1000 POPULATION** | | | | | |
| Total Population (in thousands) | 5,509 | 5,451 | 5,383 | 5,312 | 5,255 |
| **Inpatient** | | | | | |
| Beds | 2.1 | 2.1 | 2.1 | 2.1 | 2.2 |
| Admissions | 117.1 | 116.5 | 113.0 | 110.5 | 109.7 |
| Inpatient Days | 574.9 | 559.5 | 553.7 | 563.6 | 575.4 |
| Inpatient Surgeries | 33.7 | 34.1 | 34.0 | 33.6 | 33.4 |
| Births | 12.0 | 11.7 | 11.9 | 12.1 | 11.8 |
| **Outpatient** | | | | | |
| Emergency Outpatient Visits | 377.5 | 356.6 | 344.5 | 332.4 | 317.4 |
| Other Outpatient Visits | 806.5 | 829.4 | 819.5 | 800.5 | 813.7 |
| Total Outpatient Visits | 1,184.0 | 1,186.0 | 1,164.0 | 1,132.9 | 1,131.0 |
| Outpatient Surgeries | 63.1 | 63.8 | 61.4 | 63.2 | 61.1 |
| **Expense per Capita (per person)** | $1,379.8 | $1,279.1 | $1,178.7 | $1,105.6 | $1,038.6 |

# TABLE 6

# MASSACHUSETTS

*U.S. Registered Community Hospitals*
*(Nonfederal, short-term general and other special hospitals)*

## Overview 1999–2003

| | 2003 | 2002 | 2001 | 2000 | 1999 |
|---|---|---|---|---|---|
| **Total Community Hospitals in Massachusetts** | **79** | **78** | **80** | **80** | **79** |
| **Bed Size Category** | | | | | |
| 6-24 | 3 | 4 | 2 | 2 | 3 |
| 25-49 | 10 | 9 | 13 | 13 | 12 |
| 50-99 | 9 | 7 | 6 | 6 | 6 |
| 100-199 | 28 | 27 | 28 | 27 | 29 |
| 200-299 | 17 | 18 | 16 | 16 | 12 |
| 300-399 | 5 | 6 | 8 | 9 | 10 |
| 400-499 | 1 | 1 | 1 | 1 | 1 |
| 500 + | 6 | 6 | 6 | 6 | 6 |
| **Location** | | | | | |
| Hospitals Urban | 68 | 67 | 69 | 69 | 68 |
| Hospitals Rural | 11 | 11 | 11 | 11 | 11 |
| **Control** | | | | | |
| State and Local Government | 3 | 4 | 4 | 4 | 4 |
| Not for Profit | 68 | 68 | 70 | 70 | 69 |
| Investor owned | 8 | 6 | 6 | 6 | 6 |
| **Physician Models** | | | | | |
| Independent Practice Association | 33 | 34 | 31 | 31 | 37 |
| Group Practice without Walls | 7 | 8 | 10 | 9 | 9 |
| Open Physician-Hospital Organization | 15 | 17 | 18 | 19 | 21 |
| Closed Physician-Hospital Organization | 10 | 11 | 10 | 10 | 10 |
| Management Service Organization | 12 | 14 | 17 | 17 | 24 |
| Integrated Salary Model | 35 | 30 | 28 | 28 | 24 |
| Equity Model | 4 | 3 | 1 | 1 | 2 |
| Foundation | 5 | 6 | 5 | 6 | 10 |
| **Insurance Products** | | | | | |
| Health Maintenance Organization | 10 | 9 | 8 | 9 | 8 |
| Preferred Provider Organization | 6 | 6 | 4 | 5 | 6 |
| Indemnity Fee for Service | 4 | 1 | 1 | 1 | 2 |
| **Managed Care Contracts** | | | | | |
| Health Maintenance Organization | 62 | 62 | 60 | 56 | 62 |
| Preferred Provider Organization | 61 | 58 | 57 | 53 | 57 |
| **Affiliations** | | | | | |
| Hospitals in a System* | 39 | 38 | 42 | 43 | 39 |
| Hospitals in a Network | 20 | 21 | 22 | 21 | 22 |
| Hospitals in a Group Purchasing Organization | 62 | 54 | 55 | 50 | 53 |

* Please note that system affiliate information for hospitals is derived from AHA membership. In years prior to 2003 the affiliation was derived from a question on the AHA Annual Survey of hospitals; therefore, non-responding hospitals were not included in the system affiliation counts. Years prior to 2003 have been updated to reflect this change, which now include affiliation for non-reporting hospitals.

# MASSACHUSETTS

*U.S. Registered Community Hospitals*
*(Nonfederal, short-term general and other special hospitals)*

## Utilization, Personnel, Revenue and Expenses, Community Health Indicators 1999–2003

| | 2003 | 2002 | 2001 | 2000 | 1999 |
|---|---|---|---|---|---|
| **TOTAL FACILITY (Includes Hospital and Nursing Home Units)** | | | | | |
| **Utilization - Inpatient** | | | | | |
| Beds | 16,001 | 16,033 | 16,504 | 16,586 | 16,309 |
| Admissions | 784,618 | 765,820 | 766,708 | 740,286 | 739,375 |
| Inpatient Days | 4,372,515 | 4,348,099 | 4,382,048 | 4,289,840 | 4,210,454 |
| Average Length of Stay | 5.6 | 5.7 | 5.7 | 5.8 | 5.7 |
| Inpatient Surgeries | 211,618 | 205,077 | 212,539 | 217,649 | 214,009 |
| Births | 80,016 | 80,034 | 79,908 | 81,640 | 79,484 |
| **Utilization - Outpatient** | | | | | |
| Emergency Outpatient Visits | 2,929,681 | 2,882,602 | 2,717,815 | 2,715,812 | 2,726,113 |
| Other Outpatient Visits | 16,703,465 | 16,141,885 | 16,060,322 | 13,994,541 | 12,982,756 |
| Total Outpatient Visits | 19,633,146 | 19,024,487 | 18,778,137 | 16,710,353 | 15,708,869 |
| Outpatient Surgeries | 484,786 | 486,143 | 467,917 | 458,544 | 440,958 |
| **Personnel** | | | | | |
| Full Time RNs | 16,736 | 16,799 | 18,018 | 16,359 | 14,936 |
| Full Time LPNs | 974 | 1,206 | 1,236 | 1,207 | 854 |
| Part Time RNs | 17,473 | 15,846 | 16,968 | 18,591 | 17,782 |
| Part Time LPNs | 984 | 961 | 1,067 | 1,171 | 1,111 |
| Total Full Time | 96,845 | 99,089 | 101,474 | 93,354 | 87,466 |
| Total Part Time | 55,781 | 51,096 | 52,916 | 56,902 | 56,698 |
| **Revenue - Inpatient** | | | | | |
| Gross Inpatient Revenue | $14,495,247,329 | $12,947,175,259 | $12,173,968,661 | $11,247,798,711 | $9,839,772,237 |
| **Revenue - Outpatient** | | | | | |
| Gross Outpatient Revenue | $12,932,344,645 | $10,988,975,820 | $9,610,590,844 | $8,231,186,269 | $7,625,652,302 |
| **Revenue and Expenses - Totals (Includes Inpatient and Outpatient)** | | | | | |
| Total Gross Revenue | $27,427,591,974 | $23,936,151,079 | $21,784,559,505 | $19,478,984,980 | $17,465,424,539 |
| Deductions from Revenue | 15,140,167,010 | 12,756,840,606 | 11,457,845,346 | 10,026,437,014 | 8,646,920,813 |
| Net Patient Revenue | 12,287,424,964 | 11,179,310,473 | 10,326,714,159 | 9,452,547,966 | 8,818,503,726 |
| Other Operating Revenue | 2,515,283,376 | 1,822,811,119 | 1,636,890,502 | 1,232,552,918 | 1,299,771,155 |
| Other Nonoperating Revenue | 122,250,355 | -20,027,456 | 124,637,693 | 365,783,979 | 341,554,169 |
| Total Net Revenue | 14,924,958,695 | 12,982,094,136 | 12,088,242,354 | 11,050,884,863 | 10,459,829,050 |
| Total Expenses | 14,000,779,782 | 12,979,804,604 | 12,055,797,429 | 11,148,180,478 | 10,518,160,942 |
| **HOSPITAL UNIT (Excludes Separate Nursing Home Units)** | | | | | |
| **Utilization - Inpatient** | | | | | |
| Beds | 15,255 | 15,301 | 15,814 | 15,662 | 15,515 |
| Admissions | 768,485 | 754,165 | 757,011 | 725,509 | 720,669 |
| Inpatient Days | 4,130,356 | 4,118,738 | 4,140,284 | 3,993,613 | 3,980,792 |
| Average Length of Stay | 5.4 | 5.5 | 5.5 | 5.5 | 5.5 |
| **Personnel** | | | | | |
| Total Full Time | 96,223 | 98,795 | 101,143 | 92,938 | 86,618 |
| Total Part Time | 55,245 | 50,699 | 52,480 | 56,327 | 55,971 |
| **Revenue and Expenses - Totals (Includes Inpatient and Outpatient)** | | | | | |
| Total Net Revenue | $14,864,520,506 | $12,931,336,845 | $12,032,855,996 | $10,993,289,677 | $10,367,408,392 |
| Total Expenses | 13,946,133,825 | 12,931,961,619 | 12,015,811,316 | 11,098,723,636 | 10,444,538,511 |
| **COMMUNITY HEALTH INDICATORS PER 1000 POPULATION** | | | | | |
| Total Population (in thousands) | 6,433 | 6,422 | 6,400 | 6,362 | 6,317 |
| **Inpatient** | | | | | |
| Beds | 2.5 | 2.5 | 2.6 | 2.6 | 2.6 |
| Admissions | 122.0 | 119.3 | 119.8 | 116.4 | 117.0 |
| Inpatient Days | 679.7 | 677.1 | 684.7 | 674.3 | 666.5 |
| Inpatient Surgeries | 32.9 | 31.9 | 33.2 | 34.2 | 33.9 |
| Births | 12.4 | 12.5 | 12.5 | 12.8 | 12.6 |
| **Outpatient** | | | | | |
| Emergency Outpatient Visits | 455.4 | 448.9 | 424.7 | 426.9 | 431.5 |
| Other Outpatient Visits | 2,596.4 | 2,513.6 | 2,509.5 | 2,199.7 | 2,055.1 |
| Total Outpatient Visits | 3,051.7 | 2,962.5 | 2,934.1 | 2,626.6 | 2,486.6 |
| Outpatient Surgeries | 75.4 | 75.7 | 73.1 | 72.1 | 69.8 |
| **Expense per Capita (per person)** | $2,176.3 | $2,021.2 | $1,883.8 | $1,752.3 | $1,665.0 |

# TABLE 6

## MICHIGAN

*U.S. Registered Community Hospitals*
*(Nonfederal, short-term general and other special hospitals)*

## Overview 1999–2003

| | 2003 | 2002 | 2001 | 2000 | 1999 |
|---|---|---|---|---|---|
| **Total Community Hospitals in Michigan** | **144** | **145** | **145** | **146** | **145** |
| **Bed Size Category** | | | | | |
| 6-24 | 8 | 7 | 7 | 7 | 10 |
| 25-49 | 22 | 24 | 23 | 20 | 17 |
| 50-99 | 47 | 47 | 50 | 51 | 51 |
| 100-199 | 20 | 19 | 17 | 18 | 19 |
| 200-299 | 16 | 16 | 17 | 21 | 18 |
| 300-399 | 16 | 16 | 16 | 13 | 14 |
| 400-499 | 6 | 7 | 7 | 7 | 7 |
| 500 + | 9 | 9 | 8 | 9 | 9 |
| **Location** | | | | | |
| Hospitals Urban | 85 | 86 | 86 | 88 | 87 |
| Hospitals Rural | 59 | 59 | 59 | 58 | 58 |
| **Control** | | | | | |
| State and Local Government | 18 | 19 | 20 | 19 | 19 |
| Not for Profit | 122 | 122 | 122 | 124 | 122 |
| Investor owned | 4 | 4 | 3 | 3 | 4 |
| **Physician Models** | | | | | |
| Independent Practice Association | 24 | 23 | 22 | 23 | 25 |
| Group Practice without Walls | 11 | 12 | 13 | 13 | 7 |
| Open Physician-Hospital Organization | 53 | 55 | 58 | 55 | 44 |
| Closed Physician-Hospital Organization | 19 | 17 | 14 | 20 | 23 |
| Management Service Organization | 24 | 22 | 27 | 26 | 23 |
| Integrated Salary Model | 65 | 60 | 59 | 68 | 56 |
| Equity Model | 0 | 0 | 1 | 1 | 3 |
| Foundation | 8 | 5 | 4 | 5 | 6 |
| **Insurance Products** | | | | | |
| Health Maintenance Organization | 50 | 44 | 45 | 52 | 47 |
| Preferred Provider Organization | 57 | 52 | 52 | 66 | 60 |
| Indemnity Fee for Service | 16 | 13 | 11 | 18 | 14 |
| **Managed Care Contracts** | | | | | |
| Health Maintenance Organization | 117 | 111 | 117 | 114 | 106 |
| Preferred Provider Organization | 121 | 116 | 125 | 123 | 122 |
| **Affiliations** | | | | | |
| Hospitals in a System* | 77 | 73 | 74 | 69 | 68 |
| Hospitals in a Network | 57 | 50 | 50 | 56 | 46 |
| Hospitals in a Group Purchasing Organization | 129 | 124 | 124 | 125 | 119 |

* Please note that system affiliate information for hospitals is derived from AHA membership. In years prior to 2003 the affiliation was derived from a question on the AHA Annual Survey of hospitals; therefore, non-responding hospitals were not included in the system affiliation counts. Years prior to 2003 have been updated to reflect this change, which now include affiliation for non-reporting hospitals.

# TABLE 6

## MICHIGAN

*U.S. Registered Community Hospitals*
*(Nonfederal, short-term general and other special hospitals)*

## Utilization, Personnel, Revenue and Expenses, Community Health Indicators 1999–2003

| | 2003 | 2002 | 2001 | 2000 | 1999 |
|---|---|---|---|---|---|
| **TOTAL FACILITY (Includes Hospital and Nursing Home Units)** | | | | | |
| **Utilization - Inpatient** | | | | | |
| Beds | 25,820 | 26,130 | 25,630 | 26,074 | 26,144 |
| Admissions | 1,168,359 | 1,163,157 | 1,122,004 | 1,106,045 | 1,084,277 |
| Inpatient Days | 6,223,908 | 6,296,654 | 6,108,896 | 6,176,230 | 6,295,931 |
| Average Length of Stay | 5.3 | 5.4 | 5.4 | 5.6 | 5.8 |
| Inpatient Surgeries | 355,235 | 346,641 | 321,558 | 334,190 | 323,881 |
| Births | 128,886 | 127,754 | 126,846 | 131,092 | 128,720 |
| **Utilization - Outpatient** | | | | | |
| Emergency Outpatient Visits | 3,990,117 | 4,029,309 | 3,753,945 | 3,703,509 | 3,528,497 |
| Other Outpatient Visits | 23,184,923 | 21,837,056 | 22,230,144 | 21,157,782 | 18,843,667 |
| Total Outpatient Visits | 27,175,040 | 25,866,365 | 25,984,089 | 24,861,291 | 22,372,164 |
| Outpatient Surgeries | 792,887 | 739,878 | 702,275 | 650,872 | 661,422 |
| **Personnel** | | | | | |
| Full Time RNs | 25,864 | 25,067 | 25,106 | 25,678 | 24,608 |
| Full Time LPNs | 2,190 | 2,292 | 2,768 | 2,631 | 2,657 |
| Part Time RNs | 18,604 | 19,095 | 17,888 | 16,721 | 17,554 |
| Part Time LPNs | 1,568 | 1,750 | 2,420 | 1,764 | 2,068 |
| Total Full Time | 125,290 | 122,075 | 120,138 | 122,715 | 119,054 |
| Total Part Time | 61,194 | 63,009 | 60,068 | 54,816 | 58,407 |
| **Revenue - Inpatient** | | | | | |
| Gross Inpatient Revenue | $19,821,173,066 | $18,067,876,124 | $15,269,814,888 | $14,753,771,125 | $13,703,264,931 |
| **Revenue - Outpatient** | | | | | |
| Gross Outpatient Revenue | $15,428,984,110 | $13,502,108,253 | $12,008,967,077 | $10,951,098,666 | $9,612,610,858 |
| **Revenue and Expenses - Totals (Includes Inpatient and Outpatient)** | | | | | |
| Total Gross Revenue | $35,250,157,176 | $31,569,984,377 | $27,278,781,965 | $25,704,869,791 | $23,315,875,789 |
| Deductions from Revenue | 19,419,489,941 | 16,694,090,957 | 13,827,622,183 | 12,700,091,926 | 10,906,847,788 |
| Net Patient Revenue | 15,830,667,235 | 14,875,893,420 | 13,451,159,782 | 13,004,777,865 | 12,409,028,001 |
| Other Operating Revenue | 784,324,482 | 700,959,929 | 634,303,135 | 647,130,579 | 581,407,288 |
| Other Nonoperating Revenue | 113,029,604 | 19,519,553 | 122,735,458 | 687,142,951 | 515,479,497 |
| Total Net Revenue | 16,728,021,321 | 15,596,372,902 | 14,208,198,375 | 14,339,051,395 | 13,505,914,786 |
| Total Expenses | 16,333,925,475 | 15,321,064,736 | 13,891,061,790 | 13,456,111,469 | 12,897,935,106 |
| **HOSPITAL UNIT (Excludes Separate Nursing Home Units)** | | | | | |
| **Utilization - Inpatient** | | | | | |
| Beds | 23,985 | 24,354 | 23,868 | 24,012 | 23,841 |
| Admissions | 1,163,656 | 1,159,116 | 1,117,366 | 1,100,448 | 1,077,852 |
| Inpatient Days | 5,641,185 | 5,724,932 | 5,539,802 | 5,510,749 | 5,582,723 |
| Average Length of Stay | 4.8 | 4.9 | 5.0 | 5.0 | 5.2 |
| **Personnel** | | | | | |
| Total Full Time | 124,127 | 120,860 | 118,969 | 121,360 | 117,733 |
| Total Part Time | 60,504 | 62,308 | 59,286 | 54,005 | 57,651 |
| **Revenue and Expenses - Totals (Includes Inpatient and Outpatient)** | | | | | |
| Total Net Revenue | $16,618,881,265 | $15,477,617,658 | $14,113,345,021 | $14,241,432,247 | $13,399,295,963 |
| Total Expenses | 16,267,781,536 | 15,232,840,934 | 13,820,531,836 | 13,364,180,983 | 12,804,079,036 |
| **COMMUNITY HEALTH INDICATORS PER 1000 POPULATION** | | | | | |
| Total Population (in thousands) | 10,080 | 10,043 | 10,005 | 9,956 | 9,897 |
| **Inpatient** | | | | | |
| Beds | 2.6 | 2.6 | 2.6 | 2.6 | 2.6 |
| Admissions | 115.9 | 115.8 | 112.1 | 111.1 | 109.6 |
| Inpatient Days | 617.5 | 627.0 | 610.6 | 620.4 | 636.1 |
| Inpatient Surgeries | 35.2 | 34.5 | 32.1 | 33.6 | 32.7 |
| Births | 12.8 | 12.7 | 12.7 | 13.2 | 13.0 |
| **Outpatient** | | | | | |
| Emergency Outpatient Visits | 395.8 | 401.2 | 375.2 | 372.0 | 356.5 |
| Other Outpatient Visits | 2,300.1 | 2,174.3 | 2,221.9 | 2,125.2 | 1,904.0 |
| Total Outpatient Visits | 2,695.9 | 2,575.5 | 2,597.1 | 2,497.2 | 2,260.5 |
| Outpatient Surgeries | 78.7 | 73.7 | 70.2 | 65.4 | 66.8 |
| **Expense per Capita (per person)** | $1,620.4 | $1,525.5 | $1,388.4 | $1,351.6 | $1,303.2 |

# TABLE 6

## MINNESOTA

*U.S. Registered Community Hospitals*
*(Nonfederal, short-term general and other special hospitals)*

## Overview 1999–2003

| | 2003 | 2002 | 2001 | 2000 | 1999 |
|---|---|---|---|---|---|
| **Total Community Hospitals in Minnesota** | **131** | **133** | **133** | **135** | **134** |
| **Bed Size Category** | | | | | |
| 6-24 | 15 | 18 | 16 | 16 | 16 |
| 25-49 | 25 | 20 | 23 | 25 | 25 |
| 50-99 | 36 | 38 | 39 | 38 | 40 |
| 100-199 | 38 | 41 | 38 | 39 | 37 |
| 200-299 | 5 | 4 | 6 | 6 | 5 |
| 300-399 | 5 | 3 | 3 | 3 | 6 |
| 400-499 | 3 | 5 | 4 | 4 | 1 |
| 500 + | 4 | 4 | 4 | 4 | 4 |
| **Location** | | | | | |
| Hospitals Urban | 45 | 46 | 45 | 45 | 44 |
| Hospitals Rural | 86 | 87 | 88 | 90 | 90 |
| **Control** | | | | | |
| State and Local Government | 42 | 44 | 43 | 44 | 42 |
| Not for Profit | 89 | 89 | 90 | 91 | 92 |
| Investor owned | 0 | 0 | 0 | 0 | 0 |
| **Physician Models** | | | | | |
| Independent Practice Association | 29 | 24 | 24 | 21 | 15 |
| Group Practice without Walls | 6 | 2 | 2 | 1 | 1 |
| Open Physician-Hospital Organization | 13 | 8 | 9 | 8 | 7 |
| Closed Physician-Hospital Organization | 7 | 7 | 5 | 4 | 10 |
| Management Service Organization | 5 | 3 | 3 | 3 | 3 |
| Integrated Salary Model | 46 | 40 | 37 | 28 | 31 |
| Equity Model | 1 | 1 | 2 | 2 | 1 |
| Foundation | 2 | 2 | 3 | 1 | 5 |
| **Insurance Products** | | | | | |
| Health Maintenance Organization | 16 | 13 | 19 | 19 | 26 |
| Preferred Provider Organization | 16 | 16 | 18 | 22 | 20 |
| Indemnity Fee for Service | 5 | 5 | 3 | 5 | 9 |
| **Managed Care Contracts** | | | | | |
| Health Maintenance Organization | 65 | 64 | 70 | 62 | 60 |
| Preferred Provider Organization | 76 | 72 | 78 | 68 | 66 |
| **Affiliations** | | | | | |
| Hospitals in a System* | 64 | 64 | 61 | 63 | 64 |
| Hospitals in a Network | 24 | 22 | 21 | 17 | 14 |
| Hospitals in a Group Purchasing Organization | 103 | 95 | 104 | 94 | 75 |

* Please note that system affiliate information for hospitals is derived from AHA membership. In years prior to 2003 the affiliation was derived from a question on the AHA Annual Survey of hospitals; therefore, non-responding hospitals were not included in the system affiliation counts. Years prior to 2003 have been updated to reflect this change, which now include affiliation for non-reporting hospitals.

# TABLE 6

## MINNESOTA

*U.S. Registered Community Hospitals*
*(Nonfederal, short-term general and other special hospitals)*

## Utilization, Personnel, Revenue and Expenses, Community Health Indicators 1999–2003

| | 2003 | 2002 | 2001 | 2000 | 1999 |
|---|---|---|---|---|---|
| **TOTAL FACILITY (Includes Hospital and Nursing Home Units)** | | | | | |
| **Utilization - Inpatient** | | | | | |
| Beds | 16,439 | 16,659 | 16,508 | 16,705 | 16,458 |
| Admissions | 614,867 | 598,852 | 586,016 | 570,672 | 534,692 |
| Inpatient Days | 4,113,264 | 4,162,994 | 4,102,576 | 4,089,075 | 4,046,050 |
| Average Length of Stay | 6.7 | 7.0 | 7.0 | 7.2 | 7.6 |
| Inpatient Surgeries | 175,001 | 178,443 | 173,787 | 162,709 | 158,632 |
| Births | 68,492 | 68,220 | 67,706 | 61,900 | 65,535 |
| **Utilization - Outpatient** | | | | | |
| Emergency Outpatient Visits | 1,581,734 | 1,605,237 | 1,506,825 | 1,454,970 | 1,364,802 |
| Other Outpatient Visits | 7,602,634 | 7,296,661 | 7,059,035 | 5,880,642 | 5,085,822 |
| Total Outpatient Visits | 9,184,368 | 8,901,898 | 8,565,860 | 7,335,612 | 6,450,624 |
| Outpatient Surgeries | 288,902 | 279,781 | 269,459 | 265,564 | 267,683 |
| **Personnel** | | | | | |
| Full Time RNs | 8,322 | 7,750 | 7,296 | 7,235 | 8,404 |
| Full Time LPNs | 1,525 | 1,383 | 1,463 | 1,420 | 1,857 |
| Part Time RNs | 19,140 | 18,637 | 18,377 | 16,856 | 14,906 |
| Part Time LPNs | 2,605 | 2,452 | 2,612 | 2,614 | 2,845 |
| Total Full Time | 45,873 | 45,546 | 42,981 | 40,907 | 44,027 |
| Total Part Time | 56,699 | 56,063 | 56,308 | 52,536 | 47,798 |
| **Revenue - Inpatient** | | | | | |
| Gross Inpatient Revenue | $11,089,213,807 | $10,100,747,850 | $8,594,174,827 | $7,576,893,093 | $6,735,210,305 |
| **Revenue - Outpatient** | | | | | |
| Gross Outpatient Revenue | $6,771,151,253 | $6,116,730,184 | $5,096,222,863 | $4,321,208,532 | $3,755,772,176 |
| **Revenue and Expenses - Totals (Includes Inpatient and Outpatient)** | | | | | |
| Total Gross Revenue | $17,860,365,060 | $16,217,478,034 | $13,690,397,690 | $11,898,101,625 | $10,490,982,481 |
| Deductions from Revenue | 9,421,711,537 | 8,364,782,672 | 6,733,859,329 | 5,560,355,139 | 4,745,177,001 |
| Net Patient Revenue | 8,438,653,523 | 7,852,695,362 | 6,956,538,361 | 6,337,746,486 | 5,745,805,480 |
| Other Operating Revenue | 454,629,698 | 448,432,311 | 371,921,708 | 325,155,610 | 312,210,657 |
| Other Nonoperating Revenue | 96,685,979 | 42,923,367 | 77,288,116 | 160,470,734 | 137,362,929 |
| Total Net Revenue | 8,989,969,200 | 8,344,051,040 | 7,405,748,185 | 6,823,372,830 | 6,195,379,066 |
| Total Expenses | 8,522,793,912 | 7,883,926,731 | 7,067,072,024 | 6,411,848,478 | 5,807,149,050 |
| **HOSPITAL UNIT (Excludes Separate Nursing Home Units)** | | | | | |
| **Utilization - Inpatient** | | | | | |
| Beds | 12,304 | 13,078 | 12,558 | 12,669 | 12,737 |
| Admissions | 608,772 | 594,971 | 581,569 | 565,919 | 528,535 |
| Inpatient Days | 2,674,779 | 2,918,600 | 2,715,146 | 2,714,883 | 2,789,190 |
| Average Length of Stay | 4.4 | 4.9 | 4.7 | 4.8 | 5.3 |
| **Personnel** | | | | | |
| Total Full Time | 43,727 | 43,905 | 40,988 | 38,802 | 42,095 |
| Total Part Time | 53,056 | 53,701 | 53,557 | 49,441 | 45,255 |
| **Revenue and Expenses - Totals (Includes Inpatient and Outpatient)** | | | | | |
| Total Net Revenue | $8,766,867,394 | $8,180,139,592 | $7,227,917,429 | $6,659,630,244 | $6,039,668,626 |
| Total Expenses | 8,297,651,895 | 7,729,649,102 | 6,891,386,470 | 6,245,744,327 | 5,647,638,456 |
| **COMMUNITY HEALTH INDICATORS PER 1000 POPULATION** | | | | | |
| Total Population (in thousands) | 5,059 | 5,025 | 4,985 | 4,934 | 4,873 |
| **Inpatient** | | | | | |
| Beds | 3.2 | 3.3 | 3.3 | 3.4 | 3.4 |
| Admissions | 121.5 | 119.2 | 117.6 | 115.7 | 109.7 |
| Inpatient Days | 813.0 | 828.5 | 823.0 | 828.8 | 830.2 |
| Inpatient Surgeries | 34.6 | 35.5 | 34.9 | 33.0 | 32.6 |
| Births | 13.5 | 13.6 | 13.6 | 12.5 | 13.4 |
| **Outpatient** | | | | | |
| Emergency Outpatient Visits | 312.6 | 319.5 | 302.3 | 294.9 | 280.0 |
| Other Outpatient Visits | 1,502.7 | 1,452.1 | 1,416.0 | 1,191.9 | 1,043.6 |
| Total Outpatient Visits | 1,815.3 | 1,771.6 | 1,718.3 | 1,486.9 | 1,323.6 |
| Outpatient Surgeries | 57.1 | 55.7 | 54.1 | 53.8 | 54.9 |
| **Expense per Capita (per person)** | $1,684.6 | $1,569.0 | $1,417.6 | $1,299.6 | $1,191.6 |

# TABLE 6

# MISSISSIPPI

*U.S. Registered Community Hospitals*
*(Nonfederal, short-term general and other special hospitals)*

## Overview 1999–2003

| | 2003 | 2002 | 2001 | 2000 | 1999 |
|---|---|---|---|---|---|
| **Total Community Hospitals in Mississippi** | **92** | **91** | **96** | **95** | **96** |
| **Bed Size Category** | | | | | |
| 6-24 | 2 | 2 | 2 | 1 | 1 |
| 25-49 | 22 | 19 | 17 | 18 | 18 |
| 50-99 | 25 | 26 | 29 | 29 | 34 |
| 100-199 | 28 | 29 | 33 | 31 | 27 |
| 200-299 | 4 | 4 | 6 | 8 | 7 |
| 300-399 | 4 | 4 | 2 | 1 | 4 |
| 400-499 | 2 | 2 | 2 | 2 | 0 |
| 500 + | 5 | 5 | 5 | 5 | 5 |
| **Location** | | | | | |
| Hospitals Urban | 19 | 18 | 20 | 19 | 20 |
| Hospitals Rural | 73 | 73 | 76 | 76 | 76 |
| **Control** | | | | | |
| State and Local Government | 42 | 42 | 45 | 45 | 46 |
| Not for Profit | 26 | 25 | 27 | 26 | 28 |
| Investor owned | 24 | 24 | 24 | 24 | 22 |
| **Physician Models** | | | | | |
| Independent Practice Association | 8 | 11 | 5 | 13 | 11 |
| Group Practice without Walls | 4 | 10 | 4 | 9 | 8 |
| Open Physician-Hospital Organization | 20 | 21 | 18 | 22 | 27 |
| Closed Physician-Hospital Organization | 5 | 5 | 5 | 10 | 9 |
| Management Service Organization | 8 | 10 | 6 | 9 | 8 |
| Integrated Salary Model | 20 | 19 | 14 | 16 | 15 |
| Equity Model | 1 | 0 | 3 | 3 | 3 |
| Foundation | 8 | 11 | 11 | 12 | 13 |
| **Insurance Products** | | | | | |
| Health Maintenance Organization | 9 | 12 | 12 | 13 | 13 |
| Preferred Provider Organization | 45 | 50 | 47 | 48 | 53 |
| Indemnity Fee for Service | 13 | 15 | 15 | 15 | 15 |
| **Managed Care Contracts** | | | | | |
| Health Maintenance Organization | 2 | 10 | 2 | 0 | 1 |
| Preferred Provider Organization | 5 | 39 | 38 | 3 | 0 |
| **Affiliations** | | | | | |
| Hospitals in a System* | 35 | 36 | 40 | 42 | 42 |
| Hospitals in a Network | 34 | 35 | 32 | 35 | 32 |
| Hospitals in a Group Purchasing Organization | 7 | 8 | 1 | — | — |

States

* Please note that system affiliate information for hospitals is derived from AHA membership. In years prior to 2003 the affiliation was derived from a question on the AHA Annual Survey of hospitals; therefore, non-responding hospitals were not included in the system affiliation counts. Years prior to 2003 have been updated to reflect this change, which now include affiliation for non-reporting hospitals.

## TABLE 6

# MISSISSIPPI

*U.S. Registered Community Hospitals*
*(Nonfederal, short-term general and other special hospitals)*

## Utilization, Personnel, Revenue and Expenses, Community Health Indicators 1999–2003

| | 2003 | 2002 | 2001 | 2000 | 1999 |
|---|---|---|---|---|---|
| **TOTAL FACILITY (Includes Hospital and Nursing Home Units)** | | | | | |
| **Utilization - Inpatient** | | | | | |
| Beds | 13,040 | 13,144 | 13,670 | 13,598 | 13,217 |
| Admissions | 415,909 | 416,815 | 436,100 | 424,772 | 415,776 |
| Inpatient Days | 2,696,522 | 2,745,516 | 2,990,906 | 2,929,248 | 2,916,549 |
| Average Length of Stay | 6.5 | 6.6 | 6.9 | 6.9 | 7.0 |
| Inpatient Surgeries | 123,033 | 121,710 | 116,292 | 111,465 | 120,663 |
| Births | 39,540 | 39,553 | 42,049 | 42,199 | 40,410 |
| **Utilization - Outpatient** | | | | | |
| Emergency Outpatient Visits | 1,597,509 | 1,556,488 | 1,501,052 | 1,478,883 | 1,429,819 |
| Other Outpatient Visits | 2,401,457 | 2,439,892 | 2,601,447 | 2,228,914 | 2,027,658 |
| Total Outpatient Visits | 3,998,966 | 3,996,380 | 4,102,499 | 3,707,797 | 3,457,477 |
| Outpatient Surgeries | 142,791 | 152,172 | 154,317 | 151,832 | 145,593 |
| **Personnel** | | | | | |
| Full Time RNs | 9,529 | 9,091 | 9,467 | 9,424 | 9,594 |
| Full Time LPNs | 1,951 | 1,923 | 2,025 | 2,001 | 2,170 |
| Part Time RNs | 3,763 | 3,906 | 3,636 | 3,185 | 2,728 |
| Part Time LPNs | 611 | 615 | 648 | 583 | 626 |
| Total Full Time | 41,081 | 40,107 | 40,936 | 39,550 | 40,398 |
| Total Part Time | 11,821 | 11,478 | 11,627 | 11,597 | 10,122 |
| **Revenue - Inpatient** | | | | | |
| Gross Inpatient Revenue | $6,235,537,687 | $5,702,037,800 | $5,203,288,483 | $4,486,744,256 | $4,219,185,699 |
| **Revenue - Outpatient** | | | | | |
| Gross Outpatient Revenue | $3,630,142,778 | $3,320,188,769 | $2,891,655,269 | $2,471,664,887 | $2,196,978,616 |
| **Revenue and Expenses - Totals (Includes Inpatient and Outpatient)** | | | | | |
| Total Gross Revenue | $9,865,680,465 | $9,022,226,569 | $8,094,943,752 | $6,958,409,143 | $6,416,164,315 |
| Deductions from Revenue | 5,715,365,284 | 4,977,500,289 | 4,344,923,458 | 3,645,598,561 | 3,165,780,811 |
| Net Patient Revenue | 4,150,315,181 | 4,044,726,280 | 3,750,020,294 | 3,312,810,582 | 3,250,383,504 |
| Other Operating Revenue | 167,113,664 | 164,171,241 | 137,215,985 | 191,115,070 | 116,160,034 |
| Other Nonoperating Revenue | 66,551,838 | 60,542,992 | 52,257,480 | 67,563,680 | 50,570,163 |
| Total Net Revenue | 4,383,980,683 | 4,269,440,513 | 3,939,493,759 | 3,571,489,332 | 3,417,113,701 |
| Total Expenses | 4,056,824,801 | 3,907,203,934 | 3,614,544,722 | 3,327,375,432 | 3,202,825,608 |
| **HOSPITAL UNIT (Excludes Separate Nursing Home Units)** | | | | | |
| **Utilization - Inpatient** | | | | | |
| Beds | 11,510 | 11,579 | 12,000 | 11,995 | 11,633 |
| Admissions | 414,762 | 415,182 | 434,827 | 423,739 | 414,619 |
| Inpatient Days | 2,206,104 | 2,217,217 | 2,400,974 | 2,358,912 | 2,355,643 |
| Average Length of Stay | 5.3 | 5.3 | 5.5 | 5.6 | 5.7 |
| **Personnel** | | | | | |
| Total Full Time | 39,851 | 39,009 | 39,670 | 38,528 | 39,375 |
| Total Part Time | 11,510 | 11,212 | 11,254 | 11,248 | 9,815 |
| **Revenue and Expenses - Totals (Includes Inpatient and Outpatient)** | | | | | |
| Total Net Revenue | $4,326,841,865 | $4,211,247,202 | $3,896,587,199 | $3,515,536,637 | $3,377,670,317 |
| Total Expenses | 4,010,876,381 | 3,866,957,946 | 3,583,850,640 | 3,293,094,874 | 3,174,354,952 |
| **COMMUNITY HEALTH INDICATORS PER 1000 POPULATION** | | | | | |
| Total Population (in thousands) | 2,881 | 2,867 | 2,858 | 2,848 | 2,828 |
| **Inpatient** | | | | | |
| Beds | 4.5 | 4.6 | 4.8 | 4.8 | 4.7 |
| Admissions | 144.3 | 145.4 | 152.6 | 149.1 | 147.0 |
| Inpatient Days | 935.9 | 957.7 | 1,046.6 | 1,028.4 | 1,031.2 |
| Inpatient Surgeries | 42.7 | 42.5 | 40.7 | 39.1 | 42.7 |
| Births | 13.7 | 13.8 | 14.7 | 14.8 | 14.3 |
| **Outpatient** | | | | | |
| Emergency Outpatient Visits | 554.4 | 542.9 | 525.3 | 519.2 | 505.5 |
| Other Outpatient Visits | 833.5 | 851.1 | 910.3 | 782.5 | 716.9 |
| Total Outpatient Visits | 1,387.9 | 1,394.1 | 1,435.6 | 1,301.7 | 1,222.4 |
| Outpatient Surgeries | 49.6 | 53.1 | 54.0 | 53.3 | 51.5 |
| **Expense per Capita (per person)** | $1,408.0 | $1,362.9 | $1,264.8 | $1,168.1 | $1,132.4 |

# TABLE 6

## MISSOURI

*U.S. Registered Community Hospitals*
*(Nonfederal, short-term general and other special hospitals)*

## Overview 1999–2003

| | 2003 | 2002 | 2001 | 2000 | 1999 |
|---|---|---|---|---|---|
| **Total Community Hospitals in Missouri** | **119** | **119** | **117** | **119** | **118** |
| **Bed Size Category** | | | | | |
| 6-24 | 6 | 6 | 4 | 4 | 4 |
| 25-49 | 31 | 31 | 31 | 33 | 29 |
| 50-99 | 25 | 25 | 25 | 24 | 28 |
| 100-199 | 22 | 22 | 22 | 21 | 21 |
| 200-299 | 15 | 17 | 16 | 17 | 13 |
| 300-399 | 8 | 9 | 8 | 9 | 13 |
| 400-499 | 6 | 4 | 5 | 4 | 2 |
| 500 + | 6 | 5 | 6 | 7 | 8 |
| **Location** | | | | | |
| Hospitals Urban | 61 | 61 | 60 | 61 | 60 |
| Hospitals Rural | 58 | 58 | 57 | 58 | 58 |
| **Control** | | | | | |
| State and Local Government | 36 | 36 | 36 | 37 | 35 |
| Not for Profit | 67 | 68 | 69 | 71 | 71 |
| Investor owned | 16 | 15 | 12 | 11 | 12 |
| **Physician Models** | | | | | |
| Independent Practice Association | 18 | 17 | 17 | 22 | 19 |
| Group Practice without Walls | 5 | 2 | 4 | 8 | 8 |
| Open Physician-Hospital Organization | 19 | 21 | 26 | 30 | 32 |
| Closed Physician-Hospital Organization | 14 | 13 | 16 | 17 | 23 |
| Management Service Organization | 7 | 10 | 10 | 9 | 17 |
| Integrated Salary Model | 52 | 52 | 50 | 49 | 50 |
| Equity Model | 0 | 2 | 1 | 3 | 2 |
| Foundation | 1 | 1 | 4 | 3 | 2 |
| **Insurance Products** | | | | | |
| Health Maintenance Organization | 21 | 28 | 31 | 48 | 57 |
| Preferred Provider Organization | 13 | 22 | 22 | 29 | 35 |
| Indemnity Fee for Service | 6 | 11 | 12 | 11 | 14 |
| **Managed Care Contracts** | | | | | |
| Health Maintenance Organization | 102 | 100 | 99 | 105 | 104 |
| Preferred Provider Organization | 109 | 108 | 106 | 112 | 99 |
| **Affiliations** | | | | | |
| Hospitals in a System* | 67 | 66 | 66 | 63 | 58 |
| Hospitals in a Network | 33 | 39 | 43 | 44 | 40 |
| Hospitals in a Group Purchasing Organization | 110 | 107 | 103 | 105 | 100 |

* Please note that system affiliate information for hospitals is derived from AHA membership. In years prior to 2003 the affiliation was derived from a question on the AHA Annual Survey of hospitals; therefore, non-responding hospitals were not included in the system affiliation counts. Years prior to 2003 have been updated to reflect this change, which now include affiliation for non-reporting hospitals.

# TABLE 6

## MISSOURI

*U.S. Registered Community Hospitals*
*(Nonfederal, short-term general and other special hospitals)*

## Utilization, Personnel, Revenue and Expenses, Community Health Indicators 1999–2003

| | 2003 | 2002 | 2001 | 2000 | 1999 |
|---|---|---|---|---|---|
| **TOTAL FACILITY (Includes Hospital and Nursing Home Units)** | | | | | |
| **Utilization - Inpatient** | | | | | |
| Beds | 19,346 | 18,891 | 19,257 | 20,140 | 20,253 |
| Admissions | 831,210 | 809,355 | 800,648 | 773,261 | 742,867 |
| Inpatient Days | 4,342,987 | 4,235,298 | 4,219,659 | 4,269,800 | 4,247,921 |
| Average Length of Stay | 5.2 | 5.2 | 5.3 | 5.5 | 5.7 |
| Inpatient Surgeries | 205,270 | 209,739 | 210,030 | 207,476 | 200,706 |
| Births | 78,564 | 74,815 | 75,350 | 77,333 | 75,625 |
| **Utilization - Outpatient** | | | | | |
| Emergency Outpatient Visits | 2,624,926 | 2,476,194 | 2,443,744 | 2,326,906 | 2,411,820 |
| Other Outpatient Visits | 13,043,778 | 12,427,894 | 11,755,063 | 12,479,871 | 12,231,541 |
| Total Outpatient Visits | 15,668,704 | 14,904,088 | 14,198,807 | 14,806,777 | 14,643,361 |
| Outpatient Surgeries | 393,167 | 393,761 | 389,098 | 381,289 | 362,462 |
| **Personnel** | | | | | |
| Full Time RNs | 19,034 | 19,236 | 18,576 | 18,689 | 18,685 |
| Full Time LPNs | 2,860 | 3,039 | 2,881 | 3,019 | 2,917 |
| Part Time RNs | 12,255 | 11,417 | 12,017 | 11,206 | 10,562 |
| Part Time LPNs | 1,192 | 1,174 | 1,171 | 1,221 | 1,162 |
| Total Full Time | 87,529 | 85,983 | 82,978 | 82,820 | 79,501 |
| Total Part Time | 37,338 | 35,177 | 35,676 | 34,263 | 31,230 |
| **Revenue - Inpatient** | | | | | |
| Gross Inpatient Revenue | $15,395,529,429 | $13,686,358,547 | $12,106,385,281 | $11,082,223,366 | $9,964,294,835 |
| **Revenue - Outpatient** | | | | | |
| Gross Outpatient Revenue | $10,090,913,418 | $8,390,580,917 | $7,685,930,325 | $6,685,962,437 | $5,791,429,121 |
| **Revenue and Expenses - Totals (Includes Inpatient and Outpatient)** | | | | | |
| Total Gross Revenue | $25,486,442,847 | $22,076,939,464 | $19,792,315,606 | $17,768,185,803 | $15,755,723,956 |
| Deductions from Revenue | 14,843,065,456 | 12,532,916,322 | 10,984,983,535 | 9,652,801,745 | 8,213,774,013 |
| Net Patient Revenue | 10,643,377,391 | 9,544,023,142 | 8,807,332,071 | 8,115,384,058 | 7,541,949,943 |
| Other Operating Revenue | 720,949,265 | 570,212,535 | 486,319,667 | 440,053,995 | 484,296,906 |
| Other Nonoperating Revenue | 266,984,711 | 89,622,933 | 154,063,942 | 196,916,165 | 197,565,929 |
| Total Net Revenue | 11,631,311,367 | 10,203,858,610 | 9,447,715,680 | 8,752,354,218 | 8,223,812,778 |
| Total Expenses | 10,852,258,947 | 9,747,670,518 | 9,118,864,692 | 8,534,174,151 | 7,953,842,591 |
| **HOSPITAL UNIT (Excludes Separate Nursing Home Units)** | | | | | |
| **Utilization - Inpatient** | | | | | |
| Beds | 17,898 | 17,396 | 17,642 | 18,096 | 18,003 |
| Admissions | 816,595 | 791,849 | 779,379 | 746,131 | 712,942 |
| Inpatient Days | 3,934,255 | 3,844,365 | 3,781,344 | 3,724,585 | 3,599,897 |
| Average Length of Stay | 4.8 | 4.9 | 4.9 | 5.0 | 5.0 |
| **Personnel** | | | | | |
| Total Full Time | 86,094 | 85,531 | 81,903 | 81,237 | 77,895 |
| Total Part Time | 36,831 | 34,767 | 35,092 | 33,437 | 30,530 |
| **Revenue and Expenses - Totals (Includes Inpatient and Outpatient)** | | | | | |
| Total Net Revenue | $11,480,749,638 | $10,043,647,885 | $9,292,053,516 | $8,558,718,897 | $8,054,357,353 |
| Total Expenses | 10,738,245,530 | 9,620,134,560 | 8,999,337,551 | 8,392,524,096 | 7,825,633,137 |
| **COMMUNITY HEALTH INDICATORS PER 1000 POPULATION** | | | | | |
| Total Population (in thousands) | 5,704 | 5,670 | 5,636 | 5,606 | 5,562 |
| **Inpatient** | | | | | |
| Beds | 3.4 | 3.3 | 3.4 | 3.6 | 3.6 |
| Admissions | 145.7 | 142.8 | 142.1 | 137.9 | 133.6 |
| Inpatient Days | 761.3 | 747.0 | 748.7 | 761.6 | 763.7 |
| Inpatient Surgeries | 36.0 | 37.0 | 37.3 | 37.0 | 36.1 |
| Births | 13.8 | 13.2 | 13.4 | 13.8 | 13.6 |
| **Outpatient** | | | | | |
| Emergency Outpatient Visits | 460.2 | 436.8 | 433.6 | 415.1 | 433.6 |
| Other Outpatient Visits | 2,286.6 | 2,192.0 | 2,085.6 | 2,226.2 | 2,199.1 |
| Total Outpatient Visits | 2,746.7 | 2,628.8 | 2,519.2 | 2,641.2 | 2,632.8 |
| Outpatient Surgeries | 68.9 | 69.5 | 69.0 | 68.0 | 65.2 |
| **Expense per Capita (per person)** | $1,902.4 | $1,719.3 | $1,617.9 | $1,522.3 | $1,430.0 |

# TABLE 6

# MONTANA

*U.S. Registered Community Hospitals*
*(Nonfederal, short-term general and other special hospitals)*

## Overview 1999–2003

| | 2003 | 2002 | 2001 | 2000 | 1999 |
|---|---|---|---|---|---|
| **Total Community Hospitals in Montana** | **53** | **53** | **53** | **52** | **53** |
| **Bed Size Category** | | | | | |
| 6-24 | 8 | 8 | 7 | 7 | 7 |
| 25-49 | 16 | 15 | 15 | 14 | 13 |
| 50-99 | 17 | 18 | 17 | 19 | 19 |
| 100-199 | 8 | 9 | 10 | 8 | 9 |
| 200-299 | 2 | 1 | 2 | 2 | 3 |
| 300-399 | 1 | 2 | 1 | 1 | 1 |
| 400-499 | 1 | 0 | 1 | 1 | 1 |
| 500 + | 0 | 0 | 0 | 0 | 0 |
| **Location** | | | | | |
| Hospitals Urban | 5 | 5 | 5 | 3 | 3 |
| Hospitals Rural | 48 | 48 | 48 | 49 | 50 |
| **Control** | | | | | |
| State and Local Government | 10 | 10 | 11 | 10 | 12 |
| Not for Profit | 43 | 43 | 42 | 42 | 41 |
| Investor owned | 0 | 0 | 0 | 0 | 0 |
| **Physician Models** | | | | | |
| Independent Practice Association | 10 | 6 | 7 | 11 | 5 |
| Group Practice without Walls | 3 | 3 | 3 | 3 | 1 |
| Open Physician-Hospital Organization | 7 | 7 | 9 | 9 | 9 |
| Closed Physician-Hospital Organization | 0 | 1 | 1 | 1 | 3 |
| Management Service Organization | 6 | 6 | 6 | 5 | 2 |
| Integrated Salary Model | 24 | 22 | 18 | 16 | 16 |
| Equity Model | 0 | 1 | 1 | 0 | 0 |
| Foundation | 0 | 2 | 2 | 5 | 1 |
| **Insurance Products** | | | | | |
| Health Maintenance Organization | 4 | 4 | 5 | 7 | 7 |
| Preferred Provider Organization | 9 | 6 | 5 | 6 | 3 |
| Indemnity Fee for Service | 7 | 3 | 2 | 2 | 2 |
| **Managed Care Contracts** | | | | | |
| Health Maintenance Organization | 12 | 13 | 12 | 14 | 15 |
| Preferred Provider Organization | 28 | 23 | 24 | 26 | 20 |
| **Affiliations** | | | | | |
| Hospitals in a System* | 14 | 16 | 16 | 15 | 16 |
| Hospitals in a Network | 22 | 25 | 23 | 22 | 21 |
| Hospitals in a Group Purchasing Organization | 47 | 47 | 47 | 48 | 42 |



* Please note that system affiliate information for hospitals is derived from AHA membership. In years prior to 2003 the affiliation was derived from a question on the AHA Annual Survey of hospitals; therefore, non-responding hospitals were not included in the system affiliation counts. Years prior to 2003 have been updated to reflect this change, which now include affiliation for non-reporting hospitals.

# Table 6

## MONTANA

*U.S. Registered Community Hospitals*
*(Nonfederal, short-term general and other special hospitals)*

## Utilization, Personnel, Revenue and Expenses, Community Health Indicators 1999–2003

| | 2003 | 2002 | 2001 | 2000 | 1999 |
|---|---|---|---|---|---|
| **TOTAL FACILITY (Includes Hospital and Nursing Home Units)** | | | | | |
| **Utilization - Inpatient** | | | | | |
| Beds | 4,326 | 4,263 | 4,463 | 4,255 | 4,668 |
| Admissions | 107,024 | 106,758 | 103,346 | 99,273 | 97,875 |
| Inpatient Days | 1,049,607 | 1,071,834 | 1,058,079 | 1,045,460 | 1,161,334 |
| Average Length of Stay | 9.8 | 10.0 | 10.2 | 10.5 | 11.9 |
| Inpatient Surgeries | 34,689 | 32,343 | 31,774 | 31,365 | 30,824 |
| Births | 10,301 | 9,963 | 9,766 | 9,828 | 9,826 |
| **Utilization - Outpatient** | | | | | |
| Emergency Outpatient Visits | 301,772 | 276,829 | 276,175 | 270,905 | 263,239 |
| Other Outpatient Visits | 2,435,962 | 2,381,906 | 2,372,170 | 2,377,671 | 2,276,174 |
| Total Outpatient Visits | 2,737,734 | 2,658,735 | 2,648,345 | 2,648,576 | 2,539,413 |
| Outpatient Surgeries | 39,301 | 38,792 | 37,544 | 38,146 | 38,123 |
| **Personnel** | | | | | |
| Full Time RNs | 2,200 | 2,233 | 2,139 | 2,262 | 2,206 |
| Full Time LPNs | 489 | 487 | 493 | 520 | 480 |
| Part Time RNs | 1,798 | 1,819 | 1,695 | 1,705 | 1,415 |
| Part Time LPNs | 344 | 322 | 347 | 375 | 263 |
| Total Full Time | 11,912 | 11,834 | 11,464 | 11,394 | 11,578 |
| Total Part Time | 6,757 | 6,893 | 6,492 | 6,319 | 5,676 |
| **Revenue - Inpatient** | | | | | |
| Gross Inpatient Revenue | $1,311,517,596 | $1,196,591,796 | $1,105,228,828 | $999,654,818 | $926,618,947 |
| **Revenue - Outpatient** | | | | | |
| Gross Outpatient Revenue | $1,029,438,041 | $928,260,803 | $835,450,580 | $737,774,057 | $667,505,475 |
| **Revenue and Expenses - Totals (Includes Inpatient and Outpatient)** | | | | | |
| Total Gross Revenue | $2,340,955,637 | $2,124,852,599 | $1,940,679,408 | $1,737,428,875 | $1,594,124,422 |
| Deductions from Revenue | 933,232,336 | 805,155,142 | 727,980,516 | 625,526,349 | 527,906,272 |
| Net Patient Revenue | 1,407,723,301 | 1,319,697,457 | 1,212,698,892 | 1,111,902,526 | 1,066,218,150 |
| Other Operating Revenue | 62,722,453 | 54,199,364 | 52,002,157 | 46,591,161 | 64,179,153 |
| Other Nonoperating Revenue | 9,609,816 | 11,449,900 | 29,771,646 | 37,823,173 | 29,299,977 |
| Total Net Revenue | 1,480,055,570 | 1,385,346,721 | 1,294,472,695 | 1,196,316,860 | 1,159,697,280 |
| Total Expenses | 1,440,703,717 | 1,328,470,349 | 1,216,570,389 | 1,145,815,779 | 1,082,320,886 |
| **HOSPITAL UNIT (Excludes Separate Nursing Home Units)** | | | | | |
| **Utilization - Inpatient** | | | | | |
| Beds | 2,414 | 2,281 | 2,591 | 2,301 | 2,665 |
| Admissions | 103,517 | 102,888 | 99,503 | 95,295 | 92,995 |
| Inpatient Days | 459,871 | 445,638 | 466,644 | 421,283 | 526,200 |
| Average Length of Stay | 4.4 | 4.3 | 4.7 | 4.4 | 5.7 |
| **Personnel** | | | | | |
| Total Full Time | 10,667 | 10,659 | 10,407 | 10,273 | 10,632 |
| Total Part Time | 5,838 | 5,944 | 5,610 | 5,566 | 4,994 |
| **Revenue and Expenses - Totals (Includes Inpatient and Outpatient)** | | | | | |
| Total Net Revenue | $1,401,772,970 | $1,312,606,078 | $1,226,159,560 | $1,133,832,079 | $1,094,400,649 |
| Total Expenses | 1,364,748,522 | 1,254,156,946 | 1,149,226,075 | 1,083,787,392 | 1,018,250,749 |
| **COMMUNITY HEALTH INDICATORS PER 1000 POPULATION** | | | | | |
| Total Population (in thousands) | 918 | 910 | 906 | 903 | 898 |
| **Inpatient** | | | | | |
| Beds | 4.7 | 4.7 | 4.9 | 4.7 | 5.2 |
| Admissions | 116.6 | 117.3 | 114.1 | 109.9 | 109.1 |
| Inpatient Days | 1,143.8 | 1,177.4 | 1,167.9 | 1,157.3 | 1,294.0 |
| Inpatient Surgeries | 37.8 | 35.5 | 35.1 | 34.7 | 34.3 |
| Births | 11.2 | 10.9 | 10.8 | 10.9 | 10.9 |
| **Outpatient** | | | | | |
| Emergency Outpatient Visits | 328.9 | 304.1 | 304.8 | 299.9 | 293.3 |
| Other Outpatient Visits | 2,654.6 | 2,616.4 | 2,618.4 | 2,632.0 | 2,536.1 |
| Total Outpatient Visits | 2,983.5 | 2,920.5 | 2,923.3 | 2,931.9 | 2,829.4 |
| Outpatient Surgeries | 42.8 | 42.6 | 41.4 | 42.2 | 42.5 |
| **Expense per Capita (per person)** | $1,570.0 | $1,459.3 | $1,342.9 | $1,268.4 | $1,205.9 |

# TABLE 6

## NEBRASKA

*U.S. Registered Community Hospitals*
*(Nonfederal, short-term general and other special hospitals)*

## Overview 1999–2003

| | 2003 | 2002 | 2001 | 2000 | 1999 |
|---|---|---|---|---|---|
| **Total Community Hospitals in Nebraska** | **85** | **86** | **84** | **85** | **85** |
| **Bed Size Category** | | | | | |
| 6-24 | 22 | 19 | 18 | 18 | 18 |
| 25-49 | 22 | 30 | 27 | 28 | 27 |
| 50-99 | 19 | 16 | 17 | 19 | 18 |
| 100-199 | 11 | 9 | 10 | 8 | 10 |
| 200-299 | 6 | 6 | 6 | 6 | 6 |
| 300-399 | 2 | 2 | 2 | 2 | 2 |
| 400-499 | 1 | 0 | 0 | 0 | 0 |
| 500 + | 2 | 4 | 4 | 4 | 4 |
| **Location** | | | | | |
| Hospitals Urban | 13 | 14 | 14 | 13 | 13 |
| Hospitals Rural | 72 | 72 | 70 | 72 | 72 |
| **Control** | | | | | |
| State and Local Government | 39 | 41 | 39 | 41 | 41 |
| Not for Profit | 44 | 43 | 43 | 43 | 43 |
| Investor owned | 2 | 2 | 2 | 1 | 1 |
| **Physician Models** | | | | | |
| Independent Practice Association | 7 | 5 | 6 | 8 | 6 |
| Group Practice without Walls | 1 | 2 | 1 | 1 | 1 |
| Open Physician-Hospital Organization | 12 | 14 | 17 | 14 | 16 |
| Closed Physician-Hospital Organization | 0 | 0 | 0 | 1 | 2 |
| Management Service Organization | 1 | 0 | 0 | 1 | 5 |
| Integrated Salary Model | 33 | 22 | 28 | 32 | 34 |
| Equity Model | 0 | 0 | 0 | 0 | 1 |
| Foundation | 2 | 1 | 1 | 2 | 4 |
| **Insurance Products** | | | | | |
| Health Maintenance Organization | 4 | 4 | 1 | 5 | 5 |
| Preferred Provider Organization | 16 | 17 | 15 | 17 | 21 |
| Indemnity Fee for Service | 2 | 2 | 2 | 5 | 3 |
| **Managed Care Contracts** | | | | | |
| Health Maintenance Organization | 25 | 21 | 24 | 31 | 28 |
| Preferred Provider Organization | 63 | 46 | 56 | 66 | 64 |
| **Affiliations** | | | | | |
| Hospitals in a System* | 26 | 26 | 21 | 17 | 17 |
| Hospitals in a Network | 45 | 33 | 40 | 45 | 41 |
| Hospitals in a Group Purchasing Organization | 71 | 50 | 63 | 73 | 67 |

States

* Please note that system affiliate information for hospitals is derived from AHA membership. In years prior to 2003 the affiliation was derived from a question on the AHA Annual Survey of hospitals; therefore, non-responding hospitals were not included in the system affiliation counts. Years prior to 2003 have been updated to reflect this change, which now include affiliation for non-reporting hospitals.

# TABLE 6

## NEBRASKA

*U.S. Registered Community Hospitals*
*(Nonfederal, short-term general and other special hospitals)*

## Utilization, Personnel, Revenue and Expenses, Community Health Indicators 1999–2003

| | 2003 | 2002 | 2001 | 2000 | 1999 |
|---|---|---|---|---|---|
| **TOTAL FACILITY (Includes Hospital and Nursing Home Units)** | | | | | |
| **Utilization - Inpatient** | | | | | |
| Beds | 7,467 | 8,106 | 8,324 | 8,161 | 8,326 |
| Admissions | 211,567 | 206,208 | 206,700 | 209,498 | 199,471 |
| Inpatient Days | 1,593,254 | 1,723,683 | 1,826,566 | 1,760,490 | 1,821,925 |
| Average Length of Stay | 7.5 | 8.4 | 8.8 | 8.4 | 9.1 |
| Inpatient Surgeries | 73,396 | 70,433 | 68,392 | 68,738 | 66,997 |
| Births | 25,796 | 24,030 | 24,313 | 23,479 | 21,877 |
| **Utilization - Outpatient** | | | | | |
| Emergency Outpatient Visits | 532,934 | 511,085 | 545,607 | 499,960 | 491,438 |
| Other Outpatient Visits | 3,143,164 | 2,955,952 | 2,884,235 | 2,905,439 | 2,510,386 |
| Total Outpatient Visits | 3,676,098 | 3,467,037 | 3,429,842 | 3,405,399 | 3,001,824 |
| Outpatient Surgeries | 131,898 | 132,704 | 129,154 | 123,042 | 114,063 |
| **Personnel** | | | | | |
| Full Time RNs | 5,592 | 5,548 | 5,456 | 5,352 | 5,185 |
| Full Time LPNs | 1,070 | 997 | 1,044 | 1,041 | 1,059 |
| Part Time RNs | 3,839 | 4,167 | 3,695 | 3,484 | 3,993 |
| Part Time LPNs | 689 | 678 | 649 | 692 | 769 |
| Total Full Time | 25,193 | 24,517 | 24,476 | 23,898 | 23,412 |
| Total Part Time | 13,994 | 14,665 | 14,398 | 13,454 | 14,887 |
| **Revenue - Inpatient** | | | | | |
| Gross Inpatient Revenue | $3,883,504,195 | $3,420,226,799 | $3,052,706,197 | $2,675,259,869 | $2,371,471,871 |
| **Revenue - Outpatient** | | | | | |
| Gross Outpatient Revenue | $2,357,540,030 | $2,180,716,982 | $1,898,195,952 | $1,561,380,290 | $1,344,021,603 |
| **Revenue and Expenses - Totals (Includes Inpatient and Outpatient)** | | | | | |
| Total Gross Revenue | $6,241,044,225 | $5,600,943,781 | $4,950,902,149 | $4,236,640,159 | $3,715,493,474 |
| Deductions from Revenue | 3,091,883,586 | 2,630,090,894 | 2,221,659,602 | 1,816,852,259 | 1,523,396,593 |
| Net Patient Revenue | 3,149,160,639 | 2,970,852,887 | 2,729,242,547 | 2,419,787,900 | 2,192,096,881 |
| Other Operating Revenue | 160,550,119 | 146,854,319 | 131,134,300 | 122,358,298 | 111,258,095 |
| Other Nonoperating Revenue | -19,986,175 | 23,940,303 | 49,150,380 | 65,215,309 | 36,446,213 |
| Total Net Revenue | 3,289,724,583 | 3,141,647,509 | 2,909,527,227 | 2,607,361,507 | 2,339,801,189 |
| Total Expenses | 3,072,367,016 | 2,892,566,453 | 2,645,027,198 | 2,327,404,184 | 2,156,055,667 |
| **HOSPITAL UNIT (Excludes Separate Nursing Home Units)** | | | | | |
| **Utilization - Inpatient** | | | | | |
| Beds | 5,647 | 6,414 | 6,427 | 6,144 | 6,216 |
| Admissions | 207,183 | 200,622 | 201,225 | 203,541 | 191,227 |
| Inpatient Days | 1,058,691 | 1,180,270 | 1,223,636 | 1,104,318 | 1,114,416 |
| Average Length of Stay | 5.1 | 5.9 | 6.1 | 5.4 | 5.8 |
| **Personnel** | | | | | |
| Total Full Time | 24,008 | 23,564 | 23,330 | 22,725 | 22,230 |
| Total Part Time | 13,080 | 13,873 | 13,531 | 12,561 | 14,016 |
| **Revenue and Expenses - Totals (Includes Inpatient and Outpatient)** | | | | | |
| Total Net Revenue | $3,205,088,933 | $3,061,905,470 | $2,817,978,178 | $2,528,414,477 | $2,247,886,654 |
| Total Expenses | 2,987,801,196 | 2,805,501,875 | 2,562,442,544 | 2,243,914,541 | 2,078,619,066 |
| **COMMUNITY HEALTH INDICATORS PER 1000 POPULATION** | | | | | |
| Total Population (in thousands) | 1,739 | 1,728 | 1,719 | 1,713 | 1,705 |
| **Inpatient** | | | | | |
| Beds | 4.3 | 4.7 | 4.8 | 4.8 | 4.9 |
| Admissions | 121.6 | 119.4 | 120.2 | 122.3 | 117.0 |
| Inpatient Days | 916.0 | 997.8 | 1,062.6 | 1,027.6 | 1,068.7 |
| Inpatient Surgeries | 42.2 | 40.8 | 39.8 | 40.1 | 39.3 |
| Births | 14.8 | 13.9 | 14.1 | 13.7 | 12.8 |
| **Outpatient** | | | | | |
| Emergency Outpatient Visits | 306.4 | 295.8 | 317.4 | 291.8 | 288.3 |
| Other Outpatient Visits | 1,807.2 | 1,711.1 | 1,677.9 | 1,695.9 | 1,472.6 |
| Total Outpatient Visits | 2,113.6 | 2,006.9 | 1,995.3 | 1,987.8 | 1,760.8 |
| Outpatient Surgeries | 75.8 | 76.8 | 75.1 | 71.8 | 66.9 |
| **Expense per Capita (per person)** | $1,766.4 | $1,674.4 | $1,538.7 | $1,358.5 | $1,264.7 |

States

# TABLE 6

# NEVADA

*U.S. Registered Community Hospitals*
*(Nonfederal, short-term general and other special hospitals)*

## Overview 1999–2003

| | 2003 | 2002 | 2001 | 2000 | 1999 |
|---|---|---|---|---|---|
| **Total Community Hospitals in Nevada** | **25** | **26** | **24** | **22** | **22** |
| **Bed Size Category** | | | | | |
| 6-24 | 1 | 0 | 1 | 1 | 1 |
| 25-49 | 5 | 7 | 5 | 5 | 6 |
| 50-99 | 6 | 5 | 4 | 4 | 3 |
| 100-199 | 7 | 8 | 8 | 6 | 6 |
| 200-299 | 2 | 1 | 2 | 2 | 2 |
| 300-399 | 1 | 2 | 1 | 1 | 1 |
| 400-499 | 0 | 0 | 1 | 1 | 1 |
| 500 + | 3 | 3 | 2 | 2 | 2 |
| **Location** | | | | | |
| Hospitals Urban | 16 | 17 | 15 | 13 | 14 |
| Hospitals Rural | 9 | 9 | 9 | 9 | 8 |
| **Control** | | | | | |
| State and Local Government | 7 | 6 | 7 | 7 | 8 |
| Not for Profit | 9 | 9 | 7 | 7 | 6 |
| Investor owned | 9 | 11 | 10 | 8 | 8 |
| **Physician Models** | | | | | |
| Independent Practice Association | 3 | 5 | 2 | 2 | 4 |
| Group Practice without Walls | 1 | 0 | 0 | 0 | 0 |
| Open Physician-Hospital Organization | 2 | 1 | 1 | 1 | 0 |
| Closed Physician-Hospital Organization | 0 | 0 | 0 | 0 | 0 |
| Management Service Organization | 2 | 1 | 1 | 2 | 3 |
| Integrated Salary Model | 5 | 3 | 3 | 2 | 3 |
| Equity Model | 0 | 0 | 0 | 0 | 0 |
| Foundation | 0 | 0 | 0 | 0 | 1 |
| **Insurance Products** | | | | | |
| Health Maintenance Organization | 4 | 3 | 2 | 3 | 0 |
| Preferred Provider Organization | 4 | 4 | 2 | 3 | 0 |
| Indemnity Fee for Service | 3 | 2 | 1 | 1 | 0 |
| **Managed Care Contracts** | | | | | |
| Health Maintenance Organization | 11 | 13 | 9 | 8 | 11 |
| Preferred Provider Organization | 13 | 14 | 11 | 9 | 13 |
| **Affiliations** | | | | | |
| Hospitals in a System* | 14 | 14 | 11 | 12 | 12 |
| Hospitals in a Network | 4 | 4 | 3 | 3 | 4 |
| Hospitals in a Group Purchasing Organization | 15 | 14 | 14 | 7 | 10 |

* Please note that system affiliate information for hospitals is derived from AHA membership. In years prior to 2003 the affiliation was derived from a question on the AHA Annual Survey of hospitals; therefore, non-responding hospitals were not included in the system affiliation counts. Years prior to 2003 have been updated to reflect this change, which now include affiliation for non-reporting hospitals.

**TABLE 6**

# NEVADA

*U.S. Registered Community Hospitals*
*(Nonfederal, short-term general and other special hospitals)*

## Utilization, Personnel, Revenue and Expenses, Community Health Indicators 1999–2003

| | 2003 | 2002 | 2001 | 2000 | 1999 |
|---|---|---|---|---|---|
| **TOTAL FACILITY (Includes Hospital and Nursing Home Units)** | | | | | |
| **Utilization - Inpatient** | | | | | |
| Beds | 4,282 | 4,495 | 4,099 | 3,810 | 3,706 |
| Admissions | 212,821 | 211,657 | 207,844 | 199,455 | 197,501 |
| Inpatient Days | 1,111,624 | 1,110,583 | 1,019,835 | 984,845 | 1,000,369 |
| Average Length of Stay | 5.2 | 5.2 | 4.9 | 4.9 | 5.1 |
| Inpatient Surgeries | 66,661 | 75,406 | 76,427 | 72,090 | 78,969 |
| Births | 30,801 | 29,709 | 28,040 | 28,874 | 30,399 |
| **Utilization - Outpatient** | | | | | |
| Emergency Outpatient Visits | 626,686 | 626,330 | 548,798 | 573,220 | 527,219 |
| Other Outpatient Visits | 1,657,287 | 1,835,894 | 1,577,315 | 1,618,898 | 1,599,270 |
| Total Outpatient Visits | 2,283,973 | 2,462,224 | 2,126,113 | 2,192,118 | 2,126,489 |
| Outpatient Surgeries | 71,739 | 87,157 | 91,748 | 84,840 | 111,460 |
| **Personnel** | | | | | |
| Full Time RNs | 4,606 | 4,605 | 3,984 | 4,255 | 3,992 |
| Full Time LPNs | 460 | 422 | 429 | 455 | 581 |
| Part Time RNs | 1,552 | 1,398 | 1,523 | 1,388 | 1,160 |
| Part Time LPNs | 122 | 83 | 101 | 72 | 104 |
| Total Full Time | 16,859 | 16,340 | 15,682 | 16,173 | 14,846 |
| Total Part Time | 4,179 | 3,797 | 4,180 | 3,783 | 3,671 |
| **Revenue - Inpatient** | | | | | |
| Gross Inpatient Revenue | $5,787,996,156 | $5,183,035,024 | $3,997,307,168 | $3,384,346,250 | $3,224,856,025 |
| **Revenue - Outpatient** | | | | | |
| Gross Outpatient Revenue | $2,115,614,370 | $1,883,871,488 | $1,486,747,093 | $1,175,895,927 | $1,120,428,723 |
| **Revenue and Expenses - Totals (Includes Inpatient and Outpatient)** | | | | | |
| Total Gross Revenue | $7,903,610,526 | $7,066,906,512 | $5,484,054,261 | $4,560,242,177 | $4,345,284,748 |
| Deductions from Revenue | 5,414,900,197 | 4,672,604,272 | 3,441,708,915 | 2,795,643,699 | 2,673,121,276 |
| Net Patient Revenue | 2,488,710,329 | 2,394,302,240 | 2,042,345,346 | 1,764,598,478 | 1,672,163,472 |
| Other Operating Revenue | 141,955,261 | 179,018,832 | 95,047,287 | 77,338,480 | 45,314,641 |
| Other Nonoperating Revenue | 15,230,192 | 16,877,884 | 25,143,034 | 34,250,055 | 18,599,731 |
| Total Net Revenue | 2,645,895,782 | 2,590,198,956 | 2,162,535,667 | 1,876,187,013 | 1,736,077,844 |
| Total Expenses | 2,583,114,447 | 2,257,000,776 | 2,087,682,180 | 1,790,079,467 | 1,623,910,172 |
| **HOSPITAL UNIT (Excludes Separate Nursing Home Units)** | | | | | |
| **Utilization - Inpatient** | | | | | |
| Beds | 4,141 | 4,416 | 3,969 | 3,712 | 3,600 |
| Admissions | 212,723 | 211,562 | 207,237 | 198,904 | 197,292 |
| Inpatient Days | 1,066,782 | 1,083,111 | 977,487 | 954,823 | 959,252 |
| Average Length of Stay | 5.0 | 5.1 | 4.7 | 4.8 | 4.9 |
| **Personnel** | | | | | |
| Total Full Time | 16,767 | 16,270 | 15,611 | 16,039 | 14,788 |
| Total Part Time | 4,159 | 3,779 | 4,146 | 3,755 | 3,657 |
| **Revenue and Expenses - Totals (Includes Inpatient and Outpatient)** | | | | | |
| Total Net Revenue | $2,640,298,685 | $2,586,007,972 | $2,156,122,530 | $1,870,827,186 | $1,731,123,484 |
| Total Expenses | 2,578,395,080 | 2,254,904,246 | 2,083,886,026 | 1,787,243,271 | 1,621,429,707 |
| **COMMUNITY HEALTH INDICATORS PER 1000 POPULATION** | | | | | |
| Total Population (in thousands) | 2,241 | 2,167 | 2,095 | 2,018 | 1,935 |
| **Inpatient** | | | | | |
| Beds | 1.9 | 2.1 | 2.0 | 1.9 | 1.9 |
| Admissions | 95.0 | 97.7 | 99.2 | 98.8 | 102.1 |
| Inpatient Days | 496.0 | 512.4 | 486.9 | 488.0 | 517.1 |
| Inpatient Surgeries | 29.7 | 34.8 | 36.5 | 35.7 | 40.8 |
| Births | 13.7 | 13.7 | 13.4 | 14.3 | 15.7 |
| **Outpatient** | | | | | |
| Emergency Outpatient Visits | 279.6 | 289.0 | 262.0 | 284.0 | 272.5 |
| Other Outpatient Visits | 739.5 | 847.0 | 753.0 | 802.2 | 826.6 |
| Total Outpatient Visits | 1,019.1 | 1,136.0 | 1,015.0 | 1,086.2 | 1,099.1 |
| Outpatient Surgeries | 32.0 | 40.2 | 43.8 | 42.0 | 57.6 |
| **Expense per Capita (per person)** | $1,152.6 | $1,041.3 | $996.7 | $887.0 | $839.4 |

# TABLE 6

# NEW HAMPSHIRE

*U.S. Registered Community Hospitals*
*(Nonfederal, short-term general and other special hospitals)*

## Overview 1999–2003

| | 2003 | 2002 | 2001 | 2000 | 1999 |
|---|---|---|---|---|---|
| **Total Community Hospitals in New Hampshire** | **28** | **28** | **28** | **28** | **28** |
| **Bed Size Category** | | | | | |
| 6-24 | 1 | 1 | 1 | 1 | 0 |
| 25-49 | 7 | 6 | 6 | 6 | 6 |
| 50-99 | 10 | 11 | 11 | 11 | 12 |
| 100-199 | 7 | 6 | 7 | 7 | 6 |
| 200-299 | 2 | 3 | 2 | 2 | 3 |
| 300-399 | 1 | 1 | 1 | 1 | 1 |
| 400-499 | 0 | 0 | 0 | 0 | 0 |
| 500 + | 0 | 0 | 0 | 0 | 0 |
| **Location** | | | | | |
| Hospitals Urban | 10 | 10 | 10 | 10 | 10 |
| Hospitals Rural | 18 | 18 | 18 | 18 | 18 |
| **Control** | | | | | |
| State and Local Government | 0 | 0 | 0 | 0 | 0 |
| Not for Profit | 24 | 24 | 24 | 24 | 24 |
| Investor owned | 4 | 4 | 4 | 4 | 4 |
| **Physician Models** | | | | | |
| Independent Practice Association | 3 | 2 | 2 | 2 | 2 |
| Group Practice without Walls | 1 | 2 | 2 | 2 | 1 |
| Open Physician-Hospital Organization | 10 | 10 | 12 | 14 | 14 |
| Closed Physician-Hospital Organization | 4 | 4 | 4 | 3 | 2 |
| Management Service Organization | 3 | 4 | 2 | 3 | 3 |
| Integrated Salary Model | 12 | 12 | 12 | 11 | 12 |
| Equity Model | 0 | 0 | 0 | 0 | 0 |
| Foundation | 1 | 1 | 1 | 1 | 3 |
| **Insurance Products** | | | | | |
| Health Maintenance Organization | 3 | 2 | 1 | 1 | 2 |
| Preferred Provider Organization | 1 | 1 | 0 | 0 | 0 |
| Indemnity Fee for Service | 1 | 1 | 0 | 0 | 0 |
| **Managed Care Contracts** | | | | | |
| Health Maintenance Organization | 25 | 26 | 25 | 26 | 26 |
| Preferred Provider Organization | 25 | 25 | 23 | 22 | 23 |
| **Affiliations** | | | | | |
| Hospitals in a System* | 5 | 5 | 5 | 5 | 5 |
| Hospitals in a Network | 9 | 8 | 8 | 9 | 7 |
| Hospitals in a Group Purchasing Organization | 26 | 25 | 25 | 22 | 23 |

* Please note that system affiliate information for hospitals is derived from AHA membership. In years prior to 2003 the affiliation was derived from a question on the AHA Annual Survey of hospitals; therefore, non-responding hospitals were not included in the system affiliation counts. Years prior to 2003 have been updated to reflect this change, which now include affiliation for non-reporting hospitals.

# TABLE 6

## NEW HAMPSHIRE

*U.S. Registered Community Hospitals*
*(Nonfederal, short-term general and other special hospitals)*

## Utilization, Personnel, Revenue and Expenses, Community Health Indicators 1999–2003

| | 2003 | 2002 | 2001 | 2000 | 1999 |
|---|---|---|---|---|---|
| **TOTAL FACILITY (Includes Hospital and Nursing Home Units)** | | | | | |
| **Utilization - Inpatient** | | | | | |
| Beds | 2,796 | 2,879 | 2,853 | 2,865 | 2,974 |
| Admissions | 117,814 | 117,996 | 116,071 | 111,227 | 109,110 |
| Inpatient Days | 637,803 | 646,838 | 637,239 | 611,919 | 599,777 |
| Average Length of Stay | 5.4 | 5.5 | 5.5 | 5.5 | 5.5 |
| Inpatient Surgeries | 33,535 | 33,553 | 33,702 | 33,595 | 32,864 |
| Births | 13,634 | 13,748 | 13,919 | 13,715 | 13,470 |
| **Utilization - Outpatient** | | | | | |
| Emergency Outpatient Visits | 547,870 | 550,380 | 537,367 | 526,103 | 491,840 |
| Other Outpatient Visits | 2,523,260 | 2,472,527 | 2,392,259 | 2,237,250 | 1,908,936 |
| Total Outpatient Visits | 3,071,130 | 3,022,907 | 2,929,626 | 2,763,353 | 2,400,776 |
| Outpatient Surgeries | 87,795 | 85,056 | 75,467 | 68,807 | 60,607 |
| **Personnel** | | | | | |
| Full Time RNs | 3,248 | 3,053 | 3,130 | 2,825 | 2,643 |
| Full Time LPNs | 158 | 159 | 175 | 172 | 210 |
| Part Time RNs | 2,483 | 2,720 | 2,087 | 2,139 | 2,261 |
| Part Time LPNs | 139 | 135 | 135 | 146 | 180 |
| Total Full Time | 14,966 | 14,657 | 14,578 | 12,923 | 12,681 |
| Total Part Time | 7,981 | 8,522 | 7,571 | 7,905 | 8,186 |
| **Revenue - Inpatient** | | | | | |
| Gross Inpatient Revenue | $1,810,524,954 | $1,631,730,543 | $1,452,518,894 | $1,318,942,481 | $1,151,678,573 |
| **Revenue - Outpatient** | | | | | |
| Gross Outpatient Revenue | $2,014,053,023 | $1,730,622,946 | $1,422,018,438 | $1,189,795,594 | $991,577,915 |
| **Revenue and Expenses - Totals (Includes Inpatient and Outpatient)** | | | | | |
| Total Gross Revenue | $3,824,577,977 | $3,362,353,489 | $2,874,537,332 | $2,508,738,075 | $2,143,256,488 |
| Deductions from Revenue | 1,779,776,571 | 1,525,457,983 | 1,259,505,490 | 1,017,348,844 | 811,801,538 |
| Net Patient Revenue | 2,044,801,406 | 1,836,895,506 | 1,615,031,842 | 1,491,389,231 | 1,331,454,950 |
| Other Operating Revenue | 70,604,056 | 58,980,628 | 58,806,419 | 57,582,211 | 45,891,074 |
| Other Nonoperating Revenue | 2,981,869 | -13,731,846 | -2,412,941 | 60,358,157 | 88,389,168 |
| Total Net Revenue | 2,118,387,331 | 1,882,144,288 | 1,671,425,320 | 1,609,329,599 | 1,465,735,192 |
| Total Expenses | 1,994,793,981 | 1,830,377,475 | 1,617,994,197 | 1,466,080,802 | 1,288,450,986 |
| **HOSPITAL UNIT (Excludes Separate Nursing Home Units)** | | | | | |
| **Utilization - Inpatient** | | | | | |
| Beds | 2,616 | 2,691 | 2,665 | 2,677 | 2,786 |
| Admissions | 117,292 | 117,544 | 115,645 | 110,784 | 108,741 |
| Inpatient Days | 577,251 | 583,999 | 574,417 | 548,348 | 538,451 |
| Average Length of Stay | 4.9 | 5.0 | 5.0 | 4.9 | 5.0 |
| **Personnel** | | | | | |
| Total Full Time | 14,854 | 14,531 | 14,458 | 12,800 | 12,559 |
| Total Part Time | 7,905 | 8,468 | 7,510 | 7,856 | 8,107 |
| **Revenue and Expenses - Totals (Includes Inpatient and Outpatient)** | | | | | |
| Total Net Revenue | $2,107,902,639 | $1,871,385,906 | $1,660,849,124 | $1,598,999,933 | $1,456,900,913 |
| Total Expenses | 1,985,755,739 | 1,823,178,785 | 1,611,350,879 | 1,459,873,435 | 1,283,050,412 |
| **COMMUNITY HEALTH INDICATORS PER 1000 POPULATION** | | | | | |
| Total Population (in thousands) | 1,288 | 1,274 | 1,259 | 1,240 | 1,222 |
| **Inpatient** | | | | | |
| Beds | 2.2 | 2.3 | 2.3 | 2.3 | 2.4 |
| Admissions | 91.5 | 92.6 | 92.2 | 89.7 | 89.3 |
| Inpatient Days | 495.3 | 507.6 | 506.2 | 493.3 | 490.8 |
| Inpatient Surgeries | 26.0 | 26.3 | 26.8 | 27.1 | 26.9 |
| Births | 10.6 | 10.8 | 11.1 | 11.1 | 11.0 |
| **Outpatient** | | | | | |
| Emergency Outpatient Visits | 425.5 | 431.9 | 426.8 | 424.1 | 402.5 |
| Other Outpatient Visits | 1,959.5 | 1,940.1 | 1,900.2 | 1,803.5 | 1,562.1 |
| Total Outpatient Visits | 2,385.0 | 2,372.0 | 2,327.0 | 2,227.7 | 1,964.6 |
| Outpatient Surgeries | 68.2 | 66.7 | 59.9 | 55.5 | 49.6 |
| **Expense per Capita (per person)** | $1,549.1 | $1,436.3 | $1,285.2 | $1,181.9 | $1,054.4 |

# TABLE 6

# NEW JERSEY

*U.S. Registered Community Hospitals*
*(Nonfederal, short-term general and other special hospitals)*

## Overview 1999–2003

| | 2003 | 2002 | 2001 | 2000 | 1999 |
|---|---|---|---|---|---|
| **Total Community Hospitals in New Jersey** | **78** | **81** | **78** | **80** | **81** |
| **Bed Size Category** | | | | | |
| 6-24 | 0 | 0 | 0 | 0 | 0 |
| 25-49 | 0 | 0 | 0 | 0 | 1 |
| 50-99 | 5 | 5 | 5 | 5 | 4 |
| 100-199 | 25 | 24 | 20 | 23 | 23 |
| 200-299 | 18 | 17 | 20 | 20 | 20 |
| 300-399 | 13 | 16 | 14 | 13 | 14 |
| 400-499 | 9 | 11 | 9 | 11 | 9 |
| 500 + | 8 | 8 | 10 | 8 | 10 |
| **Location** | | | | | |
| Hospitals Urban | 78 | 81 | 78 | 80 | 81 |
| Hospitals Rural | 0 | 0 | 0 | 0 | 0 |
| **Control** | | | | | |
| State and Local Government | 1 | 2 | 2 | 2 | 2 |
| Not for Profit | 74 | 76 | 74 | 76 | 77 |
| Investor owned | 3 | 3 | 2 | 2 | 2 |
| **Physician Models** | | | | | |
| Independent Practice Association | 31 | 36 | 34 | 27 | 27 |
| Group Practice without Walls | 3 | 3 | 2 | 4 | 2 |
| Open Physician-Hospital Organization | 13 | 14 | 14 | 15 | 13 |
| Closed Physician-Hospital Organization | 4 | 5 | 5 | 7 | 7 |
| Management Service Organization | 18 | 23 | 19 | 16 | 21 |
| Integrated Salary Model | 11 | 15 | 16 | 15 | 9 |
| Equity Model | 1 | 2 | 1 | 1 | 2 |
| Foundation | 0 | 0 | 1 | 0 | 1 |
| **Insurance Products** | | | | | |
| Health Maintenance Organization | 9 | 10 | 7 | 14 | 14 |
| Preferred Provider Organization | 13 | 14 | 11 | 15 | 13 |
| Indemnity Fee for Service | 3 | 3 | 1 | 1 | 5 |
| **Managed Care Contracts** | | | | | |
| Health Maintenance Organization | 48 | 52 | 65 | 58 | 58 |
| Preferred Provider Organization | 47 | 50 | 63 | 57 | 56 |
| **Affiliations** | | | | | |
| Hospitals in a System* | 44 | 42 | 37 | 33 | 35 |
| Hospitals in a Network | 28 | 32 | 32 | 21 | 6 |
| Hospitals in a Group Purchasing Organization | 55 | 61 | 61 | 50 | 19 |

* Please note that system affiliate information for hospitals is derived from AHA membership. In years prior to 2003 the affiliation was derived from a question on the AHA Annual Survey of hospitals; therefore, non-responding hospitals were not included in the system affiliation counts. Years prior to 2003 have been updated to reflect this change, which now include affiliation for non-reporting hospitals.

# TABLE 6

## NEW JERSEY

*U.S. Registered Community Hospitals*
*(Nonfederal, short-term general and other special hospitals)*

## Utilization, Personnel, Revenue and Expenses, Community Health Indicators 1999–2003

| | 2003 | 2002 | 2001 | 2000 | 1999 |
|---|---|---|---|---|---|
| **TOTAL FACILITY (Includes Hospital and Nursing Home Units)** | | | | | |
| **Utilization - Inpatient** | | | | | |
| Beds | 22,807 | 24,094 | 24,580 | 25,307 | 24,570 |
| Admissions | 1,107,659 | 1,094,781 | 1,083,798 | 1,073,619 | 1,068,664 |
| Inpatient Days | 6,154,335 | 6,190,443 | 6,165,019 | 6,340,657 | 6,150,912 |
| Average Length of Stay | 5.6 | 5.7 | 5.7 | 5.9 | 5.8 |
| Inpatient Surgeries | 296,820 | 303,451 | 293,850 | 313,803 | 307,971 |
| Births | 113,420 | 112,900 | 109,870 | 111,057 | 109,793 |
| **Utilization - Outpatient** | | | | | |
| Emergency Outpatient Visits | 2,922,644 | 2,940,592 | 2,936,620 | 2,853,236 | 2,882,031 |
| Other Outpatient Visits | 11,763,785 | 12,957,409 | 15,507,940 | 13,454,037 | 13,244,138 |
| Total Outpatient Visits | 14,686,429 | 15,898,001 | 18,444,560 | 16,307,273 | 16,126,169 |
| Outpatient Surgeries | 419,982 | 416,709 | 399,564 | 412,229 | 414,003 |
| **Personnel** | | | | | |
| Full Time RNs | 22,984 | 21,384 | 22,522 | 23,154 | 21,826 |
| Full Time LPNs | 1,714 | 1,929 | 1,931 | 2,095 | 2,029 |
| Part Time RNs | 11,499 | 12,146 | 12,624 | 14,162 | 14,232 |
| Part Time LPNs | 662 | 770 | 799 | 955 | 1,016 |
| Total Full Time | 97,831 | 98,194 | 98,209 | 100,557 | 93,901 |
| Total Part Time | 36,109 | 38,591 | 42,406 | 43,732 | 42,774 |
| **Revenue - Inpatient** | | | | | |
| Gross Inpatient Revenue | $38,355,261,854 | $29,788,891,087 | $26,602,275,344 | $21,827,720,053 | $17,817,044,301 |
| **Revenue - Outpatient** | | | | | |
| Gross Outpatient Revenue | $12,472,208,125 | $10,149,816,977 | $8,452,299,275 | $7,310,430,959 | $5,867,036,075 |
| **Revenue and Expenses - Totals (Includes Inpatient and Outpatient)** | | | | | |
| Total Gross Revenue | $50,827,469,979 | $39,938,708,064 | $35,054,574,619 | $29,138,151,012 | $23,684,080,376 |
| Deductions from Revenue | 37,708,618,723 | 27,488,534,367 | 23,885,664,427 | 18,556,968,225 | 14,272,643,586 |
| Net Patient Revenue | 13,118,851,256 | 12,450,173,697 | 11,168,910,192 | 10,581,182,787 | 9,411,436,790 |
| Other Operating Revenue | 645,599,155 | 667,392,368 | 644,537,713 | 730,175,554 | 594,893,499 |
| Other Nonoperating Revenue | 213,933,523 | 26,399,177 | 77,244,348 | 226,655,485 | 205,235,554 |
| Total Net Revenue | 13,978,383,934 | 13,143,965,242 | 11,890,692,253 | 11,538,013,826 | 10,211,565,843 |
| Total Expenses | 13,616,125,636 | 12,841,553,561 | 11,716,951,020 | 11,253,553,740 | 10,079,107,532 |
| **HOSPITAL UNIT (Excludes Separate Nursing Home Units)** | | | | | |
| **Utilization - Inpatient** | | | | | |
| Beds | 22,384 | 23,315 | 23,716 | 24,650 | 23,754 |
| Admissions | 1,104,636 | 1,091,471 | 1,080,365 | 1,070,105 | 1,065,294 |
| Inpatient Days | 6,013,949 | 5,921,584 | 5,885,278 | 6,136,582 | 5,878,838 |
| Average Length of Stay | 5.4 | 5.4 | 5.4 | 5.7 | 5.5 |
| **Personnel** | | | | | |
| Total Full Time | 97,114 | 97,573 | 97,533 | 99,379 | 92,941 |
| Total Part Time | 35,637 | 38,411 | 42,140 | 43,215 | 42,320 |
| **Revenue and Expenses - Totals (Includes Inpatient and Outpatient)** | | | | | |
| Total Net Revenue | $13,942,159,660 | $13,070,208,862 | $11,822,055,392 | $11,496,256,093 | $10,161,679,983 |
| Total Expenses | 13,586,472,196 | 12,781,447,599 | 11,659,210,376 | 11,210,748,330 | 10,026,590,107 |
| **COMMUNITY HEALTH INDICATORS PER 1000 POPULATION** | | | | | |
| Total Population (in thousands) | 8,638 | 8,575 | 8,504 | 8,432 | 8,360 |
| **Inpatient** | | | | | |
| Beds | 2.6 | 2.8 | 2.9 | 3.0 | 2.9 |
| Admissions | 128.2 | 127.7 | 127.4 | 127.3 | 127.8 |
| Inpatient Days | 712.4 | 721.9 | 724.9 | 752.0 | 735.8 |
| Inpatient Surgeries | 34.4 | 35.4 | 34.6 | 37.2 | 36.8 |
| Births | 13.1 | 13.2 | 12.9 | 13.2 | 13.1 |
| **Outpatient** | | | | | |
| Emergency Outpatient Visits | 338.3 | 342.9 | 345.3 | 338.4 | 344.8 |
| Other Outpatient Visits | 1,361.8 | 1,511.0 | 1,823.6 | 1,595.6 | 1,584.3 |
| Total Outpatient Visits | 1,700.1 | 1,853.9 | 2,168.9 | 1,933.9 | 1,929.1 |
| Outpatient Surgeries | 48.6 | 48.6 | 47.0 | 48.9 | 49.5 |
| **Expense per Capita (per person)** | $1,576.2 | $1,497.5 | $1,377.8 | $1,334.6 | $1,205.7 |

# TABLE 6

# NEW MEXICO

*U.S. Registered Community Hospitals*
*(Nonfederal, short-term general and other special hospitals)*

## Overview 1999–2003

| | 2003 | 2002 | 2001 | 2000 | 1999 |
|---|---|---|---|---|---|
| **Total Community Hospitals in New Mexico** | **37** | **36** | **35** | **35** | **36** |
| **Bed Size Category** | | | | | |
| 6-24 | 4 | 3 | 2 | 4 | 5 |
| 25-49 | 9 | 11 | 12 | 9 | 8 |
| 50-99 | 9 | 8 | 8 | 9 | 11 |
| 100-199 | 10 | 9 | 8 | 8 | 9 |
| 200-299 | 4 | 4 | 3 | 4 | 2 |
| 300-399 | 1 | 0 | 2 | 1 | 1 |
| 400-499 | 0 | 1 | 0 | 0 | 0 |
| 500 + | 0 | 0 | 0 | 0 | 0 |
| **Location** | | | | | |
| Hospitals Urban | 15 | 14 | 13 | 13 | 13 |
| Hospitals Rural | 22 | 22 | 22 | 22 | 23 |
| **Control** | | | | | |
| State and Local Government | 9 | 9 | 10 | 9 | 11 |
| Not for Profit | 19 | 19 | 19 | 20 | 20 |
| Investor owned | 9 | 8 | 6 | 6 | 5 |
| **Physician Models** | | | | | |
| Independent Practice Association | 7 | 6 | 5 | 9 | 12 |
| Group Practice without Walls | 0 | 0 | 1 | 3 | 4 |
| Open Physician-Hospital Organization | 7 | 5 | 4 | 6 | 6 |
| Closed Physician-Hospital Organization | 1 | 2 | 1 | 2 | 4 |
| Management Service Organization | 0 | 1 | 0 | 1 | 3 |
| Integrated Salary Model | 7 | 6 | 9 | 9 | 5 |
| Equity Model | 0 | 0 | 0 | 0 | 0 |
| Foundation | 0 | 2 | 3 | 2 | 3 |
| **Insurance Products** | | | | | |
| Health Maintenance Organization | 8 | 8 | 10 | 8 | 8 |
| Preferred Provider Organization | 6 | 7 | 6 | 10 | 11 |
| Indemnity Fee for Service | 3 | 5 | 4 | 5 | 6 |
| **Managed Care Contracts** | | | | | |
| Health Maintenance Organization | 17 | 22 | 20 | 16 | 22 |
| Preferred Provider Organization | 16 | 20 | 17 | 16 | 18 |
| **Affiliations** | | | | | |
| Hospitals in a System* | 31 | 28 | 26 | 26 | 25 |
| Hospitals in a Network | 4 | 4 | 5 | 5 | 9 |
| Hospitals in a Group Purchasing Organization | 20 | 24 | 24 | 21 | 21 |



* Please note that system affiliate information for hospitals is derived from AHA membership. In years prior to 2003 the affiliation was derived from a question on the AHA Annual Survey of hospitals; therefore, non-responding hospitals were not included in the system affiliation counts. Years prior to 2003 have been updated to reflect this change, which now include affiliation for non-reporting hospitals.

# TABLE 6

# NEW MEXICO

*U.S. Registered Community Hospitals*
*(Nonfederal, short-term general and other special hospitals)*

## Utilization, Personnel, Revenue and Expenses, Community Health Indicators 1999–2003

| | 2003 | 2002 | 2001 | 2000 | 1999 |
|---|---|---|---|---|---|
| **TOTAL FACILITY (Includes Hospital and Nursing Home Units)** | | | | | |
| **Utilization - Inpatient** | | | | | |
| Beds | 3,680 | 3,602 | 3,584 | 3,481 | 3,370 |
| Admissions | 165,709 | 180,041 | 164,461 | 173,575 | 163,700 |
| Inpatient Days | 780,895 | 849,396 | 758,923 | 731,708 | 725,713 |
| Average Length of Stay | 4.7 | 4.7 | 4.6 | 4.2 | 4.4 |
| Inpatient Surgeries | 50,772 | 59,388 | 45,395 | 51,466 | 57,164 |
| Births | 27,950 | 28,178 | 24,884 | 24,329 | 25,526 |
| **Utilization - Outpatient** | | | | | |
| Emergency Outpatient Visits | 675,058 | 705,643 | 528,979 | 532,526 | 512,645 |
| Other Outpatient Visits | 3,827,511 | 3,482,019 | 2,880,249 | 2,568,108 | 2,622,325 |
| Total Outpatient Visits | 4,502,569 | 4,187,662 | 3,409,228 | 3,100,634 | 3,134,970 |
| Outpatient Surgeries | 81,825 | 103,434 | 78,047 | 78,014 | 86,506 |
| **Personnel** | | | | | |
| Full Time RNs | 4,332 | 4,300 | 4,037 | 3,722 | 3,467 |
| Full Time LPNs | 681 | 626 | 627 | 487 | 508 |
| Part Time RNs | 2,731 | 2,365 | 1,330 | 2,267 | 2,204 |
| Part Time LPNs | 282 | 260 | 150 | 225 | 258 |
| Total Full Time | 23,248 | 20,133 | 19,121 | 15,505 | 15,616 |
| Total Part Time | 8,001 | 7,114 | 4,201 | 6,429 | 7,608 |
| **Revenue - Inpatient** | | | | | |
| Gross Inpatient Revenue | $2,694,623,925 | $2,660,033,608 | $2,100,619,929 | $2,202,879,494 | $2,114,743,157 |
| **Revenue - Outpatient** | | | | | |
| Gross Outpatient Revenue | $1,853,344,484 | $1,848,890,309 | $1,530,614,098 | $1,280,932,571 | $1,235,146,668 |
| **Revenue and Expenses - Totals (Includes Inpatient and Outpatient)** | | | | | |
| Total Gross Revenue | $4,547,968,409 | $4,508,923,917 | $3,631,234,027 | $3,483,812,065 | $3,349,889,825 |
| Deductions from Revenue | 2,600,953,693 | 2,451,800,462 | 1,798,758,901 | 1,905,810,874 | 1,454,422,617 |
| Net Patient Revenue | 1,947,014,716 | 2,057,123,455 | 1,832,475,126 | 1,578,001,191 | 1,895,467,208 |
| Other Operating Revenue | 135,028,348 | 142,673,861 | 102,566,160 | 103,866,572 | 100,671,605 |
| Other Nonoperating Revenue | 32,695,504 | 30,460,788 | 32,406,351 | 30,473,501 | 33,471,257 |
| Total Net Revenue | 2,114,738,568 | 2,230,258,104 | 1,967,447,637 | 1,712,341,264 | 2,029,610,070 |
| Total Expenses | 2,175,580,509 | 2,129,702,267 | 1,868,614,170 | 1,695,651,227 | 1,847,553,034 |
| **HOSPITAL UNIT (Excludes Separate Nursing Home Units)** | | | | | |
| **Utilization - Inpatient** | | | | | |
| Beds | 3,680 | 3,592 | 3,498 | 3,426 | 3,279 |
| Admissions | 165,709 | 179,996 | 163,080 | 172,543 | 161,933 |
| Inpatient Days | 780,895 | 849,127 | 739,270 | 715,831 | 699,736 |
| Average Length of Stay | 4.7 | 4.7 | 4.5 | 4.1 | 4.3 |
| **Personnel** | | | | | |
| Total Full Time | 23,248 | 20,133 | 19,094 | 15,434 | 15,526 |
| Total Part Time | 8,001 | 7,114 | 4,196 | 6,401 | 7,573 |
| **Revenue and Expenses - Totals (Includes Inpatient and Outpatient)** | | | | | |
| Total Net Revenue | $2,114,738,568 | $2,230,225,516 | $1,961,248,667 | $1,709,281,550 | $2,023,848,425 |
| Total Expenses | 2,175,580,509 | 2,129,675,083 | 1,865,267,433 | 1,693,109,995 | 1,845,065,340 |
| **COMMUNITY HEALTH INDICATORS PER 1000 POPULATION** | | | | | |
| Total Population (in thousands) | 1,875 | 1,852 | 1,829 | 1,822 | 1,808 |
| **Inpatient** | | | | | |
| Beds | 2.0 | 1.9 | 2.0 | 1.9 | 1.9 |
| Admissions | 88.4 | 97.2 | 89.9 | 95.3 | 90.5 |
| Inpatient Days | 416.6 | 458.6 | 414.9 | 401.7 | 401.4 |
| Inpatient Surgeries | 27.1 | 32.1 | 24.8 | 28.3 | 31.6 |
| Births | 14.9 | 15.2 | 13.6 | 13.4 | 14.1 |
| **Outpatient** | | | | | |
| Emergency Outpatient Visits | 360.1 | 381.0 | 289.2 | 292.3 | 283.5 |
| Other Outpatient Visits | 2,041.8 | 1,880.1 | 1,574.7 | 1,409.9 | 1,450.3 |
| Total Outpatient Visits | 2,401.9 | 2,261.1 | 1,863.9 | 1,702.2 | 1,733.9 |
| Outpatient Surgeries | 43.6 | 55.8 | 42.7 | 42.8 | 47.8 |
| **Expense per Capita (per person)** | $1,160.5 | $1,149.9 | $1,021.6 | $930.9 | $1,021.8 |

# TABLE 6

## NEW YORK

*U.S. Registered Community Hospitals*
*(Nonfederal, short-term general and other special hospitals)*

## Overview 1999–2003

| | 2003 | 2002 | 2001 | 2000 | 1999 |
|---|---|---|---|---|---|
| **Total Community Hospitals in New York** | **207** | **211** | **212** | **215** | **218** |
| **Bed Size Category** | | | | | |
| 6-24 | 5 | 4 | 4 | 4 | 2 |
| 25-49 | 7 | 8 | 8 | 8 | 12 |
| 50-99 | 21 | 23 | 23 | 25 | 21 |
| 100-199 | 51 | 53 | 51 | 50 | 50 |
| 200-299 | 47 | 46 | 49 | 53 | 54 |
| 300-399 | 24 | 25 | 24 | 23 | 27 |
| 400-499 | 18 | 18 | 21 | 20 | 19 |
| 500 + | 34 | 34 | 32 | 32 | 33 |
| **Location** | | | | | |
| Hospitals Urban | 170 | 173 | 176 | 180 | 182 |
| Hospitals Rural | 37 | 38 | 36 | 35 | 36 |
| **Control** | | | | | |
| State and Local Government | 26 | 26 | 25 | 24 | 25 |
| Not for Profit | 178 | 181 | 181 | 183 | 185 |
| Investor owned | 3 | 4 | 6 | 8 | 8 |
| **Physician Models** | | | | | |
| Independent Practice Association | 42 | 45 | 44 | 70 | 70 |
| Group Practice without Walls | 5 | 8 | 6 | 10 | 5 |
| Open Physician-Hospital Organization | 16 | 22 | 28 | 36 | 34 |
| Closed Physician-Hospital Organization | 11 | 11 | 10 | 11 | 13 |
| Management Service Organization | 12 | 13 | 21 | 32 | 36 |
| Integrated Salary Model | 55 | 46 | 30 | 44 | 31 |
| Equity Model | 2 | 3 | 2 | 2 | 3 |
| Foundation | 4 | 4 | 3 | 5 | 7 |
| **Insurance Products** | | | | | |
| Health Maintenance Organization | 52 | 47 | 38 | 51 | 51 |
| Preferred Provider Organization | 29 | 26 | 30 | 42 | 38 |
| Indemnity Fee for Service | 12 | 6 | 10 | 10 | 5 |
| **Managed Care Contracts** | | | | | |
| Health Maintenance Organization | 129 | 116 | 115 | 140 | 140 |
| Preferred Provider Organization | 118 | 107 | 108 | 128 | 117 |
| **Affiliations** | | | | | |
| Hospitals in a System* | 72 | 74 | 74 | 79 | 70 |
| Hospitals in a Network | 74 | 67 | 71 | 77 | 87 |
| Hospitals in a Group Purchasing Organization | 140 | 128 | 138 | 133 | 133 |

* Please note that system affiliate information for hospitals is derived from AHA membership. In years prior to 2003 the affiliation was derived from a question on the AHA Annual Survey of hospitals; therefore, non-responding hospitals were not included in the system affiliation counts. Years prior to 2003 have been updated to reflect this change, which now include affiliation for non-reporting hospitals.

# TABLE 6

## NEW YORK

*U.S. Registered Community Hospitals*
*(Nonfederal, short-term general and other special hospitals)*

## Utilization, Personnel, Revenue and Expenses, Community Health Indicators 1999–2003

| | 2003 | 2002 | 2001 | 2000 | 1999 |
|---|---|---|---|---|---|
| **TOTAL FACILITY (Includes Hospital and Nursing Home Units)** | | | | | |
| **Utilization - Inpatient** | | | | | |
| Beds | 64,705 | 65,570 | 67,296 | 66,434 | 68,924 |
| Admissions | 2,499,137 | 2,463,447 | 2,410,906 | 2,416,112 | 2,406,327 |
| Inpatient Days | 18,455,619 | 18,394,472 | 19,021,960 | 19,074,063 | 19,349,127 |
| Average Length of Stay | 7.4 | 7.5 | 7.9 | 7.9 | 8.0 |
| Inpatient Surgeries | 663,390 | 698,796 | 692,769 | 722,083 | 710,183 |
| Births | 253,244 | 251,311 | 249,035 | 254,165 | 256,910 |
| **Utilization - Outpatient** | | | | | |
| Emergency Outpatient Visits | 7,483,787 | 7,474,440 | 7,452,574 | 7,275,122 | 7,141,070 |
| Other Outpatient Visits | 40,752,129 | 39,286,094 | 38,193,199 | 39,096,732 | 38,601,503 |
| Total Outpatient Visits | 48,235,916 | 46,760,534 | 45,645,773 | 46,371,854 | 45,742,573 |
| Outpatient Surgeries | 1,331,027 | 1,379,645 | 1,254,924 | 1,263,783 | 1,176,107 |
| **Personnel** | | | | | |
| Full Time RNs | 63,439 | 62,771 | 63,798 | 63,283 | 62,747 |
| Full Time LPNs | 6,957 | 7,361 | 7,538 | 7,424 | 7,318 |
| Part Time RNs | 22,574 | 21,022 | 18,869 | 20,945 | 19,568 |
| Part Time LPNs | 2,288 | 2,240 | 2,094 | 2,208 | 2,188 |
| Total Full Time | 305,826 | 307,318 | 308,267 | 301,182 | 305,163 |
| Total Part Time | 76,403 | 69,818 | 65,664 | 70,536 | 66,143 |
| **Revenue - Inpatient** | | | | | |
| Gross Inpatient Revenue | $55,082,083,246 | $47,822,780,230 | $42,992,186,646 | $37,492,283,644 | $34,644,592,681 |
| **Revenue - Outpatient** | | | | | |
| Gross Outpatient Revenue | $25,788,229,994 | $22,679,522,539 | $19,539,156,438 | $16,875,958,120 | $15,564,285,898 |
| **Revenue and Expenses - Totals (Includes Inpatient and Outpatient)** | | | | | |
| Total Gross Revenue | $80,870,313,240 | $70,502,302,769 | $62,531,343,084 | $54,368,241,764 | $50,208,878,579 |
| Deductions from Revenue | 44,899,282,816 | 37,481,624,861 | 31,905,296,191 | 25,694,206,309 | 22,649,391,683 |
| Net Patient Revenue | 35,971,030,424 | 33,020,677,908 | 30,626,046,893 | 28,674,035,455 | 27,559,486,896 |
| Other Operating Revenue | 3,282,754,959 | 3,204,465,501 | 3,163,011,300 | 2,641,649,037 | 2,645,639,145 |
| Other Nonoperating Revenue | 812,355,098 | 338,322,872 | 482,220,705 | 500,659,020 | 587,485,474 |
| Total Net Revenue | 40,066,140,481 | 36,563,466,281 | 34,271,278,898 | 31,816,343,512 | 30,792,611,515 |
| Total Expenses | 39,939,711,060 | 36,549,754,047 | 34,352,757,050 | 31,963,065,624 | 31,023,119,426 |
| **HOSPITAL UNIT (Excludes Separate Nursing Home Units)** | | | | | |
| **Utilization - Inpatient** | | | | | |
| Beds | 57,780 | 57,534 | 60,609 | 58,655 | 61,313 |
| Admissions | 2,484,569 | 2,448,584 | 2,398,757 | 2,404,711 | 2,395,003 |
| Inpatient Days | 16,087,573 | 15,627,829 | 16,630,275 | 16,229,578 | 16,680,325 |
| Average Length of Stay | 6.5 | 6.4 | 6.9 | 6.7 | 7.0 |
| **Personnel** | | | | | |
| Total Full Time | 300,715 | 301,508 | 302,961 | 294,588 | 300,691 |
| Total Part Time | 74,293 | 67,801 | 63,968 | 68,570 | 64,730 |
| **Revenue and Expenses - Totals (Includes Inpatient and Outpatient)** | | | | | |
| Total Net Revenue | $39,473,173,917 | $35,990,827,886 | $33,722,096,947 | $31,324,367,381 | $30,300,120,420 |
| Total Expenses | 39,358,980,608 | 35,915,200,955 | 33,937,745,908 | 31,557,256,923 | 30,613,692,890 |
| **COMMUNITY HEALTH INDICATORS PER 1000 POPULATION** | | | | | |
| Total Population (in thousands) | 19,190 | 19,134 | 19,075 | 18,997 | 18,883 |
| **Inpatient** | | | | | |
| Beds | 3.4 | 3.4 | 3.5 | 3.5 | 3.7 |
| Admissions | 130.2 | 128.7 | 126.4 | 127.2 | 127.4 |
| Inpatient Days | 961.7 | 961.3 | 997.2 | 1,004.0 | 1,024.7 |
| Inpatient Surgeries | 34.6 | 36.5 | 36.3 | 38.0 | 37.6 |
| Births | 13.2 | 13.1 | 13.1 | 13.4 | 13.6 |
| **Outpatient** | | | | | |
| Emergency Outpatient Visits | 390.0 | 390.6 | 390.7 | 383.0 | 378.2 |
| Other Outpatient Visits | 2,123.6 | 2,053.2 | 2,002.3 | 2,058.0 | 2,044.3 |
| Total Outpatient Visits | 2,513.6 | 2,443.8 | 2,393.0 | 2,441.0 | 2,422.5 |
| Outpatient Surgeries | 69.4 | 72.1 | 65.8 | 66.5 | 62.3 |
| **Expense per Capita (per person)** | $2,081.3 | $1,910.2 | $1,800.9 | $1,682.5 | $1,642.9 |

# Table 6

# NORTH CAROLINA

*U.S. Registered Community Hospitals*
*(Nonfederal, short-term general and other special hospitals)*

## Overview 1999–2003

| | 2003 | 2002 | 2001 | 2000 | 1999 |
|---|---|---|---|---|---|
| **Total Community Hospitals in North Carolina** | **113** | **113** | **111** | **113** | **114** |
| **Bed Size Category** | | | | | |
| 6-24 | 4 | 4 | 2 | 2 | 2 |
| 25-49 | 10 | 10 | 11 | 12 | 12 |
| 50-99 | 24 | 27 | 23 | 22 | 22 |
| 100-199 | 39 | 37 | 38 | 41 | 43 |
| 200-299 | 14 | 13 | 14 | 14 | 14 |
| 300-399 | 8 | 8 | 8 | 9 | 9 |
| 400-499 | 2 | 1 | 3 | 1 | 0 |
| 500 + | 12 | 13 | 12 | 12 | 12 |
| **Location** | | | | | |
| Hospitals Urban | 51 | 51 | 50 | 51 | 52 |
| Hospitals Rural | 62 | 62 | 61 | 62 | 62 |
| **Control** | | | | | |
| State and Local Government | 29 | 30 | 32 | 32 | 33 |
| Not for Profit | 76 | 75 | 70 | 71 | 72 |
| Investor owned | 8 | 8 | 9 | 10 | 9 |
| **Physician Models** | | | | | |
| Independent Practice Association | 12 | 10 | 10 | 14 | 24 |
| Group Practice without Walls | 6 | 4 | 3 | 2 | 1 |
| Open Physician-Hospital Organization | 23 | 25 | 24 | 25 | 31 |
| Closed Physician-Hospital Organization | 7 | 4 | 5 | 3 | 7 |
| Management Service Organization | 15 | 16 | 14 | 17 | 16 |
| Integrated Salary Model | 38 | 35 | 31 | 27 | 31 |
| Equity Model | 2 | 1 | 0 | 1 | 1 |
| Foundation | 8 | 7 | 6 | 5 | 9 |
| **Insurance Products** | | | | | |
| Health Maintenance Organization | 11 | 10 | 11 | 21 | 31 |
| Preferred Provider Organization | 21 | 22 | 19 | 28 | 39 |
| Indemnity Fee for Service | 7 | 5 | 4 | 5 | 10 |
| **Managed Care Contracts** | | | | | |
| Health Maintenance Organization | 72 | 66 | 67 | 71 | 73 |
| Preferred Provider Organization | 84 | 81 | 82 | 83 | 88 |
| **Affiliations** | | | | | |
| Hospitals in a System* | 62 | 63 | 57 | 58 | 52 |
| Hospitals in a Network | 45 | 41 | 42 | 42 | 55 |
| Hospitals in a Group Purchasing Organization | 93 | 86 | 86 | 86 | 96 |

States

* Please note that system affiliate information for hospitals is derived from AHA membership. In years prior to 2003 the affiliation was derived from a question on the AHA Annual Survey of hospitals; therefore, non-responding hospitals were not included in the system affiliation counts. Years prior to 2003 have been updated to reflect this change, which now include affiliation for non-reporting hospitals.

# TABLE 6

# NORTH CAROLINA

*U.S. Registered Community Hospitals*
*(Nonfederal, short-term general and other special hospitals)*

## Utilization, Personnel, Revenue and Expenses, Community Health Indicators 1999–2003

| | 2003 | 2002 | 2001 | 2000 | 1999 |
|---|---|---|---|---|---|
| **TOTAL FACILITY (Includes Hospital and Nursing Home Units)** | | | | | |
| **Utilization - Inpatient** | | | | | |
| Beds | 23,285 | 23,583 | 23,755 | 23,081 | 23,391 |
| Admissions | 987,209 | 966,722 | 973,451 | 970,742 | 930,747 |
| Inpatient Days | 6,053,100 | 5,929,916 | 5,959,143 | 5,859,282 | 5,726,618 |
| Average Length of Stay | 6.1 | 6.1 | 6.1 | 6.0 | 6.2 |
| Inpatient Surgeries | 295,672 | 291,914 | 289,260 | 278,532 | 279,057 |
| Births | 110,364 | 108,967 | 110,585 | 112,885 | 107,946 |
| **Utilization - Outpatient** | | | | | |
| Emergency Outpatient Visits | 3,433,432 | 3,322,226 | 3,230,198 | 2,983,548 | 2,844,680 |
| Other Outpatient Visits | 11,107,315 | 10,500,582 | 10,200,478 | 9,395,105 | 8,695,722 |
| Total Outpatient Visits | 14,540,747 | 13,822,808 | 13,430,676 | 12,378,653 | 11,540,402 |
| Outpatient Surgeries | 556,577 | 519,494 | 460,545 | 435,210 | 442,859 |
| **Personnel** | | | | | |
| Full Time RNs | 26,344 | 26,990 | 25,892 | 25,047 | 25,390 |
| Full Time LPNs | 2,114 | 2,221 | 2,381 | 2,393 | 2,441 |
| Part Time RNs | 12,378 | 11,510 | 10,855 | 10,575 | 9,506 |
| Part Time LPNs | 766 | 738 | 711 | 829 | 778 |
| Total Full Time | 107,326 | 107,239 | 105,994 | 104,926 | 102,981 |
| Total Part Time | 34,498 | 32,029 | 30,745 | 31,480 | 29,055 |
| **Revenue - Inpatient** | | | | | |
| Gross Inpatient Revenue | $15,414,708,940 | $13,579,832,889 | $12,324,492,251 | $11,353,688,447 | $10,061,207,112 |
| **Revenue - Outpatient** | | | | | |
| Gross Outpatient Revenue | $9,605,613,777 | $8,591,785,373 | $7,225,934,040 | $6,225,077,316 | $5,345,769,802 |
| **Revenue and Expenses - Totals (Includes Inpatient and Outpatient)** | | | | | |
| Total Gross Revenue | $25,020,322,717 | $22,171,618,262 | $19,550,426,291 | $17,578,765,763 | $15,406,976,914 |
| Deductions from Revenue | 12,727,067,302 | 10,719,115,151 | 8,934,901,143 | 7,748,738,093 | 6,466,123,700 |
| Net Patient Revenue | 12,293,255,415 | 11,452,503,111 | 10,615,525,148 | 9,830,027,670 | 8,940,853,214 |
| Other Operating Revenue | 678,356,147 | 645,286,961 | 651,522,219 | 604,076,521 | 516,615,284 |
| Other Nonoperating Revenue | 385,414,921 | 81,728,986 | 181,114,779 | 376,862,714 | 311,116,988 |
| Total Net Revenue | 13,357,026,483 | 12,179,519,058 | 11,448,162,146 | 10,810,966,905 | 9,768,585,486 |
| Total Expenses | 12,369,931,674 | 11,563,648,159 | 10,625,022,294 | 10,028,178,236 | 8,980,841,368 |
| **HOSPITAL UNIT (Excludes Separate Nursing Home Units)** | | | | | |
| **Utilization - Inpatient** | | | | | |
| Beds | 20,759 | 20,627 | 21,040 | 20,047 | 20,130 |
| Admissions | 977,527 | 957,259 | 964,357 | 961,312 | 919,616 |
| Inpatient Days | 5,215,187 | 4,968,309 | 5,064,097 | 4,881,713 | 4,623,084 |
| Average Length of Stay | 5.3 | 5.2 | 5.3 | 5.1 | 5.0 |
| **Personnel** | | | | | |
| Total Full Time | 105,215 | 105,030 | 103,658 | 102,369 | 100,023 |
| Total Part Time | 33,515 | 31,000 | 29,819 | 30,453 | 28,139 |
| **Revenue and Expenses - Totals (Includes Inpatient and Outpatient)** | | | | | |
| Total Net Revenue | $13,232,487,962 | $12,041,087,073 | $11,322,622,945 | $10,665,778,056 | $9,617,095,929 |
| Total Expenses | 12,242,509,865 | 11,418,905,299 | 10,504,024,494 | 9,896,919,542 | 8,840,059,827 |
| **COMMUNITY HEALTH INDICATORS PER 1000 POPULATION** | | | | | |
| Total Population (in thousands) | 8,407 | 8,306 | 8,195 | 8,078 | 7,949 |
| **Inpatient** | | | | | |
| Beds | 2.8 | 2.8 | 2.9 | 2.9 | 2.9 |
| Admissions | 117.4 | 116.4 | 118.8 | 120.2 | 117.1 |
| Inpatient Days | 720.0 | 713.9 | 727.1 | 725.4 | 720.4 |
| Inpatient Surgeries | 35.2 | 35.1 | 35.3 | 34.5 | 35.1 |
| Births | 13.1 | 13.1 | 13.5 | 14.0 | 13.6 |
| **Outpatient** | | | | | |
| Emergency Outpatient Visits | 408.4 | 400.0 | 394.2 | 369.4 | 357.9 |
| Other Outpatient Visits | 1,321.2 | 1,264.2 | 1,244.7 | 1,163.1 | 1,093.9 |
| Total Outpatient Visits | 1,729.5 | 1,664.2 | 1,638.8 | 1,532.5 | 1,451.7 |
| Outpatient Surgeries | 66.2 | 62.5 | 56.2 | 53.9 | 55.7 |
| **Expense per Capita (per person)** | $1,471.3 | $1,392.2 | $1,296.5 | $1,241.5 | $1,129.8 |

# TABLE 6

# NORTH DAKOTA

*U.S. Registered Community Hospitals*
*(Nonfederal, short-term general and other special hospitals)*

## Overview 1999–2003

| | 2003 | 2002 | 2001 | 2000 | 1999 |
|---|---|---|---|---|---|
| **Total Community Hospitals in North Dakota** | **40** | **42** | **40** | **42** | **41** |
| **Bed Size Category** | | | | | |
| 6-24 | 7 | 7 | 7 | 7 | 6 |
| 25-49 | 14 | 11 | 11 | 10 | 11 |
| 50-99 | 11 | 16 | 14 | 15 | 13 |
| 100-199 | 4 | 2 | 1 | 3 | 4 |
| 200-299 | 2 | 4 | 5 | 5 | 5 |
| 300-399 | 0 | 0 | 1 | 1 | 1 |
| 400-499 | 1 | 1 | 0 | 1 | 1 |
| 500 + | 1 | 1 | 1 | 0 | 0 |
| **Location** | | | | | |
| Hospitals Urban | 6 | 7 | 7 | 6 | 6 |
| Hospitals Rural | 34 | 35 | 33 | 36 | 35 |
| **Control** | | | | | |
| State and Local Government | 0 | 0 | 0 | 0 | 0 |
| Not for Profit | 40 | 41 | 39 | 40 | 39 |
| Investor owned | 0 | 1 | 1 | 2 | 2 |
| **Physician Models** | | | | | |
| Independent Practice Association | 4 | 4 | 4 | 5 | 7 |
| Group Practice without Walls | 1 | 1 | 0 | 1 | 1 |
| Open Physician-Hospital Organization | 1 | 2 | 1 | 1 | 2 |
| Closed Physician-Hospital Organization | 3 | 2 | 3 | 1 | 1 |
| Management Service Organization | 0 | 0 | 0 | 1 | 1 |
| Integrated Salary Model | 10 | 13 | 13 | 15 | 10 |
| Equity Model | 1 | 1 | 0 | 0 | 1 |
| Foundation | 1 | 2 | 1 | 0 | 1 |
| **Insurance Products** | | | | | |
| Health Maintenance Organization | 0 | 0 | 0 | 1 | 1 |
| Preferred Provider Organization | 6 | 4 | 3 | 4 | 5 |
| Indemnity Fee for Service | 2 | 1 | 1 | 2 | 1 |
| **Managed Care Contracts** | | | | | |
| Health Maintenance Organization | 4 | 5 | 7 | 8 | 9 |
| Preferred Provider Organization | 16 | 19 | 21 | 21 | 19 |
| **Affiliations** | | | | | |
| Hospitals in a System* | 13 | 12 | 10 | 11 | 15 |
| Hospitals in a Network | 11 | 9 | 10 | 8 | 7 |
| Hospitals in a Group Purchasing Organization | 25 | 27 | 28 | 28 | 28 |

States

* Please note that system affiliate information for hospitals is derived from AHA membership. In years prior to 2003 the affiliation was derived from a question on the AHA Annual Survey of hospitals; therefore, non-responding hospitals were not included in the system affiliation counts. Years prior to 2003 have been updated to reflect this change, which now include affiliation for non-reporting hospitals.

# Table 6

## NORTH DAKOTA

*U.S. Registered Community Hospitals*
*(Nonfederal, short-term general and other special hospitals)*

## Utilization, Personnel, Revenue and Expenses, Community Health Indicators 1999–2003

| | 2003 | 2002 | 2001 | 2000 | 1999 |
|---|---|---|---|---|---|
| **TOTAL FACILITY (Includes Hospital and Nursing Home Units)** | | | | | |
| **Utilization - Inpatient** | | | | | |
| Beds | 3,595 | 3,880 | 3,717 | 3,865 | 3,884 |
| Admissions | 88,132 | 94,630 | 91,530 | 89,219 | 86,931 |
| Inpatient Days | 774,175 | 845,194 | 787,722 | 841,256 | 852,457 |
| Average Length of Stay | 8.8 | 8.9 | 8.6 | 9.4 | 9.8 |
| Inpatient Surgeries | 28,325 | 27,650 | 23,814 | 25,052 | 29,603 |
| Births | 9,143 | 9,337 | 8,691 | 8,282 | 8,366 |
| **Utilization - Outpatient** | | | | | |
| Emergency Outpatient Visits | 261,714 | 295,074 | 259,673 | 248,562 | 249,955 |
| Other Outpatient Visits | 1,551,282 | 1,621,700 | 1,599,065 | 1,446,407 | 1,381,484 |
| Total Outpatient Visits | 1,812,996 | 1,916,774 | 1,858,738 | 1,694,969 | 1,631,439 |
| Outpatient Surgeries | 47,969 | 48,213 | 45,718 | 43,764 | 42,656 |
| **Personnel** | | | | | |
| Full Time RNs | 1,836 | 1,884 | 1,734 | 2,075 | 1,634 |
| Full Time LPNs | 534 | 531 | 524 | 458 | 438 |
| Part Time RNs | 2,145 | 2,453 | 2,409 | 1,910 | 2,191 |
| Part Time LPNs | 538 | 583 | 524 | 376 | 560 |
| Total Full Time | 10,892 | 11,676 | 11,343 | 10,921 | 9,834 |
| Total Part Time | 8,236 | 9,379 | 8,618 | 7,529 | 7,749 |
| **Revenue - Inpatient** | | | | | |
| Gross Inpatient Revenue | $1,104,753,788 | $1,302,289,738 | $1,068,649,264 | $1,003,041,889 | $919,295,692 |
| **Revenue - Outpatient** | | | | | |
| Gross Outpatient Revenue | $1,127,663,697 | $1,134,691,244 | $879,815,286 | $766,845,547 | $759,586,932 |
| **Revenue and Expenses - Totals (Includes Inpatient and Outpatient)** | | | | | |
| Total Gross Revenue | $2,232,417,485 | $2,436,980,982 | $1,948,464,550 | $1,769,887,436 | $1,678,882,624 |
| Deductions from Revenue | 941,238,095 | 1,094,215,330 | 798,865,633 | 705,636,353 | 648,667,094 |
| Net Patient Revenue | 1,291,179,390 | 1,342,765,652 | 1,149,598,917 | 1,064,251,083 | 1,030,215,530 |
| Other Operating Revenue | 64,972,544 | 63,807,911 | 65,081,910 | 66,992,430 | 66,044,016 |
| Other Nonoperating Revenue | 22,182,704 | 8,085,712 | 20,055,117 | 32,833,000 | 20,696,900 |
| Total Net Revenue | 1,378,334,638 | 1,414,659,275 | 1,234,735,944 | 1,164,076,513 | 1,116,956,446 |
| Total Expenses | 1,347,844,373 | 1,351,763,031 | 1,220,687,431 | 1,111,495,262 | 1,063,751,582 |
| **HOSPITAL UNIT (Excludes Separate Nursing Home Units)** | | | | | |
| **Utilization - Inpatient** | | | | | |
| Beds | 2,656 | 2,883 | 2,762 | 3,099 | 2,935 |
| Admissions | 85,822 | 92,446 | 90,169 | 87,453 | 84,780 |
| Inpatient Days | 466,368 | 515,332 | 479,300 | 606,974 | 536,949 |
| Average Length of Stay | 5.4 | 5.6 | 5.3 | 6.9 | 6.3 |
| **Personnel** | | | | | |
| Total Full Time | 10,281 | 11,066 | 10,726 | 10,496 | 9,077 |
| Total Part Time | 7,671 | 8,878 | 8,119 | 7,126 | 7,134 |
| **Revenue and Expenses - Totals (Includes Inpatient and Outpatient)** | | | | | |
| Total Net Revenue | $1,329,671,873 | $1,365,837,644 | $1,196,091,770 | $1,136,148,987 | $1,075,514,346 |
| Total Expenses | 1,307,814,219 | 1,314,789,098 | 1,188,642,681 | 1,088,906,965 | 1,032,134,787 |
| **COMMUNITY HEALTH INDICATORS PER 1000 POPULATION** | | | | | |
| Total Population (in thousands) | 634 | 634 | 636 | 641 | 644 |
| **Inpatient** | | | | | |
| Beds | 5.7 | 6.1 | 5.8 | 6.0 | 6.0 |
| Admissions | 139.0 | 149.3 | 143.9 | 139.2 | 134.9 |
| Inpatient Days | 1,221.4 | 1,333.3 | 1,238.0 | 1,312.2 | 1,323.2 |
| Inpatient Surgeries | 44.7 | 43.6 | 37.4 | 39.1 | 45.9 |
| Births | 14.4 | 14.7 | 13.7 | 12.9 | 13.0 |
| **Outpatient** | | | | | |
| Emergency Outpatient Visits | 412.9 | 465.5 | 408.1 | 387.7 | 388.0 |
| Other Outpatient Visits | 2,447.4 | 2,558.2 | 2,513.1 | 2,256.2 | 2,144.3 |
| Total Outpatient Visits | 2,860.4 | 3,023.7 | 2,921.2 | 2,643.9 | 2,532.3 |
| Outpatient Surgeries | 75.7 | 76.1 | 71.9 | 68.3 | 66.2 |
| **Expense per Capita (per person)** | $2,126.5 | $2,132.4 | $1,918.5 | $1,733.8 | $1,651.1 |

# TABLE 6

# OHIO

*U.S. Registered Community Hospitals*
*(Nonfederal, short-term general and other special hospitals)*

## Overview 1999–2003

| | 2003 | 2002 | 2001 | 2000 | 1999 |
|---|---|---|---|---|---|
| **Total Community Hospitals in Ohio** | **163** | **168** | **166** | **163** | **167** |
| **Bed Size Category** | | | | | |
| 6-24 | 0 | 2 | 2 | 2 | 3 |
| 25-49 | 29 | 27 | 22 | 21 | 21 |
| 50-99 | 26 | 27 | 33 | 31 | 33 |
| 100-199 | 49 | 50 | 50 | 50 | 52 |
| 200-299 | 24 | 27 | 26 | 24 | 23 |
| 300-399 | 16 | 16 | 14 | 15 | 14 |
| 400-499 | 9 | 9 | 9 | 9 | 10 |
| 500 + | 10 | 10 | 10 | 11 | 11 |
| **Location** | | | | | |
| Hospitals Urban | 113 | 116 | 114 | 111 | 114 |
| Hospitals Rural | 50 | 52 | 52 | 52 | 53 |
| **Control** | | | | | |
| State and Local Government | 23 | 23 | 23 | 22 | 23 |
| Not for Profit | 136 | 141 | 139 | 137 | 139 |
| Investor owned | 4 | 4 | 4 | 4 | 5 |
| **Physician Models** | | | | | |
| Independent Practice Association | 20 | 17 | 23 | 15 | 19 |
| Group Practice without Walls | 9 | 11 | 12 | 10 | 11 |
| Open Physician-Hospital Organization | 43 | 47 | 46 | 51 | 63 |
| Closed Physician-Hospital Organization | 25 | 18 | 26 | 19 | 20 |
| Management Service Organization | 35 | 33 | 33 | 39 | 44 |
| Integrated Salary Model | 55 | 44 | 53 | 44 | 52 |
| Equity Model | 2 | 7 | 9 | 7 | 7 |
| Foundation | 20 | 14 | 21 | 18 | 21 |
| **Insurance Products** | | | | | |
| Health Maintenance Organization | 28 | 27 | 32 | 38 | 45 |
| Preferred Provider Organization | 34 | 32 | 36 | 37 | 44 |
| Indemnity Fee for Service | 14 | 12 | 12 | 11 | 12 |
| **Managed Care Contracts** | | | | | |
| Health Maintenance Organization | 114 | 104 | 110 | 110 | 112 |
| Preferred Provider Organization | 123 | 112 | 115 | 116 | 118 |
| **Affiliations** | | | | | |
| Hospitals in a System* | 83 | 84 | 81 | 75 | 73 |
| Hospitals in a Network | 67 | 60 | 68 | 52 | 54 |
| Hospitals in a Group Purchasing Organization | 140 | 126 | 134 | 130 | 133 |

States

* Please note that system affiliate information for hospitals is derived from AHA membership. In years prior to 2003 the affiliation was derived from a question on the AHA Annual Survey of hospitals; therefore, non-responding hospitals were not included in the system affiliation counts. Years prior to 2003 have been updated to reflect this change, which now include affiliation for non-reporting hospitals.

# OHIO

*U.S. Registered Community Hospitals*
*(Nonfederal, short-term general and other special hospitals)*

## Utilization, Personnel, Revenue and Expenses, Community Health Indicators 1999–2003

| | 2003 | 2002 | 2001 | 2000 | 1999 |
|---|---|---|---|---|---|
| **TOTAL FACILITY (Includes Hospital and Nursing Home Units)** | | | | | |
| **Utilization - Inpatient** | | | | | |
| Beds | 32,981 | 33,706 | 33,310 | 33,849 | 34,164 |
| Admissions | 1,457,933 | 1,475,630 | 1,439,252 | 1,404,467 | 1,358,662 |
| Inpatient Days | 7,501,323 | 7,657,394 | 7,483,873 | 7,556,261 | 7,362,468 |
| Average Length of Stay | 5.1 | 5.2 | 5.2 | 5.4 | 5.4 |
| Inpatient Surgeries | 416,945 | 431,329 | 417,023 | 400,999 | 390,732 |
| Births | 147,253 | 150,298 | 151,371 | 149,565 | 147,506 |
| **Utilization - Outpatient** | | | | | |
| Emergency Outpatient Visits | 5,354,136 | 5,125,829 | 5,124,561 | 5,133,276 | 4,906,178 |
| Other Outpatient Visits | 24,668,217 | 23,229,558 | 23,252,713 | 21,724,028 | 19,980,036 |
| Total Outpatient Visits | 30,022,353 | 28,355,387 | 28,377,274 | 26,857,304 | 24,886,214 |
| Outpatient Surgeries | 798,612 | 810,253 | 793,989 | 798,907 | 765,459 |
| **Personnel** | | | | | |
| Full Time RNs | 38,391 | 35,036 | 34,676 | 33,921 | 34,424 |
| Full Time LPNs | 4,319 | 4,011 | 3,961 | 3,644 | 4,039 |
| Part Time RNs | 22,823 | 22,467 | 22,713 | 22,568 | 19,371 |
| Part Time LPNs | 2,227 | 2,211 | 2,123 | 2,028 | 2,140 |
| Total Full Time | 168,483 | 161,392 | 159,239 | 151,382 | 151,875 |
| Total Part Time | 69,146 | 66,399 | 66,944 | 66,769 | 60,642 |
| **Revenue - Inpatient** | | | | | |
| Gross Inpatient Revenue | $25,399,812,064 | $23,112,708,865 | $20,613,914,515 | $17,881,757,694 | $15,806,982,496 |
| **Revenue - Outpatient** | | | | | |
| Gross Outpatient Revenue | $19,459,508,400 | $16,391,385,950 | $14,224,448,482 | $11,888,253,297 | $10,278,820,338 |
| **Revenue and Expenses - Totals (Includes Inpatient and Outpatient)** | | | | | |
| Total Gross Revenue | $44,859,320,464 | $39,504,094,815 | $34,838,362,997 | $29,770,010,991 | $26,085,802,834 |
| Deductions from Revenue | 24,821,741,430 | 20,841,549,318 | 17,753,807,229 | 14,553,540,678 | 11,859,000,198 |
| Net Patient Revenue | 20,037,579,034 | 18,662,545,497 | 17,084,555,768 | 15,216,470,313 | 14,226,802,636 |
| Other Operating Revenue | 1,114,390,509 | 1,069,165,656 | 1,084,169,641 | 727,705,267 | 834,560,047 |
| Other Nonoperating Revenue | 252,611,257 | 60,979,408 | 132,770,316 | 558,247,388 | 446,576,015 |
| Total Net Revenue | 21,404,580,800 | 19,792,690,561 | 18,301,495,725 | 16,502,422,968 | 15,507,938,698 |
| Total Expenses | 20,465,149,310 | 19,132,292,794 | 17,866,114,856 | 15,550,349,910 | 14,881,546,876 |
| **HOSPITAL UNIT (Excludes Separate Nursing Home Units)** | | | | | |
| **Utilization - Inpatient** | | | | | |
| Beds | 31,260 | 31,729 | 31,471 | 31,413 | 31,118 |
| Admissions | 1,440,323 | 1,458,479 | 1,421,435 | 1,381,778 | 1,328,866 |
| Inpatient Days | 6,977,632 | 7,051,923 | 6,925,175 | 6,775,436 | 6,471,288 |
| Average Length of Stay | 4.8 | 4.8 | 4.9 | 4.9 | 4.9 |
| **Personnel** | | | | | |
| Total Full Time | 167,029 | 159,965 | 157,884 | 149,237 | 149,246 |
| Total Part Time | 68,267 | 65,646 | 66,306 | 65,817 | 59,403 |
| **Revenue and Expenses - Totals (Includes Inpatient and Outpatient)** | | | | | |
| Total Net Revenue | $21,161,469,394 | $19,619,443,053 | $18,146,551,602 | $16,331,999,691 | $15,247,381,253 |
| Total Expenses | 20,242,498,362 | 18,970,939,986 | 17,752,957,340 | 15,427,132,070 | 14,660,321,444 |
| **COMMUNITY HEALTH INDICATORS PER 1000 POPULATION** | | | | | |
| Total Population (in thousands) | 11,436 | 11,409 | 11,386 | 11,363 | 11,335 |
| **Inpatient** | | | | | |
| Beds | 2.9 | 3.0 | 2.9 | 3.0 | 3.0 |
| Admissions | 127.5 | 129.3 | 126.4 | 123.6 | 119.9 |
| Inpatient Days | 656.0 | 671.2 | 657.3 | 665.0 | 649.5 |
| Inpatient Surgeries | 36.5 | 37.8 | 36.6 | 35.3 | 34.5 |
| Births | 12.9 | 13.2 | 13.3 | 13.2 | 13.0 |
| **Outpatient** | | | | | |
| Emergency Outpatient Visits | 468.2 | 449.3 | 450.1 | 451.7 | 432.8 |
| Other Outpatient Visits | 2,157.1 | 2,036.1 | 2,042.2 | 1,911.8 | 1,762.6 |
| Total Outpatient Visits | 2,625.3 | 2,485.4 | 2,492.3 | 2,363.5 | 2,195.4 |
| Outpatient Surgeries | 69.8 | 71.0 | 69.7 | 70.3 | 67.5 |
| **Expense per Capita (per person)** | $1,789.6 | $1,677.0 | $1,569.2 | $1,368.5 | $1,312.8 |

# TABLE 6

## OKLAHOMA

*U.S. Registered Community Hospitals*
*(Nonfederal, short-term general and other special hospitals)*

## Overview 1999–2003

| | 2003 | 2002 | 2001 | 2000 | 1999 |
|---|---|---|---|---|---|
| **Total Community Hospitals in Oklahoma** | **108** | **105** | **108** | **108** | **109** |
| **Bed Size Category** | | | | | |
| 6-24 | 17 | 15 | 15 | 14 | 15 |
| 25-49 | 40 | 36 | 38 | 41 | 40 |
| 50-99 | 21 | 24 | 22 | 22 | 21 |
| 100-199 | 16 | 15 | 18 | 15 | 17 |
| 200-299 | 6 | 6 | 7 | 8 | 8 |
| 300-399 | 2 | 3 | 2 | 2 | 3 |
| 400-499 | 1 | 2 | 3 | 3 | 1 |
| 500 + | 5 | 4 | 3 | 3 | 4 |
| **Location** | | | | | |
| Hospitals Urban | 41 | 38 | 40 | 40 | 41 |
| Hospitals Rural | 67 | 67 | 68 | 68 | 68 |
| **Control** | | | | | |
| State and Local Government | 47 | 44 | 45 | 45 | 50 |
| Not for Profit | 46 | 46 | 48 | 49 | 44 |
| Investor owned | 15 | 15 | 15 | 14 | 15 |
| **Physician Models** | | | | | |
| Independent Practice Association | 16 | 14 | 12 | 16 | 16 |
| Group Practice without Walls | 3 | 3 | 1 | 3 | 3 |
| Open Physician-Hospital Organization | 16 | 15 | 14 | 22 | 23 |
| Closed Physician-Hospital Organization | 8 | 8 | 10 | 6 | 8 |
| Management Service Organization | 14 | 11 | 11 | 15 | 11 |
| Integrated Salary Model | 34 | 22 | 16 | 16 | 19 |
| Equity Model | 1 | 0 | 1 | 2 | 1 |
| Foundation | 4 | 0 | 4 | 4 | 2 |
| **Insurance Products** | | | | | |
| Health Maintenance Organization | 11 | 11 | 18 | 26 | 28 |
| Preferred Provider Organization | 24 | 17 | 18 | 32 | 32 |
| Indemnity Fee for Service | 10 | 6 | 5 | 6 | 6 |
| **Managed Care Contracts** | | | | | |
| Health Maintenance Organization | 39 | 37 | 40 | 42 | 55 |
| Preferred Provider Organization | 65 | 54 | 61 | 65 | 82 |
| **Affiliations** | | | | | |
| Hospitals in a System* | 56 | 55 | 58 | 53 | 56 |
| Hospitals in a Network | 22 | 17 | 18 | 22 | 29 |
| Hospitals in a Group Purchasing Organization | 80 | 66 | 67 | 63 | — |

States

* Please note that system affiliate information for hospitals is derived from AHA membership. In years prior to 2003 the affiliation was derived from a question on the AHA Annual Survey of hospitals; therefore, non-responding hospitals were not included in the system affiliation counts. Years prior to 2003 have been updated to reflect this change, which now include affiliation for non-reporting hospitals.

## TABLE 6

# OKLAHOMA

*U.S. Registered Community Hospitals*
*(Nonfederal, short-term general and other special hospitals)*

## Utilization, Personnel, Revenue and Expenses, Community Health Indicators 1999–2003

| | 2003 | 2002 | 2001 | 2000 | 1999 |
|---|---|---|---|---|---|
| **TOTAL FACILITY (Includes Hospital and Nursing Home Units)** | | | | | |
| **Utilization - Inpatient** | | | | | |
| Beds | 11,018 | 11,122 | 11,207 | 11,112 | 11,075 |
| Admissions | 449,936 | 445,952 | 434,831 | 428,927 | 411,025 |
| Inpatient Days | 2,380,232 | 2,371,009 | 2,360,979 | 2,280,050 | 2,273,850 |
| Average Length of Stay | 5.3 | 5.3 | 5.4 | 5.3 | 5.5 |
| Inpatient Surgeries | 116,951 | 109,770 | 120,417 | 117,785 | 123,765 |
| Births | 44,736 | 43,564 | 43,053 | 43,461 | 44,295 |
| **Utilization - Outpatient** | | | | | |
| Emergency Outpatient Visits | 1,386,848 | 1,292,652 | 1,226,716 | 1,134,337 | 1,172,259 |
| Other Outpatient Visits | 4,102,880 | 3,510,111 | 3,343,188 | 3,567,619 | 3,452,578 |
| Total Outpatient Visits | 5,489,728 | 4,802,763 | 4,569,904 | 4,701,956 | 4,624,837 |
| Outpatient Surgeries | 180,442 | 173,030 | 173,752 | 182,488 | 186,624 |
| **Personnel** | | | | | |
| Full Time RNs | 8,867 | 8,738 | 8,403 | 8,194 | 8,054 |
| Full Time LPNs | 2,393 | 2,302 | 2,422 | 2,087 | 2,312 |
| Part Time RNs | 3,110 | 3,469 | 3,708 | 3,453 | 3,041 |
| Part Time LPNs | 769 | 698 | 758 | 618 | 701 |
| Total Full Time | 42,527 | 41,470 | 43,342 | 41,964 | 39,901 |
| Total Part Time | 12,063 | 13,105 | 12,815 | 11,583 | 11,864 |
| **Revenue - Inpatient** | | | | | |
| Gross Inpatient Revenue | $7,071,793,695 | $6,358,250,635 | $5,478,614,594 | $5,218,973,104 | $4,678,294,998 |
| **Revenue - Outpatient** | | | | | |
| Gross Outpatient Revenue | $3,555,834,680 | $3,123,729,308 | $2,830,596,281 | $2,560,162,792 | $2,337,006,164 |
| **Revenue and Expenses - Totals (Includes Inpatient and Outpatient)** | | | | | |
| Total Gross Revenue | $10,627,628,375 | $9,481,979,943 | $8,309,210,875 | $7,779,135,896 | $7,015,301,162 |
| Deductions from Revenue | 6,294,574,391 | 5,455,901,182 | 4,548,324,907 | 4,263,955,656 | 3,677,580,563 |
| Net Patient Revenue | 4,333,053,984 | 4,026,078,761 | 3,760,885,968 | 3,515,180,240 | 3,337,720,599 |
| Other Operating Revenue | 336,044,566 | 253,147,564 | 234,843,029 | 268,105,178 | 238,136,668 |
| Other Nonoperating Revenue | 55,328,125 | 26,110,536 | 39,695,513 | 28,871,537 | 64,910,590 |
| Total Net Revenue | 4,724,426,675 | 4,305,336,861 | 4,035,424,510 | 3,812,156,955 | 3,640,767,857 |
| Total Expenses | 4,427,836,412 | 3,986,180,785 | 3,722,315,467 | 3,689,668,282 | 3,433,636,312 |
| **HOSPITAL UNIT (Excludes Separate Nursing Home Units)** | | | | | |
| **Utilization - Inpatient** | | | | | |
| Beds | 10,669 | 10,877 | 10,857 | 10,788 | 10,577 |
| Admissions | 445,825 | 443,327 | 431,093 | 423,287 | 406,459 |
| Inpatient Days | 2,274,063 | 2,295,445 | 2,248,489 | 2,179,541 | 2,123,082 |
| Average Length of Stay | 5.1 | 5.2 | 5.2 | 5.1 | 5.2 |
| **Personnel** | | | | | |
| Total Full Time | 42,093 | 41,248 | 42,873 | 41,541 | 39,636 |
| Total Part Time | 11,939 | 13,022 | 12,693 | 11,436 | 11,809 |
| **Revenue and Expenses - Totals (Includes Inpatient and Outpatient)** | | | | | |
| Total Net Revenue | $4,704,868,435 | $4,290,663,306 | $4,008,168,171 | $3,774,861,696 | $3,624,098,673 |
| Total Expenses | 4,411,790,782 | 3,977,214,712 | 3,697,330,894 | 3,669,710,412 | 3,421,100,441 |
| **COMMUNITY HEALTH INDICATORS PER 1000 POPULATION** | | | | | |
| Total Population (in thousands) | 3,512 | 3,490 | 3,467 | 3,454 | 3,437 |
| **Inpatient** | | | | | |
| Beds | 3.1 | 3.2 | 3.2 | 3.2 | 3.2 |
| Admissions | 128.1 | 127.8 | 125.4 | 124.2 | 119.6 |
| Inpatient Days | 677.8 | 679.4 | 681.0 | 660.1 | 661.6 |
| Inpatient Surgeries | 33.3 | 31.5 | 34.7 | 34.1 | 36.0 |
| Births | 12.7 | 12.5 | 12.4 | 12.6 | 12.9 |
| **Outpatient** | | | | | |
| Emergency Outpatient Visits | 394.9 | 370.4 | 353.8 | 328.4 | 341.1 |
| Other Outpatient Visits | 1,168.4 | 1,005.8 | 964.2 | 1,032.9 | 1,004.5 |
| Total Outpatient Visits | 1,563.3 | 1,376.3 | 1,318.0 | 1,361.3 | 1,345.5 |
| Outpatient Surgeries | 51.4 | 49.6 | 50.1 | 52.8 | 54.3 |
| **Expense per Capita (per person)** | $1,260.9 | $1,142.3 | $1,073.6 | $1,068.2 | $999.0 |

# TABLE 6

# OREGON

*U.S. Registered Community Hospitals*
*(Nonfederal, short-term general and other special hospitals)*

## Overview 1999–2003

| | 2003 | 2002 | 2001 | 2000 | 1999 |
|---|---|---|---|---|---|
| **Total Community Hospitals in Oregon** | **58** | **60** | **60** | **59** | **59** |
| **Bed Size Category** | | | | | |
| 6-24 | 6 | 5 | 5 | 5 | 5 |
| 25-49 | 20 | 18 | 19 | 21 | 21 |
| 50-99 | 12 | 17 | 17 | 13 | 11 |
| 100-199 | 10 | 11 | 10 | 10 | 12 |
| 200-299 | 4 | 3 | 3 | 4 | 4 |
| 300-399 | 1 | 3 | 3 | 3 | 4 |
| 400-499 | 5 | 3 | 3 | 3 | 2 |
| 500 + | 0 | 0 | 0 | 0 | 0 |
| **Location** | | | | | |
| Hospitals Urban | 27 | 29 | 28 | 27 | 27 |
| Hospitals Rural | 31 | 31 | 32 | 32 | 32 |
| **Control** | | | | | |
| State and Local Government | 12 | 12 | 12 | 15 | 15 |
| Not for Profit | 43 | 44 | 44 | 41 | 41 |
| Investor owned | 3 | 4 | 4 | 3 | 3 |
| **Physician Models** | | | | | |
| Independent Practice Association | 14 | 26 | 26 | 22 | 19 |
| Group Practice without Walls | 4 | 3 | 3 | 0 | 1 |
| Open Physician-Hospital Organization | 6 | 4 | 7 | 3 | 7 |
| Closed Physician-Hospital Organization | 4 | 4 | 5 | 3 | 4 |
| Management Service Organization | 5 | 7 | 8 | 7 | 6 |
| Integrated Salary Model | 17 | 21 | 24 | 23 | 21 |
| Equity Model | 0 | 0 | 0 | 0 | 0 |
| Foundation | 1 | 2 | 2 | 1 | 1 |
| **Insurance Products** | | | | | |
| Health Maintenance Organization | 12 | 14 | 13 | 12 | 17 |
| Preferred Provider Organization | 15 | 15 | 12 | 12 | 13 |
| Indemnity Fee for Service | 6 | 2 | 2 | 1 | 1 |
| **Managed Care Contracts** | | | | | |
| Health Maintenance Organization | 30 | 41 | 44 | 40 | 41 |
| Preferred Provider Organization | 35 | 47 | 49 | 43 | 42 |
| **Affiliations** | | | | | |
| Hospitals in a System* | 34 | 35 | 35 | 31 | 33 |
| Hospitals in a Network | 12 | 19 | 21 | 16 | 17 |
| Hospitals in a Group Purchasing Organization | 39 | 53 | 56 | 48 | 49 |

* Please note that system affiliate information for hospitals is derived from AHA membership. In years prior to 2003 the affiliation was derived from a question on the AHA Annual Survey of hospitals; therefore, non-responding hospitals were not included in the system affiliation counts. Years prior to 2003 have been updated to reflect this change, which now include affiliation for non-reporting hospitals.

# TABLE 6

# OREGON

*U.S. Registered Community Hospitals*
*(Nonfederal, short-term general and other special hospitals)*

## Utilization, Personnel, Revenue and Expenses, Community Health Indicators 1999–2003

| | 2003 | 2002 | 2001 | 2000 | 1999 |
|---|---|---|---|---|---|
| **TOTAL FACILITY (Includes Hospital and Nursing Home Units)** | | | | | |
| **Utilization - Inpatient** | | | | | |
| Beds | 6,757 | 6,798 | 6,660 | 6,631 | 6,643 |
| Admissions | 342,282 | 345,193 | 334,862 | 329,932 | 317,808 |
| Inpatient Days | 1,455,069 | 1,511,420 | 1,449,556 | 1,435,545 | 1,409,906 |
| Average Length of Stay | 4.3 | 4.4 | 4.3 | 4.4 | 4.4 |
| Inpatient Surgeries | 114,111 | 113,669 | 108,024 | 105,967 | 103,162 |
| Births | 45,704 | 45,409 | 45,279 | 46,065 | 45,328 |
| **Utilization - Outpatient** | | | | | |
| Emergency Outpatient Visits | 1,113,166 | 1,117,313 | 1,098,201 | 1,008,428 | 921,414 |
| Other Outpatient Visits | 7,073,918 | 7,058,865 | 6,559,929 | 6,264,342 | 5,736,216 |
| Total Outpatient Visits | 8,187,084 | 8,176,178 | 7,658,130 | 7,272,770 | 6,657,630 |
| Outpatient Surgeries | 196,364 | 191,717 | 172,400 | 167,938 | 163,147 |
| **Personnel** | | | | | |
| Full Time RNs | 8,074 | 7,114 | 7,975 | 8,054 | 6,426 |
| Full Time LPNs | 532 | 547 | 420 | 448 | 409 |
| Part Time RNs | 6,582 | 7,454 | 6,588 | 6,224 | 6,315 |
| Part Time LPNs | 287 | 568 | 314 | 285 | 349 |
| Total Full Time | 33,648 | 32,765 | 32,473 | 31,121 | 26,971 |
| Total Part Time | 18,250 | 22,952 | 18,793 | 17,828 | 17,324 |
| **Revenue - Inpatient** | | | | | |
| Gross Inpatient Revenue | $5,042,552,776 | $4,563,875,879 | $3,859,967,211 | $3,485,892,570 | $3,113,689,297 |
| **Revenue - Outpatient** | | | | | |
| Gross Outpatient Revenue | $3,652,443,825 | $3,183,571,829 | $2,728,455,375 | $2,350,061,380 | $2,048,806,236 |
| **Revenue and Expenses - Totals (Includes Inpatient and Outpatient)** | | | | | |
| Total Gross Revenue | $8,694,996,601 | $7,747,447,708 | $6,588,422,586 | $5,835,953,950 | $5,162,495,533 |
| Deductions from Revenue | 3,877,092,481 | 3,206,030,580 | 2,617,704,367 | 2,306,496,669 | 1,947,905,128 |
| Net Patient Revenue | 4,817,904,120 | 4,541,417,128 | 3,970,718,219 | 3,529,457,281 | 3,214,590,405 |
| Other Operating Revenue | 245,884,763 | 220,287,872 | 225,753,818 | 233,238,786 | 201,378,271 |
| Other Nonoperating Revenue | 21,294,360 | 6,824,416 | 63,051,233 | 69,416,016 | 75,147,493 |
| Total Net Revenue | 5,085,083,243 | 4,768,529,416 | 4,259,523,270 | 3,832,112,083 | 3,491,116,169 |
| Total Expenses | 4,806,543,508 | 4,468,834,030 | 3,951,387,339 | 3,600,487,783 | 3,286,343,045 |
| **HOSPITAL UNIT (Excludes Separate Nursing Home Units)** | | | | | |
| **Utilization - Inpatient** | | | | | |
| Beds | 6,460 | 6,452 | 6,184 | 6,111 | 6,027 |
| Admissions | 341,317 | 344,564 | 331,985 | 326,453 | 313,845 |
| Inpatient Days | 1,380,053 | 1,406,690 | 1,325,563 | 1,294,908 | 1,251,063 |
| Average Length of Stay | 4.0 | 4.1 | 4.0 | 4.0 | 4.0 |
| **Personnel** | | | | | |
| Total Full Time | 33,506 | 32,601 | 32,229 | 30,783 | 26,646 |
| Total Part Time | 18,131 | 22,777 | 18,651 | 17,669 | 17,145 |
| **Revenue and Expenses - Totals (Includes Inpatient and Outpatient)** | | | | | |
| Total Net Revenue | $5,075,462,319 | $4,756,252,635 | $4,234,725,706 | $3,810,739,241 | $3,469,658,693 |
| Total Expenses | 4,796,593,445 | 4,455,142,703 | 3,927,287,050 | 3,582,438,850 | 3,271,980,437 |
| **COMMUNITY HEALTH INDICATORS PER 1000 POPULATION** | | | | | |
| Total Population (in thousands) | 3,560 | 3,520 | 3,473 | 3,431 | 3,394 |
| **Inpatient** | | | | | |
| Beds | 1.9 | 1.9 | 1.9 | 1.9 | 2.0 |
| Admissions | 96.2 | 98.1 | 96.4 | 96.2 | 93.6 |
| Inpatient Days | 408.8 | 429.3 | 417.4 | 418.4 | 415.4 |
| Inpatient Surgeries | 32.1 | 32.3 | 31.1 | 30.9 | 30.4 |
| Births | 12.8 | 12.9 | 13.0 | 13.4 | 13.4 |
| **Outpatient** | | | | | |
| Emergency Outpatient Visits | 312.7 | 317.4 | 316.2 | 293.9 | 271.5 |
| Other Outpatient Visits | 1,987.3 | 2,005.2 | 1,889.0 | 1,826.0 | 1,690.1 |
| Total Outpatient Visits | 2,300.0 | 2,322.5 | 2,205.3 | 2,119.9 | 1,961.6 |
| Outpatient Surgeries | 55.2 | 54.5 | 49.6 | 49.0 | 48.1 |
| **Expense per Capita (per person)** | $1,350.3 | $1,269.4 | $1,137.9 | $1,049.5 | $968.3 |

# TABLE 6

# PENNSYLVANIA

*U.S. Registered Community Hospitals*
*(Nonfederal, short-term general and other special hospitals)*

## Overview 1999–2003

| | 2003 | 2002 | 2001 | 2000 | 1999 |
|---|---|---|---|---|---|
| **Total Community Hospitals in Pennsylvania** . . . | **201** | **201** | **205** | **207** | **210** |
| **Bed Size Category** | | | | | |
| 6-24 | 4 | 4 | 3 | 4 | 5 |
| 25-49 | 15 | 13 | 14 | 12 | 12 |
| 50-99 | 35 | 36 | 33 | 34 | 34 |
| 100-199 | 68 | 71 | 74 | 79 | 78 |
| 200-299 | 42 | 40 | 42 | 39 | 42 |
| 300-399 | 14 | 14 | 14 | 11 | 11 |
| 400-499 | 12 | 11 | 12 | 15 | 13 |
| 500 + | 11 | 12 | 13 | 13 | 15 |
| **Location** | | | | | |
| Hospitals Urban | 158 | 158 | 161 | 163 | 165 |
| Hospitals Rural | 43 | 43 | 44 | 44 | 45 |
| **Control** | | | | | |
| State and Local Government | 2 | 2 | 2 | 2 | 1 |
| Not for Profit | 177 | 184 | 189 | 194 | 199 |
| Investor owned | 22 | 15 | 14 | 11 | 10 |
| **Physician Models** | | | | | |
| Independent Practice Association | 19 | 18 | 20 | 23 | 29 |
| Group Practice without Walls | 14 | 10 | 12 | 12 | 13 |
| Open Physician-Hospital Organization | 41 | 40 | 39 | 53 | 54 |
| Closed Physician-Hospital Organization | 4 | 10 | 10 | 15 | 24 |
| Management Service Organization | 26 | 28 | 32 | 41 | 39 |
| Integrated Salary Model | 66 | 57 | 53 | 53 | 53 |
| Equity Model | 6 | 4 | 3 | 11 | 8 |
| Foundation | 8 | 7 | 5 | 9 | 9 |
| **Insurance Products** | | | | | |
| Health Maintenance Organization | 26 | 25 | 25 | 32 | 36 |
| Preferred Provider Organization | 43 | 39 | 38 | 41 | 46 |
| Indemnity Fee for Service | 9 | 8 | 6 | 4 | 5 |
| **Managed Care Contracts** | | | | | |
| Health Maintenance Organization | 142 | 149 | 150 | 153 | 153 |
| Preferred Provider Organization | 139 | 143 | 144 | 147 | 148 |
| **Affiliations** | | | | | |
| Hospitals in a System* | 104 | 99 | 100 | 99 | 96 |
| Hospitals in a Network | 45 | 53 | 45 | 57 | 53 |
| Hospitals in a Group Purchasing Organization | 156 | 161 | 151 | 151 | 137 |

* Please note that system affiliate information for hospitals is derived from AHA membership. In years prior to 2003 the affiliation was derived from a question on the AHA Annual Survey of hospitals; therefore, non-responding hospitals were not included in the system affiliation counts. Years prior to 2003 have been updated to reflect this change, which now include affiliation for non-reporting hospitals.

# TABLE 6

# PENNSYLVANIA

*U.S. Registered Community Hospitals*
*(Nonfederal, short-term general and other special hospitals)*

## Utilization, Personnel, Revenue and Expenses, Community Health Indicators 1999–2003

| | 2003 | 2002 | 2001 | 2000 | 1999 |
|---|---|---|---|---|---|
| **TOTAL FACILITY (Includes Hospital and Nursing Home Units)** | | | | | |
| **Utilization - Inpatient** | | | | | |
| Beds | 40,908 | 40,534 | 42,131 | 42,303 | 42,999 |
| Admissions | 1,824,132 | 1,798,243 | 1,808,531 | 1,796,081 | 1,755,029 |
| Inpatient Days | 10,300,758 | 10,340,276 | 10,395,360 | 10,558,152 | 10,652,791 |
| Average Length of Stay | 5.6 | 5.8 | 5.7 | 5.9 | 6.1 |
| Inpatient Surgeries | 531,212 | 537,857 | 544,254 | 534,894 | 555,367 |
| Births | 137,718 | 139,489 | 143,463 | 139,408 | 139,888 |
| **Utilization - Outpatient** | | | | | |
| Emergency Outpatient Visits | 5,160,713 | 5,059,150 | 4,873,595 | 4,727,149 | 4,615,588 |
| Other Outpatient Visits | 28,124,567 | 27,349,887 | 27,189,829 | 27,122,027 | 24,653,538 |
| Total Outpatient Visits | 33,285,280 | 32,409,037 | 32,063,424 | 31,849,176 | 29,269,126 |
| Outpatient Surgeries | 966,727 | 983,477 | 1,034,191 | 997,911 | 969,895 |
| **Personnel** | | | | | |
| Full Time RNs | 41,791 | 40,679 | 39,444 | 39,290 | 39,819 |
| Full Time LPNs | 4,803 | 4,910 | 4,962 | 4,807 | 5,287 |
| Part Time RNs | 25,123 | 24,880 | 23,733 | 22,678 | 22,707 |
| Part Time LPNs | 2,494 | 2,557 | 2,515 | 2,541 | 2,735 |
| Total Full Time | 186,132 | 185,944 | 181,276 | 178,775 | 179,851 |
| Total Part Time | 73,239 | 74,311 | 71,386 | 68,530 | 70,841 |
| **Revenue - Inpatient** | | | | | |
| Gross Inpatient Revenue | $46,206,502,599 | $36,887,336,442 | $33,160,635,367 | $29,235,892,623 | $27,097,518,634 |
| **Revenue - Outpatient** | | | | | |
| Gross Outpatient Revenue | $24,363,370,431 | $20,349,623,193 | $17,751,314,945 | $15,605,206,965 | $13,919,316,631 |
| **Revenue and Expenses - Totals (Includes Inpatient and Outpatient)** | | | | | |
| Total Gross Revenue | $70,569,873,030 | $57,236,959,635 | $50,911,950,312 | $44,841,099,588 | $41,016,835,265 |
| Deductions from Revenue | 48,563,663,012 | 36,862,617,072 | 31,902,707,556 | 27,167,023,083 | 24,081,858,092 |
| Net Patient Revenue | 22,006,210,018 | 20,374,342,563 | 19,009,242,756 | 17,674,076,505 | 16,934,977,173 |
| Other Operating Revenue | 1,114,923,665 | 1,073,805,639 | 1,050,625,699 | 1,001,303,780 | 918,424,356 |
| Other Nonoperating Revenue | 154,346,224 | 109,263,545 | 320,138,109 | 473,372,882 | 436,390,618 |
| Total Net Revenue | 23,275,479,907 | 21,557,411,747 | 20,380,006,564 | 19,148,753,167 | 18,289,792,147 |
| Total Expenses | 22,496,486,008 | 20,669,545,292 | 19,668,618,568 | 18,449,395,399 | 17,762,016,623 |
| **HOSPITAL UNIT (Excludes Separate Nursing Home Units)** | | | | | |
| **Utilization - Inpatient** | | | | | |
| Beds | 38,155 | 37,613 | 38,652 | 38,642 | 38,320 |
| Admissions | 1,793,209 | 1,765,118 | 1,772,168 | 1,753,702 | 1,704,806 |
| Inpatient Days | 9,470,572 | 9,427,742 | 9,322,503 | 9,424,533 | 9,224,935 |
| Average Length of Stay | 5.3 | 5.3 | 5.3 | 5.4 | 5.4 |
| **Personnel** | | | | | |
| Total Full Time | 183,977 | 183,198 | 178,633 | 175,754 | 176,561 |
| Total Part Time | 71,902 | 72,709 | 69,755 | 66,833 | 69,104 |
| **Revenue and Expenses - Totals (Includes Inpatient and Outpatient)** | | | | | |
| Total Net Revenue | $23,039,479,349 | $21,296,239,697 | $20,087,923,397 | $18,857,929,952 | $17,920,002,342 |
| Total Expenses | 22,296,561,994 | 20,474,291,752 | 19,453,873,721 | 18,267,250,601 | 17,508,949,084 |
| **COMMUNITY HEALTH INDICATORS PER 1000 POPULATION** | | | | | |
| Total Population (in thousands) | 12,365 | 12,329 | 12,298 | 12,285 | 12,264 |
| **Inpatient** | | | | | |
| Beds | 3.3 | 3.3 | 3.4 | 3.4 | 3.5 |
| Admissions | 147.5 | 145.9 | 147.1 | 146.2 | 143.1 |
| Inpatient Days | 833.0 | 838.7 | 845.3 | 859.4 | 868.6 |
| Inpatient Surgeries | 43.0 | 43.6 | 44.3 | 43.5 | 45.3 |
| Births | 11.1 | 11.3 | 11.7 | 11.3 | 11.4 |
| **Outpatient** | | | | | |
| Emergency Outpatient Visits | 417.3 | 410.4 | 396.3 | 384.8 | 376.4 |
| Other Outpatient Visits | 2,274.4 | 2,218.4 | 2,210.8 | 2,207.6 | 2,010.3 |
| Total Outpatient Visits | 2,691.8 | 2,628.7 | 2,607.1 | 2,592.4 | 2,386.6 |
| Outpatient Surgeries | 78.2 | 79.8 | 84.1 | 81.2 | 79.1 |
| **Expense per Capita (per person)** | $1,819.3 | $1,676.5 | $1,599.3 | $1,501.7 | $1,448.3 |

# TABLE 6

# RHODE ISLAND

*U.S. Registered Community Hospitals*
*(Nonfederal, short-term general and other special hospitals)*

## Overview 1999–2003

| | 2003 | 2002 | 2001 | 2000 | 1999 |
|---|---|---|---|---|---|
| **Total Community Hospitals in Rhode Island** . . . | **11** | **11** | **11** | **11** | **11** |
| **Bed Size Category** | | | | | |
| 6-24 | 0 | 0 | 0 | 0 | 0 |
| 25-49 | 0 | 0 | 0 | 0 | 0 |
| 50-99 | 1 | 1 | 1 | 1 | 1 |
| 100-199 | 6 | 5 | 5 | 5 | 6 |
| 200-299 | 2 | 3 | 3 | 3 | 2 |
| 300-399 | 1 | 1 | 1 | 1 | 1 |
| 400-499 | 0 | 0 | 0 | 0 | 0 |
| 500 + | 1 | 1 | 1 | 1 | 1 |
| **Location** | | | | | |
| Hospitals Urban | 10 | 10 | 10 | 10 | 10 |
| Hospitals Rural | 1 | 1 | 1 | 1 | 1 |
| **Control** | | | | | |
| State and Local Government | 0 | 0 | 0 | 0 | 0 |
| Not for Profit | 11 | 11 | 11 | 11 | 11 |
| Investor owned | 0 | 0 | 0 | 0 | 0 |
| **Physician Models** | | | | | |
| Independent Practice Association | 7 | 7 | 7 | 3 | 3 |
| Group Practice without Walls | 1 | 1 | 1 | 0 | 0 |
| Open Physician-Hospital Organization | 6 | 6 | 6 | 7 | 8 |
| Closed Physician-Hospital Organization | 1 | 2 | 3 | 2 | 1 |
| Management Service Organization | 1 | 2 | 3 | 2 | 3 |
| Integrated Salary Model | 5 | 4 | 5 | 4 | 5 |
| Equity Model | 1 | 1 | 1 | 1 | 0 |
| Foundation | 3 | 3 | 4 | 4 | 4 |
| **Insurance Products** | | | | | |
| Health Maintenance Organization | 2 | 2 | 2 | 0 | 0 |
| Preferred Provider Organization | 2 | 2 | 2 | 0 | 0 |
| Indemnity Fee for Service | 1 | 1 | 1 | 0 | 0 |
| **Managed Care Contracts** | | | | | |
| Health Maintenance Organization | 9 | 10 | 11 | 11 | 11 |
| Preferred Provider Organization | 8 | 8 | 9 | 10 | 10 |
| **Affiliations** | | | | | |
| Hospitals in a System* | 5 | 5 | 5 | 5 | 5 |
| Hospitals in a Network | 1 | 1 | 1 | 3 | 2 |
| Hospitals in a Group Purchasing Organization | 9 | 10 | 11 | 11 | 9 |

States

* Please note that system affiliate information for hospitals is derived from AHA membership. In years prior to 2003 the affiliation was derived from a question on the AHA Annual Survey of hospitals; therefore, non-responding hospitals were not included in the system affiliation counts. Years prior to 2003 have been updated to reflect this change, which now include affiliation for non-reporting hospitals.

# RHODE ISLAND

*U.S. Registered Community Hospitals*
*(Nonfederal, short-term general and other special hospitals)*

## Utilization, Personnel, Revenue and Expenses, Community Health Indicators 1999–2003

| | 2003 | 2002 | 2001 | 2000 | 1999 |
|---|---|---|---|---|---|
| **TOTAL FACILITY (Includes Hospital and Nursing Home Units)** | | | | | |
| **Utilization - Inpatient** | | | | | |
| Beds | 2,410 | 2,428 | 2,449 | 2,400 | 2,400 |
| Admissions | 122,692 | 122,741 | 120,901 | 119,070 | 117,163 |
| Inpatient Days | 657,057 | 649,451 | 638,571 | 625,939 | 623,306 |
| Average Length of Stay | 5.4 | 5.3 | 5.3 | 5.3 | 5.3 |
| Inpatient Surgeries | 38,196 | 36,943 | 35,543 | 35,483 | 35,116 |
| Births | 13,681 | 13,328 | 13,375 | 13,064 | 13,320 |
| **Utilization - Outpatient** | | | | | |
| Emergency Outpatient Visits | 463,961 | 468,530 | 451,325 | 440,098 | 421,667 |
| Other Outpatient Visits | 1,647,644 | 1,743,459 | 1,699,915 | 1,640,847 | 1,489,890 |
| Total Outpatient Visits | 2,111,605 | 2,211,989 | 2,151,240 | 2,080,945 | 1,911,557 |
| Outpatient Surgeries | 99,075 | 105,833 | 99,423 | 94,146 | 86,783 |
| **Personnel** | | | | | |
| Full Time RNs | 1,799 | 1,583 | 1,539 | 1,630 | 1,545 |
| Full Time LPNs | 180 | 183 | 184 | 183 | 161 |
| Part Time RNs | 2,703 | 2,720 | 3,056 | 3,087 | 3,145 |
| Part Time LPNs | 191 | 200 | 221 | 206 | 197 |
| Total Full Time | 11,265 | 11,440 | 10,793 | 10,894 | 10,491 |
| Total Part Time | 8,036 | 8,071 | 8,620 | 8,409 | 8,558 |
| **Revenue - Inpatient** | | | | | |
| Gross Inpatient Revenue | $2,217,386,561 | $1,954,502,575 | $1,738,042,664 | $1,512,132,670 | $1,415,053,397 |
| **Revenue - Outpatient** | | | | | |
| Gross Outpatient Revenue | $1,867,182,587 | $1,625,894,089 | $1,342,251,100 | $1,154,392,267 | $1,041,727,122 |
| **Revenue and Expenses - Totals (Includes Inpatient and Outpatient)** | | | | | |
| Total Gross Revenue | $4,084,569,148 | $3,580,396,664 | $3,080,293,764 | $2,666,524,937 | $2,456,780,519 |
| Deductions from Revenue | 2,318,336,255 | 1,965,189,964 | 1,626,498,267 | 1,338,811,208 | 1,230,336,909 |
| Net Patient Revenue | 1,766,232,893 | 1,615,206,700 | 1,453,795,497 | 1,327,713,729 | 1,226,443,610 |
| Other Operating Revenue | 177,983,705 | 113,085,707 | 97,199,257 | 101,392,569 | 84,757,555 |
| Other Nonoperating Revenue | 7,490,446 | 45,373,163 | 18,363,394 | 48,479,673 | 28,358,285 |
| Total Net Revenue | 1,951,707,044 | 1,773,665,570 | 1,569,358,148 | 1,477,585,971 | 1,339,559,450 |
| Total Expenses | 1,941,065,141 | 1,791,383,545 | 1,592,333,629 | 1,488,194,792 | 1,362,140,752 |
| **HOSPITAL UNIT (Excludes Separate Nursing Home Units)** | | | | | |
| **Utilization - Inpatient** | | | | | |
| Beds | 2,348 | 2,373 | 2,405 | 2,337 | 2,361 |
| Admissions | 121,235 | 121,485 | 119,649 | 117,446 | 116,370 |
| Inpatient Days | 639,795 | 633,715 | 622,075 | 604,416 | 612,307 |
| Average Length of Stay | 5.3 | 5.2 | 5.2 | 5.1 | 5.3 |
| **Personnel** | | | | | |
| Total Full Time | 11,240 | 11,421 | 10,718 | 10,811 | 10,485 |
| Total Part Time | 7,996 | 8,010 | 8,538 | 8,315 | 8,520 |
| **Revenue and Expenses - Totals (Includes Inpatient and Outpatient)** | | | | | |
| Total Net Revenue | $1,936,762,614 | $1,761,520,237 | $1,557,626,889 | $1,465,522,013 | $1,333,633,808 |
| Total Expenses | 1,925,735,374 | 1,780,279,260 | 1,582,522,184 | 1,479,990,940 | 1,356,396,823 |
| **COMMUNITY HEALTH INDICATORS PER 1000 POPULATION** | | | | | |
| Total Population (in thousands) | 1,076 | 1,068 | 1,059 | 1,051 | 1,040 |
| **Inpatient** | | | | | |
| Beds | 2.2 | 2.3 | 2.3 | 2.3 | 2.3 |
| Admissions | 114.0 | 114.9 | 114.2 | 113.3 | 112.6 |
| Inpatient Days | 610.6 | 607.9 | 603.0 | 595.8 | 599.1 |
| Inpatient Surgeries | 35.5 | 34.6 | 33.6 | 33.8 | 33.8 |
| Births | 12.7 | 12.5 | 12.6 | 12.4 | 12.8 |
| **Outpatient** | | | | | |
| Emergency Outpatient Visits | 431.1 | 438.6 | 426.2 | 418.9 | 405.3 |
| Other Outpatient Visits | 1,531.0 | 1,632.0 | 1,605.2 | 1,561.7 | 1,432.0 |
| Total Outpatient Visits | 1,962.2 | 2,070.5 | 2,031.4 | 1,980.6 | 1,837.3 |
| Outpatient Surgeries | 92.1 | 99.1 | 93.9 | 89.6 | 83.4 |
| **Expense per Capita (per person)** | $1,803.7 | $1,676.8 | $1,503.6 | $1,416.4 | $1,309.2 |

# TABLE 6

# SOUTH CAROLINA

*U.S. Registered Community Hospitals*
*(Nonfederal, short-term general and other special hospitals)*

## Overview 1999–2003

| | 2003 | 2002 | 2001 | 2000 | 1999 |
|---|---|---|---|---|---|
| **Total Community Hospitals in South Carolina...** | **61** | **62** | **62** | **63** | **64** |
| **Bed Size Category** | | | | | |
| 6-24 | 2 | 2 | 1 | 1 | 1 |
| 25-49 | 9 | 10 | 9 | 11 | 9 |
| 50-99 | 14 | 14 | 13 | 12 | 13 |
| 100-199 | 15 | 14 | 16 | 15 | 18 |
| 200-299 | 11 | 13 | 14 | 14 | 12 |
| 300-399 | 4 | 4 | 4 | 4 | 6 |
| 400-499 | 3 | 2 | 2 | 3 | 2 |
| 500 + | 3 | 3 | 3 | 3 | 3 |
| **Location** | | | | | |
| Hospitals Urban | 35 | 35 | 35 | 35 | 36 |
| Hospitals Rural | 26 | 27 | 27 | 28 | 28 |
| **Control** | | | | | |
| State and Local Government | 20 | 21 | 22 | 23 | 24 |
| Not for Profit | 23 | 23 | 20 | 20 | 20 |
| Investor owned | 18 | 18 | 20 | 20 | 20 |
| **Physician Models** | | | | | |
| Independent Practice Association | 1 | 3 | 6 | 6 | 4 |
| Group Practice without Walls | 0 | 0 | 0 | 0 | 0 |
| Open Physician-Hospital Organization | 11 | 11 | 13 | 13 | 11 |
| Closed Physician-Hospital Organization | 1 | 1 | 1 | 4 | 7 |
| Management Service Organization | 6 | 8 | 9 | 9 | 4 |
| Integrated Salary Model | 10 | 8 | 6 | 9 | 8 |
| Equity Model | 1 | 5 | 1 | 7 | 6 |
| Foundation | 0 | 0 | 1 | 1 | 1 |
| **Insurance Products** | | | | | |
| Health Maintenance Organization | 0 | 4 | 4 | 8 | 10 |
| Preferred Provider Organization | 1 | 10 | 11 | 11 | 14 |
| Indemnity Fee for Service | 0 | 1 | 1 | 1 | 1 |
| **Managed Care Contracts** | | | | | |
| Health Maintenance Organization | 2 | 37 | 34 | 38 | 41 |
| Preferred Provider Organization | 2 | 42 | 38 | 41 | 46 |
| **Affiliations** | | | | | |
| Hospitals in a System* | 39 | 41 | 41 | 42 | 40 |
| Hospitals in a Network | 21 | 22 | 20 | 22 | 23 |
| Hospitals in a Group Purchasing Organization | 1 | 0 | 0 | 0 | — |

States

* Please note that system affiliate information for hospitals is derived from AHA membership. In years prior to 2003 the affiliation was derived from a question on the AHA Annual Survey of hospitals; therefore, non-responding hospitals were not included in the system affiliation counts. Years prior to 2003 have been updated to reflect this change, which now include affiliation for non-reporting hospitals.

# TABLE 6

# SOUTH CAROLINA

*U.S. Registered Community Hospitals*
*(Nonfederal, short-term general and other special hospitals)*

## Utilization, Personnel, Revenue and Expenses, Community Health Indicators 1999–2003

| | 2003 | 2002 | 2001 | 2000 | 1999 |
|---|---|---|---|---|---|
| **TOTAL FACILITY (Includes Hospital and Nursing Home Units)** | | | | | |
| **Utilization - Inpatient** | | | | | |
| Beds | 11,115 | 11,107 | 11,282 | 11,520 | 11,629 |
| Admissions | 506,488 | 513,136 | 505,294 | 495,410 | 478,936 |
| Inpatient Days | 2,949,736 | 2,914,964 | 2,940,707 | 2,916,386 | 2,816,481 |
| Average Length of Stay | 5.8 | 5.7 | 5.8 | 5.9 | 5.9 |
| Inpatient Surgeries | 180,301 | 179,098 | 173,046 | 173,645 | 150,556 |
| Births | 48,497 | 48,864 | 50,304 | 51,355 | 48,875 |
| **Utilization - Outpatient** | | | | | |
| Emergency Outpatient Visits | 1,807,580 | 1,799,127 | 1,840,819 | 1,831,462 | 1,675,252 |
| Other Outpatient Visits | 5,593,826 | 5,467,718 | 5,788,476 | 5,947,571 | 4,684,820 |
| Total Outpatient Visits | 7,401,406 | 7,266,845 | 7,629,295 | 7,779,033 | 6,360,072 |
| Outpatient Surgeries | 288,576 | 278,897 | 262,308 | 253,389 | 220,015 |
| **Personnel** | | | | | |
| Full Time RNs | 13,113 | 12,161 | 11,674 | 10,921 | 11,437 |
| Full Time LPNs | 1,603 | 1,545 | 1,689 | 1,623 | 1,687 |
| Part Time RNs | 5,570 | 5,116 | 5,366 | 4,911 | 5,061 |
| Part Time LPNs | 1,593 | 648 | 622 | 585 | 599 |
| Total Full Time | 50,477 | 48,661 | 48,615 | 45,230 | 46,006 |
| Total Part Time | 17,938 | 15,356 | 15,342 | 14,772 | 13,878 |
| **Revenue - Inpatient** | | | | | |
| Gross Inpatient Revenue | $10,349,908,301 | $9,137,079,254 | $7,754,863,580 | $6,462,086,026 | $6,267,433,167 |
| **Revenue - Outpatient** | | | | | |
| Gross Outpatient Revenue | $5,396,627,841 | $4,772,097,600 | $4,036,284,822 | $3,446,830,663 | $3,111,764,599 |
| **Revenue and Expenses - Totals (Includes Inpatient and Outpatient)** | | | | | |
| Total Gross Revenue | $15,746,536,142 | $13,909,176,854 | $11,791,148,402 | $9,908,916,689 | $9,379,197,766 |
| Deductions from Revenue | 9,466,073,391 | 7,966,264,098 | 6,352,960,698 | 4,892,874,213 | 4,637,273,635 |
| Net Patient Revenue | 6,280,462,751 | 5,942,912,756 | 5,438,187,704 | 5,016,042,476 | 4,741,924,131 |
| Other Operating Revenue | 331,921,316 | 221,416,734 | 214,469,378 | 198,031,960 | 206,800,122 |
| Other Nonoperating Revenue | 137,051,311 | 48,721,284 | 60,313,151 | 85,852,895 | 55,842,812 |
| Total Net Revenue | 6,749,435,378 | 6,213,050,774 | 5,712,970,233 | 5,299,927,331 | 5,004,567,065 |
| Total Expenses | 6,271,306,129 | 5,829,536,908 | 5,211,814,991 | 5,017,991,441 | 4,714,616,676 |
| **HOSPITAL UNIT (Excludes Separate Nursing Home Units)** | | | | | |
| **Utilization - Inpatient** | | | | | |
| Beds | 10,190 | 10,182 | 10,229 | 10,411 | 10,676 |
| Admissions | 500,406 | 506,957 | 499,396 | 488,626 | 472,693 |
| Inpatient Days | 2,636,965 | 2,603,383 | 2,600,069 | 2,570,557 | 2,512,213 |
| Average Length of Stay | 5.3 | 5.1 | 5.2 | 5.3 | 5.3 |
| **Personnel** | | | | | |
| Total Full Time | 49,634 | 47,852 | 47,744 | 44,175 | 45,228 |
| Total Part Time | 17,694 | 15,120 | 15,057 | 14,394 | 13,615 |
| **Revenue and Expenses - Totals (Includes Inpatient and Outpatient)** | | | | | |
| Total Net Revenue | $6,614,628,560 | $6,100,277,342 | $5,647,774,666 | $4,478,643,578 | $4,912,849,352 |
| Total Expenses | 6,191,999,092 | 5,764,072,107 | 5,160,720,870 | 4,960,782,656 | 4,658,570,962 |
| **COMMUNITY HEALTH INDICATORS PER 1000 POPULATION** | | | | | |
| Total Population (in thousands) | 4,147 | 4,104 | 4,060 | 4,023 | 3,975 |
| **Inpatient** | | | | | |
| Beds | 2.7 | 2.7 | 2.8 | 2.9 | 2.9 |
| Admissions | 122.1 | 125.0 | 124.5 | 123.1 | 120.5 |
| Inpatient Days | 711.3 | 710.3 | 724.3 | 724.9 | 708.6 |
| Inpatient Surgeries | 43.5 | 43.6 | 42.6 | 43.2 | 37.9 |
| Births | 11.7 | 11.9 | 12.4 | 12.8 | 12.3 |
| **Outpatient** | | | | | |
| Emergency Outpatient Visits | 435.9 | 438.4 | 453.4 | 455.2 | 421.5 |
| Other Outpatient Visits | 1,348.8 | 1,332.4 | 1,425.8 | 1,478.3 | 1,178.7 |
| Total Outpatient Visits | 1,784.7 | 1,770.8 | 1,879.2 | 1,933.6 | 1,600.1 |
| Outpatient Surgeries | 69.6 | 68.0 | 64.6 | 63.0 | 55.4 |
| **Expense per Capita (per person)** | $1,512.2 | $1,420.5 | $1,283.8 | $1,247.3 | $1,186.2 |

# Table 6

# SOUTH DAKOTA

*U.S. Registered Community Hospitals*
*(Nonfederal, short-term general and other special hospitals)*

## Overview 1999–2003

| | 2003 | 2002 | 2001 | 2000 | 1999 |
|---|---|---|---|---|---|
| **Total Community Hospitals in South Dakota** | **50** | **51** | **50** | **48** | **48** |
| **Bed Size Category** | | | | | |
| 6-24 | 13 | 12 | 13 | 13 | 13 |
| 25-49 | 12 | 13 | 10 | 10 | 10 |
| 50-99 | 12 | 12 | 13 | 11 | 11 |
| 100-199 | 7 | 9 | 8 | 9 | 9 |
| 200-299 | 3 | 2 | 3 | 1 | 2 |
| 300-399 | 1 | 1 | 1 | 2 | 1 |
| 400-499 | 1 | 1 | 1 | 1 | 1 |
| 500 + | 1 | 1 | 1 | 1 | 1 |
| **Location** | | | | | |
| Hospitals Urban | 6 | 6 | 6 | 5 | 5 |
| Hospitals Rural | 44 | 45 | 44 | 43 | 43 |
| **Control** | | | | | |
| State and Local Government | 6 | 6 | 6 | 7 | 8 |
| Not for Profit | 43 | 44 | 43 | 41 | 40 |
| Investor owned | 1 | 1 | 1 | 0 | 0 |
| **Physician Models** | | | | | |
| Independent Practice Association | 9 | 9 | 11 | 9 | 7 |
| Group Practice without Walls | 3 | 3 | 2 | 3 | 2 |
| Open Physician-Hospital Organization | 4 | 5 | 4 | 6 | 5 |
| Closed Physician-Hospital Organization | 2 | 2 | 2 | 4 | 3 |
| Management Service Organization | 2 | 3 | 3 | 4 | 4 |
| Integrated Salary Model | 18 | 17 | 13 | 14 | 12 |
| Equity Model | 0 | 1 | 1 | 1 | 0 |
| Foundation | 0 | 1 | 1 | 0 | 2 |
| **Insurance Products** | | | | | |
| Health Maintenance Organization | 15 | 14 | 13 | 13 | 13 |
| Preferred Provider Organization | 20 | 21 | 17 | 17 | 14 |
| Indemnity Fee for Service | 5 | 6 | 6 | 5 | 6 |
| **Managed Care Contracts** | | | | | |
| Health Maintenance Organization | 23 | 24 | 21 | 21 | 22 |
| Preferred Provider Organization | 36 | 39 | 34 | 35 | 36 |
| **Affiliations** | | | | | |
| Hospitals in a System* | 38 | 38 | 34 | 28 | 27 |
| Hospitals in a Network | 16 | 22 | 17 | 17 | 15 |
| Hospitals in a Group Purchasing Organization | 46 | 46 | 46 | 43 | 38 |

States

* Please note that system affiliate information for hospitals is derived from AHA membership. In years prior to 2003 the affiliation was derived from a question on the AHA Annual Survey of hospitals; therefore, non-responding hospitals were not included in the system affiliation counts. Years prior to 2003 have been updated to reflect this change, which now include affiliation for non-reporting hospitals.

# TABLE 6

## SOUTH DAKOTA

*U.S. Registered Community Hospitals*
*(Nonfederal, short-term general and other special hospitals)*

## Utilization, Personnel, Revenue and Expenses, Community Health Indicators 1999–2003

| | 2003 | 2002 | 2001 | 2000 | 1999 |
|---|---|---|---|---|---|
| **TOTAL FACILITY (Includes Hospital and Nursing Home Units)** | | | | | |
| **Utilization - Inpatient** | | | | | |
| Beds | 4,418 | 4,624 | 4,465 | 4,339 | 4,344 |
| Admissions | 102,984 | 100,141 | 103,907 | 98,508 | 97,316 |
| Inpatient Days | 994,529 | 1,001,800 | 1,046,760 | 1,035,027 | 1,052,039 |
| Average Length of Stay | 9.7 | 10.0 | 10.1 | 10.5 | 10.8 |
| Inpatient Surgeries | 35,226 | 38,478 | 32,462 | 32,993 | 32,627 |
| Births | 10,588 | 9,537 | 10,261 | 10,006 | 9,363 |
| **Utilization - Outpatient** | | | | | |
| Emergency Outpatient Visits | 214,831 | 208,068 | 211,200 | 196,054 | 192,035 |
| Other Outpatient Visits | 1,321,893 | 1,296,030 | 1,616,898 | 1,522,147 | 1,361,718 |
| Total Outpatient Visits | 1,536,724 | 1,504,098 | 1,828,098 | 1,718,201 | 1,553,753 |
| Outpatient Surgeries | 49,522 | 46,159 | 44,596 | 43,642 | 46,065 |
| **Personnel** | | | | | |
| Full Time RNs | 2,610 | 3,070 | 2,719 | 2,486 | 2,147 |
| Full Time LPNs | 234 | 307 | 267 | 226 | 186 |
| Part Time RNs | 1,851 | 1,390 | 1,508 | 1,822 | 2,058 |
| Part Time LPNs | 164 | 122 | 142 | 201 | 197 |
| Total Full Time | 11,432 | 12,760 | 12,093 | 10,774 | 9,989 |
| Total Part Time | 7,286 | 6,209 | 6,074 | 7,124 | 7,034 |
| **Revenue - Inpatient** | | | | | |
| Gross Inpatient Revenue | $1,452,307,627 | $1,261,059,667 | $1,134,749,973 | $1,000,043,131 | $925,396,063 |
| **Revenue - Outpatient** | | | | | |
| Gross Outpatient Revenue | $863,523,142 | $695,088,937 | $613,055,802 | $550,896,116 | $457,270,200 |
| **Revenue and Expenses - Totals (Includes Inpatient and Outpatient)** | | | | | |
| Total Gross Revenue | $2,315,830,769 | $1,956,148,604 | $1,747,805,775 | $1,550,939,247 | $1,382,666,263 |
| Deductions from Revenue | 980,153,650 | 772,856,470 | 647,480,234 | 527,471,606 | 434,728,043 |
| Net Patient Revenue | 1,335,677,119 | 1,183,292,134 | 1,100,325,541 | 1,023,467,641 | 947,938,220 |
| Other Operating Revenue | 92,587,786 | 86,084,094 | 77,627,200 | 60,933,637 | 57,779,801 |
| Other Nonoperating Revenue | 28,979,794 | 4,988,767 | 11,008,624 | 43,912,340 | 28,755,729 |
| Total Net Revenue | 1,457,244,699 | 1,274,364,995 | 1,188,961,365 | 1,128,313,618 | 1,034,473,750 |
| Total Expenses | 1,340,422,400 | 1,195,193,697 | 1,106,276,599 | 1,058,129,155 | 942,471,403 |
| **HOSPITAL UNIT (Excludes Separate Nursing Home Units)** | | | | | |
| **Utilization - Inpatient** | | | | | |
| Beds | 2,679 | 2,937 | 2,763 | 2,619 | 2,659 |
| Admissions | 101,431 | 98,694 | 102,468 | 97,152 | 96,048 |
| Inpatient Days | 446,442 | 519,705 | 503,878 | 475,240 | 485,592 |
| Average Length of Stay | 4.4 | 5.3 | 4.9 | 4.9 | 5.1 |
| **Personnel** | | | | | |
| Total Full Time | 10,472 | 11,801 | 11,146 | 9,803 | 9,299 |
| Total Part Time | 6,345 | 5,369 | 5,249 | 6,324 | 6,271 |
| **Revenue and Expenses - Totals (Includes Inpatient and Outpatient)** | | | | | |
| Total Net Revenue | $1,390,873,445 | $1,210,167,076 | $1,129,594,457 | $1,075,161,508 | $979,061,301 |
| Total Expenses | 1,279,520,564 | 1,142,543,091 | 1,048,181,427 | 1,010,362,656 | 895,701,751 |
| **COMMUNITY HEALTH INDICATORS PER 1000 POPULATION** | | | | | |
| Total Population (in thousands) | 764 | 760 | 758 | 756 | 750 |
| **Inpatient** | | | | | |
| Beds | 5.8 | 6.1 | 5.9 | 5.7 | 5.8 |
| Admissions | 134.7 | 131.7 | 137.1 | 130.4 | 129.7 |
| Inpatient Days | 1,301.2 | 1,317.4 | 1,380.7 | 1,369.7 | 1,401.9 |
| Inpatient Surgeries | 46.1 | 50.6 | 42.8 | 43.7 | 43.5 |
| Births | 13.9 | 12.5 | 13.5 | 13.2 | 12.5 |
| **Outpatient** | | | | | |
| Emergency Outpatient Visits | 281.1 | 273.6 | 278.6 | 259.4 | 255.9 |
| Other Outpatient Visits | 1,729.5 | 1,704.3 | 2,132.7 | 2,014.3 | 1,814.6 |
| Total Outpatient Visits | 2,010.6 | 1,977.9 | 2,411.2 | 2,273.7 | 2,070.5 |
| Outpatient Surgeries | 64.8 | 60.7 | 58.8 | 57.8 | 61.4 |
| **Expense per Capita (per person)** | $1,753.8 | $1,571.7 | $1,459.2 | $1,400.2 | $1,255.9 |

# TABLE 6

# TENNESSEE

*U.S. Registered Community Hospitals*
*(Nonfederal, short-term general and other special hospitals)*

## Overview 1999–2003

| | 2003 | 2002 | 2001 | 2000 | 1999 |
|---|---|---|---|---|---|
| **Total Community Hospitals in Tennessee** | **125** | **125** | **123** | **121** | **121** |
| **Bed Size Category** | | | | | |
| 6-24 | 4 | 5 | 1 | 0 | 0 |
| 25-49 | 28 | 28 | 26 | 25 | 20 |
| 50-99 | 33 | 29 | 30 | 33 | 39 |
| 100-199 | 29 | 33 | 36 | 34 | 33 |
| 200-299 | 13 | 11 | 11 | 10 | 11 |
| 300-399 | 5 | 6 | 6 | 7 | 5 |
| 400-499 | 3 | 4 | 5 | 3 | 3 |
| 500 + | 10 | 9 | 8 | 9 | 10 |
| **Location** | | | | | |
| Hospitals Urban | 61 | 61 | 60 | 58 | 58 |
| Hospitals Rural | 64 | 64 | 63 | 63 | 63 |
| **Control** | | | | | |
| State and Local Government | 25 | 26 | 26 | 27 | 27 |
| Not for Profit | 63 | 64 | 61 | 57 | 56 |
| Investor owned | 37 | 35 | 36 | 37 | 38 |
| **Physician Models** | | | | | |
| Independent Practice Association | 16 | 27 | 21 | 19 | 22 |
| Group Practice without Walls | 2 | 2 | 1 | 0 | 1 |
| Open Physician-Hospital Organization | 17 | 24 | 25 | 15 | 19 |
| Closed Physician-Hospital Organization | 9 | 9 | 5 | 4 | 3 |
| Management Service Organization | 26 | 32 | 31 | 23 | 24 |
| Integrated Salary Model | 19 | 22 | 18 | 11 | 12 |
| Equity Model | 0 | 2 | 0 | 0 | 2 |
| Foundation | 5 | 2 | 3 | 4 | 4 |
| **Insurance Products** | | | | | |
| Health Maintenance Organization | 14 | 19 | 17 | 16 | 21 |
| Preferred Provider Organization | 35 | 44 | 35 | 27 | 36 |
| Indemnity Fee for Service | 10 | 13 | 11 | 10 | 10 |
| **Managed Care Contracts** | | | | | |
| Health Maintenance Organization | 74 | 82 | 80 | 62 | 65 |
| Preferred Provider Organization | 81 | 93 | 92 | 70 | 71 |
| **Affiliations** | | | | | |
| Hospitals in a System* | 93 | 89 | 86 | 79 | 74 |
| Hospitals in a Network | 39 | 41 | 44 | 24 | 30 |
| Hospitals in a Group Purchasing Organization | 88 | 83 | 90 | 69 | 69 |

* Please note that system affiliate information for hospitals is derived from AHA membership. In years prior to 2003 the affiliation was derived from a question on the AHA Annual Survey of hospitals; therefore, non-responding hospitals were not included in the system affiliation counts. Years prior to 2003 have been updated to reflect this change, which now include affiliation for non-reporting hospitals.

# TENNESSEE

*U.S. Registered Community Hospitals*
*(Nonfederal, short-term general and other special hospitals)*

## Utilization, Personnel, Revenue and Expenses, Community Health Indicators 1999–2003

| | 2003 | 2002 | 2001 | 2000 | 1999 |
|---|---|---|---|---|---|
| **TOTAL FACILITY (Includes Hospital and Nursing Home Units)** | | | | | |
| **Utilization - Inpatient** | | | | | |
| Beds | 20,313 | 20,446 | 20,600 | 20,561 | 20,627 |
| Admissions | 812,915 | 797,318 | 751,495 | 737,313 | 751,523 |
| Inpatient Days | 4,533,373 | 4,473,786 | 4,122,419 | 4,225,812 | 4,296,679 |
| Average Length of Stay | 5.6 | 5.6 | 5.5 | 5.7 | 5.7 |
| Inpatient Surgeries | 233,939 | 227,882 | 238,914 | 241,938 | 236,298 |
| Births | 79,022 | 77,090 | 76,722 | 71,854 | 76,194 |
| **Utilization - Outpatient** | | | | | |
| Emergency Outpatient Visits | 2,947,003 | 2,815,655 | 2,710,481 | 2,601,659 | 2,589,171 |
| Other Outpatient Visits | 7,209,449 | 7,136,086 | 6,826,446 | 7,673,605 | 6,890,695 |
| Total Outpatient Visits | 10,156,452 | 9,951,741 | 9,536,927 | 10,275,264 | 9,479,866 |
| Outpatient Surgeries | 393,996 | 391,725 | 406,248 | 399,184 | 378,646 |
| **Personnel** | | | | | |
| Full Time RNs | 19,389 | 18,073 | 16,806 | 18,265 | 19,220 |
| Full Time LPNs | 3,880 | 3,895 | 3,799 | 3,273 | 3,388 |
| Part Time RNs | 7,451 | 7,661 | 6,683 | 6,880 | 5,037 |
| Part Time LPNs | 1,051 | 1,154 | 1,070 | 916 | 723 |
| Total Full Time | 80,655 | 78,261 | 79,904 | 78,784 | 80,276 |
| Total Part Time | 20,875 | 23,695 | 18,899 | 20,550 | 15,446 |
| **Revenue - Inpatient** | | | | | |
| Gross Inpatient Revenue | $13,868,325,538 | $11,947,904,647 | $11,374,599,693 | $10,080,668,101 | $9,327,573,723 |
| **Revenue - Outpatient** | | | | | |
| Gross Outpatient Revenue | $8,306,909,117 | $7,268,386,224 | $6,608,725,588 | $5,810,556,366 | $5,004,878,950 |
| **Revenue and Expenses - Totals (Includes Inpatient and Outpatient)** | | | | | |
| Total Gross Revenue | $22,175,234,655 | $19,216,290,871 | $17,983,325,281 | $15,891,224,467 | $14,332,452,673 |
| Deductions from Revenue | 13,155,043,109 | 10,705,040,668 | 10,088,328,741 | 8,531,972,395 | 7,456,932,016 |
| Net Patient Revenue | 9,020,191,546 | 8,511,250,203 | 7,894,996,540 | 7,359,252,072 | 6,875,520,657 |
| Other Operating Revenue | 606,002,225 | 340,382,627 | 395,634,694 | 361,920,349 | 419,276,199 |
| Other Nonoperating Revenue | 122,126,401 | 63,525,859 | 310,696,758 | 328,615,366 | 163,624,734 |
| Total Net Revenue | 9,748,320,172 | 8,915,158,689 | 8,601,327,992 | 8,049,787,787 | 7,458,421,590 |
| Total Expenses | 9,206,522,220 | 8,386,650,030 | 8,143,131,226 | 7,554,623,035 | 7,233,873,814 |
| **HOSPITAL UNIT (Excludes Separate Nursing Home Units)** | | | | | |
| **Utilization - Inpatient** | | | | | |
| Beds | 18,695 | 18,928 | 19,170 | 19,273 | 19,104 |
| Admissions | 798,996 | 784,003 | 739,360 | 726,271 | 738,689 |
| Inpatient Days | 4,022,663 | 3,902,204 | 3,621,415 | 3,801,360 | 3,827,904 |
| Average Length of Stay | 5.0 | 5.0 | 4.9 | 5.2 | 5.2 |
| **Personnel** | | | | | |
| Total Full Time | 79,171 | 76,883 | 78,783 | 77,416 | 78,259 |
| Total Part Time | 20,510 | 23,351 | 18,561 | 20,230 | 15,095 |
| **Revenue and Expenses - Totals (Includes Inpatient and Outpatient)** | | | | | |
| Total Net Revenue | $9,652,030,897 | $8,781,164,810 | $8,500,355,125 | $7,950,369,293 | $7,321,010,015 |
| Total Expenses | 9,116,779,809 | 8,276,736,830 | 8,058,017,723 | 7,475,659,236 | 7,128,551,841 |
| **COMMUNITY HEALTH INDICATORS PER 1000 POPULATION** | | | | | |
| Total Population (in thousands) | 5,842 | 5,790 | 5,746 | 5,703 | 5,639 |
| **Inpatient** | | | | | |
| Beds | 3.5 | 3.5 | 3.6 | 3.6 | 3.7 |
| Admissions | 139.2 | 137.7 | 130.8 | 129.3 | 133.3 |
| Inpatient Days | 776.0 | 772.7 | 717.5 | 741.0 | 762.0 |
| Inpatient Surgeries | 40.0 | 39.4 | 41.6 | 42.4 | 41.9 |
| Births | 13.5 | 13.3 | 13.4 | 12.6 | 13.5 |
| **Outpatient** | | | | | |
| Emergency Outpatient Visits | 504.5 | 486.3 | 471.7 | 456.2 | 459.2 |
| Other Outpatient Visits | 1,234.1 | 1,232.5 | 1,188.1 | 1,345.6 | 1,222.0 |
| Total Outpatient Visits | 1,738.6 | 1,718.8 | 1,659.8 | 1,801.8 | 1,681.2 |
| Outpatient Surgeries | 67.4 | 67.7 | 70.7 | 70.0 | 67.2 |
| **Expense per Capita (per person)** | $1,576.0 | $1,448.5 | $1,417.2 | $1,324.8 | $1,282.9 |

# Table 6

# TEXAS

*U.S. Registered Community Hospitals*
*(Nonfederal, short-term general and other special hospitals)*

## Overview 1999–2003

| | 2003 | 2002 | 2001 | 2000 | 1999 |
|---|---|---|---|---|---|
| **Total Community Hospitals in Texas** | **414** | **416** | **411** | **403** | **408** |
| **Bed Size Category** | | | | | |
| 6-24 | 51 | 51 | 48 | 48 | 54 |
| 25-49 | 114 | 110 | 111 | 108 | 101 |
| 50-99 | 74 | 78 | 75 | 68 | 70 |
| 100-199 | 83 | 87 | 88 | 86 | 91 |
| 200-299 | 41 | 39 | 34 | 41 | 40 |
| 300-399 | 27 | 27 | 31 | 28 | 26 |
| 400-499 | 8 | 9 | 8 | 7 | 9 |
| 500 + | 16 | 15 | 16 | 17 | 17 |
| **Location** | | | | | |
| Hospitals Urban | 253 | 255 | 250 | 241 | 245 |
| Hospitals Rural | 161 | 161 | 161 | 162 | 163 |
| **Control** | | | | | |
| State and Local Government | 129 | 129 | 128 | 130 | 131 |
| Not for Profit | 152 | 155 | 146 | 142 | 143 |
| Investor owned | 133 | 132 | 137 | 131 | 134 |
| **Physician Models** | | | | | |
| Independent Practice Association | 84 | 79 | 76 | 82 | 103 |
| Group Practice without Walls | 15 | 14 | 18 | 20 | 18 |
| Open Physician-Hospital Organization | 90 | 91 | 96 | 104 | 109 |
| Closed Physician-Hospital Organization | 17 | 20 | 21 | 23 | 30 |
| Management Service Organization | 50 | 53 | 53 | 79 | 98 |
| Integrated Salary Model | 69 | 62 | 58 | 55 | 64 |
| Equity Model | 7 | 7 | 8 | 15 | 22 |
| Foundation | 29 | 30 | 34 | 41 | 50 |
| **Insurance Products** | | | | | |
| Health Maintenance Organization | 52 | 59 | 60 | 73 | 100 |
| Preferred Provider Organization | 87 | 85 | 76 | 95 | 118 |
| Indemnity Fee for Service | 16 | 23 | 22 | 27 | 39 |
| **Managed Care Contracts** | | | | | |
| Health Maintenance Organization | 304 | 311 | 311 | 309 | 330 |
| Preferred Provider Organization | 353 | 352 | 351 | 350 | 370 |
| **Affiliations** | | | | | |
| Hospitals in a System* | 245 | 242 | 244 | 232 | 228 |
| Hospitals in a Network | 94 | 94 | 93 | 102 | 121 |
| Hospitals in a Group Purchasing Organization | 348 | 344 | 335 | 326 | 306 |

States

* Please note that system affiliate information for hospitals is derived from AHA membership. In years prior to 2003 the affiliation was derived from a question on the AHA Annual Survey of hospitals; therefore, non-responding hospitals were not included in the system affiliation counts. Years prior to 2003 have been updated to reflect this change, which now include affiliation for non-reporting hospitals.

# TABLE 6

# TEXAS

*U.S. Registered Community Hospitals*
*(Nonfederal, short-term general and other special hospitals)*

## Utilization, Personnel, Revenue and Expenses, Community Health Indicators 1999–2003

| | 2003 | 2002 | 2001 | 2000 | 1999 |
|---|---|---|---|---|---|
| **TOTAL FACILITY (Includes Hospital and Nursing Home Units)** | | | | | |
| **Utilization - Inpatient** | | | | | |
| Beds | 57,374 | 56,833 | 56,354 | 55,877 | 56,824 |
| Admissions | 2,550,314 | 2,533,821 | 2,461,016 | 2,366,652 | 2,302,892 |
| Inpatient Days | 13,296,596 | 13,187,000 | 12,650,063 | 12,122,361 | 12,015,612 |
| Average Length of Stay | 5.2 | 5.2 | 5.1 | 5.1 | 5.2 |
| Inpatient Surgeries | 770,184 | 752,465 | 725,998 | 716,990 | 695,394 |
| Births | 370,572 | 371,677 | 366,373 | 357,906 | 339,105 |
| **Utilization - Outpatient** | | | | | |
| Emergency Outpatient Visits | 8,315,483 | 8,243,642 | 7,806,334 | 7,375,580 | 7,071,236 |
| Other Outpatient Visits | 24,379,552 | 25,258,993 | 23,647,614 | 22,017,896 | 21,187,640 |
| Total Outpatient Visits | 32,695,035 | 33,502,635 | 31,453,948 | 29,393,476 | 28,258,876 |
| Outpatient Surgeries | 1,094,832 | 1,093,705 | 1,049,923 | 1,043,853 | 1,033,349 |
| **Personnel** | | | | | |
| Full Time RNs | 60,518 | 58,370 | 55,139 | 52,889 | 53,028 |
| Full Time LPNs | 12,546 | 12,137 | 11,908 | 11,420 | 12,738 |
| Part Time RNs | 18,134 | 18,458 | 18,430 | 17,165 | 16,782 |
| Part Time LPNs | 3,396 | 3,396 | 3,484 | 3,197 | 3,199 |
| Total Full Time | 252,229 | 243,520 | 235,495 | 227,471 | 231,401 |
| Total Part Time | 57,159 | 58,389 | 57,901 | 53,904 | 53,137 |
| **Revenue - Inpatient** | | | | | |
| Gross Inpatient Revenue | $55,923,623,627 | $48,954,346,337 | $42,086,234,028 | $36,110,028,792 | $32,577,994,295 |
| **Revenue - Outpatient** | | | | | |
| Gross Outpatient Revenue | $28,032,723,560 | $24,518,438,912 | $20,856,680,055 | $17,722,021,020 | $15,630,753,126 |
| **Revenue and Expenses - Totals (Includes Inpatient and Outpatient)** | | | | | |
| Total Gross Revenue | $83,956,347,187 | $73,472,785,249 | $62,942,914,083 | $53,832,049,812 | $48,168,747,421 |
| Deductions from Revenue | 54,205,639,586 | 45,004,634,205 | 37,784,174,261 | 31,935,698,552 | 27,344,870,806 |
| Net Patient Revenue | 29,750,707,601 | 28,468,151,044 | 25,158,739,822 | 21,896,351,260 | 20,823,876,615 |
| Other Operating Revenue | 2,888,147,540 | 2,760,139,848 | 2,466,963,729 | 2,311,583,837 | 2,071,860,033 |
| Other Nonoperating Revenue | 561,783,689 | 162,526,064 | 397,849,826 | 476,653,999 | 457,181,324 |
| Total Net Revenue | 33,200,638,830 | 31,390,816,956 | 28,023,553,377 | 24,684,589,096 | 23,352,917,972 |
| Total Expenses | 30,644,006,743 | 28,457,791,824 | 25,906,399,927 | 23,494,693,306 | 21,811,587,994 |
| **HOSPITAL UNIT (Excludes Separate Nursing Home Units)** | | | | | |
| **Utilization - Inpatient** | | | | | |
| Beds | 55,387 | 55,040 | 54,430 | 53,335 | 53,570 |
| Admissions | 2,527,209 | 2,508,127 | 2,427,696 | 2,323,817 | 2,246,168 |
| Inpatient Days | 12,803,387 | 12,719,345 | 12,142,510 | 11,498,881 | 11,180,783 |
| Average Length of Stay | 5.1 | 5.1 | 5.0 | 4.9 | 5.0 |
| **Personnel** | | | | | |
| Total Full Time | 250,202 | 241,964 | 233,563 | 225,255 | 228,566 |
| Total Part Time | 56,556 | 57,963 | 57,471 | 53,479 | 52,351 |
| **Revenue and Expenses - Totals (Includes Inpatient and Outpatient)** | | | | | |
| Total Net Revenue | $32,978,132,120 | $31,211,712,467 | $27,788,903,511 | $24,508,683,378 | $23,037,586,558 |
| Total Expenses | 30,437,055,194 | 28,313,376,914 | 25,757,452,142 | 23,374,693,756 | 21,595,696,612 |
| **COMMUNITY HEALTH INDICATORS PER 1000 POPULATION** | | | | | |
| Total Population (in thousands) | 22,119 | 21,737 | 21,341 | 20,949 | 20,558 |
| **Inpatient** | | | | | |
| Beds | 2.6 | 2.6 | 2.6 | 2.7 | 2.8 |
| Admissions | 115.3 | 116.6 | 115.3 | 113.0 | 112.0 |
| Inpatient Days | 601.2 | 606.7 | 592.8 | 578.7 | 584.5 |
| Inpatient Surgeries | 34.8 | 34.6 | 34.0 | 34.2 | 33.8 |
| Births | 16.8 | 17.1 | 17.2 | 17.1 | 16.5 |
| **Outpatient** | | | | | |
| Emergency Outpatient Visits | 376.0 | 379.2 | 365.8 | 352.1 | 344.0 |
| Other Outpatient Visits | 1,102.2 | 1,162.0 | 1,108.1 | 1,051.0 | 1,030.6 |
| Total Outpatient Visits | 1,478.2 | 1,541.3 | 1,473.9 | 1,403.1 | 1,374.6 |
| Outpatient Surgeries | 49.5 | 50.3 | 49.2 | 49.8 | 50.3 |
| **Expense per Capita (per person)** | $1,385.4 | $1,309.2 | $1,213.9 | $1,121.5 | $1,061.0 |

# TABLE 6

# UTAH

*U.S. Registered Community Hospitals*
*(Nonfederal, short-term general and other special hospitals)*

## Overview 1999–2003

| | 2003 | 2002 | 2001 | 2000 | 1999 |
|---|---|---|---|---|---|
| **Total Community Hospitals in Utah** | **42** | **42** | **42** | **42** | **42** |
| **Bed Size Category** | | | | | |
| 6-24 | 7 | 6 | 8 | 7 | 7 |
| 25-49 | 12 | 13 | 11 | 14 | 12 |
| 50-99 | 8 | 8 | 8 | 5 | 7 |
| 100-199 | 9 | 9 | 9 | 10 | 11 |
| 200-299 | 3 | 3 | 3 | 3 | 2 |
| 300-399 | 2 | 2 | 1 | 2 | 2 |
| 400-499 | 1 | 1 | 2 | 1 | 1 |
| 500 + | 0 | 0 | 0 | 0 | 0 |
| **Location** | | | | | |
| Hospitals Urban | 20 | 21 | 21 | 20 | 20 |
| Hospitals Rural | 22 | 21 | 21 | 22 | 22 |
| **Control** | | | | | |
| State and Local Government | 6 | 6 | 7 | 7 | 9 |
| Not for Profit | 22 | 22 | 22 | 22 | 20 |
| Investor owned | 14 | 14 | 13 | 13 | 13 |
| **Physician Models** | | | | | |
| Independent Practice Association | 5 | 8 | 11 | 16 | 15 |
| Group Practice without Walls | 0 | 2 | 1 | 1 | 1 |
| Open Physician-Hospital Organization | 3 | 4 | 4 | 5 | 3 |
| Closed Physician-Hospital Organization | 1 | 0 | 0 | 0 | 1 |
| Management Service Organization | 2 | 2 | 2 | 4 | 5 |
| Integrated Salary Model | 19 | 13 | 17 | 18 | 16 |
| Equity Model | 1 | 0 | 0 | 0 | 0 |
| Foundation | 0 | 0 | 0 | 0 | 1 |
| **Insurance Products** | | | | | |
| Health Maintenance Organization | 19 | 15 | 18 | 19 | 15 |
| Preferred Provider Organization | 18 | 15 | 20 | 20 | 16 |
| Indemnity Fee for Service | 8 | 8 | 12 | 11 | 6 |
| **Managed Care Contracts** | | | | | |
| Health Maintenance Organization | 25 | 17 | 21 | 25 | 24 |
| Preferred Provider Organization | 25 | 20 | 23 | 28 | 26 |
| **Affiliations** | | | | | |
| Hospitals in a System* | 35 | 36 | 38 | 37 | 38 |
| Hospitals in a Network | 18 | 10 | 11 | 14 | 8 |
| Hospitals in a Group Purchasing Organization | 31 | 26 | 33 | 32 | 24 |

States

* Please note that system affiliate information for hospitals is derived from AHA membership. In years prior to 2003 the affiliation was derived from a question on the AHA Annual Survey of hospitals; therefore, non-responding hospitals were not included in the system affiliation counts. Years prior to 2003 have been updated to reflect this change, which now include affiliation for non-reporting hospitals.

# TABLE 6

## UTAH

*U.S. Registered Community Hospitals*
*(Nonfederal, short-term general and other special hospitals)*

## Utilization, Personnel, Revenue and Expenses, Community Health Indicators 1999–2003

| | 2003 | 2002 | 2001 | 2000 | 1999 |
|---|---|---|---|---|---|
| **TOTAL FACILITY (Includes Hospital and Nursing Home Units)** | | | | | |
| **Utilization - Inpatient** | | | | | |
| Beds | 4,406 | 4,403 | 4,437 | 4,330 | 4,170 |
| Admissions | 215,158 | 206,344 | 203,037 | 194,047 | 189,430 |
| Inpatient Days | 921,001 | 876,524 | 902,313 | 886,846 | 871,864 |
| Average Length of Stay | 4.3 | 4.2 | 4.4 | 4.6 | 4.6 |
| Inpatient Surgeries | 59,864 | 72,489 | 59,425 | 58,729 | 56,992 |
| Births | 49,824 | 48,792 | 47,319 | 47,389 | 45,831 |
| **Utilization - Outpatient** | | | | | |
| Emergency Outpatient Visits | 740,160 | 797,951 | 699,934 | 697,703 | 687,822 |
| Other Outpatient Visits | 3,805,509 | 4,016,360 | 3,718,415 | 3,771,285 | 3,677,904 |
| Total Outpatient Visits | 4,545,669 | 4,814,311 | 4,418,349 | 4,468,988 | 4,365,726 |
| Outpatient Surgeries | 155,803 | 156,769 | 122,692 | 125,430 | 120,031 |
| **Personnel** | | | | | |
| Full Time RNs | 5,506 | 4,939 | 4,442 | 4,143 | 4,405 |
| Full Time LPNs | 520 | 627 | 566 | 413 | 493 |
| Part Time RNs | 3,164 | 3,145 | 2,749 | 3,426 | 3,134 |
| Part Time LPNs | 381 | 405 | 387 | 359 | 326 |
| Total Full Time | 21,693 | 21,063 | 20,005 | 18,807 | 18,880 |
| Total Part Time | 11,760 | 10,564 | 10,822 | 11,987 | 9,852 |
| **Revenue - Inpatient** | | | | | |
| Gross Inpatient Revenue | $3,082,671,800 | $3,062,158,326 | $2,559,345,455 | $2,168,015,062 | $2,124,901,031 |
| **Revenue - Outpatient** | | | | | |
| Gross Outpatient Revenue | $2,102,021,110 | $1,897,673,822 | $1,582,419,304 | $1,347,153,458 | $1,328,671,681 |
| **Revenue and Expenses - Totals (Includes Inpatient and Outpatient)** | | | | | |
| Total Gross Revenue | $5,184,692,910 | $4,959,832,148 | $4,141,764,759 | $3,515,168,520 | $3,453,572,712 |
| Deductions from Revenue | 2,355,358,986 | 2,384,893,655 | 1,865,061,006 | 1,391,174,618 | 1,439,113,434 |
| Net Patient Revenue | 2,829,333,924 | 2,574,938,493 | 2,276,703,753 | 2,123,993,902 | 2,014,459,278 |
| Other Operating Revenue | 123,232,186 | 139,121,419 | 158,563,665 | 115,758,563 | 105,790,033 |
| Other Nonoperating Revenue | 25,696,305 | 23,585,217 | 21,198,879 | 12,177,408 | 16,489,703 |
| Total Net Revenue | 2,978,262,415 | 2,737,645,129 | 2,456,466,297 | 2,251,929,873 | 2,136,739,014 |
| Total Expenses | 2,682,023,991 | 2,505,242,473 | 2,242,551,322 | 2,069,630,397 | 1,927,577,263 |
| **HOSPITAL UNIT (Excludes Separate Nursing Home Units)** | | | | | |
| **Utilization - Inpatient** | | | | | |
| Beds | 4,326 | 4,257 | 4,283 | 4,187 | 3,967 |
| Admissions | 213,834 | 204,612 | 200,838 | 191,941 | 187,940 |
| Inpatient Days | 898,863 | 831,512 | 857,332 | 844,301 | 825,693 |
| Average Length of Stay | 4.2 | 4.1 | 4.3 | 4.4 | 4.4 |
| **Personnel** | | | | | |
| Total Full Time | 21,616 | 21,007 | 19,858 | 18,739 | 18,803 |
| Total Part Time | 11,658 | 10,462 | 10,689 | 11,891 | 9,772 |
| **Revenue and Expenses - Totals (Includes Inpatient and Outpatient)** | | | | | |
| Total Net Revenue | $2,972,748,366 | $2,728,571,258 | $2,435,680,792 | $2,239,569,389 | $2,124,836,350 |
| Total Expenses | 2,678,937,711 | 2,500,424,658 | 2,230,611,574 | 2,064,796,222 | 1,921,753,908 |
| **COMMUNITY HEALTH INDICATORS PER 1000 POPULATION** | | | | | |
| Total Population (in thousands) | 2,351 | 2,319 | 2,280 | 2,243 | 2,203 |
| **Inpatient** | | | | | |
| Beds | 1.9 | 1.9 | 1.9 | 1.9 | 1.9 |
| Admissions | 91.5 | 89.0 | 89.1 | 86.5 | 86.0 |
| Inpatient Days | 391.7 | 378.0 | 395.8 | 395.4 | 395.7 |
| Inpatient Surgeries | 25.5 | 31.3 | 26.1 | 26.2 | 25.9 |
| Births | 21.2 | 21.0 | 20.8 | 21.1 | 20.8 |
| **Outpatient** | | | | | |
| Emergency Outpatient Visits | 314.8 | 344.1 | 307.0 | 311.0 | 312.2 |
| Other Outpatient Visits | 1,618.4 | 1,732.1 | 1,631.2 | 1,681.3 | 1,669.1 |
| Total Outpatient Visits | 1,933.1 | 2,076.2 | 1,938.2 | 1,992.3 | 1,981.3 |
| Outpatient Surgeries | 66.3 | 67.6 | 53.8 | 55.9 | 54.5 |
| **Expense per Capita (per person)** | $1,140.6 | $1,080.4 | $983.8 | $922.7 | $874.8 |

# TABLE 6

# VERMONT

*U.S. Registered Community Hospitals*
*(Nonfederal, short-term general and other special hospitals)*

## Overview 1999–2003

| | 2003 | 2002 | 2001 | 2000 | 1999 |
|---|---|---|---|---|---|
| **Total Community Hospitals in Vermont** | **14** | **14** | **14** | **14** | **14** |
| **Bed Size Category** | | | | | |
| 6-24 | 0 | 0 | 0 | 0 | 0 |
| 25-49 | 7 | 6 | 5 | 5 | 5 |
| 50-99 | 4 | 5 | 5 | 4 | 5 |
| 100-199 | 1 | 1 | 2 | 3 | 2 |
| 200-299 | 1 | 1 | 1 | 1 | 1 |
| 300-399 | 0 | 0 | 0 | 0 | 0 |
| 400-499 | 0 | 0 | 0 | 0 | 0 |
| 500 + | 1 | 1 | 1 | 1 | 1 |
| **Location** | | | | | |
| Hospitals Urban | 2 | 2 | 2 | 2 | 2 |
| Hospitals Rural | 12 | 12 | 12 | 12 | 12 |
| **Control** | | | | | |
| State and Local Government | 0 | 0 | 0 | 0 | 0 |
| Not for Profit | 14 | 14 | 14 | 14 | 14 |
| Investor owned | 0 | 0 | 0 | 0 | 0 |
| **Physician Models** | | | | | |
| Independent Practice Association | 0 | 1 | 1 | 1 | 1 |
| Group Practice without Walls | 1 | 2 | 2 | 0 | 1 |
| Open Physician-Hospital Organization | 6 | 5 | 6 | 5 | 5 |
| Closed Physician-Hospital Organization | 0 | 1 | 1 | 2 | 2 |
| Management Service Organization | 2 | 3 | 3 | 2 | 3 |
| Integrated Salary Model | 8 | 7 | 8 | 5 | 6 |
| Equity Model | 0 | 0 | 0 | 0 | 0 |
| Foundation | 0 | 1 | 1 | 0 | 0 |
| **Insurance Products** | | | | | |
| Health Maintenance Organization | 5 | 5 | 6 | 6 | 6 |
| Preferred Provider Organization | 6 | 4 | 3 | 2 | 2 |
| Indemnity Fee for Service | 2 | 0 | 1 | 2 | 1 |
| **Managed Care Contracts** | | | | | |
| Health Maintenance Organization | 9 | 9 | 11 | 8 | 11 |
| Preferred Provider Organization | 11 | 7 | 9 | 8 | 10 |
| **Affiliations** | | | | | |
| Hospitals in a System* | 1 | 1 | 1 | 2 | 2 |
| Hospitals in a Network | 5 | 2 | 3 | 3 | 4 |
| Hospitals in a Group Purchasing Organization | 12 | 11 | 13 | 9 | 7 |

States

* Please note that system affiliate information for hospitals is derived from AHA membership. In years prior to 2003 the affiliation was derived from a question on the AHA Annual Survey of hospitals; therefore, non-responding hospitals were not included in the system affiliation counts. Years prior to 2003 have been updated to reflect this change, which now include affiliation for non-reporting hospitals.

# TABLE 6

# VERMONT

*U.S. Registered Community Hospitals*
*(Nonfederal, short-term general and other special hospitals)*

## Utilization, Personnel, Revenue and Expenses, Community Health Indicators 1999–2003

| | 2003 | 2002 | 2001 | 2000 | 1999 |
|---|---|---|---|---|---|
| **TOTAL FACILITY (Includes Hospital and Nursing Home Units)** | | | | | |
| **Utilization - Inpatient** | | | | | |
| Beds | 1,506 | 1,576 | 1,694 | 1,674 | 1,669 |
| Admissions | 51,852 | 52,236 | 54,701 | 52,413 | 50,820 |
| Inpatient Days | 341,581 | 348,528 | 403,993 | 407,915 | 394,752 |
| Average Length of Stay | 6.6 | 6.7 | 7.4 | 7.8 | 7.8 |
| Inpatient Surgeries | 14,499 | 14,971 | 14,507 | 14,677 | 15,890 |
| Births | 6,028 | 6,003 | 5,982 | 6,086 | 6,521 |
| **Utilization - Outpatient** | | | | | |
| Emergency Outpatient Visits | 251,346 | 230,643 | 237,773 | 236,337 | 220,500 |
| Other Outpatient Visits | 1,960,218 | 1,239,885 | 1,053,731 | 1,006,715 | 1,193,334 |
| Total Outpatient Visits | 2,211,564 | 1,470,528 | 1,291,504 | 1,243,052 | 1,413,834 |
| Outpatient Surgeries | 54,857 | 39,468 | 37,983 | 34,739 | 33,443 |
| **Personnel** | | | | | |
| Full Time RNs | 1,016 | 1,040 | 939 | 977 | 948 |
| Full Time LPNs | 219 | 216 | 202 | 167 | 170 |
| Part Time RNs | 1,619 | 1,770 | 1,201 | 1,651 | 1,505 |
| Part Time LPNs | 227 | 240 | 216 | 265 | 222 |
| Total Full Time | 7,224 | 7,981 | 7,317 | 5,977 | 5,911 |
| Total Part Time | 4,977 | 5,589 | 4,134 | 5,307 | 4,958 |
| **Revenue - Inpatient** | | | | | |
| Gross Inpatient Revenue | $669,226,956 | $632,612,094 | $594,629,834 | $574,346,167 | $518,323,168 |
| **Revenue - Outpatient** | | | | | |
| Gross Outpatient Revenue | $1,056,083,809 | $683,857,958 | $583,052,967 | $496,200,352 | $435,098,015 |
| **Revenue and Expenses - Totals (Includes Inpatient and Outpatient)** | | | | | |
| Total Gross Revenue | $1,725,310,765 | $1,316,470,052 | $1,177,682,801 | $1,070,546,519 | $953,421,183 |
| Deductions from Revenue | 705,626,932 | 514,087,762 | 406,248,096 | 373,526,131 | 321,690,952 |
| Net Patient Revenue | 1,019,683,833 | 802,382,290 | 771,434,705 | 697,020,388 | 631,730,231 |
| Other Operating Revenue | 22,305,529 | 17,504,386 | 16,049,961 | 15,403,343 | 15,793,813 |
| Other Nonoperating Revenue | 10,299,848 | 260,503 | -17,559,247 | 27,208,270 | 15,736,174 |
| Total Net Revenue | 1,052,289,210 | 820,147,179 | 769,925,419 | 739,632,001 | 663,260,218 |
| Total Expenses | 1,012,039,974 | 812,757,084 | 771,202,476 | 696,036,667 | 646,945,630 |
| **HOSPITAL UNIT (Excludes Separate Nursing Home Units)** | | | | | |
| **Utilization - Inpatient** | | | | | |
| Beds | 1,258 | 1,325 | 1,318 | 1,425 | 1,302 |
| Admissions | 51,454 | 51,785 | 54,016 | 52,048 | 50,270 |
| Inpatient Days | 255,263 | 263,456 | 275,686 | 320,624 | 270,279 |
| Average Length of Stay | 5.0 | 5.1 | 5.1 | 6.2 | 5.4 |
| **Personnel** | | | | | |
| Total Full Time | 6,965 | 7,778 | 7,062 | 5,844 | 5,712 |
| Total Part Time | 4,765 | 5,469 | 3,936 | 5,192 | 4,753 |
| **Revenue and Expenses - Totals (Includes Inpatient and Outpatient)** | | | | | |
| Total Net Revenue | $1,034,057,663 | $807,750,162 | $749,316,386 | $727,972,770 | $645,310,922 |
| Total Expenses | 994,881,487 | 798,095,694 | 751,409,578 | 685,479,802 | 629,980,592 |
| **COMMUNITY HEALTH INDICATORS PER 1000 POPULATION** | | | | | |
| Total Population (in thousands) | 619 | 616 | 613 | 610 | 605 |
| **Inpatient** | | | | | |
| Beds | 2.4 | 2.6 | 2.8 | 2.7 | 2.8 |
| Admissions | 83.8 | 84.7 | 89.2 | 85.9 | 84.0 |
| Inpatient Days | 551.7 | 565.4 | 659.1 | 668.8 | 652.8 |
| Inpatient Surgeries | 23.4 | 24.3 | 23.7 | 24.1 | 26.3 |
| Births | 9.7 | 9.7 | 9.8 | 10.0 | 10.8 |
| **Outpatient** | | | | | |
| Emergency Outpatient Visits | 406.0 | 374.2 | 387.9 | 387.5 | 364.7 |
| Other Outpatient Visits | 3,166.2 | 2,011.5 | 1,719.2 | 1,650.5 | 1,973.5 |
| Total Outpatient Visits | 3,572.2 | 2,385.6 | 2,107.1 | 2,038.0 | 2,338.1 |
| Outpatient Surgeries | 88.6 | 64.0 | 62.0 | 57.0 | 55.3 |
| **Expense per Capita (per person)** | $1,634.7 | $1,318.5 | $1,258.2 | $1,141.2 | $1,069.9 |

# TABLE 6

# VIRGINIA

*U.S. Registered Community Hospitals*
*(Nonfederal, short-term general and other special hospitals)*

## Overview 1999–2003

| | 2003 | 2002 | 2001 | 2000 | 1999 |
|---|---|---|---|---|---|
| **Total Community Hospitals in Virginia** | **84** | **86** | **87** | **88** | **89** |
| **Bed Size Category** | | | | | |
| 6-24 | 1 | 1 | 2 | 4 | 2 |
| 25-49 | 11 | 11 | 10 | 7 | 7 |
| 50-99 | 17 | 18 | 18 | 17 | 20 |
| 100-199 | 25 | 25 | 25 | 29 | 28 |
| 200-299 | 14 | 15 | 17 | 15 | 16 |
| 300-399 | 6 | 5 | 5 | 7 | 8 |
| 400-499 | 2 | 3 | 3 | 3 | 2 |
| 500 + | 8 | 8 | 7 | 6 | 6 |
| **Location** | | | | | |
| Hospitals Urban | 50 | 51 | 52 | 53 | 54 |
| Hospitals Rural | 34 | 35 | 35 | 35 | 35 |
| **Control** | | | | | |
| State and Local Government | 4 | 5 | 5 | 5 | 5 |
| Not for Profit | 63 | 67 | 67 | 66 | 68 |
| Investor owned | 17 | 14 | 15 | 17 | 16 |
| **Physician Models** | | | | | |
| Independent Practice Association | 12 | 8 | 6 | 11 | 11 |
| Group Practice without Walls | 7 | 1 | 1 | 6 | 10 |
| Open Physician-Hospital Organization | 14 | 20 | 22 | 24 | 30 |
| Closed Physician-Hospital Organization | 3 | 3 | 2 | 4 | 8 |
| Management Service Organization | 5 | 6 | 9 | 11 | 21 |
| Integrated Salary Model | 28 | 28 | 23 | 28 | 32 |
| Equity Model | 7 | 2 | 1 | 3 | 6 |
| Foundation | 2 | 5 | 3 | 4 | 4 |
| **Insurance Products** | | | | | |
| Health Maintenance Organization | 22 | 26 | 23 | 25 | 31 |
| Preferred Provider Organization | 29 | 33 | 30 | 37 | 41 |
| Indemnity Fee for Service | 14 | 9 | 7 | 13 | 17 |
| **Managed Care Contracts** | | | | | |
| Health Maintenance Organization | 55 | 56 | 51 | 55 | 55 |
| Preferred Provider Organization | 63 | 64 | 57 | 64 | 64 |
| **Affiliations** | | | | | |
| Hospitals in a System* | 51 | 51 | 56 | 54 | 54 |
| Hospitals in a Network | 27 | 28 | 28 | 32 | 29 |
| Hospitals in a Group Purchasing Organization | 67 | 66 | 60 | 65 | 62 |

States

* Please note that system affiliate information for hospitals is derived from AHA membership. In years prior to 2003 the affiliation was derived from a question on the AHA Annual Survey of hospitals; therefore, non-responding hospitals were not included in the system affiliation counts. Years prior to 2003 have been updated to reflect this change, which now include affiliation for non-reporting hospitals.

# TABLE 6

# VIRGINIA

*U.S. Registered Community Hospitals*
*(Nonfederal, short-term general and other special hospitals)*

## Utilization, Personnel, Revenue and Expenses, Community Health Indicators 1999–2003

| | 2003 | 2002 | 2001 | 2000 | 1999 |
|---|---|---|---|---|---|
| **TOTAL FACILITY (Includes Hospital and Nursing Home Units)** | | | | | |
| **Utilization - Inpatient** | | | | | |
| Beds | 17,225 | 17,241 | 16,775 | 16,869 | 17,295 |
| Admissions | 758,258 | 746,686 | 743,992 | 726,772 | 723,803 |
| Inpatient Days | 4,367,997 | 4,278,445 | 4,239,227 | 4,161,981 | 4,133,834 |
| Average Length of Stay | 5.8 | 5.7 | 5.7 | 5.7 | 5.7 |
| Inpatient Surgeries | 233,220 | 236,774 | 235,109 | 221,837 | 215,568 |
| Births | 92,014 | 90,401 | 90,043 | 88,419 | 87,384 |
| **Utilization - Outpatient** | | | | | |
| Emergency Outpatient Visits | 2,759,886 | 2,606,320 | 2,482,380 | 2,476,006 | 2,291,867 |
| Other Outpatient Visits | 8,431,492 | 8,183,177 | 7,266,153 | 7,067,468 | 6,439,017 |
| Total Outpatient Visits | 11,191,378 | 10,789,497 | 9,748,533 | 9,543,474 | 8,730,884 |
| Outpatient Surgeries | 489,438 | 503,094 | 468,427 | 424,570 | 399,995 |
| **Personnel** | | | | | |
| Full Time RNs | 18,335 | 18,038 | 17,572 | 17,875 | 17,243 |
| Full Time LPNs | 2,833 | 2,764 | 2,690 | 2,704 | 2,778 |
| Part Time RNs | 9,614 | 8,110 | 7,902 | 7,432 | 6,990 |
| Part Time LPNs | 939 | 844 | 865 | 861 | 1,090 |
| Total Full Time | 71,709 | 72,397 | 72,228 | 71,430 | 68,276 |
| Total Part Time | 26,516 | 23,323 | 24,196 | 23,153 | 22,200 |
| **Revenue - Inpatient** | | | | | |
| Gross Inpatient Revenue | $13,740,614,713 | $12,167,189,859 | $10,850,288,232 | $9,441,736,067 | $8,879,124,657 |
| **Revenue - Outpatient** | | | | | |
| Gross Outpatient Revenue | $8,210,447,929 | $7,232,253,089 | $6,253,409,826 | $5,348,095,706 | $4,761,310,776 |
| **Revenue and Expenses - Totals (Includes Inpatient and Outpatient)** | | | | | |
| Total Gross Revenue | $21,951,062,642 | $19,399,442,948 | $17,103,698,058 | $14,789,831,773 | $13,640,435,433 |
| Deductions from Revenue | 12,410,069,628 | 10,621,457,968 | 8,992,877,116 | 7,349,786,545 | 6,565,622,328 |
| Net Patient Revenue | 9,540,993,014 | 8,777,984,980 | 8,110,820,942 | 7,440,045,228 | 7,074,813,105 |
| Other Operating Revenue | 266,650,457 | 241,242,013 | 302,761,541 | 273,304,634 | 261,032,965 |
| Other Nonoperating Revenue | 185,982,334 | -14,532,952 | 131,168,071 | 126,490,381 | 226,795,432 |
| Total Net Revenue | 9,993,625,805 | 9,004,694,041 | 8,544,750,554 | 7,839,840,243 | 7,562,641,502 |
| Total Expenses | 9,225,809,610 | 8,779,480,958 | 7,961,019,921 | 7,109,751,133 | 6,637,854,513 |
| **HOSPITAL UNIT (Excludes Separate Nursing Home Units)** | | | | | |
| **Utilization - Inpatient** | | | | | |
| Beds | 15,890 | 15,938 | 15,866 | 15,709 | 15,872 |
| Admissions | 754,821 | 743,372 | 740,997 | 723,853 | 720,497 |
| Inpatient Days | 3,919,369 | 3,875,511 | 3,927,254 | 3,769,912 | 3,653,766 |
| Average Length of Stay | 5.2 | 5.2 | 5.3 | 5.2 | 5.1 |
| **Personnel** | | | | | |
| Total Full Time | 70,682 | 71,403 | 71,289 | 70,525 | 67,346 |
| Total Part Time | 26,126 | 23,004 | 23,845 | 22,889 | 21,770 |
| **Revenue and Expenses - Totals (Includes Inpatient and Outpatient)** | | | | | |
| Total Net Revenue | $9,930,690,590 | $8,947,350,583 | $8,501,564,931 | $7,795,125,327 | $7,500,435,588 |
| Total Expenses | 9,167,578,607 | 8,727,817,754 | 7,921,569,817 | 7,069,123,980 | 6,592,027,665 |
| **COMMUNITY HEALTH INDICATORS PER 1000 POPULATION** | | | | | |
| Total Population (in thousands) | 7,386 | 7,288 | 7,193 | 7,105 | 7,000 |
| **Inpatient** | | | | | |
| Beds | 2.3 | 2.4 | 2.3 | 2.4 | 2.5 |
| Admissions | 102.7 | 102.5 | 103.4 | 102.3 | 103.4 |
| Inpatient Days | 591.4 | 587.1 | 589.4 | 585.8 | 590.5 |
| Inpatient Surgeries | 31.6 | 32.5 | 32.7 | 31.2 | 30.8 |
| Births | 12.5 | 12.4 | 12.5 | 12.4 | 12.5 |
| **Outpatient** | | | | | |
| Emergency Outpatient Visits | 373.6 | 357.6 | 345.1 | 348.5 | 327.4 |
| Other Outpatient Visits | 1,141.5 | 1,122.9 | 1,010.2 | 994.7 | 919.8 |
| Total Outpatient Visits | 1,515.1 | 1,480.5 | 1,355.3 | 1,343.2 | 1,247.2 |
| Outpatient Surgeries | 66.3 | 69.0 | 65.1 | 59.8 | 57.1 |
| **Expense per Capita (per person)** | $1,249.0 | $1,204.7 | $1,106.8 | $1,000.7 | $948.2 |

# TABLE 6

## WASHINGTON

*U.S. Registered Community Hospitals*
*(Nonfederal, short-term general and other special hospitals)*

## Overview 1999–2003

| | 2003 | 2002 | 2001 | 2000 | 1999 |
|---|---|---|---|---|---|
| **Total Community Hospitals in Washington** | **85** | **86** | **84** | **84** | **86** |
| **Bed Size Category** | | | | | |
| 6-24 | 9 | 9 | 5 | 6 | 8 |
| 25-49 | 24 | 20 | 22 | 22 | 22 |
| 50-99 | 12 | 18 | 18 | 17 | 17 |
| 100-199 | 18 | 16 | 17 | 16 | 18 |
| 200-299 | 13 | 14 | 12 | 15 | 13 |
| 300-399 | 7 | 6 | 7 | 6 | 6 |
| 400-499 | 0 | 1 | 1 | 0 | 0 |
| 500 + | 2 | 2 | 2 | 2 | 2 |
| **Location** | | | | | |
| Hospitals Urban | 45 | 45 | 44 | 44 | 46 |
| Hospitals Rural | 40 | 41 | 40 | 40 | 40 |
| **Control** | | | | | |
| State and Local Government | 39 | 40 | 39 | 38 | 40 |
| Not for Profit | 41 | 42 | 41 | 42 | 43 |
| Investor owned | 5 | 4 | 4 | 4 | 3 |
| **Physician Models** | | | | | |
| Independent Practice Association | 7 | 3 | 9 | 9 | 11 |
| Group Practice without Walls | 2 | 3 | 5 | 2 | 2 |
| Open Physician-Hospital Organization | 5 | 11 | 10 | 13 | 14 |
| Closed Physician-Hospital Organization | 4 | 1 | 3 | 3 | 6 |
| Management Service Organization | 5 | 6 | 7 | 7 | 9 |
| Integrated Salary Model | 37 | 36 | 22 | 22 | 20 |
| Equity Model | 0 | 0 | 1 | 2 | 2 |
| Foundation | 1 | 0 | 2 | 3 | 3 |
| **Insurance Products** | | | | | |
| Health Maintenance Organization | 5 | 9 | 6 | 7 | 13 |
| Preferred Provider Organization | 8 | 12 | 9 | 11 | 17 |
| Indemnity Fee for Service | 3 | 3 | 3 | 4 | 6 |
| **Managed Care Contracts** | | | | | |
| Health Maintenance Organization | 40 | 41 | 35 | 37 | 43 |
| Preferred Provider Organization | 49 | 54 | 39 | 43 | 48 |
| **Affiliations** | | | | | |
| Hospitals in a System* | 28 | 28 | 29 | 28 | 31 |
| Hospitals in a Network | 16 | 16 | 19 | 15 | 17 |
| Hospitals in a Group Purchasing Organization | 64 | 62 | 53 | 49 | 52 |

States

* Please note that system affiliate information for hospitals is derived from AHA membership. In years prior to 2003 the affiliation was derived from a question on the AHA Annual Survey of hospitals; therefore, non-responding hospitals were not included in the system affiliation counts. Years prior to 2003 have been updated to reflect this change, which now include affiliation for non-reporting hospitals.

# TABLE 6

# WASHINGTON

*U.S. Registered Community Hospitals*
*(Nonfederal, short-term general and other special hospitals)*

## Utilization, Personnel, Revenue and Expenses, Community Health Indicators 1999–2003

| | 2003 | 2002 | 2001 | 2000 | 1999 |
|---|---|---|---|---|---|
| **TOTAL FACILITY (Includes Hospital and Nursing Home Units)** | | | | | |
| **Utilization - Inpatient** | | | | | |
| Beds | 11,190 | 11,338 | 11,382 | 11,136 | 11,092 |
| Admissions | 515,939 | 518,562 | 522,624 | 504,836 | 490,659 |
| Inpatient Days | 2,477,079 | 2,486,925 | 2,501,066 | 2,432,089 | 2,375,711 |
| Average Length of Stay | 4.8 | 4.8 | 4.8 | 4.8 | 4.8 |
| Inpatient Surgeries | 172,130 | 162,809 | 163,263 | 163,298 | 164,275 |
| Births | 72,453 | 72,586 | 74,134 | 73,816 | 72,814 |
| **Utilization - Outpatient** | | | | | |
| Emergency Outpatient Visits | 2,030,209 | 1,936,458 | 2,063,313 | 1,932,238 | 1,887,881 |
| Other Outpatient Visits | 8,261,544 | 7,811,926 | 7,369,191 | 7,656,940 | 8,072,113 |
| Total Outpatient Visits | 10,291,753 | 9,748,384 | 9,432,504 | 9,589,178 | 9,959,994 |
| Outpatient Surgeries | 268,924 | 280,786 | 312,357 | 261,219 | 247,937 |
| **Personnel** | | | | | |
| Full Time RNs | 10,475 | 10,214 | 10,991 | 10,083 | 8,427 |
| Full Time LPNs | 913 | 1,060 | 1,098 | 1,175 | 932 |
| Part Time RNs | 12,041 | 11,477 | 9,567 | 11,165 | 11,467 |
| Part Time LPNs | 950 | 866 | 595 | 1,155 | 1,176 |
| Total Full Time | 51,107 | 53,490 | 54,672 | 50,106 | 45,373 |
| Total Part Time | 35,276 | 32,880 | 27,551 | 33,201 | 33,715 |
| **Revenue - Inpatient** | | | | | |
| Gross Inpatient Revenue | $9,520,850,529 | $8,210,414,712 | $7,463,136,201 | $6,558,652,349 | $5,936,579,978 |
| **Revenue - Outpatient** | | | | | |
| Gross Outpatient Revenue | $7,359,274,143 | $6,583,605,589 | $5,100,762,752 | $4,446,084,034 | $3,979,924,518 |
| **Revenue and Expenses - Totals (Includes Inpatient and Outpatient)** | | | | | |
| Total Gross Revenue | $16,880,124,672 | $14,794,020,301 | $12,563,898,953 | $11,004,736,383 | $9,916,504,496 |
| Deductions from Revenue | 8,552,487,105 | 7,178,544,115 | 5,870,547,412 | 4,776,586,811 | 3,981,377,196 |
| Net Patient Revenue | 8,327,637,567 | 7,615,476,186 | 6,693,351,541 | 6,228,149,572 | 5,935,127,300 |
| Other Operating Revenue | 469,719,678 | 473,047,880 | 438,253,314 | 344,678,358 | 329,844,922 |
| Other Nonoperating Revenue | 130,473,550 | 45,762,585 | 81,540,504 | 160,620,397 | 127,455,356 |
| Total Net Revenue | 8,927,830,795 | 8,134,286,651 | 7,213,145,359 | 6,733,448,327 | 6,392,427,578 |
| Total Expenses | 8,358,507,505 | 7,830,121,368 | 6,971,690,572 | 6,384,423,283 | 6,091,763,363 |
| **HOSPITAL UNIT (Excludes Separate Nursing Home Units)** | | | | | |
| **Utilization - Inpatient** | | | | | |
| Beds | 10,475 | 10,494 | 10,696 | 10,326 | 10,217 |
| Admissions | 511,844 | 513,922 | 516,955 | 501,157 | 484,728 |
| Inpatient Days | 2,237,474 | 2,219,549 | 2,292,820 | 2,211,500 | 2,125,679 |
| Average Length of Stay | 4.4 | 4.3 | 4.4 | 4.4 | 4.4 |
| **Personnel** | | | | | |
| Total Full Time | 50,508 | 52,927 | 54,120 | 49,627 | 44,769 |
| Total Part Time | 34,926 | 32,525 | 27,177 | 32,905 | 33,403 |
| **Revenue and Expenses - Totals (Includes Inpatient and Outpatient)** | | | | | |
| Total Net Revenue | $8,875,530,733 | $8,082,984,927 | $7,171,721,867 | $6,697,390,270 | $6,346,757,006 |
| Total Expenses | 8,315,286,786 | 7,788,632,966 | 6,932,850,141 | 6,352,247,750 | 6,054,313,545 |
| **COMMUNITY HEALTH INDICATORS PER 1000 POPULATION** | | | | | |
| Total Population (in thousands) | 6,131 | 6,067 | 5,993 | 5,911 | 5,843 |
| **Inpatient** | | | | | |
| Beds | 1.8 | 1.9 | 1.9 | 1.9 | 1.9 |
| Admissions | 84.1 | 85.5 | 87.2 | 85.4 | 84.0 |
| Inpatient Days | 404.0 | 409.9 | 417.3 | 411.4 | 406.6 |
| Inpatient Surgeries | 28.1 | 26.8 | 27.2 | 27.6 | 28.1 |
| Births | 11.8 | 12.0 | 12.4 | 12.5 | 12.5 |
| **Outpatient** | | | | | |
| Emergency Outpatient Visits | 331.1 | 319.2 | 344.3 | 326.9 | 323.1 |
| Other Outpatient Visits | 1,347.4 | 1,287.6 | 1,229.7 | 1,295.4 | 1,381.6 |
| Total Outpatient Visits | 1,678.5 | 1,606.8 | 1,574.0 | 1,622.2 | 1,704.7 |
| Outpatient Surgeries | 43.9 | 46.3 | 52.1 | 44.2 | 42.4 |
| **Expense per Capita (per person)** | $1,363.2 | $1,290.6 | $1,163.4 | $1,080.1 | $1,042.7 |

# TABLE 6

# WEST VIRGINIA

*U.S. Registered Community Hospitals*
*(Nonfederal, short-term general and other special hospitals)*

## Overview 1999–2003

| | 2003 | 2002 | 2001 | 2000 | 1999 |
|---|---|---|---|---|---|
| **Total Community Hospitals in West Virginia** | **57** | **57** | **57** | **57** | **58** |
| **Bed Size Category** | | | | | |
| 6-24 | 4 | 4 | 3 | 3 | 3 |
| 25-49 | 11 | 11 | 13 | 13 | 13 |
| 50-99 | 17 | 17 | 16 | 16 | 16 |
| 100-199 | 12 | 12 | 10 | 10 | 10 |
| 200-299 | 7 | 8 | 10 | 10 | 10 |
| 300-399 | 4 | 3 | 3 | 2 | 3 |
| 400-499 | 1 | 1 | 1 | 2 | 2 |
| 500 + | 1 | 1 | 1 | 1 | 1 |
| **Location** | | | | | |
| Hospitals Urban | 18 | 18 | 18 | 18 | 18 |
| Hospitals Rural | 39 | 39 | 39 | 39 | 40 |
| **Control** | | | | | |
| State and Local Government | 10 | 10 | 10 | 10 | 10 |
| Not for Profit | 31 | 33 | 33 | 33 | 34 |
| Investor owned | 16 | 14 | 14 | 14 | 14 |
| **Physician Models** | | | | | |
| Independent Practice Association | 6 | 3 | 3 | 3 | 0 |
| Group Practice without Walls | 2 | 1 | 2 | 2 | 3 |
| Open Physician-Hospital Organization | 15 | 16 | 17 | 17 | 19 |
| Closed Physician-Hospital Organization | 2 | 1 | 1 | 3 | 1 |
| Management Service Organization | 4 | 4 | 4 | 7 | 10 |
| Integrated Salary Model | 25 | 21 | 20 | 17 | 14 |
| Equity Model | 2 | 1 | 1 | 1 | 1 |
| Foundation | 0 | 0 | 0 | 0 | 1 |
| **Insurance Products** | | | | | |
| Health Maintenance Organization | 5 | 6 | 4 | 8 | 7 |
| Preferred Provider Organization | 9 | 9 | 8 | 12 | 12 |
| Indemnity Fee for Service | 5 | 5 | 4 | 6 | 4 |
| **Managed Care Contracts** | | | | | |
| Health Maintenance Organization | 32 | 34 | 35 | 37 | 38 |
| Preferred Provider Organization | 45 | 48 | 45 | 47 | 46 |
| **Affiliations** | | | | | |
| Hospitals in a System* | 23 | 24 | 23 | 26 | 28 |
| Hospitals in a Network | 28 | 30 | 28 | 28 | 26 |
| Hospitals in a Group Purchasing Organization | 52 | 52 | 52 | 48 | 45 |

* Please note that system affiliate information for hospitals is derived from AHA membership. In years prior to 2003 the affiliation was derived from a question on the AHA Annual Survey of hospitals; therefore, non-responding hospitals were not included in the system affiliation counts. Years prior to 2003 have been updated to reflect this change, which now include affiliation for non-reporting hospitals.

# WEST VIRGINIA

*U.S. Registered Community Hospitals*
*(Nonfederal, short-term general and other special hospitals)*

## Utilization, Personnel, Revenue and Expenses, Community Health Indicators 1999–2003

| | 2003 | 2002 | 2001 | 2000 | 1999 |
|---|---|---|---|---|---|
| **TOTAL FACILITY (Includes Hospital and Nursing Home Units)** | | | | | |
| **Utilization - Inpatient** | | | | | |
| Beds | 7,779 | 7,821 | 7,906 | 7,966 | 8,109 |
| Admissions | 296,089 | 295,011 | 297,079 | 288,095 | 289,427 |
| Inpatient Days | 1,770,290 | 1,775,869 | 1,806,411 | 1,772,580 | 1,792,038 |
| Average Length of Stay | 6.0 | 6.0 | 6.1 | 6.2 | 6.2 |
| Inpatient Surgeries | 77,583 | 79,711 | 82,783 | 81,969 | 100,693 |
| Births | 21,302 | 20,659 | 20,775 | 20,917 | 20,785 |
| **Utilization - Outpatient** | | | | | |
| Emergency Outpatient Visits | 1,112,496 | 1,100,258 | 1,057,155 | 1,007,028 | 1,002,071 |
| Other Outpatient Visits | 4,644,732 | 4,585,150 | 4,705,105 | 4,188,510 | 4,093,375 |
| Total Outpatient Visits | 5,757,228 | 5,685,408 | 5,762,260 | 5,195,538 | 5,095,446 |
| Outpatient Surgeries | 200,952 | 201,288 | 203,775 | 185,222 | 196,421 |
| **Personnel** | | | | | |
| Full Time RNs | 6,459 | 6,836 | 7,005 | 7,013 | 6,869 |
| Full Time LPNs | 1,559 | 1,599 | 1,656 | 1,639 | 1,599 |
| Part Time RNs | 3,641 | 3,191 | 3,019 | 2,435 | 2,426 |
| Part Time LPNs | 514 | 532 | 452 | 512 | 468 |
| Total Full Time | 29,264 | 29,733 | 29,730 | 29,191 | 29,397 |
| Total Part Time | 9,749 | 9,691 | 9,679 | 8,528 | 8,212 |
| **Revenue - Inpatient** | | | | | |
| Gross Inpatient Revenue | $3,679,723,811 | $3,247,995,766 | $3,059,121,057 | $2,738,379,228 | $2,558,226,357 |
| **Revenue - Outpatient** | | | | | |
| Gross Outpatient Revenue | $2,738,672,867 | $2,395,425,269 | $2,108,241,241 | $1,896,927,001 | $1,702,148,428 |
| **Revenue and Expenses - Totals (Includes Inpatient and Outpatient)** | | | | | |
| Total Gross Revenue | $6,418,396,678 | $5,643,421,035 | $5,167,362,298 | $4,635,306,229 | $4,260,374,785 |
| Deductions from Revenue | 3,177,374,702 | 2,606,272,014 | 2,318,812,349 | 2,018,286,724 | 1,717,929,145 |
| Net Patient Revenue | 3,241,021,976 | 3,037,149,021 | 2,848,549,949 | 2,617,019,505 | 2,542,445,640 |
| Other Operating Revenue | 99,592,313 | 87,401,673 | 94,610,622 | 83,958,168 | 67,331,452 |
| Other Nonoperating Revenue | 34,650,258 | 16,381,152 | 42,442,849 | 62,118,544 | 73,508,215 |
| Total Net Revenue | 3,375,264,547 | 3,140,931,846 | 2,985,603,420 | 2,763,096,217 | 2,683,285,307 |
| Total Expenses | 3,286,535,065 | 3,068,384,987 | 2,867,459,406 | 2,672,667,972 | 2,569,940,576 |
| **HOSPITAL UNIT (Excludes Separate Nursing Home Units)** | | | | | |
| **Utilization - Inpatient** | | | | | |
| Beds | 6,756 | 6,756 | 6,835 | 6,904 | 7,063 |
| Admissions | 288,258 | 286,752 | 288,941 | 279,560 | 280,887 |
| Inpatient Days | 1,439,093 | 1,435,794 | 1,475,652 | 1,442,082 | 1,463,906 |
| Average Length of Stay | 5.0 | 5.0 | 5.1 | 5.2 | 5.2 |
| **Personnel** | | | | | |
| Total Full Time | 28,411 | 28,849 | 28,817 | 28,286 | 28,402 |
| Total Part Time | 9,393 | 9,386 | 9,398 | 8,251 | 7,907 |
| **Revenue and Expenses - Totals (Includes Inpatient and Outpatient)** | | | | | |
| Total Net Revenue | $3,303,564,652 | $3,073,370,762 | $2,917,661,986 | $2,707,349,521 | $2,628,108,392 |
| Total Expenses | 3,230,266,642 | 3,005,319,455 | 2,818,658,157 | 2,625,906,089 | 2,521,864,295 |
| **COMMUNITY HEALTH INDICATORS PER 1000 POPULATION** | | | | | |
| Total Population (in thousands) | 1,810 | 1,805 | 1,802 | 1,807 | 1,812 |
| **Inpatient** | | | | | |
| Beds | 4.3 | 4.3 | 4.4 | 4.4 | 4.5 |
| Admissions | 163.6 | 163.5 | 164.9 | 159.4 | 159.7 |
| Inpatient Days | 977.9 | 983.9 | 1,002.6 | 980.8 | 989.1 |
| Inpatient Surgeries | 42.9 | 44.2 | 45.9 | 45.4 | 55.6 |
| Births | 11.8 | 11.4 | 11.5 | 11.6 | 11.5 |
| **Outpatient** | | | | | |
| Emergency Outpatient Visits | 614.5 | 609.6 | 586.8 | 557.2 | 553.1 |
| Other Outpatient Visits | 2,565.6 | 2,540.4 | 2,611.6 | 2,317.5 | 2,259.3 |
| Total Outpatient Visits | 3,180.2 | 3,150.0 | 3,198.3 | 2,874.7 | 2,812.4 |
| Outpatient Surgeries | 111.0 | 111.5 | 113.1 | 102.5 | 108.4 |
| **Expense per Capita (per person)** | $1,815.4 | $1,700.0 | $1,591.6 | $1,478.8 | $1,418.4 |

# TABLE 6

## WISCONSIN

*U.S. Registered Community Hospitals*
*(Nonfederal, short-term general and other special hospitals)*

## Overview 1999–2003

| | 2003 | 2002 | 2001 | 2000 | 1999 |
|---|---|---|---|---|---|
| **Total Community Hospitals in Wisconsin** | **121** | **120** | **121** | **118** | **123** |
| **Bed Size Category** | | | | | |
| 6-24 | 8 | 8 | 5 | 5 | 6 |
| 25-49 | 26 | 29 | 30 | 27 | 26 |
| 50-99 | 30 | 27 | 29 | 26 | 29 |
| 100-199 | 35 | 36 | 35 | 40 | 40 |
| 200-299 | 14 | 14 | 15 | 13 | 15 |
| 300-399 | 4 | 4 | 2 | 2 | 2 |
| 400-499 | 3 | 1 | 3 | 3 | 3 |
| 500 + | 1 | 1 | 2 | 2 | 2 |
| **Location** | | | | | |
| Hospitals Urban | 57 | 55 | 56 | 56 | 57 |
| Hospitals Rural | 64 | 65 | 65 | 62 | 66 |
| **Control** | | | | | |
| State and Local Government | 2 | 2 | 2 | 2 | 2 |
| Not for Profit | 117 | 117 | 118 | 115 | 120 |
| Investor owned | 2 | 1 | 1 | 1 | 1 |
| **Physician Models** | | | | | |
| Independent Practice Association | 12 | 12 | 12 | 16 | 14 |
| Group Practice without Walls | 11 | 9 | 10 | 8 | 11 |
| Open Physician-Hospital Organization | 8 | 8 | 12 | 17 | 14 |
| Closed Physician-Hospital Organization | 8 | 8 | 6 | 8 | 5 |
| Management Service Organization | 6 | 7 | 6 | 9 | 7 |
| Integrated Salary Model | 49 | 42 | 36 | 35 | 38 |
| Equity Model | 4 | 2 | 3 | 7 | 3 |
| Foundation | 3 | 2 | 2 | 6 | 2 |
| **Insurance Products** | | | | | |
| Health Maintenance Organization | 21 | 28 | 30 | 22 | 25 |
| Preferred Provider Organization | 21 | 21 | 20 | 27 | 35 |
| Indemnity Fee for Service | 8 | 5 | 5 | 7 | 10 |
| **Managed Care Contracts** | | | | | |
| Health Maintenance Organization | 113 | 102 | 106 | 93 | 112 |
| Preferred Provider Organization | 116 | 108 | 113 | 101 | 115 |
| **Affiliations** | | | | | |
| Hospitals in a System* | 68 | 66 | 66 | 62 | 67 |
| Hospitals in a Network | 46 | 41 | 39 | 38 | 41 |
| Hospitals in a Group Purchasing Organization | 116 | 109 | 107 | 93 | 61 |



* Please note that system affiliate information for hospitals is derived from AHA membership. In years prior to 2003 the affiliation was derived from a question on the AHA Annual Survey of hospitals; therefore, non-responding hospitals were not included in the system affiliation counts. Years prior to 2003 have been updated to reflect this change, which now include affiliation for non-reporting hospitals.

# Table 6

# WISCONSIN

*U.S. Registered Community Hospitals*
*(Nonfederal, short-term general and other special hospitals)*

## Utilization, Personnel, Revenue and Expenses, Community Health Indicators 1999–2003

| | 2003 | 2002 | 2001 | 2000 | 1999 |
|---|---|---|---|---|---|
| **TOTAL FACILITY (Includes Hospital and Nursing Home Units)** | | | | | |
| **Utilization - Inpatient** | | | | | |
| Beds | 14,829 | 14,610 | 15,597 | 15,329 | 15,870 |
| Admissions | 588,466 | 579,830 | 579,089 | 558,357 | 553,337 |
| Inpatient Days | 3,355,918 | 3,396,381 | 3,455,633 | 3,331,095 | 3,394,502 |
| Average Length of Stay | 5.7 | 5.9 | 6.0 | 6.0 | 6.1 |
| Inpatient Surgeries | 190,192 | 181,674 | 184,704 | 181,028 | 179,457 |
| Births | 65,669 | 65,588 | 67,772 | 66,406 | 65,961 |
| **Utilization - Outpatient** | | | | | |
| Emergency Outpatient Visits | 1,813,690 | 1,833,344 | 1,866,201 | 1,785,771 | 1,723,490 |
| Other Outpatient Visits | 10,001,511 | 9,778,893 | 9,163,082 | 9,068,481 | 8,787,589 |
| Total Outpatient Visits | 11,815,201 | 11,612,237 | 11,029,283 | 10,854,252 | 10,511,079 |
| Outpatient Surgeries | 416,065 | 388,879 | 358,874 | 346,742 | 329,008 |
| **Personnel** | | | | | |
| Full Time RNs | 10,729 | 10,225 | 9,873 | 9,982 | 10,002 |
| Full Time LPNs | 842 | 794 | 751 | 689 | 712 |
| Part Time RNs | 14,302 | 12,915 | 13,772 | 13,399 | 12,989 |
| Part Time LPNs | 1,010 | 1,125 | 1,114 | 1,139 | 1,163 |
| Total Full Time | 55,058 | 53,737 | 51,379 | 49,099 | 50,249 |
| Total Part Time | 44,896 | 42,826 | 43,352 | 41,266 | 42,222 |
| **Revenue - Inpatient** | | | | | |
| Gross Inpatient Revenue | $8,686,033,584 | $7,802,749,118 | $6,991,429,425 | $6,098,946,220 | $5,948,871,964 |
| **Revenue - Outpatient** | | | | | |
| Gross Outpatient Revenue | $7,135,965,468 | $6,112,204,146 | $5,291,918,670 | $4,468,653,347 | $4,013,180,391 |
| **Revenue and Expenses - Totals (Includes Inpatient and Outpatient)** | | | | | |
| Total Gross Revenue | $15,821,999,052 | $13,914,953,264 | $12,283,348,095 | $10,567,599,567 | $9,962,052,355 |
| Deductions from Revenue | 7,007,752,524 | 5,950,993,178 | 5,054,991,610 | 3,975,769,894 | 3,784,662,896 |
| Net Patient Revenue | 8,814,246,528 | 7,963,960,086 | 7,228,356,485 | 6,591,829,673 | 6,177,389,459 |
| Other Operating Revenue | 473,220,938 | 437,318,773 | 330,549,912 | 318,938,842 | 308,659,328 |
| Other Nonoperating Revenue | 89,274,796 | 92,711,281 | 132,446,055 | 153,176,880 | 139,860,357 |
| Total Net Revenue | 9,376,742,262 | 8,493,990,140 | 7,691,352,452 | 7,063,945,395 | 6,625,909,144 |
| Total Expenses | 8,797,685,529 | 7,917,744,877 | 7,182,972,349 | 6,662,561,165 | 6,232,856,297 |
| **HOSPITAL UNIT (Excludes Separate Nursing Home Units)** | | | | | |
| **Utilization - Inpatient** | | | | | |
| Beds | 12,634 | 12,413 | 13,124 | 13,069 | 13,455 |
| Admissions | 584,556 | 576,456 | 575,849 | 555,586 | 549,946 |
| Inpatient Days | 2,628,162 | 2,653,543 | 2,656,174 | 2,587,690 | 2,596,699 |
| Average Length of Stay | 4.5 | 4.6 | 4.6 | 4.7 | 4.7 |
| **Personnel** | | | | | |
| Total Full Time | 54,308 | 53,066 | 50,535 | 47,736 | 49,158 |
| Total Part Time | 43,929 | 41,988 | 42,513 | 40,098 | 41,046 |
| **Revenue and Expenses - Totals (Includes Inpatient and Outpatient)** | | | | | |
| Total Net Revenue | $9,306,678,467 | $8,402,275,478 | $7,614,643,256 | $7,003,452,628 | $6,535,271,256 |
| Total Expenses | 8,729,956,837 | 7,837,518,200 | 7,116,127,111 | 6,570,298,128 | 6,157,416,203 |
| **COMMUNITY HEALTH INDICATORS PER 1000 POPULATION** | | | | | |
| Total Population (in thousands) | 5,472 | 5,440 | 5,405 | 5,374 | 5,333 |
| **Inpatient** | | | | | |
| Beds | 2.7 | 2.7 | 2.9 | 2.9 | 3.0 |
| Admissions | 107.5 | 106.6 | 107.1 | 103.9 | 103.8 |
| Inpatient Days | 613.3 | 624.4 | 639.3 | 619.9 | 636.5 |
| Inpatient Surgeries | 34.8 | 33.4 | 34.2 | 33.7 | 33.7 |
| Births | 12.0 | 12.1 | 12.5 | 12.4 | 12.4 |
| **Outpatient** | | | | | |
| Emergency Outpatient Visits | 331.4 | 337.0 | 345.3 | 332.3 | 323.2 |
| Other Outpatient Visits | 1,827.7 | 1,797.7 | 1,695.3 | 1,687.5 | 1,647.9 |
| Total Outpatient Visits | 2,159.1 | 2,134.7 | 2,040.5 | 2,019.8 | 1,971.1 |
| Outpatient Surgeries | 76.0 | 71.5 | 66.4 | 64.5 | 61.7 |
| **Expense per Capita (per person)** | $1,607.7 | $1,455.6 | $1,328.9 | $1,239.8 | $1,168.8 |

# TABLE 6

## WYOMING

*U.S. Registered Community Hospitals*
*(Nonfederal, short-term general and other special hospitals)*

## Overview 1999–2003

| | 2003 | 2002 | 2001 | 2000 | 1999 |
|---|---|---|---|---|---|
| **Total Community Hospitals in Wyoming** | **23** | **24** | **24** | **24** | **23** |
| **Bed Size Category** | | | | | |
| 6-24 | 1 | 0 | 0 | 0 | 0 |
| 25-49 | 8 | 9 | 9 | 9 | 9 |
| 50-99 | 9 | 10 | 10 | 9 | 8 |
| 100-199 | 4 | 4 | 4 | 4 | 5 |
| 200-299 | 1 | 1 | 1 | 2 | 1 |
| 300-399 | 0 | 0 | 0 | 0 | 0 |
| 400-499 | 0 | 0 | 0 | 0 | 0 |
| 500 + | 0 | 0 | 0 | 0 | 0 |
| **Location** | | | | | |
| Hospitals Urban | 2 | 2 | 2 | 2 | 2 |
| Hospitals Rural | 21 | 22 | 22 | 22 | 21 |
| **Control** | | | | | |
| State and Local Government | 15 | 16 | 16 | 16 | 15 |
| Not for Profit | 5 | 5 | 5 | 5 | 5 |
| Investor owned | 3 | 3 | 3 | 3 | 3 |
| **Physician Models** | | | | | |
| Independent Practice Association | 3 | 2 | 2 | 2 | 3 |
| Group Practice without Walls | 0 | 0 | 0 | 0 | 0 |
| Open Physician-Hospital Organization | 2 | 2 | 1 | 1 | 2 |
| Closed Physician-Hospital Organization | 1 | 1 | 1 | 1 | 1 |
| Management Service Organization | 2 | 1 | 1 | 1 | 1 |
| Integrated Salary Model | 9 | 7 | 5 | 4 | 3 |
| Equity Model | 0 | 0 | 0 | 0 | 0 |
| Foundation | 0 | 0 | 0 | 1 | 0 |
| **Insurance Products** | | | | | |
| Health Maintenance Organization | 1 | 1 | 0 | 1 | 1 |
| Preferred Provider Organization | 1 | 1 | 3 | 4 | 4 |
| Indemnity Fee for Service | 1 | 1 | 1 | 1 | 0 |
| **Managed Care Contracts** | | | | | |
| Health Maintenance Organization | 4 | 3 | 3 | 2 | 3 |
| Preferred Provider Organization | 13 | 12 | 10 | 10 | 10 |
| **Affiliations** | | | | | |
| Hospitals in a System* | 10 | 10 | 9 | 8 | 8 |
| Hospitals in a Network | 4 | 2 | 2 | 2 | 0 |
| Hospitals in a Group Purchasing Organization | 22 | 21 | 22 | 20 | 17 |

States

* Please note that system affiliate information for hospitals is derived from AHA membership. In years prior to 2003 the affiliation was derived from a question on the AHA Annual Survey of hospitals; therefore, non-responding hospitals were not included in the system affiliation counts. Years prior to 2003 have been updated to reflect this change, which now include affiliation for non-reporting hospitals.

# Table 6

# WYOMING

*U.S. Registered Community Hospitals*
*(Nonfederal, short-term general and other special hospitals)*

## Utilization, Personnel, Revenue and Expenses, Community Health Indicators 1999–2003

| | 2003 | 2002 | 2001 | 2000 | 1999 |
|---|---|---|---|---|---|
| **TOTAL FACILITY (Includes Hospital and Nursing Home Units)** | | | | | |
| **Utilization - Inpatient** | | | | | |
| Beds | 1,773 | 1,882 | 1,920 | 1,920 | 1,830 |
| Admissions | 52,612 | 49,201 | 47,587 | 47,852 | 45,212 |
| Inpatient Days | 342,260 | 370,143 | 379,674 | 392,856 | 350,011 |
| Average Length of Stay | 6.5 | 7.5 | 8.0 | 8.2 | 7.7 |
| Inpatient Surgeries | 13,178 | 13,393 | 13,020 | 13,277 | 13,788 |
| Births | 6,048 | 5,945 | 5,779 | 5,668 | 5,376 |
| **Utilization - Outpatient** | | | | | |
| Emergency Outpatient Visits | 212,562 | 212,868 | 196,723 | 198,691 | 184,370 |
| Other Outpatient Visits | 655,482 | 676,043 | 621,299 | 679,917 | 681,309 |
| Total Outpatient Visits | 868,044 | 888,911 | 818,022 | 878,608 | 865,679 |
| Outpatient Surgeries | 28,912 | 28,197 | 27,168 | 26,600 | 24,333 |
| **Personnel** | | | | | |
| Full Time RNs | 1,453 | 1,424 | 1,385 | 1,250 | 1,346 |
| Full Time LPNs | 177 | 185 | 251 | 254 | 237 |
| Part Time RNs | 443 | 426 | 440 | 461 | 339 |
| Part Time LPNs | 61 | 47 | 86 | 78 | 56 |
| Total Full Time | 6,003 | 6,224 | 6,265 | 5,693 | 5,719 |
| Total Part Time | 1,666 | 1,798 | 1,905 | 2,075 | 1,532 |
| **Revenue - Inpatient** | | | | | |
| Gross Inpatient Revenue | $591,634,445 | $539,374,103 | $490,186,370 | $459,146,586 | $391,557,628 |
| **Revenue - Outpatient** | | | | | |
| Gross Outpatient Revenue | $478,863,281 | $429,084,211 | $370,431,371 | $341,692,739 | $286,160,208 |
| **Revenue and Expenses - Totals (Includes Inpatient and Outpatient)** | | | | | |
| Total Gross Revenue | $1,070,497,726 | $968,458,314 | $860,617,741 | $800,839,325 | $677,717,836 |
| Deductions from Revenue | 429,180,139 | 371,291,521 | 307,942,802 | 270,948,291 | 213,650,230 |
| Net Patient Revenue | 641,317,587 | 597,166,793 | 552,674,939 | 529,891,034 | 464,067,606 |
| Other Operating Revenue | 32,237,152 | 28,889,946 | 26,930,485 | 26,084,236 | 23,737,455 |
| Other Nonoperating Revenue | 19,937,176 | 16,008,231 | 16,580,965 | 17,942,529 | 12,176,866 |
| Total Net Revenue | 693,491,915 | 642,064,970 | 596,186,389 | 573,917,799 | 499,981,927 |
| Total Expenses | 635,488,902 | 610,888,942 | 558,590,503 | 514,916,805 | 445,760,593 |
| **HOSPITAL UNIT (Excludes Separate Nursing Home Units)** | | | | | |
| **Utilization - Inpatient** | | | | | |
| Beds | 1,236 | 1,271 | 1,298 | 1,296 | 1,275 |
| Admissions | 51,509 | 47,931 | 46,489 | 46,687 | 44,283 |
| Inpatient Days | 172,278 | 178,227 | 183,768 | 194,293 | 175,560 |
| Average Length of Stay | 3.3 | 3.7 | 4.0 | 4.2 | 4.0 |
| **Personnel** | | | | | |
| Total Full Time | 5,592 | 5,750 | 5,740 | 5,248 | 5,351 |
| Total Part Time | 1,534 | 1,636 | 1,743 | 1,937 | 1,440 |
| **Revenue and Expenses - Totals (Includes Inpatient and Outpatient)** | | | | | |
| Total Net Revenue | $669,886,380 | $617,051,893 | $568,830,781 | $548,439,718 | $480,479,888 |
| Total Expenses | 613,975,806 | 589,286,951 | 533,736,510 | 494,194,490 | 427,158,396 |
| **COMMUNITY HEALTH INDICATORS PER 1000 POPULATION** | | | | | |
| Total Population (in thousands) | 501 | 499 | 494 | 494 | 492 |
| **Inpatient** | | | | | |
| Beds | 3.5 | 3.8 | 3.9 | 3.9 | 3.7 |
| Admissions | 105.0 | 98.6 | 96.4 | 96.9 | 91.9 |
| Inpatient Days | 682.8 | 742.0 | 769.0 | 795.1 | 711.7 |
| Inpatient Surgeries | 26.3 | 26.8 | 26.4 | 26.9 | 28.0 |
| Births | 12.1 | 11.9 | 11.7 | 11.5 | 10.9 |
| **Outpatient** | | | | | |
| Emergency Outpatient Visits | 424.1 | 426.7 | 398.5 | 402.1 | 374.9 |
| Other Outpatient Visits | 1,307.7 | 1,355.3 | 1,258.4 | 1,376.1 | 1,385.4 |
| Total Outpatient Visits | 1,731.8 | 1,782.0 | 1,656.9 | 1,778.3 | 1,760.3 |
| Outpatient Surgeries | 57.7 | 56.5 | 55.0 | 53.8 | 49.5 |
| **Expense per Capita (per person)** | $1,267.8 | $1,224.6 | $1,131.4 | $1,042.2 | $906.4 |

# Table 7

| Table | | Page |
|---|---|---|
| **7** | **Facilities and Services in the U. S. Census Divisions and States for 2003** | 153 |

The facilities and services presented in Table 7 are listed below in alphabetical order by major heading (where applicable).

Table

# 7

## 2003 Facilities and Services in the U.S. Census Divisions and States

*These data include only hospital-based facilities and services as reported by responding hospitals in Section C of the 2003 AHA Annual Survey, beginning on page 205. All hospitals are represented with Community Hospitals listed separately under United States. No estimates have been made for nonresponding hospitals. Definitions of facilities and services are listed in the Glossary, page 193.*

| CLASSIFICATION | HOSPITALS REPORTING | GENERAL MEDICAL SURGICAL CARE | | | | OBSTETRICS INPATIENT CARE | | NEONATAL INTERMEDIATE CARE | | INTENSIVE CARE | | | | | | | | | |
|---|---|---|---|---|---|---|---|---|---|---|---|---|---|---|---|---|---|---|---|
| | | ADULT | | PEDIATRIC | | | | | | NEONATAL | | PEDIATRIC | | CARDIAC | | MEDICAL SURGICAL | | OTHER | |
| | | UNITS | | UNITS | | UNITS | | UNITS | | UNITS | | UNITS | | UNITS | | UNITS | | UNITS | |
| | | Number | Percent | Number | Percent | Number | Percent | Number | Percent | Number | Percent | Number | Percent | Number | Percent | Number | Percent | Number | Percent |
| **UNITED STATES** | 4,946 | 4,146 | 83.8 | 2,280 | 46.1 | 2,947 | 59.6 | 743 | 15.0 | 921 | 18.6 | 506 | 10.2 | 1,588 | 32.1 | 3,138 | 63.4 | 533 | 10.8 |
| COMMUNITY HOSPITALS | 4,320 | 3,959 | 91.6 | 2,240 | 51.9 | 2,917 | 67.5 | 731 | 16.9 | 908 | 21.0 | 498 | 11.5 | 1,541 | 35.7 | 3,007 | 69.6 | 508 | 11.8 |
| **CENSUS DIVISION 1, NEW ENGLAND** | 228 | 186 | 81.6 | 125 | 54.8 | 146 | 64.0 | 24 | 10.5 | 38 | 16.7 | 18 | 7.9 | 76 | 33.3 | 170 | 74.6 | 12 | 5.3 |
| Connecticut | 36 | 31 | 86.1 | 24 | 66.7 | 28 | 77.8 | 2 | 5.6 | 14 | 38.9 | 2 | 5.6 | 16 | 44.4 | 30 | 83.3 | 1 | 2.8 |
| Maine | 39 | 35 | 89.7 | 17 | 43.6 | 30 | 76.9 | 3 | 7.7 | 4 | 10.3 | 4 | 10.3 | 10 | 25.6 | 33 | 84.6 | 3 | 7.7 |
| Massachusetts | 95 | 70 | 73.7 | 53 | 55.8 | 47 | 49.5 | 13 | 13.7 | 15 | 15.8 | 7 | 7.4 | 32 | 33.7 | 62 | 65.3 | 6 | 6.3 |
| New Hampshire | 30 | 26 | 86.7 | 18 | 60.0 | 25 | 83.3 | 1 | 3.3 | 3 | 10.0 | 3 | 10.0 | 8 | 26.7 | 25 | 83.3 | 0 | 0.0 |
| Rhode Island | 12 | 10 | 83.3 | 5 | 41.7 | 5 | 41.7 | 2 | 16.7 | 1 | 8.3 | 1 | 8.3 | 4 | 33.3 | 8 | 66.7 | 2 | 16.7 |
| Vermont | 16 | 14 | 87.5 | 8 | 50.0 | 11 | 68.8 | 3 | 18.8 | 1 | 6.3 | 1 | 6.3 | 6 | 37.5 | 12 | 75.0 | 0 | 0.0 |
| **CENSUS DIVISION 2, MIDDLE ATLANTIC** | 442 | 380 | 86.0 | 241 | 54.5 | 285 | 64.5 | 113 | 25.6 | 109 | 24.7 | 59 | 13.3 | 196 | 44.3 | 349 | 79.0 | 53 | 12.0 |
| New Jersey | 72 | 62 | 86.1 | 50 | 69.4 | 52 | 72.2 | 40 | 55.6 | 17 | 23.6 | 11 | 15.3 | 43 | 59.7 | 61 | 84.7 | 9 | 12.5 |
| New York | 180 | 158 | 87.8 | 107 | 59.4 | 117 | 65.0 | 48 | 26.7 | 51 | 28.3 | 36 | 20.0 | 84 | 46.7 | 142 | 78.9 | 25 | 13.9 |
| Pennsylvania | 190 | 160 | 84.2 | 84 | 44.2 | 116 | 61.1 | 25 | 13.2 | 41 | 21.6 | 12 | 6.3 | 69 | 36.3 | 146 | 76.8 | 19 | 10.0 |
| **CENSUS DIVISION 3, SOUTH ATLANTIC** | 714 | 617 | 86.4 | 355 | 49.7 | 424 | 59.4 | 135 | 18.9 | 157 | 22.0 | 84 | 11.8 | 267 | 37.4 | 519 | 72.7 | 115 | 16.1 |
| Delaware | 8 | 6 | 75.0 | 4 | 50.0 | 5 | 62.5 | 1 | 12.5 | 4 | 50.0 | 3 | 37.5 | 3 | 37.5 | 6 | 75.0 | 2 | 25.0 |
| District of Columbia | 13 | 8 | 61.5 | 6 | 46.2 | 6 | 46.2 | 3 | 23.1 | 6 | 46.2 | 3 | 23.1 | 6 | 46.2 | 7 | 53.8 | 2 | 15.4 |
| Florida | 158 | 143 | 90.5 | 71 | 44.9 | 83 | 52.5 | 26 | 16.5 | 43 | 27.2 | 27 | 17.1 | 72 | 45.6 | 125 | 79.1 | 23 | 14.6 |
| Georgia | 147 | 127 | 86.4 | 70 | 47.6 | 84 | 57.1 | 33 | 22.4 | 30 | 20.4 | 10 | 6.8 | 43 | 29.3 | 93 | 63.3 | 17 | 11.6 |
| Maryland | 61 | 49 | 80.3 | 35 | 57.4 | 33 | 54.1 | 6 | 9.8 | 17 | 27.9 | 8 | 13.1 | 27 | 44.3 | 48 | 78.7 | 6 | 9.8 |
| North Carolina | 111 | 100 | 90.1 | 55 | 49.5 | 78 | 70.3 | 27 | 24.3 | 21 | 18.9 | 11 | 9.9 | 29 | 26.1 | 87 | 78.4 | 19 | 17.1 |
| South Carolina | 67 | 58 | 86.6 | 51 | 76.1 | 46 | 68.7 | 21 | 31.3 | 13 | 19.4 | 10 | 14.9 | 39 | 58.2 | 48 | 71.6 | 29 | 43.3 |
| Virginia | 84 | 70 | 83.3 | 36 | 42.9 | 57 | 67.9 | 13 | 15.5 | 18 | 21.4 | 8 | 9.5 | 29 | 34.5 | 66 | 78.6 | 13 | 15.5 |
| West Virginia | 65 | 56 | 86.2 | 27 | 41.5 | 32 | 49.2 | 5 | 7.7 | 5 | 7.7 | 4 | 6.2 | 19 | 29.2 | 39 | 60.0 | 4 | 6.2 |
| **CENSUS DIVISION 4, EAST NORTH CENTRAL** | 749 | 662 | 88.4 | 442 | 59.0 | 513 | 68.5 | 97 | 13.0 | 138 | 18.4 | 95 | 12.7 | 291 | 38.9 | 543 | 72.5 | 130 | 17.4 |
| Illinois | 186 | 172 | 92.5 | 119 | 64.0 | 126 | 67.7 | 42 | 22.6 | 40 | 21.5 | 25 | 13.4 | 59 | 31.7 | 144 | 77.4 | 13 | 7.0 |
| Indiana | 107 | 90 | 84.1 | 53 | 49.5 | 79 | 73.8 | 16 | 15.0 | 19 | 17.8 | 9 | 8.4 | 30 | 28.0 | 74 | 69.2 | 8 | 7.5 |
| Michigan | 154 | 134 | 87.0 | 85 | 55.2 | 95 | 61.7 | 10 | 6.5 | 24 | 15.6 | 11 | 7.1 | 53 | 34.4 | 99 | 64.3 | 13 | 8.4 |
| Ohio | 161 | 145 | 90.1 | 73 | 45.3 | 111 | 68.9 | 29 | 18.0 | 33 | 20.5 | 11 | 6.8 | 58 | 36.0 | 130 | 80.7 | 18 | 11.2 |
| Wisconsin | 141 | 121 | 85.8 | 112 | 79.4 | 102 | 72.3 | 0 | 0.0 | 22 | 15.6 | 39 | 27.7 | 91 | 64.5 | 96 | 68.1 | 78 | 55.3 |
| **CENSUS DIVISION 5, EAST SOUTH CENTRAL** | 438 | 382 | 87.2 | 215 | 49.1 | 227 | 51.8 | 69 | 15.8 | 62 | 14.2 | 43 | 9.8 | 145 | 33.1 | 260 | 59.4 | 45 | 10.3 |
| Alabama | 97 | 86 | 88.7 | 43 | 44.3 | 51 | 52.6 | 9 | 9.3 | 15 | 15.5 | 10 | 10.3 | 28 | 28.9 | 60 | 61.9 | 13 | 13.4 |
| Kentucky | 102 | 92 | 90.2 | 42 | 41.2 | 54 | 52.9 | 17 | 16.7 | 13 | 12.7 | 3 | 2.9 | 33 | 32.4 | 70 | 68.6 | 8 | 7.8 |
| Mississippi | 104 | 95 | 91.3 | 80 | 76.9 | 50 | 48.1 | 29 | 27.9 | 17 | 16.3 | 20 | 19.2 | 51 | 49.0 | 54 | 51.9 | 7 | 6.7 |
| Tennessee | 135 | 109 | 80.7 | 50 | 37.0 | 72 | 53.3 | 14 | 10.4 | 17 | 12.6 | 10 | 7.4 | 33 | 24.4 | 76 | 56.3 | 17 | 12.6 |
| **CENSUS DIVISION 6, WEST NORTH CENTRAL** | 695 | 633 | 91.1 | 303 | 43.6 | 417 | 60.0 | 72 | 10.4 | 84 | 12.1 | 45 | 6.5 | 174 | 25.0 | 370 | 53.2 | 36 | 5.2 |
| Iowa | 125 | 118 | 94.4 | 60 | 48.0 | 88 | 70.4 | 9 | 7.2 | 17 | 13.6 | 8 | 6.4 | 28 | 22.4 | 79 | 63.2 | 5 | 4.0 |
| Kansas | 145 | 132 | 91.0 | 41 | 28.3 | 67 | 46.2 | 10 | 6.9 | 10 | 6.9 | 4 | 2.8 | 14 | 9.7 | 51 | 35.2 | 6 | 4.1 |
| Minnesota | 117 | 108 | 92.3 | 60 | 51.3 | 91 | 77.8 | 16 | 13.7 | 16 | 13.7 | 13 | 11.1 | 44 | 37.6 | 67 | 57.3 | 9 | 7.7 |
| Missouri | 143 | 117 | 81.8 | 72 | 50.3 | 73 | 51.0 | 22 | 15.4 | 21 | 14.7 | 9 | 6.3 | 39 | 27.3 | 92 | 64.3 | 12 | 8.4 |
| Nebraska | 75 | 71 | 94.7 | 33 | 44.0 | 48 | 64.0 | 6 | 8.0 | 10 | 13.3 | 4 | 5.3 | 21 | 28.0 | 36 | 48.0 | 3 | 4.0 |
| North Dakota | 32 | 32 | 100.0 | 18 | 56.3 | 20 | 62.5 | 6 | 18.8 | 7 | 21.9 | 3 | 9.4 | 17 | 53.1 | 18 | 56.3 | 1 | 3.1 |
| South Dakota | 58 | 55 | 94.8 | 19 | 32.8 | 30 | 51.7 | 3 | 5.2 | 3 | 5.2 | 4 | 6.9 | 11 | 19.0 | 27 | 46.6 | 0 | 0.0 |
| **CENSUS DIVISION 7, WEST SOUTH CENTRAL** | 784 | 603 | 76.9 | 267 | 34.1 | 396 | 50.5 | 113 | 14.4 | 134 | 17.1 | 66 | 8.4 | 174 | 22.2 | 409 | 52.2 | 60 | 7.7 |
| Arkansas | 104 | 81 | 77.9 | 26 | 25.0 | 52 | 50.0 | 17 | 16.3 | 15 | 14.4 | 5 | 4.8 | 35 | 33.7 | 50 | 48.1 | 10 | 9.6 |
| Louisiana | 111 | 86 | 77.5 | 48 | 43.2 | 48 | 43.2 | 12 | 10.8 | 25 | 22.5 | 16 | 14.4 | 23 | 20.7 | 65 | 58.6 | 8 | 7.2 |
| Oklahoma | 108 | 88 | 81.5 | 41 | 38.0 | 56 | 51.9 | 13 | 12.0 | 11 | 10.2 | 7 | 6.5 | 28 | 25.9 | 52 | 48.1 | 10 | 9.3 |
| Texas | 461 | 348 | 75.5 | 152 | 33.0 | 240 | 52.1 | 71 | 15.4 | 83 | 18.0 | 38 | 8.2 | 88 | 19.1 | 242 | 52.5 | 32 | 6.9 |
| **CENSUS DIVISION 8, MOUNTAIN** | 320 | 288 | 90.0 | 137 | 42.8 | 219 | 68.4 | 60 | 18.8 | 57 | 17.8 | 37 | 11.6 | 90 | 28.1 | 195 | 60.9 | 32 | 10.0 |
| Arizona | 55 | 47 | 85.5 | 20 | 36.4 | 31 | 56.4 | 8 | 14.5 | 10 | 18.2 | 6 | 10.9 | 17 | 30.9 | 40 | 72.7 | 3 | 5.5 |
| Colorado | 56 | 52 | 92.9 | 29 | 51.8 | 42 | 75.0 | 13 | 23.2 | 15 | 26.8 | 7 | 12.5 | 14 | 25.0 | 38 | 67.9 | 8 | 14.3 |
| Idaho | 30 | 27 | 90.0 | 13 | 43.3 | 23 | 76.7 | 2 | 6.7 | 5 | 16.7 | 2 | 6.7 | 8 | 26.7 | 17 | 56.7 | 2 | 6.7 |
| Montana | 54 | 52 | 96.3 | 22 | 40.7 | 33 | 61.1 | 7 | 13.0 | 6 | 11.1 | 7 | 13.0 | 17 | 31.5 | 26 | 48.1 | 3 | 5.6 |
| Nevada | 22 | 17 | 77.3 | 9 | 40.9 | 13 | 59.1 | 5 | 22.7 | 6 | 27.3 | 5 | 22.7 | 7 | 31.8 | 13 | 59.1 | 7 | 31.8 |
| New Mexico | 34 | 30 | 88.2 | 17 | 50.0 | 24 | 70.6 | 5 | 14.7 | 3 | 8.8 | 4 | 11.8 | 7 | 20.6 | 18 | 52.9 | 5 | 14.7 |
| Utah | 41 | 36 | 87.8 | 18 | 43.9 | 34 | 82.9 | 17 | 41.5 | 12 | 29.3 | 5 | 12.2 | 18 | 43.9 | 24 | 58.5 | 4 | 9.8 |
| Wyoming | 28 | 27 | 96.4 | 9 | 32.1 | 19 | 67.9 | 3 | 10.7 | 0 | 0.0 | 1 | 3.6 | 2 | 7.1 | 19 | 67.9 | 0 | 0.0 |
| **CENSUS DIVISION 9, PACIFIC** | 576 | 395 | 68.6 | 195 | 33.9 | 320 | 55.6 | 60 | 10.4 | 142 | 24.7 | 59 | 10.2 | 175 | 30.4 | 323 | 56.1 | 50 | 8.7 |
| Alaska | 15 | 14 | 93.3 | 7 | 46.7 | 13 | 86.7 | 2 | 13.3 | 3 | 20.0 | 1 | 6.7 | 3 | 20.0 | 10 | 66.7 | 1 | 6.7 |
| California | 402 | 234 | 58.2 | 127 | 31.6 | 191 | 47.5 | 37 | 9.2 | 114 | 28.4 | 42 | 10.4 | 122 | 30.3 | 207 | 51.5 | 29 | 7.2 |
| Hawaii | 18 | 15 | 83.3 | 4 | 22.2 | 10 | 55.6 | 1 | 5.6 | 2 | 11.1 | 2 | 11.1 | 6 | 33.3 | 9 | 50.0 | 1 | 5.6 |
| Oregon | 59 | 58 | 98.3 | 23 | 39.0 | 52 | 88.1 | 5 | 8.5 | 6 | 10.2 | 3 | 5.1 | 17 | 28.8 | 49 | 83.1 | 6 | 10.2 |
| Washington | 82 | 74 | 90.2 | 34 | 41.5 | 54 | 65.9 | 15 | 18.3 | 17 | 20.7 | 11 | 13.4 | 27 | 32.9 | 48 | 58.5 | 13 | 15.9 |

## Table 7 (Continued)

*These data include only hospital-based facilities and services as reported by responding hospitals in Section C of the 2003 AHA Annual Survey, beginning on page 205. All hospitals are represented with Community Hospitals listed separately under United States. No estimates have been made for nonresponding hospitals. Definitions of facilities and services are listed in the Glossary, page 193.*

| CLASSIFICATION | HOSPITALS REPORTING | BURN CARE UNITS | | LONG-TERM CARE: ACUTE LONG-TERM CARE UNITS | | LONG-TERM CARE: SKILLED NURSING CARE UNITS | | LONG-TERM CARE: INTERMEDIATE CARE UNITS | | LONG-TERM CARE: OTHER LONG-TERM CARE UNITS | | PSYCHIATRIC INPATIENT CARE UNITS | | ALCOHOL/DRUG ABUSE OR DEPENDENCY INPATIENT CARE UNITS | | OTHER SPECIAL CARE UNITS | | PHYSICAL REHABILITATION INPATIENT CARE UNITS | |
|---|---|---|---|---|---|---|---|---|---|---|---|---|---|---|---|---|---|---|---|
| | | Number | Percent | Number | Percent | Number | Percent | Number | Percent | Number | Percent | Number | Percent | Number | Percent | Number | Percent | Number | Percent |
| **UNITED STATES** | 4,946 | 216 | 4.4 | 339 | 6.9 | 1,650 | 33.4 | 506 | 10.2 | 701 | 14.2 | 1,779 | 36.0 | 598 | 12.1 | 748 | 15.1 | 1,434 | 29.0 |
| COMMUNITY HOSPITALS | 4,320 | 208 | 4.8 | 237 | 5.5 | 1,540 | 35.6 | 445 | 10.3 | 616 | 14.3 | 1,404 | 32.5 | 452 | 10.5 | 706 | 16.3 | 1,356 | 31.4 |
| **CENSUS DIVISION 1, NEW ENGLAND** | 228 | 7 | 3.1 | 13 | 5.7 | 61 | 26.8 | 25 | 11.0 | 28 | 12.3 | 119 | 52.2 | 27 | 11.8 | 23 | 10.1 | 50 | 21.9 |
| Connecticut | 36 | 1 | 2.8 | 3 | 8.3 | 3 | 8.3 | 2 | 5.6 | 5 | 13.9 | 27 | 75.0 | 6 | 16.7 | 5 | 13.9 | 11 | 30.6 |
| Maine | 39 | 2 | 5.1 | 2 | 5.1 | 16 | 41.0 | 8 | 20.5 | 3 | 7.7 | 14 | 35.9 | 7 | 17.9 | 4 | 10.3 | 8 | 20.5 |
| Massachusetts | 95 | 4 | 4.2 | 8 | 8.4 | 28 | 29.5 | 6 | 6.3 | 14 | 14.7 | 49 | 51.6 | 12 | 12.6 | 10 | 10.5 | 16 | 16.8 |
| New Hampshire | 30 | 0 | 0.0 | 0 | 0.0 | 9 | 30.0 | 8 | 26.7 | 4 | 13.3 | 13 | 43.3 | 1 | 3.3 | 2 | 6.7 | 7 | 23.3 |
| Rhode Island | 12 | 0 | 0.0 | 0 | 0.0 | 3 | 25.0 | 1 | 8.3 | 0 | 0.0 | 9 | 75.0 | 1 | 8.3 | 1 | 8.3 | 4 | 33.3 |
| Vermont | 16 | 0 | 0.0 | 0 | 0.0 | 2 | 12.5 | 0 | 0.0 | 2 | 12.5 | 7 | 43.8 | 0 | 0.0 | 1 | 6.3 | 4 | 25.0 |
| **CENSUS DIVISION 2, MIDDLE ATLANTIC** | 442 | 26 | 5.9 | 21 | 4.8 | 148 | 33.5 | 27 | 6.1 | 68 | 15.4 | 264 | 59.7 | 97 | 21.9 | 72 | 16.3 | 158 | 35.7 |
| New Jersey | 72 | 4 | 5.6 | 3 | 4.2 | 15 | 20.8 | 5 | 6.9 | 11 | 15.3 | 46 | 63.9 | 11 | 15.3 | 11 | 15.3 | 13 | 18.1 |
| New York | 180 | 12 | 6.7 | 8 | 4.4 | 57 | 31.7 | 9 | 5.0 | 33 | 18.3 | 110 | 61.1 | 59 | 32.8 | 30 | 16.7 | 67 | 37.2 |
| Pennsylvania | 190 | 10 | 5.3 | 10 | 5.3 | 76 | 40.0 | 13 | 6.8 | 24 | 12.6 | 108 | 56.8 | 27 | 14.2 | 31 | 16.3 | 78 | 41.1 |
| **CENSUS DIVISION 3, SOUTH ATLANTIC** | 714 | 31 | 4.3 | 67 | 9.4 | 247 | 34.6 | 70 | 9.8 | 130 | 18.2 | 275 | 38.5 | 98 | 13.7 | 146 | 20.4 | 202 | 28.3 |
| Delaware | 8 | 0 | 0.0 | 0 | 0.0 | 5 | 62.5 | 4 | 50.0 | 3 | 37.5 | 4 | 50.0 | 1 | 12.5 | 2 | 25.0 | 4 | 50.0 |
| District of Columbia | 13 | 2 | 15.4 | 0 | 0.0 | 3 | 23.1 | 2 | 15.4 | 3 | 23.1 | 11 | 84.6 | 2 | 15.4 | 2 | 15.4 | 6 | 46.2 |
| Florida | 158 | 7 | 4.4 | 6 | 3.8 | 29 | 18.4 | 7 | 4.4 | 21 | 13.3 | 51 | 32.3 | 21 | 13.3 | 41 | 25.9 | 36 | 22.8 |
| Georgia | 147 | 6 | 4.1 | 13 | 8.8 | 50 | 34.0 | 15 | 10.2 | 28 | 19.0 | 42 | 28.6 | 17 | 11.6 | 23 | 15.6 | 43 | 29.3 |
| Maryland | 61 | 4 | 6.6 | 5 | 8.2 | 22 | 36.1 | 5 | 8.2 | 17 | 27.9 | 39 | 63.9 | 10 | 16.4 | 17 | 27.9 | 17 | 27.9 |
| North Carolina | 111 | 3 | 2.7 | 4 | 3.6 | 45 | 40.5 | 14 | 12.6 | 15 | 13.5 | 50 | 45.0 | 13 | 11.7 | 20 | 18.0 | 27 | 24.3 |
| South Carolina | 67 | 3 | 4.5 | 35 | 52.2 | 40 | 59.7 | 0 | 0.0 | 20 | 29.9 | 21 | 31.3 | 15 | 22.4 | 20 | 29.9 | 39 | 58.2 |
| Virginia | 84 | 5 | 6.0 | 4 | 4.8 | 20 | 23.8 | 15 | 17.9 | 14 | 16.7 | 39 | 46.4 | 14 | 16.7 | 17 | 20.2 | 23 | 27.4 |
| West Virginia | 65 | 1 | 1.5 | 0 | 0.0 | 33 | 50.8 | 8 | 12.3 | 9 | 13.8 | 18 | 27.7 | 5 | 7.7 | 4 | 6.2 | 7 | 10.8 |
| **CENSUS DIVISION 4, EAST NORTH CENTRAL** | 749 | 47 | 6.3 | 49 | 6.5 | 247 | 33.0 | 76 | 10.1 | 99 | 13.2 | 321 | 42.9 | 136 | 18.2 | 187 | 25.0 | 275 | 36.7 |
| Illinois | 186 | 7 | 3.8 | 8 | 4.3 | 71 | 38.2 | 18 | 9.7 | 15 | 8.1 | 78 | 41.9 | 29 | 15.6 | 18 | 9.7 | 54 | 29.0 |
| Indiana | 107 | 6 | 5.6 | 9 | 8.4 | 39 | 36.4 | 11 | 10.3 | 24 | 22.4 | 41 | 38.3 | 15 | 14.0 | 15 | 14.0 | 31 | 29.0 |
| Michigan | 154 | 8 | 5.2 | 10 | 6.5 | 35 | 22.7 | 9 | 5.8 | 20 | 13.0 | 62 | 40.3 | 14 | 9.1 | 16 | 10.4 | 55 | 35.7 |
| Ohio | 161 | 9 | 5.6 | 7 | 4.3 | 65 | 40.4 | 13 | 8.1 | 25 | 15.5 | 86 | 53.4 | 28 | 17.4 | 22 | 13.7 | 57 | 35.4 |
| Wisconsin | 141 | 17 | 12.1 | 15 | 10.6 | 37 | 26.2 | 25 | 17.7 | 15 | 10.6 | 54 | 38.3 | 50 | 35.5 | 116 | 82.3 | 78 | 55.3 |
| **CENSUS DIVISION 5, EAST SOUTH CENTRAL** | 438 | 17 | 3.9 | 13 | 3.0 | 132 | 30.1 | 25 | 5.7 | 79 | 18.0 | 153 | 34.9 | 47 | 10.7 | 69 | 15.8 | 124 | 28.3 |
| Alabama | 97 | 5 | 5.2 | 4 | 4.1 | 18 | 18.6 | 5 | 5.2 | 16 | 16.5 | 32 | 33.0 | 8 | 8.2 | 13 | 13.4 | 17 | 17.5 |
| Kentucky | 102 | 4 | 3.9 | 4 | 3.9 | 43 | 42.2 | 8 | 7.8 | 13 | 12.7 | 30 | 29.4 | 7 | 6.9 | 17 | 16.7 | 24 | 23.5 |
| Mississippi | 104 | 4 | 3.8 | 0 | 0.0 | 30 | 28.8 | 0 | 0.0 | 23 | 22.1 | 49 | 47.1 | 20 | 19.2 | 17 | 16.3 | 47 | 45.2 |
| Tennessee | 135 | 4 | 3.0 | 5 | 3.7 | 41 | 30.4 | 12 | 8.9 | 27 | 20.0 | 42 | 31.1 | 12 | 8.9 | 22 | 16.3 | 36 | 26.7 |
| **CENSUS DIVISION 6, WEST NORTH CENTRAL** | 695 | 24 | 3.5 | 39 | 5.6 | 362 | 52.1 | 143 | 20.6 | 126 | 18.1 | 184 | 26.5 | 56 | 8.1 | 73 | 10.5 | 181 | 26.0 |
| Iowa | 125 | 4 | 3.2 | 4 | 3.2 | 64 | 51.2 | 39 | 31.2 | 17 | 13.6 | 41 | 32.8 | 11 | 8.8 | 12 | 9.6 | 22 | 17.6 |
| Kansas | 145 | 3 | 2.1 | 6 | 4.1 | 75 | 51.7 | 43 | 29.7 | 20 | 13.8 | 29 | 20.0 | 2 | 1.4 | 5 | 3.4 | 30 | 20.7 |
| Minnesota | 117 | 7 | 6.0 | 10 | 8.5 | 67 | 57.3 | 9 | 7.7 | 19 | 16.2 | 29 | 24.8 | 15 | 12.8 | 14 | 12.0 | 27 | 23.1 |
| Missouri | 143 | 7 | 4.9 | 9 | 6.3 | 65 | 45.5 | 16 | 11.2 | 32 | 22.4 | 60 | 42.0 | 18 | 12.6 | 32 | 22.4 | 72 | 50.3 |
| Nebraska | 75 | 2 | 2.7 | 4 | 5.3 | 47 | 62.7 | 19 | 25.3 | 13 | 17.3 | 10 | 13.3 | 5 | 6.7 | 4 | 5.3 | 13 | 17.3 |
| North Dakota | 32 | 0 | 0.0 | 3 | 9.4 | 13 | 40.6 | 5 | 15.6 | 7 | 21.9 | 8 | 25.0 | 4 | 12.5 | 2 | 6.3 | 8 | 25.0 |
| South Dakota | 58 | 1 | 1.7 | 3 | 5.2 | 31 | 53.4 | 12 | 20.7 | 18 | 31.0 | 7 | 12.1 | 1 | 1.7 | 4 | 6.9 | 9 | 15.5 |
| **CENSUS DIVISION 7, WEST SOUTH CENTRAL** | 784 | 25 | 3.2 | 84 | 10.7 | 169 | 21.6 | 50 | 6.4 | 72 | 9.2 | 226 | 28.8 | 56 | 7.1 | 89 | 11.4 | 234 | 29.8 |
| Arkansas | 104 | 5 | 4.8 | 10 | 9.6 | 32 | 30.8 | 8 | 7.7 | 14 | 13.5 | 40 | 38.5 | 7 | 6.7 | 7 | 6.7 | 34 | 32.7 |
| Louisiana | 111 | 3 | 2.7 | 13 | 11.7 | 36 | 32.4 | 9 | 8.1 | 13 | 11.7 | 58 | 52.3 | 7 | 6.3 | 6 | 5.4 | 38 | 34.2 |
| Oklahoma | 108 | 5 | 4.6 | 10 | 9.3 | 27 | 25.0 | 12 | 11.1 | 13 | 12.0 | 33 | 30.6 | 5 | 4.6 | 10 | 9.3 | 32 | 29.6 |
| Texas | 461 | 12 | 2.6 | 51 | 11.1 | 74 | 16.1 | 21 | 4.6 | 32 | 6.9 | 95 | 20.6 | 37 | 8.0 | 66 | 14.3 | 130 | 28.2 |
| **CENSUS DIVISION 8, MOUNTAIN** | 320 | 14 | 4.4 | 20 | 6.3 | 126 | 39.4 | 47 | 14.7 | 46 | 14.4 | 89 | 27.8 | 37 | 11.6 | 30 | 9.4 | 86 | 26.9 |
| Arizona | 55 | 2 | 3.6 | 3 | 5.5 | 7 | 12.7 | 6 | 10.9 | 7 | 12.7 | 19 | 34.5 | 2 | 3.6 | 2 | 3.6 | 20 | 36.4 |
| Colorado | 56 | 4 | 7.1 | 3 | 5.4 | 25 | 44.6 | 4 | 7.1 | 8 | 14.3 | 17 | 30.4 | 9 | 16.1 | 9 | 16.1 | 23 | 41.1 |
| Idaho | 30 | 0 | 0.0 | 0 | 0.0 | 15 | 50.0 | 1 | 3.3 | 3 | 10.0 | 9 | 30.0 | 2 | 6.7 | 2 | 6.7 | 6 | 20.0 |
| Montana | 54 | 1 | 1.9 | 8 | 14.8 | 44 | 81.5 | 12 | 22.2 | 11 | 20.4 | 11 | 20.4 | 7 | 13.0 | 4 | 7.4 | 12 | 22.2 |
| Nevada | 22 | 3 | 13.6 | 4 | 18.2 | 5 | 22.7 | 3 | 13.6 | 6 | 27.3 | 6 | 27.3 | 4 | 18.2 | 5 | 22.7 | 6 | 27.3 |
| New Mexico | 34 | 1 | 2.9 | 1 | 2.9 | 6 | 17.6 | 3 | 8.8 | 5 | 14.7 | 8 | 23.5 | 3 | 8.8 | 4 | 11.8 | 5 | 14.7 |
| Utah | 41 | 3 | 7.3 | 1 | 2.4 | 15 | 36.6 | 11 | 26.8 | 3 | 7.3 | 14 | 34.1 | 7 | 17.1 | 3 | 7.3 | 9 | 22.0 |
| Wyoming | 28 | 0 | 0.0 | 0 | 0.0 | 9 | 32.1 | 7 | 25.0 | 3 | 10.7 | 5 | 17.9 | 3 | 10.7 | 1 | 3.6 | 5 | 17.9 |
| **CENSUS DIVISION 9, PACIFIC** | 576 | 25 | 4.3 | 33 | 5.7 | 158 | 27.4 | 43 | 7.5 | 53 | 9.2 | 148 | 25.7 | 44 | 7.6 | 59 | 10.2 | 124 | 21.5 |
| Alaska | 15 | 1 | 6.7 | 1 | 6.7 | 4 | 26.7 | 3 | 20.0 | 1 | 6.7 | 6 | 40.0 | 0 | 0.0 | 1 | 6.7 | 3 | 20.0 |
| California | 402 | 17 | 4.2 | 22 | 5.5 | 108 | 26.9 | 19 | 4.7 | 31 | 7.7 | 90 | 22.4 | 24 | 6.0 | 36 | 9.0 | 84 | 20.9 |
| Hawaii | 18 | 1 | 5.6 | 3 | 16.7 | 9 | 50.0 | 6 | 33.3 | 3 | 16.7 | 6 | 33.3 | 1 | 5.6 | 2 | 11.1 | 1 | 5.6 |
| Oregon | 59 | 2 | 3.4 | 3 | 5.1 | 14 | 23.7 | 9 | 15.3 | 4 | 6.8 | 18 | 30.5 | 5 | 8.5 | 7 | 11.9 | 8 | 13.6 |
| Washington | 82 | 4 | 4.9 | 4 | 4.9 | 23 | 28.0 | 6 | 7.3 | 14 | 17.1 | 28 | 34.1 | 14 | 17.1 | 13 | 15.9 | 28 | 34.1 |

## Table 7 (Continued)

*These data include only hospital-based facilities and services as reported by responding hospitals in Section C of the 2003 AHA Annual Survey, beginning on page 205. All hospitals are represented with Community Hospitals listed separately under United States. No estimates have been made for nonresponding hospitals. Definitions of facilities and services are listed in the Glossary, page 193.*

| CLASSIFICATION | HOSPITALS REPORTING | ADULT DAY CARE PROGRAM | | AIRBORNE INFECTION ISOLATION ROOM | | ALCOHOL/DRUG ABUSE OR DEPENDENCY OUTPATIENT SERVICES | | ALZHEIMER CENTER | | AMBULANCE SERVICES | | ANGIOPLASTY | | ARTHRITIS TREATMENT CENTER | | ASSISTED LIVING | | AUXILIARY | |
|---|---|---|---|---|---|---|---|---|---|---|---|---|---|---|---|---|---|---|---|
| | | Number | Percent | Number | Percent | Number | Percent | Number | Percent | Number | Percent | Number | Percent | Number | Percent | Number | Percent | Number | Percent |
| **UNITED STATES** | 4,946 | 400 | 8.1 | 2,863 | 57.9 | 908 | 18.4 | 135 | 2.7 | 869 | 17.6 | 1,289 | 26.1 | 303 | 6.1 | 263 | 5.3 | 3,020 | 61.1 |
| COMMUNITY HOSPITALS | 4,320 | 346 | 8.0 | 2,638 | 61.1 | 696 | 16.1 | 103 | 2.4 | 818 | 18.9 | 1,238 | 28.7 | 275 | 6.4 | 241 | 5.6 | 2,935 | 67.9 |
| **CENSUS DIVISION 1, NEW ENGLAND** | 228 | 30 | 13.2 | 135 | 59.2 | 80 | 35.1 | 14 | 6.1 | 33 | 14.5 | 47 | 20.6 | 22 | 9.6 | 16 | 7.0 | 131 | 57.5 |
| Connecticut | 36 | 5 | 13.9 | 29 | 80.6 | 19 | 52.8 | 2 | 5.6 | 4 | 11.1 | 8 | 22.2 | 4 | 11.1 | 2 | 5.6 | 24 | 66.7 |
| Maine | 39 | 3 | 7.7 | 23 | 59.0 | 15 | 38.5 | 4 | 10.3 | 10 | 25.6 | 7 | 17.9 | 0 | 0.0 | 4 | 10.3 | 25 | 64.1 |
| Massachusetts | 95 | 12 | 12.6 | 50 | 52.6 | 37 | 38.9 | 7 | 7.4 | 6 | 6.3 | 21 | 22.1 | 12 | 12.6 | 3 | 3.2 | 48 | 50.5 |
| New Hampshire | 30 | 7 | 23.3 | 18 | 60.0 | 2 | 6.7 | 0 | 0.0 | 7 | 23.3 | 7 | 23.3 | 3 | 10.0 | 2 | 6.7 | 18 | 60.0 |
| Rhode Island | 12 | 1 | 8.3 | 5 | 41.7 | 3 | 25.0 | 0 | 0.0 | 3 | 25.0 | 2 | 16.7 | 1 | 8.3 | 2 | 16.7 | 6 | 50.0 |
| Vermont | 16 | 2 | 12.5 | 10 | 62.5 | 4 | 25.0 | 1 | 6.3 | 3 | 18.8 | 2 | 12.5 | 2 | 12.5 | 3 | 18.8 | 10 | 62.5 |
| **CENSUS DIVISION 2, MIDDLE ATLANTIC** | 442 | 61 | 13.8 | 301 | 68.1 | 131 | 29.6 | 22 | 5.0 | 83 | 18.8 | 123 | 27.8 | 53 | 12.0 | 23 | 5.2 | 299 | 67.6 |
| New Jersey | 72 | 18 | 25.0 | 54 | 75.0 | 29 | 40.3 | 4 | 5.6 | 15 | 20.8 | 21 | 29.2 | 10 | 13.9 | 2 | 2.8 | 56 | 77.8 |
| New York | 180 | 29 | 16.1 | 114 | 63.3 | 70 | 38.9 | 12 | 6.7 | 36 | 20.0 | 41 | 22.8 | 24 | 13.3 | 8 | 4.4 | 113 | 62.8 |
| Pennsylvania | 190 | 14 | 7.4 | 133 | 70.0 | 32 | 16.8 | 6 | 3.2 | 32 | 16.8 | 61 | 32.1 | 19 | 10.0 | 13 | 6.8 | 130 | 68.4 |
| **CENSUS DIVISION 3, SOUTH ATLANTIC** | 714 | 40 | 5.6 | 470 | 65.8 | 139 | 19.5 | 25 | 3.5 | 126 | 17.6 | 210 | 29.4 | 46 | 6.4 | 27 | 3.8 | 464 | 65.0 |
| Delaware | 8 | 2 | 25.0 | 6 | 75.0 | 2 | 25.0 | 1 | 12.5 | 0 | 0.0 | 4 | 50.0 | 1 | 12.5 | 0 | 0.0 | 7 | 87.5 |
| District of Columbia | 13 | 0 | 0.0 | 11 | 84.6 | 6 | 46.2 | 1 | 7.7 | 4 | 30.8 | 7 | 53.8 | 6 | 46.2 | 1 | 7.7 | 3 | 23.1 |
| Florida | 158 | 6 | 3.8 | 100 | 63.3 | 22 | 13.9 | 9 | 5.7 | 19 | 12.0 | 62 | 39.2 | 10 | 6.3 | 3 | 1.9 | 101 | 63.9 |
| Georgia | 147 | 9 | 6.1 | 87 | 59.2 | 27 | 18.4 | 4 | 2.7 | 38 | 25.9 | 24 | 16.3 | 2 | 1.4 | 9 | 6.1 | 91 | 61.9 |
| Maryland | 61 | 5 | 8.2 | 44 | 72.1 | 16 | 26.2 | 4 | 6.6 | 6 | 9.8 | 21 | 34.4 | 7 | 11.5 | 5 | 8.2 | 48 | 78.7 |
| North Carolina | 111 | 8 | 7.2 | 75 | 67.6 | 22 | 19.8 | 3 | 2.7 | 27 | 24.3 | 28 | 25.2 | 9 | 8.1 | 1 | 0.9 | 77 | 69.4 |
| South Carolina | 67 | 2 | 3.0 | 44 | 65.7 | 13 | 19.4 | 0 | 0.0 | 14 | 20.9 | 17 | 25.4 | 0 | 0.0 | 3 | 4.5 | 41 | 61.2 |
| Virginia | 84 | 7 | 8.3 | 68 | 81.0 | 23 | 27.4 | 3 | 3.6 | 12 | 14.3 | 36 | 42.9 | 6 | 7.1 | 4 | 4.8 | 60 | 71.4 |
| West Virginia | 65 | 1 | 1.5 | 35 | 53.8 | 8 | 12.3 | 0 | 0.0 | 6 | 9.2 | 11 | 16.9 | 5 | 7.7 | 1 | 1.5 | 36 | 55.4 |
| **CENSUS DIVISION 4, EAST NORTH CENTRAL** | 749 | 73 | 9.7 | 494 | 66.0 | 210 | 28.0 | 20 | 2.7 | 132 | 17.6 | 228 | 30.4 | 85 | 11.3 | 42 | 5.6 | 503 | 67.2 |
| Illinois | 186 | 27 | 14.5 | 129 | 69.4 | 53 | 28.5 | 11 | 5.9 | 38 | 20.4 | 75 | 40.3 | 24 | 12.9 | 10 | 5.4 | 131 | 70.4 |
| Indiana | 107 | 7 | 6.5 | 71 | 66.4 | 26 | 24.3 | 0 | 0.0 | 33 | 30.8 | 27 | 25.2 | 7 | 6.5 | 4 | 3.7 | 56 | 52.3 |
| Michigan | 154 | 12 | 7.8 | 98 | 63.6 | 38 | 24.7 | 4 | 2.6 | 17 | 11.0 | 38 | 24.7 | 12 | 7.8 | 10 | 6.5 | 104 | 67.5 |
| Ohio | 161 | 8 | 5.0 | 109 | 67.7 | 48 | 29.8 | 5 | 3.1 | 26 | 16.1 | 55 | 34.2 | 20 | 12.4 | 8 | 5.0 | 121 | 75.2 |
| Wisconsin | 141 | 19 | 13.5 | 87 | 61.7 | 45 | 31.9 | 0 | 0.0 | 18 | 12.8 | 33 | 23.4 | 22 | 15.6 | 10 | 7.1 | 91 | 64.5 |
| **CENSUS DIVISION 5, EAST SOUTH CENTRAL** | 438 | 14 | 3.2 | 181 | 41.3 | 48 | 11.0 | 2 | 0.5 | 62 | 14.2 | 85 | 19.4 | 14 | 3.2 | 10 | 2.3 | 186 | 42.5 |
| Alabama | 97 | 3 | 3.1 | 41 | 42.3 | 7 | 7.2 | 0 | 0.0 | 15 | 15.5 | 27 | 27.8 | 4 | 4.1 | 5 | 5.2 | 55 | 56.7 |
| Kentucky | 102 | 6 | 5.9 | 67 | 65.7 | 14 | 13.7 | 1 | 1.0 | 13 | 12.7 | 25 | 24.5 | 5 | 4.9 | 1 | 1.0 | 67 | 65.7 |
| Mississippi | 104 | 2 | 1.9 | 5 | 4.8 | 11 | 10.6 | 1 | 1.0 | 4 | 3.8 | 1 | 1.0 | 1 | 1.0 | 1 | 1.0 | 5 | 4.8 |
| Tennessee | 135 | 3 | 2.2 | 68 | 50.4 | 16 | 11.9 | 0 | 0.0 | 30 | 22.2 | 32 | 23.7 | 4 | 3.0 | 3 | 2.2 | 59 | 43.7 |
| **CENSUS DIVISION 6, WEST NORTH CENTRAL** | 695 | 90 | 12.9 | 344 | 49.5 | 105 | 15.1 | 26 | 3.7 | 194 | 27.9 | 125 | 18.0 | 29 | 4.2 | 88 | 12.7 | 501 | 72.1 |
| Iowa | 125 | 13 | 10.4 | 50 | 40.0 | 26 | 20.8 | 3 | 2.4 | 54 | 43.2 | 19 | 15.2 | 4 | 3.2 | 10 | 8.0 | 108 | 86.4 |
| Kansas | 145 | 18 | 12.4 | 70 | 48.3 | 8 | 5.5 | 4 | 2.8 | 27 | 18.6 | 17 | 11.7 | 2 | 1.4 | 11 | 7.6 | 86 | 59.3 |
| Minnesota | 117 | 29 | 24.8 | 56 | 47.9 | 25 | 21.4 | 9 | 7.7 | 45 | 38.5 | 18 | 15.4 | 4 | 3.4 | 23 | 19.7 | 87 | 74.4 |
| Missouri | 143 | 6 | 4.2 | 104 | 72.7 | 23 | 16.1 | 4 | 2.8 | 34 | 23.8 | 48 | 33.6 | 12 | 8.4 | 5 | 3.5 | 104 | 72.7 |
| Nebraska | 75 | 13 | 17.3 | 28 | 37.3 | 9 | 12.0 | 3 | 4.0 | 15 | 20.0 | 12 | 16.0 | 1 | 1.3 | 13 | 17.3 | 55 | 73.3 |
| North Dakota | 32 | 3 | 9.4 | 17 | 53.1 | 8 | 25.0 | 0 | 0.0 | 8 | 25.0 | 6 | 18.8 | 5 | 15.6 | 5 | 15.6 | 26 | 81.3 |
| South Dakota | 58 | 8 | 13.8 | 19 | 32.8 | 6 | 10.3 | 3 | 5.2 | 11 | 19.0 | 5 | 8.6 | 1 | 1.7 | 21 | 36.2 | 35 | 60.3 |
| **CENSUS DIVISION 7, WEST SOUTH CENTRAL** | 784 | 24 | 3.1 | 479 | 61.1 | 66 | 8.4 | 10 | 1.3 | 124 | 15.8 | 203 | 25.9 | 19 | 2.4 | 23 | 2.9 | 456 | 58.2 |
| Arkansas | 104 | 7 | 6.7 | 73 | 70.2 | 6 | 5.8 | 1 | 1.0 | 20 | 19.2 | 25 | 24.0 | 2 | 1.9 | 1 | 1.0 | 71 | 68.3 |
| Louisiana | 111 | 6 | 5.4 | 52 | 46.8 | 12 | 10.8 | 4 | 3.6 | 13 | 11.7 | 33 | 29.7 | 4 | 3.6 | 1 | 0.9 | 60 | 54.1 |
| Oklahoma | 108 | 3 | 2.8 | 76 | 70.4 | 8 | 7.4 | 2 | 1.9 | 20 | 18.5 | 23 | 21.3 | 2 | 1.9 | 5 | 4.6 | 67 | 62.0 |
| Texas | 461 | 8 | 1.7 | 278 | 60.3 | 40 | 8.7 | 3 | 0.7 | 71 | 15.4 | 122 | 26.5 | 11 | 2.4 | 16 | 3.5 | 258 | 56.0 |
| **CENSUS DIVISION 8, MOUNTAIN** | 320 | 34 | 10.6 | 191 | 59.7 | 58 | 18.1 | 11 | 3.4 | 64 | 20.0 | 104 | 32.5 | 12 | 3.8 | 19 | 5.9 | 201 | 62.8 |
| Arizona | 55 | 2 | 3.6 | 38 | 69.1 | 11 | 20.0 | 4 | 7.3 | 5 | 9.1 | 32 | 58.2 | 1 | 1.8 | 2 | 3.6 | 31 | 56.4 |
| Colorado | 56 | 4 | 7.1 | 38 | 67.9 | 13 | 23.2 | 1 | 1.8 | 15 | 26.8 | 20 | 35.7 | 4 | 7.1 | 2 | 3.6 | 41 | 73.2 |
| Idaho | 30 | 6 | 20.0 | 18 | 60.0 | 3 | 10.0 | 0 | 0.0 | 8 | 26.7 | 5 | 16.7 | 2 | 6.7 | 1 | 3.3 | 24 | 80.0 |
| Montana | 54 | 17 | 31.5 | 25 | 46.3 | 4 | 7.4 | 3 | 5.6 | 16 | 29.6 | 8 | 14.8 | 1 | 1.9 | 13 | 24.1 | 34 | 63.0 |
| Nevada | 22 | 0 | 0.0 | 10 | 45.5 | 5 | 22.7 | 0 | 0.0 | 2 | 9.1 | 9 | 40.9 | 1 | 4.5 | 0 | 0.0 | 11 | 50.0 |
| New Mexico | 34 | 1 | 2.9 | 17 | 50.0 | 5 | 14.7 | 0 | 0.0 | 6 | 17.6 | 9 | 26.5 | 2 | 5.9 | 0 | 0.0 | 20 | 58.8 |
| Utah | 41 | 2 | 4.9 | 31 | 75.6 | 9 | 22.0 | 0 | 0.0 | 4 | 9.8 | 16 | 39.0 | 1 | 2.4 | 0 | 0.0 | 22 | 53.7 |
| Wyoming | 28 | 2 | 7.1 | 14 | 50.0 | 8 | 28.6 | 3 | 10.7 | 8 | 28.6 | 5 | 17.9 | 0 | 0.0 | 1 | 3.6 | 18 | 64.3 |
| **CENSUS DIVISION 9, PACIFIC** | 576 | 34 | 5.9 | 268 | 46.5 | 71 | 12.3 | 5 | 0.9 | 51 | 8.9 | 164 | 28.5 | 23 | 4.0 | 15 | 2.6 | 279 | 48.4 |
| Alaska | 15 | 1 | 6.7 | 10 | 66.7 | 5 | 33.3 | 0 | 0.0 | 4 | 26.7 | 2 | 13.3 | 0 | 0.0 | 1 | 6.7 | 9 | 60.0 |
| California | 402 | 22 | 5.5 | 168 | 41.8 | 38 | 9.5 | 4 | 1.0 | 25 | 6.2 | 114 | 28.4 | 17 | 4.2 | 3 | 0.7 | 168 | 41.8 |
| Hawaii | 18 | 1 | 5.6 | 10 | 55.6 | 3 | 16.7 | 0 | 0.0 | 1 | 5.6 | 4 | 22.2 | 1 | 5.6 | 0 | 0.0 | 8 | 44.4 |
| Oregon | 59 | 5 | 8.5 | 38 | 64.4 | 8 | 13.6 | 0 | 0.0 | 7 | 11.9 | 17 | 28.8 | 3 | 5.1 | 4 | 6.8 | 45 | 76.3 |
| Washington | 82 | 5 | 6.1 | 42 | 51.2 | 17 | 20.7 | 1 | 1.2 | 14 | 17.1 | 27 | 32.9 | 2 | 2.4 | 7 | 8.5 | 49 | 59.8 |

## Table 7 (Continued)

*These data include only hospital-based facilities and services as reported by responding hospitals in Section C of the 2003 AHA Annual Survey, beginning on page 205. All hospitals are represented with Community Hospitals listed separately under United States. No estimates have been made for nonresponding hospitals. Definitions of facilities and services are listed in the Glossary, page 193.*

| CLASSIFICATION | HOSPITALS REPORTING | BARIATRIC/WEIGHT CONTROL SERVICES | | BIRTHING/LDR/ LDRP ROOM | | BREAST CANCER SCREENING | | CARDIOLOGY SERVICES | | CARDIAC CATHETERIZATION LABORATORY | | CASE MANAGEMENT | | CHAPLAINCY/ PASTORAL CARE SERVICES | | CHEMOTHERAPY | | CHILDREN WELLNESS PROGRAM | | CHIROPRACTIC SERVICES | | COMMUNITY OUTREACH | |
|---|---|---|---|---|---|---|---|---|---|---|---|---|---|---|---|---|---|---|---|---|---|---|---|
| | | Number | Percent | Number | Percent | Number | Percent | Number | Percent | Number | Percent | Number | Percent | Number | Percent | Number | Percent | Number | Percent | Number | Percent | Number | Percent |
| **UNITED STATES** | 4,946 | 855 | 17.3 | 2,886 | 58.4 | 3,487 | 70.5 | 2,004 | 40.5 | 1,745 | 35.3 | 3,733 | 75.5 | 2,934 | 59.3 | 2,220 | 44.9 | 918 | 18.6 | 109 | 2.2 | 3,125 | 63.2 |
| COMMUNITY HOSPITALS | 4,320 | 821 | 19.0 | 2,860 | 66.2 | 3,408 | 78.9 | 1,915 | 44.3 | 1,678 | 38.8 | 3,371 | 78.0 | 2,670 | 61.8 | 2,133 | 49.4 | 884 | 20.5 | 95 | 2.2 | 2,907 | 67.3 |
| **CENSUS DIVISION 1, NEW ENGLAND** | 228 | 51 | 22.4 | 144 | 63.2 | 175 | 76.8 | 112 | 49.1 | 85 | 37.3 | 186 | 81.6 | 150 | 65.8 | 133 | 58.3 | 71 | 31.1 | 10 | 4.4 | 181 | 79.4 |
| Connecticut | 36 | 15 | 41.7 | 28 | 77.8 | 31 | 86.1 | 26 | 72.2 | 19 | 52.8 | 32 | 88.9 | 31 | 86.1 | 25 | 69.4 | 15 | 41.7 | 3 | 8.3 | 32 | 88.9 |
| Maine | 39 | 5 | 12.8 | 29 | 74.4 | 31 | 79.5 | 11 | 28.2 | 11 | 28.2 | 31 | 79.5 | 24 | 61.5 | 23 | 59.0 | 10 | 25.6 | 1 | 2.6 | 30 | 76.9 |
| Massachusetts | 95 | 21 | 22.1 | 47 | 49.5 | 67 | 70.5 | 45 | 47.4 | 35 | 36.8 | 77 | 81.1 | 56 | 58.9 | 50 | 52.6 | 25 | 26.3 | 4 | 4.2 | 71 | 74.7 |
| New Hampshire | 30 | 8 | 26.7 | 25 | 83.3 | 25 | 83.3 | 14 | 46.7 | 12 | 40.0 | 25 | 83.3 | 21 | 70.0 | 18 | 60.0 | 12 | 40.0 | 2 | 6.7 | 27 | 90.0 |
| Rhode Island | 12 | 0 | 0.0 | 5 | 41.7 | 9 | 75.0 | 7 | 58.3 | 6 | 50.0 | 10 | 83.3 | 8 | 66.7 | 8 | 66.7 | 3 | 25.0 | 0 | 0.0 | 9 | 75.0 |
| Vermont | 16 | 2 | 12.5 | 10 | 62.5 | 12 | 75.0 | 9 | 56.3 | 2 | 12.5 | 11 | 68.8 | 10 | 62.5 | 9 | 56.3 | 6 | 37.5 | 0 | 0.0 | 12 | 75.0 |
| **CENSUS DIVISION 2, MIDDLE ATLANTIC** | 442 | 127 | 28.7 | 277 | 62.7 | 354 | 80.1 | 254 | 57.5 | 185 | 41.9 | 394 | 89.1 | 337 | 76.2 | 267 | 60.4 | 154 | 34.8 | 17 | 3.8 | 359 | 81.2 |
| New Jersey | 72 | 28 | 38.9 | 50 | 69.4 | 60 | 83.3 | 46 | 63.9 | 45 | 62.5 | 64 | 88.9 | 60 | 83.3 | 51 | 70.8 | 36 | 50.0 | 6 | 8.3 | 63 | 87.5 |
| New York | 180 | 58 | 32.2 | 112 | 62.2 | 145 | 80.6 | 101 | 56.1 | 52 | 28.9 | 159 | 88.3 | 137 | 76.1 | 100 | 55.6 | 63 | 35.0 | 6 | 3.3 | 146 | 81.1 |
| Pennsylvania | 190 | 41 | 21.6 | 115 | 60.5 | 149 | 78.4 | 107 | 56.3 | 88 | 46.3 | 171 | 90.0 | 140 | 73.7 | 116 | 61.1 | 55 | 28.9 | 5 | 2.6 | 150 | 78.9 |
| **CENSUS DIVISION 3, SOUTH ATLANTIC** | 714 | 161 | 22.5 | 404 | 56.6 | 548 | 76.8 | 353 | 49.4 | 344 | 48.2 | 598 | 83.8 | 506 | 70.9 | 358 | 50.1 | 135 | 18.9 | 15 | 2.1 | 507 | 71.0 |
| Delaware | 8 | 4 | 50.0 | 5 | 62.5 | 5 | 62.5 | 5 | 62.5 | 6 | 75.0 | 7 | 87.5 | 7 | 87.5 | 5 | 62.5 | 4 | 50.0 | 0 | 0.0 | 6 | 75.0 |
| District of Columbia | 13 | 4 | 30.8 | 6 | 46.2 | 7 | 53.8 | 6 | 46.2 | 9 | 69.2 | 11 | 84.6 | 13 | 100.0 | 9 | 69.2 | 3 | 23.1 | 1 | 7.7 | 10 | 76.9 |
| Florida | 158 | 41 | 25.9 | 76 | 48.1 | 116 | 73.4 | 88 | 55.7 | 102 | 64.6 | 143 | 90.5 | 106 | 67.1 | 82 | 51.9 | 19 | 12.0 | 3 | 1.9 | 99 | 62.7 |
| Georgia | 147 | 30 | 20.4 | 80 | 54.4 | 112 | 76.2 | 54 | 36.7 | 50 | 34.0 | 117 | 79.6 | 88 | 59.9 | 55 | 37.4 | 21 | 14.3 | 2 | 1.4 | 95 | 64.6 |
| Maryland | 61 | 15 | 24.6 | 33 | 54.1 | 45 | 73.8 | 38 | 62.3 | 37 | 60.7 | 52 | 85.2 | 52 | 85.2 | 41 | 67.2 | 17 | 27.9 | 2 | 3.3 | 52 | 85.2 |
| North Carolina | 111 | 27 | 24.3 | 80 | 72.1 | 90 | 81.1 | 64 | 57.7 | 52 | 46.8 | 98 | 88.3 | 91 | 82.0 | 66 | 59.5 | 22 | 19.8 | 4 | 3.6 | 83 | 74.8 |
| South Carolina | 67 | 9 | 13.4 | 36 | 53.7 | 55 | 82.1 | 19 | 28.4 | 30 | 44.8 | 47 | 70.1 | 37 | 55.2 | 27 | 40.3 | 18 | 26.9 | 0 | 0.0 | 58 | 86.6 |
| Virginia | 84 | 21 | 25.0 | 56 | 66.7 | 69 | 82.1 | 54 | 64.3 | 41 | 48.8 | 75 | 89.3 | 73 | 86.9 | 49 | 58.3 | 14 | 16.7 | 2 | 2.4 | 63 | 75.0 |
| West Virginia | 65 | 10 | 15.4 | 32 | 49.2 | 49 | 75.4 | 25 | 38.5 | 17 | 26.2 | 48 | 73.8 | 39 | 60.0 | 24 | 36.9 | 17 | 26.2 | 1 | 1.5 | 41 | 63.1 |
| **CENSUS DIVISION 4, EAST NORTH CENTRAL** | 749 | 161 | 21.5 | 501 | 66.9 | 611 | 81.6 | 365 | 48.7 | 312 | 41.7 | 603 | 80.5 | 519 | 69.3 | 415 | 55.4 | 171 | 22.8 | 23 | 3.1 | 531 | 70.9 |
| Illinois | 186 | 48 | 25.8 | 124 | 66.7 | 163 | 87.6 | 106 | 57.0 | 88 | 47.3 | 156 | 83.9 | 147 | 79.0 | 115 | 61.8 | 51 | 27.4 | 9 | 4.8 | 141 | 75.8 |
| Indiana | 107 | 12 | 11.2 | 77 | 72.0 | 82 | 76.6 | 48 | 44.9 | 38 | 35.5 | 90 | 84.1 | 79 | 73.8 | 59 | 55.1 | 25 | 23.4 | 0 | 0.0 | 77 | 72.0 |
| Michigan | 154 | 31 | 20.1 | 92 | 59.7 | 123 | 79.9 | 83 | 53.9 | 59 | 38.3 | 118 | 76.6 | 111 | 72.1 | 86 | 55.8 | 34 | 22.1 | 4 | 2.6 | 111 | 72.1 |
| Ohio | 161 | 39 | 24.2 | 108 | 67.1 | 134 | 83.2 | 96 | 59.6 | 85 | 52.8 | 139 | 86.3 | 114 | 70.8 | 105 | 65.2 | 40 | 24.8 | 7 | 4.3 | 127 | 78.9 |
| Wisconsin | 141 | 31 | 22.0 | 100 | 70.9 | 109 | 77.3 | 32 | 22.7 | 42 | 29.8 | 100 | 70.9 | 68 | 48.2 | 50 | 35.5 | 21 | 14.9 | 3 | 2.1 | 75 | 53.2 |
| **CENSUS DIVISION 5, EAST SOUTH CENTRAL** | 438 | 49 | 11.2 | 218 | 49.8 | 310 | 70.8 | 161 | 36.8 | 123 | 28.1 | 319 | 72.8 | 199 | 45.4 | 113 | 25.8 | 36 | 8.2 | 0 | 0.0 | 252 | 57.5 |
| Alabama | 97 | 18 | 18.6 | 46 | 47.4 | 68 | 70.1 | 40 | 41.2 | 37 | 38.1 | 70 | 72.2 | 43 | 44.3 | 31 | 32.0 | 8 | 8.2 | 0 | 0.0 | 47 | 48.5 |
| Kentucky | 102 | 15 | 14.7 | 53 | 52.0 | 87 | 85.3 | 52 | 51.0 | 43 | 42.2 | 84 | 82.4 | 76 | 74.5 | 41 | 40.2 | 17 | 16.7 | 0 | 0.0 | 71 | 69.6 |
| Mississippi | 104 | 1 | 1.0 | 49 | 47.1 | 62 | 59.6 | 28 | 26.9 | 2 | 1.9 | 58 | 55.8 | 7 | 6.7 | 2 | 1.9 | 1 | 1.0 | 0 | 0.0 | 63 | 60.6 |
| Tennessee | 135 | 15 | 11.1 | 70 | 51.9 | 93 | 68.9 | 41 | 30.4 | 41 | 30.4 | 107 | 79.3 | 73 | 54.1 | 39 | 28.9 | 10 | 7.4 | 0 | 0.0 | 71 | 52.6 |
| **CENSUS DIVISION 6, WEST NORTH CENTRAL** | 695 | 83 | 11.9 | 434 | 62.4 | 488 | 70.2 | 170 | 24.5 | 146 | 21.0 | 432 | 62.2 | 348 | 50.1 | 339 | 48.8 | 101 | 14.5 | 14 | 2.0 | 411 | 59.1 |
| Iowa | 125 | 17 | 13.6 | 87 | 69.6 | 111 | 88.8 | 32 | 25.6 | 22 | 17.6 | 92 | 73.6 | 55 | 44.0 | 80 | 64.0 | 23 | 18.4 | 4 | 3.2 | 88 | 70.4 |
| Kansas | 145 | 11 | 7.6 | 77 | 53.1 | 78 | 53.8 | 29 | 20.0 | 20 | 13.8 | 76 | 52.4 | 72 | 49.7 | 39 | 26.9 | 12 | 8.3 | 0 | 0.0 | 48 | 33.1 |
| Minnesota | 117 | 22 | 18.8 | 94 | 80.3 | 89 | 76.1 | 28 | 23.9 | 20 | 17.1 | 70 | 59.8 | 59 | 50.4 | 75 | 64.1 | 19 | 16.2 | 3 | 2.6 | 84 | 71.8 |
| Missouri | 143 | 16 | 11.2 | 73 | 51.0 | 101 | 70.6 | 42 | 29.4 | 56 | 39.2 | 112 | 78.3 | 97 | 67.8 | 59 | 41.3 | 19 | 13.3 | 2 | 1.4 | 91 | 63.6 |
| Nebraska | 75 | 9 | 12.0 | 54 | 72.0 | 57 | 76.0 | 21 | 28.0 | 15 | 20.0 | 37 | 49.3 | 31 | 41.3 | 45 | 60.0 | 13 | 17.3 | 1 | 1.3 | 45 | 60.0 |
| North Dakota | 32 | 4 | 12.5 | 20 | 62.5 | 22 | 68.8 | 8 | 25.0 | 6 | 18.8 | 15 | 46.9 | 18 | 56.3 | 19 | 59.4 | 8 | 25.0 | 3 | 9.4 | 22 | 68.8 |
| South Dakota | 58 | 4 | 6.9 | 29 | 50.0 | 30 | 51.7 | 10 | 17.2 | 7 | 12.1 | 30 | 51.7 | 16 | 27.6 | 22 | 37.9 | 7 | 12.1 | 1 | 1.7 | 33 | 56.9 |
| **CENSUS DIVISION 7, WEST SOUTH CENTRAL** | 784 | 94 | 12.0 | 384 | 49.0 | 449 | 57.3 | 269 | 34.3 | 250 | 31.9 | 621 | 79.2 | 395 | 50.4 | 234 | 29.8 | 104 | 13.3 | 10 | 1.3 | 378 | 48.2 |
| Arkansas | 104 | 11 | 10.6 | 49 | 47.1 | 68 | 65.4 | 34 | 32.7 | 32 | 30.8 | 89 | 85.6 | 52 | 50.0 | 30 | 28.8 | 5 | 4.8 | 0 | 0.0 | 58 | 55.8 |
| Louisiana | 111 | 13 | 11.7 | 46 | 41.4 | 73 | 65.8 | 38 | 34.2 | 36 | 32.4 | 94 | 84.7 | 50 | 45.0 | 39 | 35.1 | 20 | 18.0 | 1 | 0.9 | 51 | 45.9 |
| Oklahoma | 108 | 12 | 11.1 | 54 | 50.0 | 57 | 52.8 | 36 | 33.3 | 30 | 27.8 | 81 | 75.0 | 58 | 53.7 | 32 | 29.6 | 14 | 13.0 | 3 | 2.8 | 52 | 48.1 |
| Texas | 461 | 58 | 12.6 | 235 | 51.0 | 251 | 54.4 | 161 | 34.9 | 152 | 33.0 | 357 | 77.4 | 235 | 51.0 | 133 | 28.9 | 65 | 14.1 | 6 | 1.3 | 217 | 47.1 |
| **CENSUS DIVISION 8, MOUNTAIN** | 320 | 39 | 12.2 | 224 | 70.0 | 234 | 73.1 | 126 | 39.4 | 111 | 34.7 | 238 | 74.4 | 180 | 56.3 | 145 | 45.3 | 59 | 18.4 | 9 | 2.8 | 208 | 65.0 |
| Arizona | 55 | 11 | 20.0 | 34 | 61.8 | 38 | 69.1 | 36 | 65.5 | 35 | 63.6 | 53 | 96.4 | 46 | 83.6 | 27 | 49.1 | 12 | 21.8 | 0 | 0.0 | 36 | 65.5 |
| Colorado | 56 | 10 | 17.9 | 43 | 76.8 | 45 | 80.4 | 28 | 50.0 | 23 | 41.1 | 46 | 82.1 | 43 | 76.8 | 39 | 69.6 | 8 | 14.3 | 4 | 7.1 | 41 | 73.2 |
| Idaho | 30 | 4 | 13.3 | 25 | 83.3 | 21 | 70.0 | 8 | 26.7 | 6 | 20.0 | 19 | 63.3 | 17 | 56.7 | 12 | 40.0 | 4 | 13.3 | 1 | 3.3 | 21 | 70.0 |
| Montana | 54 | 4 | 7.4 | 32 | 59.3 | 37 | 68.5 | 12 | 22.2 | 9 | 16.7 | 26 | 48.1 | 21 | 38.9 | 17 | 31.5 | 12 | 22.2 | 0 | 0.0 | 31 | 57.4 |
| Nevada | 22 | 3 | 13.6 | 13 | 59.1 | 14 | 63.6 | 10 | 45.5 | 9 | 40.9 | 16 | 72.7 | 13 | 59.1 | 12 | 54.5 | 3 | 13.6 | 0 | 0.0 | 16 | 72.7 |
| New Mexico | 34 | 0 | 0.0 | 22 | 64.7 | 25 | 73.5 | 9 | 26.5 | 9 | 26.5 | 25 | 73.5 | 20 | 58.8 | 7 | 20.6 | 9 | 26.5 | 2 | 5.9 | 23 | 67.6 |
| Utah | 41 | 6 | 14.6 | 34 | 82.9 | 34 | 82.9 | 20 | 48.8 | 17 | 41.5 | 34 | 82.9 | 10 | 24.4 | 16 | 39.0 | 8 | 19.5 | 1 | 2.4 | 26 | 63.4 |
| Wyoming | 28 | 1 | 3.6 | 21 | 75.0 | 20 | 71.4 | 3 | 10.7 | 3 | 10.7 | 19 | 67.9 | 10 | 35.7 | 15 | 53.6 | 3 | 10.7 | 1 | 3.6 | 14 | 50.0 |
| **CENSUS DIVISION 9, PACIFIC** | 576 | 90 | 15.6 | 300 | 52.1 | 318 | 55.2 | 194 | 33.7 | 189 | 32.8 | 342 | 59.4 | 300 | 52.1 | 216 | 37.5 | 87 | 15.1 | 11 | 1.9 | 298 | 51.7 |
| Alaska | 15 | 4 | 26.7 | 12 | 80.0 | 13 | 86.7 | 2 | 13.3 | 2 | 13.3 | 11 | 73.3 | 10 | 66.7 | 7 | 46.7 | 4 | 26.7 | 1 | 6.7 | 8 | 53.3 |
| California | 402 | 57 | 14.2 | 175 | 43.5 | 190 | 47.3 | 139 | 34.6 | 130 | 32.3 | 225 | 56.0 | 186 | 46.3 | 140 | 34.8 | 50 | 12.4 | 7 | 1.7 | 188 | 46.8 |
| Hawaii | 18 | 3 | 16.7 | 9 | 50.0 | 9 | 50.0 | 4 | 22.2 | 6 | 33.3 | 13 | 72.2 | 10 | 55.6 | 7 | 38.9 | 4 | 22.2 | 1 | 5.6 | 7 | 38.9 |
| Oregon | 59 | 12 | 20.3 | 51 | 86.4 | 50 | 84.7 | 15 | 25.4 | 18 | 30.5 | 40 | 67.8 | 40 | 67.8 | 25 | 42.4 | 14 | 23.7 | 0 | 0.0 | 42 | 71.2 |
| Washington | 82 | 14 | 17.1 | 53 | 64.6 | 56 | 68.3 | 34 | 41.5 | 33 | 40.2 | 53 | 64.6 | 54 | 65.9 | 37 | 45.1 | 15 | 18.3 | 2 | 2.4 | 53 | 64.6 |

## Table 7 (Continued)

*These data include only hospital-based facilities and services as reported by responding hospitals in Section C of the 2003 AHA Annual Survey, beginning on page 205. All hospitals are represented with Community Hospitals listed separately under United States. No estimates have been made for nonresponding hospitals. Definitions of facilities and services are listed in the Glossary, page 193.*

| CLASSIFICATION | HOSPITALS REPORTING | COMPLEMENTARY MEDICINE SERVICES | | CRISIS PREVENTION | | CT SCANNER | | DENTAL SERVICES | | DIAGNOSTIC RADIOISOTOPE FACILITY | | ELECTRON BEAM COMPUTED TOMOGRAPHY | | EMERGENCY DEPARTMENT | | ENABLING SERVICES | |
|---|---|---|---|---|---|---|---|---|---|---|---|---|---|---|---|---|---|
| | | Number | Percent | Number | Percent | Number | Percent | Number | Percent | Number | Percent | Number | Percent | Number | Percent | Number | Percent |
| **UNITED STATES** | 4,946 | 885 | 17.9 | 996 | 20.1 | 3,888 | 78.6 | 1,168 | 23.6 | 2,743 | 55.5 | 201 | 4.1 | 4,079 | 82.5 | 962 | 19.5 |
| COMMUNITY HOSPITALS | 4,320 | 830 | 19.2 | 846 | 19.6 | 3,726 | 86.3 | 954 | 22.1 | 2,646 | 61.3 | 190 | 4.4 | 3,910 | 90.5 | 884 | 20.5 |
| **CENSUS DIVISION 1, NEW ENGLAND** | 228 | 74 | 32.5 | 69 | 30.3 | 185 | 81.1 | 70 | 30.7 | 151 | 66.2 | 8 | 3.5 | 179 | 78.5 | 56 | 24.6 |
| Connecticut | 36 | 17 | 47.2 | 21 | 58.3 | 30 | 83.3 | 19 | 52.8 | 30 | 83.3 | 4 | 11.1 | 30 | 83.3 | 8 | 22.2 |
| Maine | 39 | 9 | 23.1 | 5 | 12.8 | 35 | 89.7 | 7 | 17.9 | 27 | 69.2 | 0 | 0.0 | 34 | 87.2 | 4 | 10.3 |
| Massachusetts | 95 | 31 | 32.6 | 29 | 30.5 | 69 | 72.6 | 24 | 25.3 | 56 | 58.9 | 3 | 3.2 | 65 | 68.4 | 25 | 26.3 |
| New Hampshire | 30 | 11 | 36.7 | 9 | 30.0 | 27 | 90.0 | 13 | 43.3 | 19 | 63.3 | 1 | 3.3 | 27 | 90.0 | 11 | 36.7 |
| Rhode Island | 12 | 2 | 16.7 | 3 | 25.0 | 11 | 91.7 | 4 | 33.3 | 9 | 75.0 | 0 | 0.0 | 9 | 75.0 | 2 | 16.7 |
| Vermont | 16 | 4 | 25.0 | 2 | 12.5 | 13 | 81.3 | 3 | 18.8 | 10 | 62.5 | 0 | 0.0 | 14 | 87.5 | 6 | 37.5 |
| **CENSUS DIVISION 2, MIDDLE ATLANTIC** | 442 | 139 | 31.4 | 160 | 36.2 | 376 | 85.1 | 194 | 43.9 | 321 | 72.6 | 38 | 8.6 | 369 | 83.5 | 124 | 28.1 |
| New Jersey | 72 | 29 | 40.3 | 37 | 51.4 | 62 | 86.1 | 32 | 44.4 | 56 | 77.8 | 12 | 16.7 | 61 | 84.7 | 27 | 37.5 |
| New York | 180 | 57 | 31.7 | 74 | 41.1 | 155 | 86.1 | 83 | 46.1 | 128 | 71.1 | 12 | 6.7 | 148 | 82.2 | 41 | 22.8 |
| Pennsylvania | 190 | 53 | 27.9 | 49 | 25.8 | 159 | 83.7 | 79 | 41.6 | 137 | 72.1 | 14 | 7.4 | 160 | 84.2 | 56 | 29.5 |
| **CENSUS DIVISION 3, SOUTH ATLANTIC** | 714 | 129 | 18.1 | 149 | 20.9 | 603 | 84.5 | 204 | 28.6 | 466 | 65.3 | 30 | 4.2 | 603 | 84.5 | 170 | 23.8 |
| Delaware | 8 | 3 | 37.5 | 4 | 50.0 | 7 | 87.5 | 3 | 37.5 | 5 | 62.5 | 0 | 0.0 | 7 | 87.5 | 5 | 62.5 |
| District of Columbia | 13 | 5 | 38.5 | 4 | 30.8 | 9 | 69.2 | 8 | 61.5 | 8 | 61.5 | 2 | 15.4 | 9 | 69.2 | 5 | 38.5 |
| Florida | 158 | 29 | 18.4 | 23 | 14.6 | 138 | 87.3 | 33 | 20.9 | 111 | 70.3 | 8 | 5.1 | 136 | 86.1 | 33 | 20.9 |
| Georgia | 147 | 18 | 12.2 | 25 | 17.0 | 125 | 85.0 | 39 | 26.5 | 84 | 57.1 | 3 | 2.0 | 124 | 84.4 | 35 | 23.8 |
| Maryland | 61 | 19 | 31.1 | 25 | 41.0 | 48 | 78.7 | 15 | 24.6 | 39 | 63.9 | 3 | 4.9 | 47 | 77.0 | 21 | 34.4 |
| North Carolina | 111 | 17 | 15.3 | 25 | 22.5 | 98 | 88.3 | 40 | 36.0 | 74 | 66.7 | 5 | 4.5 | 98 | 88.3 | 27 | 24.3 |
| South Carolina | 67 | 3 | 4.5 | 4 | 6.0 | 53 | 79.1 | 16 | 23.9 | 45 | 67.2 | 4 | 6.0 | 57 | 85.1 | 5 | 7.5 |
| Virginia | 84 | 25 | 29.8 | 29 | 34.5 | 70 | 83.3 | 30 | 35.7 | 61 | 72.6 | 3 | 3.6 | 70 | 83.3 | 28 | 33.3 |
| West Virginia | 65 | 10 | 15.4 | 10 | 15.4 | 55 | 84.6 | 20 | 30.8 | 39 | 60.0 | 2 | 3.1 | 55 | 84.6 | 11 | 16.9 |
| **CENSUS DIVISION 4, EAST NORTH CENTRAL** | 749 | 216 | 28.8 | 204 | 27.2 | 649 | 86.6 | 197 | 26.3 | 487 | 65.0 | 43 | 5.7 | 655 | 87.4 | 208 | 27.8 |
| Illinois | 186 | 53 | 28.5 | 58 | 31.2 | 173 | 93.0 | 53 | 28.5 | 127 | 68.3 | 11 | 5.9 | 175 | 94.1 | 52 | 28.0 |
| Indiana | 107 | 21 | 19.6 | 21 | 19.6 | 88 | 82.2 | 27 | 25.2 | 68 | 63.6 | 8 | 7.5 | 87 | 81.3 | 18 | 16.8 |
| Michigan | 154 | 48 | 31.2 | 46 | 29.9 | 128 | 83.1 | 40 | 26.0 | 102 | 66.2 | 5 | 3.2 | 129 | 83.8 | 49 | 31.8 |
| Ohio | 161 | 54 | 33.5 | 41 | 25.5 | 146 | 90.7 | 50 | 31.1 | 120 | 74.5 | 9 | 5.6 | 145 | 90.1 | 51 | 31.7 |
| Wisconsin | 141 | 40 | 28.4 | 38 | 27.0 | 114 | 80.9 | 27 | 19.1 | 70 | 49.6 | 10 | 7.1 | 119 | 84.4 | 38 | 27.0 |
| **CENSUS DIVISION 5, EAST SOUTH CENTRAL** | 438 | 31 | 7.1 | 52 | 11.9 | 362 | 82.6 | 86 | 19.6 | 247 | 56.4 | 7 | 1.6 | 364 | 83.1 | 48 | 11.0 |
| Alabama | 97 | 4 | 4.1 | 9 | 9.3 | 80 | 82.5 | 9 | 9.3 | 64 | 66.0 | 2 | 2.1 | 80 | 82.5 | 11 | 11.3 |
| Kentucky | 102 | 20 | 19.6 | 22 | 21.6 | 92 | 90.2 | 22 | 21.6 | 58 | 56.9 | 1 | 1.0 | 91 | 89.2 | 16 | 15.7 |
| Mississippi | 104 | 0 | 0.0 | 1 | 1.0 | 83 | 79.8 | 34 | 32.7 | 54 | 51.9 | 0 | 0.0 | 86 | 82.7 | 1 | 1.0 |
| Tennessee | 135 | 7 | 5.2 | 20 | 14.8 | 107 | 79.3 | 21 | 15.6 | 71 | 52.6 | 4 | 3.0 | 107 | 79.3 | 20 | 14.8 |
| **CENSUS DIVISION 6, WEST NORTH CENTRAL** | 695 | 123 | 17.7 | 125 | 18.0 | 515 | 74.1 | 127 | 18.3 | 265 | 38.1 | 15 | 2.2 | 631 | 90.8 | 122 | 17.6 |
| Iowa | 125 | 33 | 26.4 | 22 | 17.6 | 106 | 84.8 | 26 | 20.8 | 50 | 40.0 | 2 | 1.6 | 118 | 94.4 | 26 | 20.8 |
| Kansas | 145 | 8 | 5.5 | 11 | 7.6 | 91 | 62.8 | 19 | 13.1 | 47 | 32.4 | 5 | 3.4 | 125 | 86.2 | 15 | 10.3 |
| Minnesota | 117 | 29 | 24.8 | 26 | 22.2 | 93 | 79.5 | 12 | 10.3 | 42 | 35.9 | 6 | 5.1 | 109 | 93.2 | 16 | 13.7 |
| Missouri | 143 | 33 | 23.1 | 42 | 29.4 | 116 | 81.1 | 49 | 34.3 | 75 | 52.4 | 0 | 0.0 | 120 | 83.9 | 48 | 33.6 |
| Nebraska | 75 | 7 | 9.3 | 13 | 17.3 | 51 | 68.0 | 9 | 12.0 | 22 | 29.3 | 2 | 2.7 | 72 | 96.0 | 9 | 12.0 |
| North Dakota | 32 | 7 | 21.9 | 4 | 12.5 | 24 | 75.0 | 3 | 9.4 | 13 | 40.6 | 0 | 0.0 | 31 | 96.9 | 4 | 12.5 |
| South Dakota | 58 | 6 | 10.3 | 7 | 12.1 | 34 | 58.6 | 9 | 15.5 | 16 | 27.6 | 0 | 0.0 | 56 | 96.6 | 4 | 6.9 |
| **CENSUS DIVISION 7, WEST SOUTH CENTRAL** | 784 | 55 | 7.0 | 80 | 10.2 | 565 | 72.1 | 145 | 18.5 | 362 | 46.2 | 21 | 2.7 | 613 | 78.2 | 98 | 12.5 |
| Arkansas | 104 | 7 | 6.7 | 9 | 8.7 | 80 | 76.9 | 17 | 16.3 | 52 | 50.0 | 3 | 2.9 | 82 | 78.8 | 8 | 7.7 |
| Louisiana | 111 | 11 | 9.9 | 12 | 10.8 | 85 | 76.6 | 21 | 18.9 | 49 | 44.1 | 2 | 1.8 | 85 | 76.6 | 10 | 9.0 |
| Oklahoma | 108 | 6 | 5.6 | 14 | 13.0 | 78 | 72.2 | 23 | 21.3 | 47 | 43.5 | 2 | 1.9 | 90 | 83.3 | 10 | 9.3 |
| Texas | 461 | 31 | 6.7 | 45 | 9.8 | 322 | 69.8 | 84 | 18.2 | 214 | 46.4 | 14 | 3.0 | 356 | 77.2 | 70 | 15.2 |
| **CENSUS DIVISION 8, MOUNTAIN** | 320 | 56 | 17.5 | 68 | 21.3 | 260 | 81.3 | 62 | 19.4 | 164 | 51.3 | 12 | 3.8 | 286 | 89.4 | 47 | 14.7 |
| Arizona | 55 | 11 | 20.0 | 14 | 25.5 | 45 | 81.8 | 13 | 23.6 | 33 | 60.0 | 3 | 5.5 | 49 | 89.1 | 11 | 20.0 |
| Colorado | 56 | 22 | 39.3 | 10 | 17.9 | 51 | 91.1 | 15 | 26.8 | 32 | 57.1 | 4 | 7.1 | 52 | 92.9 | 10 | 17.9 |
| Idaho | 30 | 3 | 10.0 | 4 | 13.3 | 26 | 86.7 | 6 | 20.0 | 13 | 43.3 | 0 | 0.0 | 27 | 90.0 | 5 | 16.7 |
| Montana | 54 | 6 | 11.1 | 7 | 13.0 | 35 | 64.8 | 3 | 5.6 | 21 | 38.9 | 0 | 0.0 | 51 | 94.4 | 5 | 9.3 |
| Nevada | 22 | 1 | 4.5 | 6 | 27.3 | 17 | 77.3 | 4 | 18.2 | 12 | 54.5 | 0 | 0.0 | 18 | 81.8 | 2 | 9.1 |
| New Mexico | 34 | 3 | 8.8 | 7 | 20.6 | 26 | 76.5 | 7 | 20.6 | 16 | 47.1 | 1 | 2.9 | 27 | 79.4 | 2 | 5.9 |
| Utah | 41 | 6 | 14.6 | 17 | 41.5 | 36 | 87.8 | 9 | 22.0 | 23 | 56.1 | 2 | 4.9 | 36 | 87.8 | 12 | 29.3 |
| Wyoming | 28 | 4 | 14.3 | 3 | 10.7 | 24 | 85.7 | 5 | 17.9 | 14 | 50.0 | 2 | 7.1 | 26 | 92.9 | 0 | 0.0 |
| **CENSUS DIVISION 9, PACIFIC** | 576 | 62 | 10.8 | 89 | 15.5 | 373 | 64.8 | 83 | 14.4 | 280 | 48.6 | 27 | 4.7 | 379 | 65.8 | 89 | 15.5 |
| Alaska | 15 | 3 | 20.0 | 4 | 26.7 | 10 | 66.7 | 6 | 40.0 | 6 | 40.0 | 1 | 6.7 | 13 | 86.7 | 2 | 13.3 |
| California | 402 | 31 | 7.7 | 53 | 13.2 | 227 | 56.5 | 53 | 13.2 | 180 | 44.8 | 15 | 3.7 | 221 | 55.0 | 51 | 12.7 |
| Hawaii | 18 | 2 | 11.1 | 3 | 16.7 | 12 | 66.7 | 4 | 22.2 | 11 | 61.1 | 0 | 0.0 | 14 | 77.8 | 3 | 16.7 |
| Oregon | 59 | 11 | 18.6 | 11 | 18.6 | 59 | 100.0 | 7 | 11.9 | 38 | 64.4 | 3 | 5.1 | 58 | 98.3 | 17 | 28.8 |
| Washington | 82 | 15 | 18.3 | 18 | 22.0 | 65 | 79.3 | 13 | 15.9 | 45 | 54.9 | 8 | 9.8 | 73 | 89.0 | 16 | 19.5 |

## Table 7 (Continued)

*These data include only hospital-based facilities and services as reported by responding hospitals in Section C of the 2003 AHA Annual Survey, beginning on page 205. All hospitals are represented with Community Hospitals listed separately under United States. No estimates have been made for nonresponding hospitals. Definitions of facilities and services are listed in the Glossary, page 193.*

| CLASSIFICATION | HOSPITALS REPORTING | ENROLLMENT ASSISTANCE SERVICES | | EXTRACORPOREAL SHOCK WAVE LITHOTRIPTER (ESWL) | | FERTILITY CLINIC | | FITNESS CENTER | | GAMMA KNIFE | | GENETIC TESTING/ COUNSELING | | GERIATRIC SERVICES | | HEALTH FAIR | |
|---|---|---|---|---|---|---|---|---|---|---|---|---|---|---|---|---|---|---|---|
| | | Number | Percent | Number | Percent | Number | Percent | Number | Percent | Number | Percent | Number | Percent | Number | Percent | Number | Percent |
| UNITED STATES | 4,946 | 1,749 | 35.4 | 1,038 | 21.0 | 295 | 6.0 | 1,321 | 26.7 | 199 | 4.0 | 365 | 7.4 | 1,998 | 40.4 | 3,449 | 69.7 |
| COMMUNITY HOSPITALS | 4,320 | 1,608 | 37.2 | 1,012 | 23.4 | 281 | 6.5 | 1,222 | 28.3 | 190 | 4.4 | 353 | 8.2 | 1,784 | 41.3 | 3,272 | 75.7 |
| CENSUS DIVISION 1, NEW ENGLAND | 228 | 117 | 51.3 | 84 | 36.8 | 29 | 12.7 | 53 | 23.2 | 12 | 5.3 | 27 | 11.8 | 116 | 50.9 | 165 | 72.4 |
| Connecticut | 36 | 19 | 52.8 | 16 | 44.4 | 7 | 19.4 | 14 | 38.9 | 2 | 5.6 | 7 | 19.4 | 19 | 52.8 | 30 | 83.3 |
| Maine | 39 | 15 | 38.5 | 13 | 33.3 | 3 | 7.7 | 8 | 20.5 | 0 | 0.0 | 4 | 10.3 | 20 | 51.3 | 24 | 61.5 |
| Massachusetts | 95 | 48 | 50.5 | 29 | 30.5 | 11 | 11.6 | 10 | 10.5 | 6 | 6.3 | 13 | 13.7 | 47 | 49.5 | 63 | 66.3 |
| New Hampshire | 30 | 21 | 70.0 | 14 | 46.7 | 5 | 16.7 | 13 | 43.3 | 3 | 10.0 | 1 | 3.3 | 16 | 53.3 | 28 | 93.3 |
| Rhode Island | 12 | 6 | 50.0 | 8 | 66.7 | 1 | 8.3 | 2 | 16.7 | 1 | 8.3 | 1 | 8.3 | 8 | 66.7 | 9 | 75.0 |
| Vermont | 16 | 8 | 50.0 | 4 | 25.0 | 2 | 12.5 | 6 | 37.5 | 0 | 0.0 | 1 | 6.3 | 6 | 37.5 | 11 | 68.8 |
| CENSUS DIVISION 2, MIDDLE ATLANTIC | 442 | 231 | 52.3 | 114 | 25.8 | 46 | 10.4 | 125 | 28.3 | 29 | 6.6 | 70 | 15.8 | 252 | 57.0 | 356 | 80.5 |
| New Jersey | 72 | 39 | 54.2 | 17 | 23.6 | 7 | 9.7 | 28 | 38.9 | 5 | 6.9 | 16 | 22.2 | 50 | 69.4 | 64 | 88.9 |
| New York | 180 | 97 | 53.9 | 44 | 24.4 | 22 | 12.2 | 37 | 20.6 | 12 | 6.7 | 31 | 17.2 | 100 | 55.6 | 144 | 80.0 |
| Pennsylvania | 190 | 95 | 50.0 | 53 | 27.9 | 17 | 8.9 | 60 | 31.6 | 12 | 6.3 | 23 | 12.1 | 102 | 53.7 | 148 | 77.9 |
| CENSUS DIVISION 3, SOUTH ATLANTIC | 714 | 295 | 41.3 | 197 | 27.6 | 43 | 6.0 | 205 | 28.7 | 41 | 5.7 | 64 | 9.0 | 290 | 40.6 | 560 | 78.4 |
| Delaware | 8 | 6 | 75.0 | 4 | 50.0 | 0 | 0.0 | 4 | 50.0 | 0 | 0.0 | 2 | 25.0 | 3 | 37.5 | 6 | 75.0 |
| District of Columbia | 13 | 6 | 46.2 | 2 | 15.4 | 3 | 23.1 | 4 | 30.8 | 4 | 30.8 | 3 | 23.1 | 7 | 53.8 | 9 | 69.2 |
| Florida | 158 | 61 | 38.6 | 51 | 32.3 | 9 | 5.7 | 57 | 36.1 | 13 | 8.2 | 14 | 8.9 | 68 | 43.0 | 111 | 70.3 |
| Georgia | 147 | 56 | 38.1 | 36 | 24.5 | 6 | 4.1 | 32 | 21.8 | 4 | 2.7 | 6 | 4.1 | 45 | 30.6 | 110 | 74.8 |
| Maryland | 61 | 29 | 47.5 | 19 | 31.1 | 9 | 14.8 | 14 | 23.0 | 2 | 3.3 | 15 | 24.6 | 31 | 50.8 | 48 | 78.7 |
| North Carolina | 111 | 47 | 42.3 | 19 | 17.1 | 9 | 8.1 | 32 | 28.8 | 6 | 5.4 | 10 | 9.0 | 49 | 44.1 | 94 | 84.7 |
| South Carolina | 67 | 18 | 26.9 | 17 | 25.4 | 2 | 3.0 | 24 | 35.8 | 7 | 10.4 | 4 | 6.0 | 30 | 44.8 | 60 | 89.6 |
| Virginia | 84 | 47 | 56.0 | 31 | 36.9 | 4 | 4.8 | 18 | 21.4 | 3 | 3.6 | 6 | 7.1 | 34 | 40.5 | 66 | 78.6 |
| West Virginia | 65 | 25 | 38.5 | 18 | 27.7 | 1 | 1.5 | 20 | 30.8 | 2 | 3.1 | 4 | 6.2 | 23 | 35.4 | 56 | 86.2 |
| CENSUS DIVISION 4, EAST NORTH CENTRAL | 749 | 308 | 41.1 | 165 | 22.0 | 60 | 8.0 | 247 | 33.0 | 37 | 4.9 | 73 | 9.7 | 402 | 53.7 | 560 | 74.8 |
| Illinois | 186 | 82 | 44.1 | 33 | 17.7 | 17 | 9.1 | 51 | 27.4 | 9 | 4.8 | 24 | 12.9 | 90 | 48.4 | 155 | 83.3 |
| Indiana | 107 | 38 | 35.5 | 29 | 27.1 | 3 | 2.8 | 33 | 30.8 | 4 | 3.7 | 2 | 1.9 | 44 | 41.1 | 84 | 78.5 |
| Michigan | 154 | 68 | 44.2 | 29 | 18.8 | 16 | 10.4 | 48 | 31.2 | 6 | 3.9 | 12 | 7.8 | 72 | 46.8 | 111 | 72.1 |
| Ohio | 161 | 72 | 44.7 | 42 | 26.1 | 19 | 11.8 | 57 | 35.4 | 14 | 8.7 | 20 | 12.4 | 79 | 49.1 | 138 | 85.7 |
| Wisconsin | 141 | 48 | 34.0 | 32 | 22.7 | 5 | 3.5 | 58 | 41.1 | 4 | 2.8 | 15 | 10.6 | 117 | 83.0 | 72 | 51.1 |
| CENSUS DIVISION 5, EAST SOUTH CENTRAL | 438 | 104 | 23.7 | 95 | 21.7 | 14 | 3.2 | 101 | 23.1 | 9 | 2.1 | 9 | 2.1 | 143 | 32.6 | 251 | 57.3 |
| Alabama | 97 | 25 | 25.8 | 22 | 22.7 | 3 | 3.1 | 21 | 21.6 | 2 | 2.1 | 2 | 2.1 | 25 | 25.8 | 68 | 70.1 |
| Kentucky | 102 | 42 | 41.2 | 22 | 21.6 | 6 | 5.9 | 25 | 24.5 | 3 | 2.9 | 2 | 2.0 | 44 | 43.1 | 86 | 84.3 |
| Mississippi | 104 | 2 | 1.9 | 18 | 17.3 | 3 | 2.9 | 27 | 26.0 | 0 | 0.0 | 0 | 0.0 | 23 | 22.1 | 3 | 2.9 |
| Tennessee | 135 | 35 | 25.9 | 33 | 24.4 | 2 | 1.5 | 28 | 20.7 | 4 | 3.0 | 5 | 3.7 | 51 | 37.8 | 94 | 69.6 |
| CENSUS DIVISION 6, WEST NORTH CENTRAL | 695 | 182 | 26.2 | 86 | 12.4 | 29 | 4.2 | 237 | 34.1 | 13 | 1.9 | 35 | 5.0 | 266 | 38.3 | 493 | 70.9 |
| Iowa | 125 | 42 | 33.6 | 14 | 11.2 | 5 | 4.0 | 50 | 40.0 | 4 | 3.2 | 2 | 1.6 | 50 | 40.0 | 96 | 76.8 |
| Kansas | 145 | 23 | 15.9 | 19 | 13.1 | 3 | 2.1 | 41 | 28.3 | 1 | 0.7 | 0 | 0.0 | 50 | 34.5 | 88 | 60.7 |
| Minnesota | 117 | 27 | 23.1 | 14 | 12.0 | 8 | 6.8 | 35 | 29.9 | 3 | 2.6 | 12 | 10.3 | 49 | 41.9 | 77 | 65.8 |
| Missouri | 143 | 54 | 37.8 | 24 | 16.8 | 8 | 5.6 | 51 | 35.7 | 2 | 1.4 | 16 | 11.2 | 58 | 40.6 | 111 | 77.6 |
| Nebraska | 75 | 13 | 17.3 | 6 | 8.0 | 2 | 2.7 | 27 | 36.0 | 2 | 2.7 | 3 | 4.0 | 23 | 30.7 | 56 | 74.7 |
| North Dakota | 32 | 10 | 31.3 | 5 | 15.6 | 3 | 9.4 | 14 | 43.8 | 1 | 3.1 | 1 | 3.1 | 17 | 53.1 | 26 | 81.3 |
| South Dakota | 58 | 13 | 22.4 | 4 | 6.9 | 0 | 0.0 | 19 | 32.8 | 0 | 0.0 | 1 | 1.7 | 19 | 32.8 | 39 | 67.2 |
| CENSUS DIVISION 7, WEST SOUTH CENTRAL | 784 | 233 | 29.7 | 132 | 16.8 | 32 | 4.1 | 179 | 22.8 | 23 | 2.9 | 28 | 3.6 | 260 | 33.2 | 519 | 66.2 |
| Arkansas | 104 | 30 | 28.8 | 15 | 14.4 | 2 | 1.9 | 19 | 18.3 | 3 | 2.9 | 1 | 1.0 | 38 | 36.5 | 78 | 75.0 |
| Louisiana | 111 | 37 | 33.3 | 15 | 13.5 | 8 | 7.2 | 30 | 27.0 | 5 | 4.5 | 8 | 7.2 | 40 | 36.0 | 71 | 64.0 |
| Oklahoma | 108 | 23 | 21.3 | 15 | 13.9 | 3 | 2.8 | 16 | 14.8 | 3 | 2.8 | 2 | 1.9 | 32 | 29.6 | 68 | 63.0 |
| Texas | 461 | 143 | 31.0 | 87 | 18.9 | 19 | 4.1 | 114 | 24.7 | 12 | 2.6 | 17 | 3.7 | 150 | 32.5 | 302 | 65.5 |
| CENSUS DIVISION 8, MOUNTAIN | 320 | 113 | 35.3 | 64 | 20.0 | 15 | 4.7 | 81 | 25.3 | 12 | 3.8 | 17 | 5.3 | 114 | 35.6 | 243 | 75.9 |
| Arizona | 55 | 25 | 45.5 | 16 | 29.1 | 5 | 9.1 | 15 | 27.3 | 4 | 7.3 | 4 | 7.3 | 19 | 34.5 | 39 | 70.9 |
| Colorado | 56 | 26 | 46.4 | 11 | 19.6 | 5 | 8.9 | 27 | 48.2 | 3 | 5.4 | 5 | 8.9 | 25 | 44.6 | 38 | 67.9 |
| Idaho | 30 | 11 | 36.7 | 8 | 26.7 | 0 | 0.0 | 5 | 16.7 | 1 | 3.3 | 1 | 3.3 | 7 | 23.3 | 24 | 80.0 |
| Montana | 54 | 18 | 33.3 | 7 | 13.0 | 1 | 1.9 | 11 | 20.4 | 1 | 1.9 | 2 | 3.7 | 22 | 40.7 | 44 | 81.5 |
| Nevada | 22 | 5 | 22.7 | 3 | 13.6 | 0 | 0.0 | 1 | 4.5 | 1 | 4.5 | 0 | 0.0 | 7 | 31.8 | 16 | 72.7 |
| New Mexico | 34 | 6 | 17.6 | 5 | 14.7 | 1 | 2.9 | 6 | 17.6 | 1 | 2.9 | 1 | 2.9 | 6 | 17.6 | 21 | 61.8 |
| Utah | 41 | 16 | 39.0 | 10 | 24.4 | 3 | 7.3 | 11 | 26.8 | 0 | 0.0 | 4 | 9.8 | 17 | 41.5 | 35 | 85.4 |
| Wyoming | 28 | 6 | 21.4 | 4 | 14.3 | 0 | 0.0 | 5 | 17.9 | 1 | 3.6 | 0 | 0.0 | 11 | 39.3 | 26 | 92.9 |
| CENSUS DIVISION 9, PACIFIC | 576 | 166 | 28.8 | 101 | 17.5 | 27 | 4.7 | 93 | 16.1 | 23 | 4.0 | 42 | 7.3 | 155 | 26.9 | 302 | 52.4 |
| Alaska | 15 | 7 | 46.7 | 2 | 13.3 | 0 | 0.0 | 4 | 26.7 | 0 | 0.0 | 1 | 6.7 | 4 | 26.7 | 14 | 93.3 |
| California | 402 | 93 | 23.1 | 67 | 16.7 | 18 | 4.5 | 53 | 13.2 | 16 | 4.0 | 29 | 7.2 | 90 | 22.4 | 183 | 45.5 |
| Hawaii | 18 | 7 | 38.9 | 5 | 27.8 | 1 | 5.6 | 1 | 5.6 | 1 | 5.6 | 2 | 11.1 | 8 | 44.4 | 6 | 33.3 |
| Oregon | 59 | 29 | 49.2 | 10 | 16.9 | 1 | 1.7 | 18 | 30.5 | 2 | 3.4 | 1 | 1.7 | 27 | 45.8 | 48 | 81.4 |
| Washington | 82 | 30 | 36.6 | 17 | 20.7 | 7 | 8.5 | 17 | 20.7 | 4 | 4.9 | 9 | 11.0 | 26 | 31.7 | 51 | 62.2 |

## Table 7 (Continued)

*These data include only hospital-based facilities and services as reported by responding hospitals in Section C of the 2003 AHA Annual Survey, beginning on page 205. All hospitals are represented with Community Hospitals listed separately under United States. No estimates have been made for nonresponding hospitals. Definitions of facilities and services are listed in the Glossary, page 193.*

| CLASSIFICATION | HOSPITALS REPORTING | HEALTH INFORMATION CENTER | | HEALTH SCREENINGS | | HEMODIALYSIS | | HIV/AIDS SERVICES | | HOME HEALTH SERVICES | | HOSPICE | | INTENSITY-MODULATED RADIATION THERAPHY (IMRT) | | MAGNETIC RESONANCE IMAGING (MRI) | | MEALS ON WHEELS | |
|---|---|---|---|---|---|---|---|---|---|---|---|---|---|---|---|---|---|---|---|
| | | Number | Percent | Number | Percent | Number | Percent | Number | Percent | Number | Percent | Number | Percent | Number | Percent | Number | Percent | Number | Percent |
| **UNITED STATES** | 4,946 | 2,182 | 44.1 | 3,526 | 71.3 | 1,354 | 27.4 | 1,342 | 27.1 | 1,848 | 37.4 | 1,153 | 23.3 | 567 | 11.5 | 2,631 | 53.2 | 633 | 12.8 |
| COMMUNITY HOSPITALS | 4,320 | 2,017 | 46.7 | 3,317 | 76.8 | 1,276 | 29.5 | 1,206 | 27.9 | 1,761 | 40.8 | 1,070 | 24.8 | 553 | 12.8 | 2,543 | 58.9 | 620 | 14.4 |
| **CENSUS DIVISION 1, NEW ENGLAND** | 228 | 137 | 60.1 | 192 | 84.2 | 74 | 32.5 | 107 | 46.9 | 58 | 25.4 | 71 | 31.1 | 29 | 12.7 | 119 | 52.2 | 24 | 10.5 |
| Connecticut | 36 | 26 | 72.2 | 30 | 83.3 | 16 | 44.4 | 23 | 63.9 | 10 | 27.8 | 19 | 52.8 | 11 | 30.6 | 28 | 77.8 | 8 | 22.2 |
| Maine | 39 | 18 | 46.2 | 34 | 87.2 | 8 | 20.5 | 13 | 33.3 | 14 | 35.9 | 8 | 20.5 | 2 | 5.1 | 14 | 35.9 | 4 | 10.3 |
| Massachusetts | 95 | 55 | 57.9 | 76 | 80.0 | 30 | 31.6 | 42 | 44.2 | 24 | 25.3 | 24 | 25.3 | 11 | 11.6 | 45 | 47.4 | 8 | 8.4 |
| New Hampshire | 30 | 20 | 66.7 | 27 | 90.0 | 10 | 33.3 | 17 | 56.7 | 7 | 23.3 | 11 | 36.7 | 4 | 13.3 | 16 | 53.3 | 2 | 6.7 |
| Rhode Island | 12 | 9 | 75.0 | 10 | 83.3 | 8 | 66.7 | 6 | 50.0 | 2 | 16.7 | 3 | 25.0 | 0 | 0.0 | 8 | 66.7 | 1 | 8.3 |
| Vermont | 16 | 9 | 56.3 | 15 | 93.8 | 2 | 12.5 | 6 | 37.5 | 1 | 6.3 | 6 | 37.5 | 1 | 6.3 | 8 | 50.0 | 1 | 6.3 |
| **CENSUS DIVISION 2, MIDDLE ATLANTIC** | 442 | 257 | 58.1 | 371 | 83.9 | 183 | 41.4 | 203 | 45.9 | 159 | 36.0 | 124 | 28.1 | 97 | 21.9 | 270 | 61.1 | 59 | 13.3 |
| New Jersey | 72 | 47 | 65.3 | 61 | 84.7 | 43 | 59.7 | 42 | 58.3 | 24 | 33.3 | 22 | 30.6 | 24 | 33.3 | 45 | 62.5 | 17 | 23.6 |
| New York | 180 | 109 | 60.6 | 150 | 83.3 | 92 | 51.1 | 83 | 46.1 | 47 | 26.1 | 42 | 23.3 | 36 | 20.0 | 110 | 61.1 | 25 | 13.9 |
| Pennsylvania | 190 | 101 | 53.2 | 160 | 84.2 | 48 | 25.3 | 78 | 41.1 | 88 | 46.3 | 60 | 31.6 | 37 | 19.5 | 115 | 60.5 | 17 | 8.9 |
| **CENSUS DIVISION 3, SOUTH ATLANTIC** | 714 | 347 | 48.6 | 572 | 80.1 | 279 | 39.1 | 255 | 35.7 | 231 | 32.4 | 152 | 21.3 | 102 | 14.3 | 452 | 63.3 | 47 | 6.6 |
| Delaware | 8 | 4 | 50.0 | 6 | 75.0 | 6 | 75.0 | 6 | 75.0 | 5 | 62.5 | 0 | 0.0 | 2 | 25.0 | 6 | 75.0 | 0 | 0.0 |
| District of Columbia | 13 | 8 | 61.5 | 10 | 76.9 | 9 | 69.2 | 7 | 53.8 | 3 | 23.1 | 2 | 15.4 | 6 | 46.2 | 8 | 61.5 | 0 | 0.0 |
| Florida | 158 | 75 | 47.5 | 120 | 75.9 | 79 | 50.0 | 56 | 35.4 | 49 | 31.0 | 26 | 16.5 | 24 | 15.2 | 119 | 75.3 | 8 | 5.1 |
| Georgia | 147 | 60 | 40.8 | 112 | 76.2 | 43 | 29.3 | 37 | 25.2 | 29 | 19.7 | 30 | 20.4 | 12 | 8.2 | 76 | 51.7 | 4 | 2.7 |
| Maryland | 61 | 40 | 65.6 | 48 | 78.7 | 33 | 54.1 | 24 | 39.3 | 14 | 23.0 | 10 | 16.4 | 9 | 14.8 | 36 | 59.0 | 4 | 6.6 |
| North Carolina | 111 | 59 | 53.2 | 92 | 82.9 | 38 | 34.2 | 35 | 31.5 | 47 | 42.3 | 26 | 23.4 | 22 | 19.8 | 66 | 59.5 | 13 | 11.7 |
| South Carolina | 67 | 26 | 38.8 | 58 | 86.6 | 24 | 35.8 | 37 | 55.2 | 15 | 22.4 | 13 | 19.4 | 10 | 14.9 | 46 | 68.7 | 5 | 7.5 |
| Virginia | 84 | 47 | 56.0 | 71 | 84.5 | 35 | 41.7 | 38 | 45.2 | 38 | 45.2 | 33 | 39.3 | 13 | 15.5 | 63 | 75.0 | 9 | 10.7 |
| West Virginia | 65 | 28 | 43.1 | 55 | 84.6 | 12 | 18.5 | 15 | 23.1 | 31 | 47.7 | 12 | 18.5 | 4 | 6.2 | 32 | 49.2 | 4 | 6.2 |
| **CENSUS DIVISION 4, EAST NORTH CENTRAL** | 749 | 438 | 58.5 | 599 | 80.0 | 227 | 30.3 | 208 | 27.8 | 307 | 41.0 | 215 | 28.7 | 119 | 15.9 | 437 | 58.3 | 185 | 24.7 |
| Illinois | 186 | 107 | 57.5 | 159 | 85.5 | 61 | 32.8 | 66 | 35.5 | 80 | 43.0 | 60 | 32.3 | 35 | 18.8 | 110 | 59.1 | 51 | 27.4 |
| Indiana | 107 | 53 | 49.5 | 88 | 82.2 | 21 | 19.6 | 21 | 19.6 | 55 | 51.4 | 38 | 35.5 | 12 | 11.2 | 76 | 71.0 | 32 | 29.9 |
| Michigan | 154 | 86 | 55.8 | 126 | 81.8 | 46 | 29.9 | 54 | 35.1 | 63 | 40.9 | 51 | 33.1 | 26 | 16.9 | 70 | 45.5 | 20 | 13.0 |
| Ohio | 161 | 96 | 59.6 | 146 | 90.7 | 66 | 41.0 | 56 | 34.8 | 78 | 48.4 | 49 | 30.4 | 22 | 13.7 | 114 | 70.8 | 36 | 22.4 |
| Wisconsin | 141 | 96 | 68.1 | 80 | 56.7 | 33 | 23.4 | 11 | 7.8 | 31 | 22.0 | 17 | 12.1 | 24 | 17.0 | 67 | 47.5 | 46 | 32.6 |
| **CENSUS DIVISION 5, EAST SOUTH CENTRAL** | 438 | 122 | 27.9 | 236 | 53.9 | 78 | 17.8 | 95 | 21.7 | 155 | 35.4 | 54 | 12.3 | 27 | 6.2 | 221 | 50.5 | 15 | 3.4 |
| Alabama | 97 | 32 | 33.0 | 61 | 62.9 | 28 | 28.9 | 21 | 21.6 | 44 | 45.4 | 15 | 15.5 | 11 | 11.3 | 56 | 57.7 | 6 | 6.2 |
| Kentucky | 102 | 55 | 53.9 | 82 | 80.4 | 17 | 16.7 | 19 | 18.6 | 45 | 44.1 | 16 | 15.7 | 4 | 3.9 | 47 | 46.1 | 6 | 5.9 |
| Mississippi | 104 | 1 | 1.0 | 2 | 1.9 | 1 | 1.0 | 28 | 26.9 | 21 | 20.2 | 1 | 1.0 | 1 | 1.0 | 38 | 36.5 | 2 | 1.9 |
| Tennessee | 135 | 34 | 25.2 | 91 | 67.4 | 32 | 23.7 | 27 | 20.0 | 45 | 33.3 | 22 | 16.3 | 11 | 8.1 | 80 | 59.3 | 1 | 0.7 |
| **CENSUS DIVISION 6, WEST NORTH CENTRAL** | 695 | 276 | 39.7 | 521 | 75.0 | 126 | 18.1 | 151 | 21.7 | 359 | 51.7 | 228 | 32.8 | 48 | 6.9 | 309 | 44.5 | 190 | 27.3 |
| Iowa | 125 | 63 | 50.4 | 115 | 92.0 | 27 | 21.6 | 29 | 23.2 | 72 | 57.6 | 58 | 46.4 | 7 | 5.6 | 57 | 45.6 | 55 | 44.0 |
| Kansas | 145 | 32 | 22.1 | 72 | 49.7 | 11 | 7.6 | 23 | 15.9 | 62 | 42.8 | 24 | 16.6 | 10 | 6.9 | 51 | 35.2 | 41 | 28.3 |
| Minnesota | 117 | 46 | 39.3 | 87 | 74.4 | 18 | 15.4 | 21 | 17.9 | 68 | 58.1 | 53 | 45.3 | 13 | 11.1 | 52 | 44.4 | 35 | 29.9 |
| Missouri | 143 | 80 | 55.9 | 116 | 81.1 | 37 | 25.9 | 53 | 37.1 | 61 | 42.7 | 27 | 18.9 | 11 | 7.7 | 90 | 62.9 | 24 | 16.8 |
| Nebraska | 75 | 21 | 28.0 | 54 | 72.0 | 14 | 18.7 | 10 | 13.3 | 44 | 58.7 | 27 | 36.0 | 3 | 4.0 | 27 | 36.0 | 14 | 18.7 |
| North Dakota | 32 | 16 | 50.0 | 29 | 90.6 | 7 | 21.9 | 6 | 18.8 | 18 | 56.3 | 15 | 46.9 | 3 | 9.4 | 14 | 43.8 | 8 | 25.0 |
| South Dakota | 58 | 18 | 31.0 | 48 | 82.8 | 12 | 20.7 | 9 | 15.5 | 34 | 58.6 | 24 | 41.4 | 1 | 1.7 | 18 | 31.0 | 13 | 22.4 |
| **CENSUS DIVISION 7, WEST SOUTH CENTRAL** | 784 | 253 | 32.3 | 488 | 62.2 | 161 | 20.5 | 133 | 17.0 | 276 | 35.2 | 104 | 13.3 | 44 | 5.6 | 370 | 47.2 | 52 | 6.6 |
| Arkansas | 104 | 30 | 28.8 | 77 | 74.0 | 19 | 18.3 | 16 | 15.4 | 63 | 60.6 | 25 | 24.0 | 1 | 1.0 | 50 | 48.1 | 7 | 6.7 |
| Louisiana | 111 | 39 | 35.1 | 66 | 59.5 | 32 | 28.8 | 23 | 20.7 | 32 | 28.8 | 12 | 10.8 | 9 | 8.1 | 49 | 44.1 | 4 | 3.6 |
| Oklahoma | 108 | 34 | 31.5 | 62 | 57.4 | 19 | 17.6 | 14 | 13.0 | 54 | 50.0 | 19 | 17.6 | 6 | 5.6 | 45 | 41.7 | 19 | 17.6 |
| Texas | 461 | 150 | 32.5 | 283 | 61.4 | 91 | 19.7 | 80 | 17.4 | 127 | 27.5 | 48 | 10.4 | 28 | 6.1 | 226 | 49.0 | 22 | 4.8 |
| **CENSUS DIVISION 8, MOUNTAIN** | 320 | 136 | 42.5 | 229 | 71.6 | 79 | 24.7 | 68 | 21.3 | 127 | 39.7 | 93 | 29.1 | 32 | 10.0 | 187 | 58.4 | 30 | 9.4 |
| Arizona | 55 | 30 | 54.5 | 38 | 69.1 | 25 | 45.5 | 16 | 29.1 | 14 | 25.5 | 11 | 20.0 | 7 | 12.7 | 36 | 65.5 | 6 | 10.9 |
| Colorado | 56 | 28 | 50.0 | 41 | 73.2 | 15 | 26.8 | 14 | 25.0 | 27 | 48.2 | 13 | 23.2 | 11 | 19.6 | 39 | 69.6 | 7 | 12.5 |
| Idaho | 30 | 13 | 43.3 | 21 | 70.0 | 4 | 13.3 | 5 | 16.7 | 16 | 53.3 | 12 | 40.0 | 3 | 10.0 | 14 | 46.7 | 3 | 10.0 |
| Montana | 54 | 17 | 31.5 | 43 | 79.6 | 8 | 14.8 | 9 | 16.7 | 26 | 48.1 | 25 | 46.3 | 1 | 1.9 | 20 | 37.0 | 9 | 16.7 |
| Nevada | 22 | 8 | 36.4 | 16 | 72.7 | 5 | 22.7 | 9 | 40.9 | 7 | 31.8 | 2 | 9.1 | 1 | 4.5 | 15 | 68.2 | 0 | 0.0 |
| New Mexico | 34 | 9 | 26.5 | 21 | 61.8 | 7 | 20.6 | 5 | 14.7 | 11 | 32.4 | 7 | 20.6 | 3 | 8.8 | 18 | 52.9 | 2 | 5.9 |
| Utah | 41 | 24 | 58.5 | 30 | 73.2 | 8 | 19.5 | 7 | 17.1 | 12 | 29.3 | 13 | 31.7 | 4 | 9.8 | 31 | 75.6 | 1 | 2.4 |
| Wyoming | 28 | 7 | 25.0 | 19 | 67.9 | 7 | 25.0 | 3 | 10.7 | 14 | 50.0 | 10 | 35.7 | 2 | 7.1 | 14 | 50.0 | 2 | 7.1 |
| **CENSUS DIVISION 9, PACIFIC** | 576 | 216 | 37.5 | 318 | 55.2 | 147 | 25.5 | 122 | 21.2 | 176 | 30.6 | 112 | 19.4 | 69 | 12.0 | 266 | 46.2 | 31 | 5.4 |
| Alaska | 15 | 6 | 40.0 | 11 | 73.3 | 3 | 20.0 | 2 | 13.3 | 9 | 60.0 | 0 | 0.0 | 0 | 0.0 | 8 | 53.3 | 0 | 0.0 |
| California | 402 | 131 | 32.6 | 187 | 46.5 | 103 | 25.6 | 76 | 18.9 | 95 | 23.6 | 61 | 15.2 | 45 | 11.2 | 171 | 42.5 | 24 | 6.0 |
| Hawaii | 18 | 5 | 27.8 | 11 | 61.1 | 4 | 22.2 | 6 | 33.3 | 5 | 27.8 | 2 | 11.1 | 1 | 5.6 | 10 | 55.6 | 3 | 16.7 |
| Oregon | 59 | 35 | 59.3 | 51 | 86.4 | 13 | 22.0 | 15 | 25.4 | 43 | 72.9 | 28 | 47.5 | 11 | 18.6 | 36 | 61.0 | 1 | 1.7 |
| Washington | 82 | 39 | 47.6 | 58 | 70.7 | 24 | 29.3 | 23 | 28.0 | 24 | 29.3 | 21 | 25.6 | 12 | 14.6 | 41 | 50.0 | 3 | 3.7 |

## Table 7 (Continued)

*These data include only hospital-based facilities and services as reported by responding hospitals in Section C of the 2003 AHA Annual Survey, beginning on page 205. All hospitals are represented with Community Hospitals listed separately under United States. No estimates have been made for nonresponding hospitals. Definitions of facilities and services are listed in the Glossary, page 193.*

| CLASSIFICATION | HOSPITALS REPORTING | MULTISLICE SPIRAL COMPUTED TOMOGRAPHY (MSCT) | | NEUROLOGICAL SERVICES | | NUTRITION PROGRAMS CENTER | | OCCUPATIONAL HEALTH SERVICES | | ONCOLOGY SERVICES | | OPEN HEART SURGERY | | ORTHOPEDIC SERVICES | | OUTPATIENT CARE CENTER (FREESTANDING) | |
|---|---|---|---|---|---|---|---|---|---|---|---|---|---|---|---|---|---|
| | | Number | Percent | Number | Percent | Number | Percent | Number | Percent | Number | Percent | Number | Percent | Number | Percent | Number | Percent |
| UNITED STATES | 4,946 | 1,302 | 26.3 | 1,951 | 39.4 | 3,474 | 70.2 | 3,061 | 61.9 | 2,589 | 52.3 | 1,011 | 20.4 | 2,938 | 59.4 | 1,289 | 26.1 |
| COMMUNITY HOSPITALS | 4,320 | 1,255 | 29.1 | 1,811 | 41.9 | 3,178 | 73.6 | 2,839 | 65.7 | 2,482 | 57.5 | 978 | 22.6 | 2,799 | 64.8 | 1,156 | 26.8 |
| CENSUS DIVISION 1, NEW ENGLAND | 228 | 73 | 32.0 | 118 | 51.8 | 195 | 85.5 | 170 | 74.6 | 173 | 75.9 | 34 | 14.9 | 154 | 67.5 | 79 | 34.6 |
| Connecticut | 36 | 20 | 55.6 | 27 | 75.0 | 32 | 88.9 | 25 | 69.4 | 28 | 77.8 | 8 | 22.2 | 28 | 77.8 | 16 | 44.4 |
| Maine | 39 | 7 | 17.9 | 13 | 33.3 | 35 | 89.7 | 30 | 76.9 | 31 | 79.5 | 3 | 7.7 | 29 | 74.4 | 13 | 33.3 |
| Massachusetts | 95 | 30 | 31.6 | 50 | 52.6 | 75 | 78.9 | 65 | 68.4 | 71 | 74.7 | 16 | 16.8 | 56 | 58.9 | 34 | 35.8 |
| New Hampshire | 30 | 11 | 36.7 | 16 | 53.3 | 29 | 96.7 | 28 | 93.3 | 23 | 76.7 | 4 | 13.3 | 24 | 80.0 | 10 | 33.3 |
| Rhode Island | 12 | 2 | 16.7 | 8 | 66.7 | 10 | 83.3 | 7 | 58.3 | 10 | 83.3 | 2 | 16.7 | 7 | 58.3 | 2 | 16.7 |
| Vermont | 16 | 3 | 18.8 | 4 | 25.0 | 14 | 87.5 | 15 | 93.8 | 10 | 62.5 | 1 | 6.3 | 10 | 62.5 | 4 | 25.0 |
| CENSUS DIVISION 2, MIDDLE ATLANTIC | 442 | 154 | 34.8 | 264 | 59.7 | 378 | 85.5 | 320 | 72.4 | 310 | 70.1 | 91 | 20.6 | 344 | 77.8 | 190 | 43.0 |
| New Jersey | 72 | 30 | 41.7 | 49 | 68.1 | 61 | 84.7 | 53 | 73.6 | 58 | 80.6 | 10 | 13.9 | 57 | 79.2 | 25 | 34.7 |
| New York | 180 | 57 | 31.7 | 106 | 58.9 | 149 | 82.8 | 126 | 70.0 | 119 | 66.1 | 29 | 16.1 | 138 | 76.7 | 94 | 52.2 |
| Pennsylvania | 190 | 67 | 35.3 | 109 | 57.4 | 168 | 88.4 | 141 | 74.2 | 133 | 70.0 | 52 | 27.4 | 149 | 78.4 | 71 | 37.4 |
| CENSUS DIVISION 3, SOUTH ATLANTIC | 714 | 261 | 36.6 | 359 | 50.3 | 532 | 74.5 | 479 | 67.1 | 401 | 56.2 | 149 | 20.9 | 517 | 72.4 | 230 | 32.2 |
| Delaware | 8 | 4 | 50.0 | 6 | 75.0 | 7 | 87.5 | 6 | 75.0 | 6 | 75.0 | 3 | 37.5 | 7 | 87.5 | 4 | 50.0 |
| District of Columbia | 13 | 6 | 46.2 | 10 | 76.9 | 11 | 84.6 | 9 | 69.2 | 9 | 69.2 | 6 | 46.2 | 11 | 84.6 | 6 | 46.2 |
| Florida | 158 | 61 | 38.6 | 94 | 59.5 | 123 | 77.8 | 105 | 66.5 | 104 | 65.8 | 51 | 32.3 | 120 | 75.9 | 57 | 36.1 |
| Georgia | 147 | 43 | 29.3 | 57 | 38.8 | 99 | 67.3 | 93 | 63.3 | 59 | 40.1 | 19 | 12.9 | 86 | 58.5 | 42 | 28.6 |
| Maryland | 61 | 25 | 41.0 | 41 | 67.2 | 48 | 78.7 | 46 | 75.4 | 43 | 70.5 | 9 | 14.8 | 51 | 83.6 | 25 | 41.0 |
| North Carolina | 111 | 45 | 40.5 | 56 | 50.5 | 82 | 73.9 | 80 | 72.1 | 72 | 64.9 | 21 | 18.9 | 86 | 77.5 | 35 | 31.5 |
| South Carolina | 67 | 26 | 38.8 | 20 | 29.9 | 44 | 65.7 | 44 | 65.7 | 22 | 32.8 | 16 | 23.9 | 47 | 70.1 | 20 | 29.9 |
| Virginia | 84 | 36 | 42.9 | 52 | 61.9 | 69 | 82.1 | 57 | 67.9 | 54 | 64.3 | 19 | 22.6 | 71 | 84.5 | 26 | 31.0 |
| West Virginia | 65 | 15 | 23.1 | 23 | 35.4 | 49 | 75.4 | 39 | 60.0 | 32 | 49.2 | 5 | 7.7 | 38 | 58.5 | 15 | 23.1 |
| CENSUS DIVISION 4, EAST NORTH CENTRAL | 749 | 240 | 32.0 | 372 | 49.7 | 622 | 83.0 | 548 | 73.2 | 506 | 67.6 | 186 | 24.8 | 535 | 71.4 | 254 | 33.9 |
| Illinois | 186 | 76 | 40.9 | 108 | 58.1 | 152 | 81.7 | 128 | 68.8 | 130 | 69.9 | 59 | 31.7 | 132 | 71.0 | 58 | 31.2 |
| Indiana | 107 | 37 | 34.6 | 46 | 43.0 | 85 | 79.4 | 79 | 73.8 | 70 | 65.4 | 22 | 20.6 | 79 | 73.8 | 30 | 28.0 |
| Michigan | 154 | 38 | 24.7 | 78 | 50.6 | 127 | 82.5 | 117 | 76.0 | 95 | 61.7 | 32 | 20.8 | 111 | 72.1 | 54 | 35.1 |
| Ohio | 161 | 66 | 41.0 | 89 | 55.3 | 139 | 86.3 | 130 | 80.7 | 122 | 75.8 | 46 | 28.6 | 135 | 83.9 | 61 | 37.9 |
| Wisconsin | 141 | 23 | 16.3 | 51 | 36.2 | 119 | 84.4 | 94 | 66.7 | 89 | 63.1 | 27 | 19.1 | 78 | 55.3 | 51 | 36.2 |
| CENSUS DIVISION 5, EAST SOUTH CENTRAL | 438 | 74 | 16.9 | 121 | 27.6 | 253 | 57.8 | 216 | 49.3 | 177 | 40.4 | 76 | 17.4 | 186 | 42.5 | 52 | 11.9 |
| Alabama | 97 | 14 | 14.4 | 39 | 40.2 | 53 | 54.6 | 43 | 44.3 | 46 | 47.4 | 21 | 21.6 | 53 | 54.6 | 13 | 13.4 |
| Kentucky | 102 | 35 | 34.3 | 43 | 42.2 | 81 | 79.4 | 60 | 58.8 | 50 | 49.0 | 19 | 18.6 | 65 | 63.7 | 16 | 15.7 |
| Mississippi | 104 | 1 | 1.0 | 2 | 1.9 | 36 | 34.6 | 30 | 28.8 | 28 | 26.9 | 17 | 16.3 | 3 | 2.9 | 0 | 0.0 |
| Tennessee | 135 | 24 | 17.8 | 37 | 27.4 | 83 | 61.5 | 83 | 61.5 | 53 | 39.3 | 19 | 14.1 | 65 | 48.1 | 23 | 17.0 |
| CENSUS DIVISION 6, WEST NORTH CENTRAL | 695 | 136 | 19.6 | 174 | 25.0 | 476 | 68.5 | 438 | 63.0 | 332 | 47.8 | 96 | 13.8 | 339 | 48.8 | 108 | 15.5 |
| Iowa | 125 | 37 | 29.6 | 28 | 22.4 | 108 | 86.4 | 92 | 73.6 | 76 | 60.8 | 12 | 9.6 | 64 | 51.2 | 16 | 12.8 |
| Kansas | 145 | 18 | 12.4 | 27 | 18.6 | 71 | 49.0 | 72 | 49.7 | 51 | 35.2 | 13 | 9.0 | 60 | 41.4 | 16 | 11.0 |
| Minnesota | 117 | 25 | 21.4 | 26 | 22.2 | 79 | 67.5 | 87 | 74.4 | 59 | 50.4 | 13 | 11.1 | 63 | 53.8 | 18 | 15.4 |
| Missouri | 143 | 31 | 21.7 | 60 | 42.0 | 112 | 78.3 | 94 | 65.7 | 72 | 50.3 | 38 | 26.6 | 93 | 65.0 | 38 | 26.6 |
| Nebraska | 75 | 12 | 16.0 | 17 | 22.7 | 52 | 69.3 | 44 | 58.7 | 43 | 57.3 | 10 | 13.3 | 36 | 48.0 | 10 | 13.3 |
| North Dakota | 32 | 8 | 25.0 | 9 | 28.1 | 23 | 71.9 | 20 | 62.5 | 15 | 46.9 | 6 | 18.8 | 8 | 25.0 | 3 | 9.4 |
| South Dakota | 58 | 5 | 8.6 | 7 | 12.1 | 31 | 53.4 | 29 | 50.0 | 16 | 27.6 | 4 | 6.9 | 15 | 25.9 | 7 | 12.1 |
| CENSUS DIVISION 7, WEST SOUTH CENTRAL | 784 | 158 | 20.2 | 232 | 29.6 | 479 | 61.1 | 394 | 50.3 | 288 | 36.7 | 174 | 22.2 | 382 | 48.7 | 168 | 21.4 |
| Arkansas | 104 | 21 | 20.2 | 30 | 28.8 | 67 | 64.4 | 51 | 49.0 | 42 | 40.4 | 22 | 21.2 | 54 | 51.9 | 20 | 19.2 |
| Louisiana | 111 | 19 | 17.1 | 37 | 33.3 | 64 | 57.7 | 58 | 52.3 | 44 | 39.6 | 28 | 25.2 | 53 | 47.7 | 26 | 23.4 |
| Oklahoma | 108 | 21 | 19.4 | 28 | 25.9 | 64 | 59.3 | 60 | 55.6 | 38 | 35.2 | 16 | 14.8 | 55 | 50.9 | 20 | 18.5 |
| Texas | 461 | 97 | 21.0 | 137 | 29.7 | 284 | 61.6 | 225 | 48.8 | 164 | 35.6 | 108 | 23.4 | 220 | 47.7 | 102 | 22.1 |
| CENSUS DIVISION 8, MOUNTAIN | 320 | 82 | 25.6 | 115 | 35.9 | 226 | 70.6 | 199 | 62.2 | 144 | 45.0 | 68 | 21.3 | 186 | 58.1 | 80 | 25.0 |
| Arizona | 55 | 20 | 36.4 | 31 | 56.4 | 43 | 78.2 | 40 | 72.7 | 31 | 56.4 | 17 | 30.9 | 38 | 69.1 | 18 | 32.7 |
| Colorado | 56 | 21 | 37.5 | 28 | 50.0 | 44 | 78.6 | 43 | 76.8 | 36 | 64.3 | 18 | 32.1 | 44 | 78.6 | 20 | 35.7 |
| Idaho | 30 | 7 | 23.3 | 8 | 26.7 | 25 | 83.3 | 23 | 76.7 | 12 | 40.0 | 4 | 13.3 | 17 | 56.7 | 9 | 30.0 |
| Montana | 54 | 8 | 14.8 | 10 | 18.5 | 27 | 50.0 | 31 | 57.4 | 17 | 31.5 | 5 | 9.3 | 23 | 42.6 | 4 | 7.4 |
| Nevada | 22 | 2 | 9.1 | 9 | 40.9 | 14 | 63.6 | 12 | 54.5 | 12 | 54.5 | 7 | 31.8 | 9 | 40.9 | 10 | 45.5 |
| New Mexico | 34 | 7 | 20.6 | 9 | 26.5 | 21 | 61.8 | 13 | 38.2 | 11 | 32.4 | 6 | 17.6 | 13 | 38.2 | 5 | 14.7 |
| Utah | 41 | 12 | 29.3 | 15 | 36.6 | 30 | 73.2 | 20 | 48.8 | 15 | 36.6 | 9 | 22.0 | 23 | 56.1 | 12 | 29.3 |
| Wyoming | 28 | 5 | 17.9 | 5 | 17.9 | 22 | 78.6 | 17 | 60.7 | 10 | 35.7 | 2 | 7.1 | 19 | 67.9 | 2 | 7.1 |
| CENSUS DIVISION 9, PACIFIC | 576 | 124 | 21.5 | 196 | 34.0 | 313 | 54.3 | 297 | 51.6 | 258 | 44.8 | 137 | 23.8 | 295 | 51.2 | 128 | 22.2 |
| Alaska | 15 | 6 | 40.0 | 5 | 33.3 | 11 | 73.3 | 10 | 66.7 | 7 | 46.7 | 2 | 13.3 | 8 | 53.3 | 2 | 13.3 |
| California | 402 | 69 | 17.2 | 130 | 32.3 | 183 | 45.5 | 184 | 45.8 | 167 | 41.5 | 99 | 24.6 | 191 | 47.5 | 79 | 19.7 |
| Hawaii | 18 | 6 | 33.3 | 6 | 33.3 | 12 | 66.7 | 12 | 66.7 | 9 | 50.0 | 4 | 22.2 | 9 | 50.0 | 5 | 27.8 |
| Oregon | 59 | 18 | 30.5 | 24 | 40.7 | 50 | 84.7 | 40 | 67.8 | 31 | 52.5 | 10 | 16.9 | 36 | 61.0 | 19 | 32.2 |
| Washington | 82 | 25 | 30.5 | 31 | 37.8 | 57 | 69.5 | 51 | 62.2 | 44 | 53.7 | 22 | 26.8 | 51 | 62.2 | 23 | 28.0 |

## Table 7 (Continued)

*These data include only hospital-based facilities and services as reported by responding hospitals in Section C of the 2003 AHA Annual Survey, beginning on page 205. All hospitals are represented with Community Hospitals listed separately under United States. No estimates have been made for nonresponding hospitals. Definitions of facilities and services are listed in the Glossary, page 193.*

| CLASSIFICATION | HOSPITALS REPORTING | OUTPATIENT CARE CENTER SERVICES (HOSPITAL BASED) | | OUTPATIENT SURGERY | | PAIN MANAGEMENT PROGRAM | | PALLIATIVE CARE PROGRAM | | PATIENT EDUCATION CENTER | | PATIENT REPRESENTATIVE SERVICES | | PHYSICAL REHABILITATION OUTPATIENT SERVICES | | POSITRON EMISSION TOMOGRAPHY (PET) | | PRIMARY CARE DEPARTMENT | |
|---|---|---|---|---|---|---|---|---|---|---|---|---|---|---|---|---|---|---|---|
| | | Number | Percent | Number | Percent | Number | Percent | Number | Percent | Number | Percent | Number | Percent | Number | Percent | Number | Percent | Number | Percent |
| UNITED STATES | 4,946 | 3,518 | 71.1 | 3,998 | 80.8 | 2,257 | 45.6 | 1,098 | 22.2 | 2,791 | 56.4 | 3,101 | 62.7 | 3,746 | 75.7 | 710 | 14.4 | 1,772 | 35.8 |
| COMMUNITY HOSPITALS | 4,320 | 3,284 | 76.0 | 3,834 | 88.8 | 2,077 | 48.1 | 979 | 22.7 | 2,526 | 58.5 | 2,798 | 64.8 | 3,548 | 82.1 | 694 | 16.1 | 1,617 | 37.4 |
| CENSUS DIVISION 1, NEW ENGLAND | 228 | 184 | 80.7 | 187 | 82.0 | 148 | 64.9 | 85 | 37.3 | 148 | 64.9 | 165 | 72.4 | 189 | 82.9 | 52 | 22.8 | 110 | 48.2 |
| Connecticut | 36 | 33 | 91.7 | 30 | 83.3 | 26 | 72.2 | 16 | 44.4 | 28 | 77.8 | 30 | 83.3 | 29 | 80.6 | 20 | 55.6 | 20 | 55.6 |
| Maine | 39 | 30 | 76.9 | 35 | 89.7 | 21 | 53.8 | 15 | 38.5 | 22 | 56.4 | 25 | 64.1 | 34 | 87.2 | 5 | 12.8 | 17 | 43.6 |
| Massachusetts | 95 | 73 | 76.8 | 70 | 73.7 | 62 | 65.3 | 25 | 26.3 | 56 | 58.9 | 68 | 71.6 | 75 | 78.9 | 16 | 16.8 | 38 | 40.0 |
| New Hampshire | 30 | 24 | 80.0 | 27 | 90.0 | 22 | 73.3 | 15 | 50.0 | 20 | 66.7 | 23 | 76.7 | 29 | 96.7 | 8 | 26.7 | 18 | 60.0 |
| Rhode Island | 12 | 9 | 75.0 | 11 | 91.7 | 6 | 50.0 | 3 | 25.0 | 9 | 75.0 | 6 | 50.0 | 8 | 66.7 | 1 | 8.3 | 8 | 66.7 |
| Vermont | 16 | 15 | 93.8 | 14 | 87.5 | 11 | 68.8 | 11 | 68.8 | 13 | 81.3 | 13 | 81.3 | 14 | 87.5 | 2 | 12.5 | 9 | 56.3 |
| CENSUS DIVISION 2, MIDDLE ATLANTIC | 442 | 360 | 81.4 | 378 | 85.5 | 305 | 69.0 | 148 | 33.5 | 309 | 69.9 | 350 | 79.2 | 373 | 84.4 | 95 | 21.5 | 237 | 53.6 |
| New Jersey | 72 | 58 | 80.6 | 63 | 87.5 | 55 | 76.4 | 31 | 43.1 | 60 | 83.3 | 66 | 91.7 | 63 | 87.5 | 17 | 23.6 | 43 | 59.7 |
| New York | 180 | 146 | 81.1 | 154 | 85.6 | 122 | 67.8 | 58 | 32.2 | 123 | 68.3 | 144 | 80.0 | 151 | 83.9 | 35 | 19.4 | 119 | 66.1 |
| Pennsylvania | 190 | 156 | 82.1 | 161 | 84.7 | 128 | 67.4 | 59 | 31.1 | 126 | 66.3 | 140 | 73.7 | 159 | 83.7 | 43 | 22.6 | 75 | 39.5 |
| CENSUS DIVISION 3, SOUTH ATLANTIC | 714 | 535 | 74.9 | 606 | 84.9 | 380 | 53.2 | 179 | 25.1 | 470 | 65.8 | 496 | 69.5 | 565 | 79.1 | 154 | 21.6 | 243 | 34.0 |
| Delaware | 8 | 7 | 87.5 | 7 | 87.5 | 5 | 62.5 | 2 | 25.0 | 5 | 62.5 | 7 | 87.5 | 7 | 87.5 | 2 | 25.0 | 5 | 62.5 |
| District of Columbia | 13 | 11 | 84.6 | 9 | 69.2 | 8 | 61.5 | 8 | 61.5 | 9 | 69.2 | 12 | 92.3 | 11 | 84.6 | 5 | 38.5 | 7 | 53.8 |
| Florida | 158 | 120 | 75.9 | 140 | 88.6 | 94 | 59.5 | 34 | 21.5 | 97 | 61.4 | 99 | 62.7 | 122 | 77.2 | 38 | 24.1 | 53 | 33.5 |
| Georgia | 147 | 96 | 65.3 | 121 | 82.3 | 65 | 44.2 | 23 | 15.6 | 85 | 57.8 | 96 | 65.3 | 110 | 74.8 | 29 | 19.7 | 44 | 29.9 |
| Maryland | 61 | 47 | 77.0 | 49 | 80.3 | 43 | 70.5 | 23 | 37.7 | 39 | 63.9 | 50 | 82.0 | 46 | 75.4 | 12 | 19.7 | 22 | 36.1 |
| North Carolina | 111 | 85 | 76.6 | 100 | 90.1 | 64 | 57.7 | 37 | 33.3 | 70 | 63.1 | 76 | 68.5 | 97 | 87.4 | 16 | 14.4 | 37 | 33.3 |
| South Carolina | 67 | 54 | 80.6 | 56 | 83.6 | 29 | 43.3 | 3 | 4.5 | 61 | 91.0 | 46 | 68.7 | 50 | 74.6 | 14 | 20.9 | 18 | 26.9 |
| Virginia | 84 | 62 | 73.8 | 71 | 84.5 | 52 | 61.9 | 27 | 32.1 | 62 | 73.8 | 70 | 83.3 | 71 | 84.5 | 24 | 28.6 | 28 | 33.3 |
| West Virginia | 65 | 53 | 81.5 | 53 | 81.5 | 20 | 30.8 | 22 | 33.8 | 42 | 64.6 | 40 | 61.5 | 51 | 78.5 | 14 | 21.5 | 29 | 44.6 |
| CENSUS DIVISION 4, EAST NORTH CENTRAL | 749 | 622 | 83.0 | 658 | 87.9 | 419 | 55.9 | 181 | 24.2 | 530 | 70.8 | 551 | 73.6 | 629 | 84.0 | 141 | 18.8 | 365 | 48.7 |
| Illinois | 186 | 151 | 81.2 | 171 | 91.9 | 112 | 60.2 | 53 | 28.5 | 115 | 61.8 | 127 | 68.3 | 162 | 87.1 | 44 | 23.7 | 87 | 46.8 |
| Indiana | 107 | 79 | 73.8 | 90 | 84.1 | 52 | 48.6 | 26 | 24.3 | 63 | 58.9 | 73 | 68.2 | 86 | 80.4 | 24 | 22.4 | 49 | 45.8 |
| Michigan | 154 | 123 | 79.9 | 129 | 83.8 | 90 | 58.4 | 50 | 32.5 | 105 | 68.2 | 113 | 73.4 | 128 | 83.1 | 19 | 12.3 | 87 | 56.5 |
| Ohio | 161 | 136 | 84.5 | 147 | 91.3 | 99 | 61.5 | 52 | 32.3 | 116 | 72.0 | 132 | 82.0 | 142 | 88.2 | 37 | 23.0 | 82 | 50.9 |
| Wisconsin | 141 | 133 | 94.3 | 121 | 85.8 | 66 | 46.8 | 0 | 0.0 | 131 | 92.9 | 106 | 75.2 | 111 | 78.7 | 17 | 12.1 | 60 | 42.6 |
| CENSUS DIVISION 5, EAST SOUTH CENTRAL | 438 | 224 | 51.1 | 340 | 77.6 | 118 | 26.9 | 47 | 10.7 | 219 | 50.0 | 268 | 61.2 | 314 | 71.7 | 51 | 11.6 | 106 | 24.2 |
| Alabama | 97 | 66 | 68.0 | 75 | 77.3 | 34 | 35.1 | 14 | 14.4 | 44 | 45.4 | 52 | 53.6 | 68 | 70.1 | 10 | 10.3 | 20 | 20.6 |
| Kentucky | 102 | 79 | 77.5 | 89 | 87.3 | 40 | 39.2 | 15 | 14.7 | 57 | 55.9 | 69 | 67.6 | 81 | 79.4 | 16 | 15.7 | 34 | 33.3 |
| Mississippi | 104 | 1 | 1.0 | 72 | 69.2 | 3 | 2.9 | 0 | 0.0 | 48 | 46.2 | 64 | 61.5 | 60 | 57.7 | 11 | 10.6 | 21 | 20.2 |
| Tennessee | 135 | 78 | 57.8 | 104 | 77.0 | 41 | 30.4 | 18 | 13.3 | 70 | 51.9 | 83 | 61.5 | 105 | 77.8 | 14 | 10.4 | 31 | 23.0 |
| CENSUS DIVISION 6, WEST NORTH CENTRAL | 695 | 530 | 76.3 | 609 | 87.6 | 267 | 38.4 | 150 | 21.6 | 359 | 51.7 | 367 | 52.8 | 558 | 80.3 | 70 | 10.1 | 242 | 34.8 |
| Iowa | 125 | 106 | 84.8 | 116 | 92.8 | 47 | 37.6 | 26 | 20.8 | 71 | 56.8 | 62 | 49.6 | 103 | 82.4 | 12 | 9.6 | 54 | 43.2 |
| Kansas | 145 | 89 | 61.4 | 118 | 81.4 | 38 | 26.2 | 27 | 18.6 | 51 | 35.2 | 59 | 40.7 | 114 | 78.6 | 7 | 4.8 | 36 | 24.8 |
| Minnesota | 117 | 99 | 84.6 | 112 | 95.7 | 45 | 38.5 | 29 | 24.8 | 61 | 52.1 | 67 | 57.3 | 104 | 88.9 | 16 | 13.7 | 39 | 33.3 |
| Missouri | 143 | 116 | 81.1 | 115 | 80.4 | 74 | 51.7 | 38 | 26.6 | 91 | 63.6 | 109 | 76.2 | 111 | 77.6 | 20 | 14.0 | 55 | 38.5 |
| Nebraska | 75 | 57 | 76.0 | 71 | 94.7 | 25 | 33.3 | 8 | 10.7 | 39 | 52.0 | 34 | 45.3 | 57 | 76.0 | 7 | 9.3 | 19 | 25.3 |
| North Dakota | 32 | 22 | 68.8 | 31 | 96.9 | 16 | 50.0 | 15 | 46.9 | 17 | 53.1 | 16 | 50.0 | 27 | 84.4 | 4 | 12.5 | 17 | 53.1 |
| South Dakota | 58 | 41 | 70.7 | 46 | 79.3 | 22 | 37.9 | 7 | 12.1 | 29 | 50.0 | 20 | 34.5 | 42 | 72.4 | 4 | 6.9 | 22 | 37.9 |
| CENSUS DIVISION 7, WEST SOUTH CENTRAL | 784 | 513 | 65.4 | 570 | 72.7 | 274 | 34.9 | 96 | 12.2 | 358 | 45.7 | 436 | 55.6 | 545 | 69.5 | 49 | 6.3 | 203 | 25.9 |
| Arkansas | 104 | 76 | 73.1 | 80 | 76.9 | 32 | 30.8 | 11 | 10.6 | 42 | 40.4 | 53 | 51.0 | 77 | 74.0 | 2 | 1.9 | 27 | 26.0 |
| Louisiana | 111 | 65 | 58.6 | 79 | 71.2 | 32 | 28.8 | 19 | 17.1 | 49 | 44.1 | 65 | 58.6 | 70 | 63.1 | 9 | 8.1 | 34 | 30.6 |
| Oklahoma | 108 | 67 | 62.0 | 84 | 77.8 | 40 | 37.0 | 15 | 13.9 | 40 | 37.0 | 54 | 50.0 | 75 | 69.4 | 7 | 6.5 | 31 | 28.7 |
| Texas | 461 | 305 | 66.2 | 327 | 70.9 | 170 | 36.9 | 51 | 11.1 | 227 | 49.2 | 264 | 57.3 | 323 | 70.1 | 31 | 6.7 | 111 | 24.1 |
| CENSUS DIVISION 8, MOUNTAIN | 320 | 221 | 69.1 | 269 | 84.1 | 144 | 45.0 | 85 | 26.6 | 158 | 49.4 | 190 | 59.4 | 246 | 76.9 | 33 | 10.3 | 122 | 38.1 |
| Arizona | 55 | 42 | 76.4 | 48 | 87.3 | 30 | 54.5 | 19 | 34.5 | 28 | 50.9 | 40 | 72.7 | 44 | 80.0 | 8 | 14.5 | 18 | 32.7 |
| Colorado | 56 | 46 | 82.1 | 52 | 92.9 | 32 | 57.1 | 16 | 28.6 | 34 | 60.7 | 46 | 82.1 | 50 | 89.3 | 7 | 12.5 | 34 | 60.7 |
| Idaho | 30 | 21 | 70.0 | 27 | 90.0 | 14 | 46.7 | 9 | 30.0 | 15 | 50.0 | 18 | 60.0 | 22 | 73.3 | 3 | 10.0 | 8 | 26.7 |
| Montana | 54 | 34 | 63.0 | 38 | 70.4 | 22 | 40.7 | 16 | 29.6 | 20 | 37.0 | 19 | 35.2 | 45 | 83.3 | 2 | 3.7 | 21 | 38.9 |
| Nevada | 22 | 14 | 63.6 | 16 | 72.7 | 7 | 31.8 | 3 | 13.6 | 9 | 40.9 | 12 | 54.5 | 16 | 72.7 | 4 | 18.2 | 9 | 40.9 |
| New Mexico | 34 | 21 | 61.8 | 27 | 79.4 | 10 | 29.4 | 7 | 20.6 | 10 | 29.4 | 17 | 50.0 | 25 | 73.5 | 1 | 2.9 | 7 | 20.6 |
| Utah | 41 | 26 | 63.4 | 37 | 90.2 | 21 | 51.2 | 11 | 26.8 | 26 | 63.4 | 23 | 56.1 | 26 | 63.4 | 7 | 17.1 | 15 | 36.6 |
| Wyoming | 28 | 17 | 60.7 | 24 | 85.7 | 8 | 28.6 | 4 | 14.3 | 16 | 57.1 | 15 | 53.6 | 18 | 64.3 | 1 | 3.6 | 10 | 35.7 |
| CENSUS DIVISION 9, PACIFIC | 576 | 329 | 57.1 | 381 | 66.1 | 202 | 35.1 | 127 | 22.0 | 240 | 41.7 | 278 | 48.3 | 327 | 56.8 | 65 | 11.3 | 144 | 25.0 |
| Alaska | 15 | 11 | 73.3 | 13 | 86.7 | 7 | 46.7 | 2 | 13.3 | 5 | 33.3 | 7 | 46.7 | 13 | 86.7 | 0 | 0.0 | 5 | 33.3 |
| California | 402 | 198 | 49.3 | 231 | 57.5 | 118 | 29.4 | 73 | 18.2 | 146 | 36.3 | 170 | 42.3 | 196 | 48.8 | 46 | 11.4 | 73 | 18.2 |
| Hawaii | 18 | 10 | 55.6 | 10 | 55.6 | 10 | 55.6 | 4 | 22.2 | 5 | 27.8 | 10 | 55.6 | 12 | 66.7 | 1 | 5.6 | 4 | 22.2 |
| Oregon | 59 | 50 | 84.7 | 57 | 96.6 | 30 | 50.8 | 21 | 35.6 | 39 | 66.1 | 39 | 66.1 | 50 | 84.7 | 5 | 8.5 | 25 | 42.4 |
| Washington | 82 | 60 | 73.2 | 70 | 85.4 | 37 | 45.1 | 27 | 32.9 | 45 | 54.9 | 52 | 63.4 | 56 | 68.3 | 13 | 15.9 | 37 | 45.1 |

## Table 7 (Continued)

*These data include only hospital-based facilities and services as reported by responding hospitals in Section C of the 2003 AHA Annual Survey, beginning on page 205. All hospitals are represented with Community Hospitals listed separately under United States. No estimates have been made for nonresponding hospitals. Definitions of facilities and services are listed in the Glossary, page 193.*

| CLASSIFICATION | HOSPITALS REPORTING | PSYCHIATRIC CHILD/ADOLESCENT SERVICES | | PSYCHIATRIC CONSULTATION/ LIAISON SERVICES | | PSYCHIATRIC EDUCATION SERVICES | | PSYCHIATRIC EMERGENCY SERVICES | | PSYCHIATRIC GERIATRIC SERVICES | | PSYCHIATRIC OUTPATIENT SERVICES | | PSYCHIATRIC PARTIAL HOSPITILIZATION PROGRAM | | RADIATION THERAPY | | RETIREMENT HOUSING | | SLEEP CENTER | |
|---|---|---|---|---|---|---|---|---|---|---|---|---|---|---|---|---|---|---|---|---|---|
| | | Number | Percent | Number | Percent | Number | Percent | Number | Percent | Number | Percent | Number | Percent | Number | Percent | Number | Percent | Number | Percent | Number | Percent |
| **UNITED STATES** | 4,946 | 936 | 18.9 | 1,589 | 32.1 | 1,243 | 25.1 | 1,671 | 33.8 | 1,505 | 30.4 | 1,327 | 26.8 | 941 | 19.0 | 1,227 | 24.8 | 184 | 3.7 | 1,862 | 37.6 |
| COMMUNITY HOSPITALS | 4,320 | 707 | 16.4 | 1,306 | 30.2 | 950 | 22.0 | 1,417 | 32.8 | 1,215 | 28.1 | 1,057 | 24.5 | 743 | 17.2 | 1,185 | 27.4 | 179 | 4.1 | 1,785 | 41.3 |
| **CENSUS DIVISION 1, NEW ENGLAND** | 228 | 76 | 33.3 | 123 | 53.9 | 94 | 41.2 | 112 | 49.1 | 113 | 49.6 | 115 | 50.4 | 91 | 39.9 | 71 | 31.1 | 10 | 4.4 | 114 | 50.0 |
| Connecticut | 36 | 20 | 55.6 | 28 | 77.8 | 27 | 75.0 | 27 | 75.0 | 28 | 77.8 | 27 | 75.0 | 21 | 58.3 | 20 | 55.6 | 3 | 8.3 | 24 | 66.7 |
| Maine | 39 | 8 | 20.5 | 14 | 35.9 | 8 | 20.5 | 15 | 38.5 | 11 | 28.2 | 15 | 38.5 | 10 | 25.6 | 6 | 15.4 | 3 | 7.7 | 16 | 41.0 |
| Massachusetts | 95 | 31 | 32.6 | 48 | 50.5 | 37 | 38.9 | 41 | 43.2 | 45 | 47.4 | 43 | 45.3 | 38 | 40.0 | 33 | 34.7 | 1 | 1.1 | 43 | 45.3 |
| New Hampshire | 30 | 10 | 33.3 | 16 | 53.3 | 10 | 33.3 | 14 | 46.7 | 15 | 50.0 | 13 | 43.3 | 9 | 30.0 | 6 | 20.0 | 1 | 3.3 | 16 | 53.3 |
| Rhode Island | 12 | 2 | 16.7 | 8 | 66.7 | 5 | 41.7 | 8 | 66.7 | 7 | 58.3 | 7 | 58.3 | 6 | 50.0 | 3 | 25.0 | 1 | 8.3 | 8 | 66.7 |
| Vermont | 16 | 5 | 31.3 | 9 | 56.3 | 7 | 43.8 | 7 | 43.8 | 7 | 43.8 | 10 | 62.5 | 7 | 43.8 | 3 | 18.8 | 1 | 6.3 | 7 | 43.8 |
| **CENSUS DIVISION 2, MIDDLE ATLANTIC** | 442 | 152 | 34.4 | 243 | 55.0 | 185 | 41.9 | 238 | 53.8 | 216 | 48.9 | 181 | 41.0 | 120 | 27.1 | 181 | 41.0 | 8 | 1.8 | 226 | 51.1 |
| New Jersey | 72 | 29 | 40.3 | 46 | 63.9 | 36 | 50.0 | 45 | 62.5 | 39 | 54.2 | 30 | 41.7 | 27 | 37.5 | 39 | 54.2 | 2 | 2.8 | 48 | 66.7 |
| New York | 180 | 67 | 37.2 | 108 | 60.0 | 79 | 43.9 | 103 | 57.2 | 81 | 45.0 | 86 | 47.8 | 50 | 27.8 | 74 | 41.1 | 3 | 1.7 | 73 | 40.6 |
| Pennsylvania | 190 | 56 | 29.5 | 89 | 46.8 | 70 | 36.8 | 90 | 47.4 | 96 | 50.5 | 65 | 34.2 | 43 | 22.6 | 68 | 35.8 | 3 | 1.6 | 105 | 55.3 |
| **CENSUS DIVISION 3, SOUTH ATLANTIC** | 714 | 144 | 20.2 | 271 | 38.0 | 208 | 29.1 | 283 | 39.6 | 231 | 32.4 | 190 | 26.6 | 154 | 21.6 | 208 | 29.1 | 10 | 1.4 | 322 | 45.1 |
| Delaware | 8 | 4 | 50.0 | 5 | 62.5 | 3 | 37.5 | 7 | 87.5 | 5 | 62.5 | 5 | 62.5 | 4 | 50.0 | 3 | 37.5 | 0 | 0.0 | 6 | 75.0 |
| District of Columbia | 13 | 5 | 38.5 | 11 | 84.6 | 7 | 53.8 | 9 | 69.2 | 9 | 69.2 | 7 | 53.8 | 7 | 53.8 | 7 | 53.8 | 0 | 0.0 | 9 | 69.2 |
| Florida | 158 | 26 | 16.5 | 50 | 31.6 | 34 | 21.5 | 55 | 34.8 | 46 | 29.1 | 37 | 23.4 | 23 | 14.6 | 57 | 36.1 | 2 | 1.3 | 65 | 41.1 |
| Georgia | 147 | 21 | 14.3 | 40 | 27.2 | 35 | 23.8 | 39 | 26.5 | 32 | 21.8 | 33 | 22.4 | 27 | 18.4 | 29 | 19.7 | 4 | 2.7 | 69 | 46.9 |
| Maryland | 61 | 23 | 37.7 | 40 | 65.6 | 28 | 45.9 | 39 | 63.9 | 28 | 45.9 | 24 | 39.3 | 26 | 42.6 | 21 | 34.4 | 0 | 0.0 | 37 | 60.7 |
| North Carolina | 111 | 25 | 22.5 | 41 | 36.9 | 38 | 34.2 | 48 | 43.2 | 46 | 41.4 | 31 | 27.9 | 24 | 21.6 | 40 | 36.0 | 2 | 1.8 | 66 | 59.5 |
| South Carolina | 67 | 15 | 22.4 | 26 | 38.8 | 21 | 31.3 | 24 | 35.8 | 20 | 29.9 | 13 | 19.4 | 11 | 16.4 | 9 | 13.4 | 1 | 1.5 | 13 | 19.4 |
| Virginia | 84 | 14 | 16.7 | 38 | 45.2 | 24 | 28.6 | 45 | 53.6 | 28 | 33.3 | 27 | 32.1 | 26 | 31.0 | 32 | 38.1 | 0 | 0.0 | 33 | 39.3 |
| West Virginia | 65 | 11 | 16.9 | 20 | 30.8 | 18 | 27.7 | 17 | 26.2 | 17 | 26.2 | 13 | 20.0 | 6 | 9.2 | 10 | 15.4 | 1 | 1.5 | 24 | 36.9 |
| **CENSUS DIVISION 4, EAST NORTH CENTRAL** | 749 | 173 | 23.8 | 304 | 40.6 | 253 | 33.8 | 321 | 42.9 | 276 | 36.8 | 271 | 36.2 | 195 | 26.0 | 232 | 31.0 | 34 | 4.5 | 368 | 49.1 |
| Illinois | 186 | 47 | 25.3 | 78 | 41.9 | 62 | 33.3 | 85 | 45.7 | 71 | 38.2 | 74 | 39.8 | 61 | 32.8 | 62 | 33.3 | 7 | 3.8 | 96 | 51.6 |
| Indiana | 107 | 23 | 21.5 | 30 | 28.0 | 32 | 29.9 | 34 | 31.8 | 35 | 32.7 | 33 | 30.8 | 23 | 21.5 | 33 | 30.8 | 3 | 2.8 | 52 | 48.6 |
| Michigan | 154 | 27 | 17.5 | 62 | 40.3 | 51 | 33.1 | 72 | 46.8 | 51 | 33.1 | 49 | 31.8 | 31 | 20.1 | 46 | 29.9 | 5 | 3.2 | 79 | 51.3 |
| Ohio | 161 | 42 | 26.1 | 75 | 46.6 | 67 | 41.6 | 78 | 48.4 | 66 | 41.0 | 66 | 41.0 | 52 | 32.3 | 60 | 37.3 | 7 | 4.3 | 89 | 55.3 |
| Wisconsin | 141 | 39 | 27.7 | 59 | 41.8 | 41 | 29.1 | 52 | 36.9 | 53 | 37.6 | 49 | 34.8 | 28 | 19.9 | 31 | 22.0 | 12 | 8.5 | 52 | 36.9 |
| **CENSUS DIVISION 5, EAST SOUTH CENTRAL** | 438 | 49 | 11.2 | 100 | 22.8 | 83 | 18.9 | 98 | 22.4 | 134 | 30.6 | 84 | 19.2 | 61 | 13.9 | 85 | 19.4 | 6 | 1.4 | 121 | 27.6 |
| Alabama | 97 | 7 | 7.2 | 21 | 21.6 | 19 | 19.6 | 22 | 22.7 | 24 | 24.7 | 16 | 16.5 | 14 | 14.4 | 27 | 27.8 | 3 | 3.1 | 36 | 37.1 |
| Kentucky | 102 | 13 | 12.7 | 26 | 25.5 | 20 | 19.6 | 27 | 26.5 | 26 | 25.5 | 24 | 23.5 | 15 | 14.7 | 21 | 20.6 | 2 | 2.0 | 33 | 32.4 |
| Mississippi | 104 | 13 | 12.5 | 21 | 20.2 | 18 | 17.3 | 18 | 17.3 | 41 | 39.4 | 20 | 19.2 | 12 | 11.5 | 4 | 3.8 | 0 | 0.0 | 3 | 2.9 |
| Tennessee | 135 | 16 | 11.9 | 32 | 23.7 | 26 | 19.3 | 31 | 23.0 | 43 | 31.9 | 24 | 17.8 | 20 | 14.8 | 33 | 24.4 | 1 | 0.7 | 49 | 36.3 |
| **CENSUS DIVISION 6, WEST NORTH CENTRAL** | 695 | 117 | 16.8 | 173 | 24.9 | 138 | 19.9 | 193 | 27.8 | 161 | 23.2 | 161 | 23.2 | 95 | 13.7 | 108 | 15.5 | 91 | 13.1 | 247 | 35.5 |
| Iowa | 125 | 33 | 26.4 | 38 | 30.4 | 34 | 27.2 | 44 | 35.2 | 32 | 25.6 | 36 | 28.8 | 26 | 20.8 | 20 | 16.0 | 19 | 15.2 | 52 | 41.6 |
| Kansas | 145 | 12 | 8.3 | 16 | 11.0 | 12 | 8.3 | 22 | 15.2 | 27 | 18.6 | 15 | 10.3 | 7 | 4.8 | 16 | 11.0 | 16 | 11.0 | 45 | 31.0 |
| Minnesota | 117 | 24 | 20.5 | 38 | 32.5 | 27 | 23.1 | 36 | 30.8 | 27 | 23.1 | 33 | 28.2 | 18 | 15.4 | 16 | 13.7 | 25 | 21.4 | 39 | 33.3 |
| Missouri | 143 | 26 | 18.2 | 55 | 38.5 | 44 | 30.8 | 58 | 40.6 | 49 | 34.3 | 44 | 30.8 | 21 | 14.7 | 29 | 20.3 | 3 | 2.1 | 68 | 47.6 |
| Nebraska | 75 | 8 | 10.7 | 12 | 16.0 | 10 | 13.3 | 15 | 20.0 | 11 | 14.7 | 15 | 20.0 | 9 | 12.0 | 15 | 20.0 | 5 | 6.7 | 24 | 32.0 |
| North Dakota | 32 | 7 | 21.9 | 6 | 18.8 | 6 | 18.8 | 9 | 28.1 | 8 | 25.0 | 10 | 31.3 | 8 | 25.0 | 5 | 15.6 | 10 | 31.3 | 8 | 25.0 |
| South Dakota | 58 | 7 | 12.1 | 8 | 13.8 | 5 | 8.6 | 9 | 15.5 | 7 | 12.1 | 8 | 13.8 | 6 | 10.3 | 7 | 12.1 | 13 | 22.4 | 11 | 19.0 |
| **CENSUS DIVISION 7, WEST SOUTH CENTRAL** | 784 | 88 | 11.2 | 148 | 18.9 | 121 | 15.4 | 164 | 20.9 | 194 | 24.7 | 121 | 15.4 | 100 | 12.8 | 135 | 17.2 | 12 | 1.5 | 229 | 29.2 |
| Arkansas | 104 | 13 | 12.5 | 23 | 22.1 | 17 | 16.3 | 20 | 19.2 | 32 | 30.8 | 16 | 15.4 | 7 | 6.7 | 12 | 11.5 | 2 | 1.9 | 36 | 34.6 |
| Louisiana | 111 | 12 | 10.8 | 26 | 23.4 | 21 | 18.9 | 33 | 29.7 | 46 | 41.4 | 21 | 18.9 | 22 | 19.8 | 20 | 18.0 | 2 | 1.8 | 35 | 31.5 |
| Oklahoma | 108 | 16 | 14.8 | 25 | 23.1 | 20 | 18.5 | 28 | 25.9 | 27 | 25.0 | 21 | 19.4 | 12 | 11.1 | 26 | 24.1 | 3 | 2.8 | 31 | 28.7 |
| Texas | 461 | 47 | 10.2 | 74 | 16.1 | 63 | 13.7 | 83 | 18.0 | 89 | 19.3 | 63 | 13.7 | 59 | 12.8 | 77 | 16.7 | 5 | 1.1 | 127 | 27.5 |
| **CENSUS DIVISION 8, MOUNTAIN** | 320 | 64 | 20.0 | 100 | 31.3 | 72 | 22.5 | 111 | 34.7 | 80 | 25.0 | 91 | 28.4 | 51 | 15.9 | 63 | 19.7 | 5 | 1.6 | 116 | 36.3 |
| Arizona | 55 | 11 | 20.0 | 22 | 40.0 | 15 | 27.3 | 20 | 36.4 | 19 | 34.5 | 22 | 40.0 | 13 | 23.6 | 11 | 20.0 | 0 | 0.0 | 18 | 32.7 |
| Colorado | 56 | 14 | 25.0 | 21 | 37.5 | 14 | 25.0 | 24 | 42.9 | 15 | 26.8 | 20 | 35.7 | 12 | 21.4 | 19 | 33.9 | 2 | 3.6 | 32 | 57.1 |
| Idaho | 30 | 5 | 16.7 | 9 | 30.0 | 7 | 23.3 | 10 | 33.3 | 7 | 23.3 | 7 | 23.3 | 2 | 6.7 | 6 | 20.0 | 0 | 0.0 | 11 | 36.7 |
| Montana | 54 | 6 | 11.1 | 10 | 18.5 | 7 | 13.0 | 15 | 27.8 | 8 | 14.8 | 10 | 18.5 | 7 | 13.0 | 6 | 11.1 | 3 | 5.6 | 12 | 22.2 |
| Nevada | 22 | 3 | 13.6 | 7 | 31.8 | 6 | 27.3 | 5 | 22.7 | 5 | 22.7 | 6 | 27.3 | 3 | 13.6 | 4 | 18.2 | 0 | 0.0 | 5 | 22.7 |
| New Mexico | 34 | 11 | 32.4 | 12 | 35.3 | 9 | 26.5 | 12 | 35.3 | 10 | 29.4 | 11 | 32.4 | 4 | 11.8 | 3 | 8.8 | 0 | 0.0 | 10 | 29.4 |
| Utah | 41 | 8 | 19.5 | 12 | 29.3 | 7 | 17.1 | 15 | 36.6 | 9 | 22.0 | 8 | 19.5 | 8 | 19.5 | 9 | 22.0 | 0 | 0.0 | 20 | 48.8 |
| Wyoming | 28 | 6 | 21.4 | 7 | 25.0 | 7 | 25.0 | 10 | 35.7 | 7 | 25.0 | 7 | 25.0 | 2 | 7.1 | 5 | 17.9 | 0 | 0.0 | 8 | 28.6 |
| **CENSUS DIVISION 9, PACIFIC** | 576 | 68 | 11.8 | 127 | 22.0 | 89 | 15.5 | 151 | 26.2 | 100 | 17.4 | 113 | 19.6 | 74 | 12.8 | 144 | 25.0 | 8 | 1.4 | 119 | 20.7 |
| Alaska | 15 | 3 | 20.0 | 8 | 53.3 | 4 | 26.7 | 10 | 66.7 | 3 | 20.0 | 7 | 46.7 | 3 | 20.0 | 2 | 13.3 | 0 | 0.0 | 4 | 26.7 |
| California | 402 | 42 | 10.4 | 75 | 18.7 | 54 | 13.4 | 86 | 21.4 | 65 | 16.2 | 66 | 16.4 | 46 | 11.4 | 95 | 23.6 | 3 | 0.7 | 63 | 15.7 |
| Hawaii | 18 | 4 | 22.2 | 4 | 22.2 | 4 | 22.2 | 5 | 27.8 | 4 | 22.2 | 5 | 27.8 | 4 | 22.2 | 3 | 16.7 | 0 | 0.0 | 3 | 16.7 |
| Oregon | 59 | 8 | 13.6 | 19 | 32.2 | 11 | 18.6 | 27 | 45.8 | 11 | 18.6 | 11 | 18.6 | 7 | 11.9 | 15 | 25.4 | 3 | 5.1 | 18 | 30.5 |
| Washington | 82 | 11 | 13.4 | 21 | 25.6 | 16 | 19.5 | 23 | 28.0 | 17 | 20.7 | 24 | 29.3 | 14 | 17.1 | 29 | 35.4 | 2 | 2.4 | 31 | 37.8 |

## Table 7 (Continued)

*These data include only hospital-based facilities and services as reported by responding hospitals in Section C of the 2003 AHA Annual Survey, beginning on page 205. All hospitals are represented with Community Hospitals listed separately under United States. No estimates have been made for nonresponding hospitals. Definitions of facilities and services are listed in the Glossary, page 193.*

| CLASSIFICATION | HOSPITALS REPORTING | SINGLE PHOTON EMISSION COMPUTED TOMOGRAPHY (SPECT) | | SOCIAL WORK SERVICES | | SPORTS MEDICINE | | SUPPORT GROUPS | | SWING BED SERVICES | | TEEN OUTREACH SERVICES | | TOBACCO TREATMENT | | TRANSPLANT SERVICES | | TRANSPORTATION TO HEALTH FACILITIES | |
|---|---|---|---|---|---|---|---|---|---|---|---|---|---|---|---|---|---|---|---|
| | | Number | Percent | Number | Percent | Number | Percent | Number | Percent | Number | Percent | Number | Percent | Number | Percent | Number | Percent | Number | Percent |
| **UNITED STATES** | 4,946 | 1,667 | 33.7 | 4,143 | 83.8 | 1,713 | 34.6 | 3,022 | 61.1 | 1,414 | 28.6 | 669 | 13.5 | 1,873 | 37.9 | 367 | 7.4 | 1,312 | 26.5 |
| COMMUNITY HOSPITALS | 4,320 | 1,612 | 37.3 | 3,673 | 85.0 | 1,680 | 38.9 | 2,757 | 63.8 | 1,383 | 32.0 | 639 | 14.8 | 1,701 | 39.4 | 348 | 8.1 | 1,115 | 25.8 |
| **CENSUS DIVISION 1, NEW ENGLAND** | 228 | 111 | 48.7 | 214 | 93.9 | 105 | 46.1 | 189 | 82.9 | 41 | 18.0 | 60 | 26.3 | 144 | 63.2 | 21 | 9.2 | 70 | 30.7 |
| Connecticut | 36 | 26 | 72.2 | 36 | 100.0 | 19 | 52.8 | 34 | 94.4 | 3 | 8.3 | 16 | 44.4 | 26 | 72.2 | 4 | 11.1 | 10 | 27.8 |
| Maine | 39 | 19 | 48.7 | 37 | 94.9 | 14 | 35.9 | 31 | 79.5 | 10 | 25.6 | 6 | 15.4 | 32 | 82.1 | 1 | 2.6 | 8 | 20.5 |
| Massachusetts | 95 | 41 | 43.2 | 83 | 87.4 | 47 | 49.5 | 73 | 76.8 | 4 | 4.2 | 29 | 30.5 | 41 | 43.2 | 11 | 11.6 | 30 | 31.6 |
| New Hampshire | 30 | 13 | 43.3 | 30 | 100.0 | 16 | 53.3 | 26 | 86.7 | 15 | 50.0 | 7 | 23.3 | 23 | 76.7 | 2 | 6.7 | 10 | 33.3 |
| Rhode Island | 12 | 6 | 50.0 | 12 | 100.0 | 3 | 25.0 | 10 | 83.3 | 1 | 8.3 | 2 | 16.7 | 8 | 66.7 | 2 | 16.7 | 4 | 33.3 |
| Vermont | 16 | 6 | 37.5 | 16 | 100.0 | 6 | 37.5 | 15 | 93.8 | 8 | 50.0 | 0 | 0.0 | 14 | 87.5 | 1 | 6.3 | 8 | 50.0 |
| **CENSUS DIVISION 2, MIDDLE ATLANTIC** | 442 | 211 | 47.7 | 422 | 95.5 | 182 | 41.2 | 355 | 80.3 | 72 | 16.3 | 125 | 28.3 | 263 | 59.5 | 46 | 10.4 | 178 | 40.3 |
| New Jersey | 72 | 47 | 65.3 | 69 | 95.8 | 32 | 44.4 | 65 | 90.3 | 8 | 11.1 | 36 | 50.0 | 42 | 58.3 | 7 | 9.7 | 47 | 65.3 |
| New York | 180 | 76 | 42.2 | 170 | 94.4 | 70 | 38.9 | 137 | 76.1 | 28 | 15.6 | 46 | 25.6 | 102 | 56.7 | 23 | 12.8 | 61 | 33.9 |
| Pennsylvania | 190 | 88 | 46.3 | 183 | 96.3 | 80 | 42.1 | 153 | 80.5 | 36 | 18.9 | 43 | 22.6 | 119 | 62.6 | 16 | 8.4 | 70 | 36.8 |
| **CENSUS DIVISION 3, SOUTH ATLANTIC** | 714 | 311 | 43.6 | 620 | 86.8 | 246 | 34.5 | 469 | 65.7 | 131 | 18.3 | 94 | 13.2 | 285 | 39.9 | 69 | 9.7 | 192 | 26.9 |
| Delaware | 8 | 5 | 62.5 | 7 | 87.5 | 4 | 50.0 | 7 | 87.5 | 0 | 0.0 | 3 | 37.5 | 5 | 62.5 | 3 | 37.5 | 2 | 25.0 |
| District of Columbia | 13 | 7 | 53.8 | 12 | 92.3 | 7 | 53.8 | 11 | 84.6 | 0 | 0.0 | 3 | 23.1 | 5 | 38.5 | 6 | 46.2 | 7 | 53.8 |
| Florida | 158 | 68 | 43.0 | 125 | 79.1 | 51 | 32.3 | 106 | 67.1 | 13 | 8.2 | 18 | 11.4 | 52 | 32.9 | 14 | 8.9 | 45 | 28.5 |
| Georgia | 147 | 39 | 26.5 | 123 | 83.7 | 43 | 29.3 | 79 | 53.7 | 47 | 32.0 | 21 | 14.3 | 53 | 36.1 | 11 | 7.5 | 38 | 25.9 |
| Maryland | 61 | 32 | 52.5 | 60 | 98.4 | 17 | 27.9 | 52 | 85.2 | 8 | 13.1 | 11 | 18.0 | 36 | 59.0 | 4 | 6.6 | 16 | 26.2 |
| North Carolina | 111 | 53 | 47.7 | 103 | 92.8 | 43 | 38.7 | 78 | 70.3 | 25 | 22.5 | 15 | 13.5 | 50 | 45.0 | 7 | 6.3 | 33 | 29.7 |
| South Carolina | 67 | 24 | 35.8 | 55 | 82.1 | 21 | 31.3 | 34 | 50.7 | 0 | 0.0 | 7 | 10.4 | 13 | 19.4 | 9 | 13.4 | 15 | 22.4 |
| Virginia | 84 | 55 | 65.5 | 74 | 88.1 | 35 | 41.7 | 63 | 75.0 | 17 | 20.2 | 10 | 11.9 | 40 | 47.6 | 11 | 13.1 | 21 | 25.0 |
| West Virginia | 65 | 28 | 43.1 | 61 | 93.8 | 25 | 38.5 | 39 | 60.0 | 21 | 32.3 | 6 | 9.2 | 31 | 47.7 | 4 | 6.2 | 15 | 23.1 |
| **CENSUS DIVISION 4, EAST NORTH CENTRAL** | 749 | 351 | 46.9 | 689 | 92.0 | 389 | 51.9 | 557 | 74.4 | 198 | 26.4 | 136 | 18.2 | 386 | 51.5 | 58 | 7.7 | 241 | 32.2 |
| Illinois | 186 | 84 | 45.2 | 170 | 91.4 | 83 | 44.6 | 141 | 75.8 | 57 | 30.6 | 31 | 16.7 | 93 | 50.0 | 15 | 8.1 | 75 | 40.3 |
| Indiana | 107 | 45 | 42.1 | 94 | 87.9 | 47 | 43.9 | 82 | 76.6 | 32 | 29.9 | 18 | 16.8 | 67 | 62.6 | 4 | 3.7 | 30 | 28.0 |
| Michigan | 154 | 69 | 44.8 | 141 | 91.6 | 77 | 50.0 | 123 | 79.9 | 35 | 22.7 | 22 | 14.3 | 74 | 48.1 | 13 | 8.4 | 45 | 29.2 |
| Ohio | 161 | 98 | 60.9 | 156 | 96.9 | 95 | 59.0 | 130 | 80.7 | 34 | 21.1 | 42 | 26.1 | 96 | 59.6 | 18 | 11.2 | 62 | 38.5 |
| Wisconsin | 141 | 55 | 39.0 | 128 | 90.8 | 87 | 61.7 | 81 | 57.4 | 40 | 28.4 | 23 | 16.3 | 56 | 39.7 | 8 | 5.7 | 29 | 20.6 |
| **CENSUS DIVISION 5, EAST SOUTH CENTRAL** | 438 | 120 | 27.4 | 376 | 85.8 | 135 | 30.8 | 219 | 50.0 | 97 | 22.1 | 43 | 9.8 | 118 | 26.9 | 24 | 5.5 | 76 | 17.4 |
| Alabama | 97 | 23 | 23.7 | 81 | 83.5 | 36 | 37.1 | 43 | 44.3 | 21 | 21.6 | 9 | 9.3 | 22 | 22.7 | 5 | 5.2 | 19 | 19.6 |
| Kentucky | 102 | 30 | 29.4 | 88 | 86.3 | 31 | 30.4 | 63 | 61.8 | 44 | 43.1 | 14 | 13.7 | 56 | 54.9 | 4 | 3.9 | 16 | 15.7 |
| Mississippi | 104 | 31 | 29.8 | 97 | 93.3 | 22 | 21.2 | 41 | 39.4 | 2 | 1.9 | 9 | 8.7 | 0 | 0.0 | 3 | 2.9 | 19 | 18.3 |
| Tennessee | 135 | 36 | 26.7 | 110 | 81.5 | 46 | 34.1 | 72 | 53.3 | 30 | 22.2 | 11 | 8.1 | 40 | 29.6 | 12 | 8.9 | 22 | 16.3 |
| **CENSUS DIVISION 6, WEST NORTH CENTRAL** | 695 | 162 | 23.3 | 560 | 80.6 | 267 | 38.4 | 406 | 58.4 | 418 | 60.1 | 68 | 9.8 | 237 | 34.1 | 30 | 4.3 | 185 | 26.6 |
| Iowa | 125 | 37 | 29.6 | 107 | 85.6 | 57 | 45.6 | 92 | 73.6 | 83 | 66.4 | 20 | 16.0 | 52 | 41.6 | 7 | 5.6 | 32 | 25.6 |
| Kansas | 145 | 21 | 14.5 | 101 | 69.7 | 35 | 24.1 | 55 | 37.9 | 92 | 63.4 | 7 | 4.8 | 22 | 15.2 | 2 | 1.4 | 33 | 22.8 |
| Minnesota | 117 | 18 | 15.4 | 101 | 86.3 | 43 | 36.8 | 81 | 69.2 | 76 | 65.0 | 12 | 10.3 | 45 | 38.5 | 3 | 2.6 | 29 | 24.8 |
| Missouri | 143 | 54 | 37.8 | 129 | 90.2 | 65 | 45.5 | 95 | 66.4 | 47 | 32.9 | 18 | 12.6 | 63 | 44.1 | 10 | 7.0 | 45 | 31.5 |
| Nebraska | 75 | 16 | 21.3 | 55 | 73.3 | 34 | 45.3 | 37 | 49.3 | 53 | 70.7 | 7 | 9.3 | 23 | 30.7 | 4 | 5.3 | 20 | 26.7 |
| North Dakota | 32 | 8 | 25.0 | 29 | 90.6 | 15 | 46.9 | 22 | 68.8 | 25 | 78.1 | 3 | 9.4 | 11 | 34.4 | 2 | 6.3 | 9 | 28.1 |
| South Dakota | 58 | 8 | 13.8 | 38 | 65.5 | 18 | 31.0 | 24 | 41.4 | 42 | 72.4 | 1 | 1.7 | 21 | 36.2 | 2 | 3.4 | 17 | 29.3 |
| **CENSUS DIVISION 7, WEST SOUTH CENTRAL** | 784 | 181 | 23.1 | 628 | 80.1 | 185 | 23.6 | 372 | 47.4 | 235 | 30.0 | 40 | 5.1 | 171 | 21.8 | 48 | 6.1 | 160 | 20.4 |
| Arkansas | 104 | 19 | 18.3 | 84 | 80.8 | 21 | 20.2 | 59 | 56.7 | 43 | 41.3 | 5 | 4.8 | 32 | 30.8 | 3 | 2.9 | 25 | 24.0 |
| Louisiana | 111 | 28 | 25.2 | 93 | 83.8 | 22 | 19.8 | 39 | 35.1 | 34 | 30.6 | 7 | 6.3 | 26 | 23.4 | 8 | 7.2 | 28 | 25.2 |
| Oklahoma | 108 | 23 | 21.3 | 80 | 74.1 | 33 | 30.6 | 44 | 40.7 | 42 | 38.9 | 5 | 4.6 | 24 | 22.2 | 8 | 7.4 | 16 | 14.8 |
| Texas | 461 | 111 | 24.1 | 371 | 80.5 | 109 | 23.6 | 230 | 49.9 | 116 | 25.2 | 23 | 5.0 | 89 | 19.3 | 29 | 6.3 | 91 | 19.7 |
| **CENSUS DIVISION 8, MOUNTAIN** | 320 | 79 | 24.7 | 265 | 82.8 | 94 | 29.4 | 168 | 52.5 | 133 | 41.6 | 47 | 14.7 | 127 | 39.7 | 23 | 7.2 | 81 | 25.3 |
| Arizona | 55 | 18 | 32.7 | 48 | 87.3 | 6 | 10.9 | 34 | 61.8 | 10 | 18.2 | 7 | 12.7 | 23 | 41.8 | 5 | 9.1 | 13 | 23.6 |
| Colorado | 56 | 24 | 42.9 | 47 | 83.9 | 26 | 46.4 | 31 | 55.4 | 26 | 46.4 | 9 | 16.1 | 26 | 46.4 | 5 | 8.9 | 17 | 30.4 |
| Idaho | 30 | 5 | 16.7 | 26 | 86.7 | 14 | 46.7 | 17 | 56.7 | 15 | 50.0 | 7 | 23.3 | 12 | 40.0 | 4 | 13.3 | 8 | 26.7 |
| Montana | 54 | 9 | 16.7 | 44 | 81.5 | 20 | 37.0 | 23 | 42.6 | 39 | 72.2 | 7 | 13.0 | 18 | 33.3 | 1 | 1.9 | 22 | 40.7 |
| Nevada | 22 | 4 | 18.2 | 18 | 81.8 | 4 | 18.2 | 10 | 45.5 | 1 | 4.5 | 3 | 13.6 | 5 | 22.7 | 2 | 9.1 | 6 | 27.3 |
| New Mexico | 34 | 5 | 14.7 | 26 | 76.5 | 4 | 11.8 | 12 | 35.3 | 9 | 26.5 | 6 | 17.6 | 13 | 38.2 | 2 | 5.9 | 4 | 11.8 |
| Utah | 41 | 9 | 22.0 | 31 | 75.6 | 13 | 31.7 | 24 | 58.5 | 14 | 34.1 | 7 | 17.1 | 15 | 36.6 | 4 | 9.8 | 3 | 7.3 |
| Wyoming | 28 | 5 | 17.9 | 25 | 89.3 | 7 | 25.0 | 17 | 60.7 | 19 | 67.9 | 1 | 3.6 | 15 | 53.6 | 0 | 0.0 | 8 | 28.6 |
| **CENSUS DIVISION 9, PACIFIC** | 576 | 141 | 24.5 | 369 | 64.1 | 110 | 19.1 | 287 | 49.8 | 89 | 15.5 | 56 | 9.7 | 142 | 24.7 | 48 | 8.3 | 129 | 22.4 |
| Alaska | 15 | 3 | 20.0 | 13 | 86.7 | 2 | 13.3 | 8 | 53.3 | 9 | 60.0 | 4 | 26.7 | 9 | 60.0 | 0 | 0.0 | 3 | 20.0 |
| California | 402 | 93 | 23.1 | 230 | 57.2 | 60 | 14.9 | 170 | 42.3 | 31 | 7.7 | 37 | 9.2 | 67 | 16.7 | 31 | 7.7 | 89 | 22.1 |
| Hawaii | 18 | 3 | 16.7 | 17 | 94.4 | 4 | 22.2 | 9 | 50.0 | 4 | 22.2 | 3 | 16.7 | 4 | 22.2 | 1 | 5.6 | 2 | 11.1 |
| Oregon | 59 | 22 | 37.3 | 47 | 79.7 | 17 | 28.8 | 50 | 84.7 | 21 | 35.6 | 5 | 8.5 | 31 | 52.5 | 7 | 11.9 | 18 | 30.5 |
| Washington | 82 | 20 | 24.4 | 62 | 75.6 | 27 | 32.9 | 50 | 61.0 | 24 | 29.3 | 7 | 8.5 | 31 | 37.8 | 9 | 11.0 | 17 | 20.7 |

## Table 7 (Continued)

*These data include only hospital-based facilities and services as reported by responding hospitals in Section C of the 2003 AHA Annual Survey, beginning on page 205. All hospitals are represented with Community Hospitals listed separately under United States. No estimates have been made for nonresponding hospitals. Definitions of facilities and services are listed in the Glossary, page 193.*

| CLASSIFICATION | HOSPITALS REPORTING | TRAUMA CENTER (CERTIFIED) | | ULTRASOUND | | URGENT CARE CENTER | | VOLUNTEER SERVICES DEPARTMENT | | WOMEN'S HEALTH SERVICES | | WOUND MANAGEMENT SERVICES | |
|---|---|---|---|---|---|---|---|---|---|---|---|---|---|
| | | Number | Percent | Number | Percent | Number | Percent | Number | Percent | Number | Percent | Number | Percent |
| UNITED STATES | 4,946 | 1,480 | 29.9 | 3,881 | 78.5 | 1,142 | 23.1 | 3,638 | 73.6 | 2,168 | 43.8 | 2,116 | 42.8 |
| COMMUNITY HOSPITALS | 4,320 | 1,453 | 33.6 | 3,707 | 85.8 | 1,047 | 24.2 | 3,345 | 77.4 | 2,031 | 47.0 | 1,921 | 44.5 |
| CENSUS DIVISION 1, NEW ENGLAND | 228 | 72 | 31.6 | 186 | 81.6 | 93 | 40.8 | 206 | 90.4 | 147 | 64.5 | 101 | 44.3 |
| Connecticut | 36 | 17 | 47.2 | 31 | 86.1 | 22 | 61.1 | 35 | 97.2 | 26 | 72.2 | 20 | 55.6 |
| Maine | 39 | 11 | 28.2 | 33 | 84.6 | 12 | 30.8 | 32 | 82.1 | 22 | 56.4 | 17 | 43.6 |
| Massachusetts | 95 | 21 | 22.1 | 72 | 75.8 | 35 | 36.8 | 84 | 88.4 | 57 | 60.0 | 41 | 43.2 |
| New Hampshire | 30 | 15 | 50.0 | 27 | 90.0 | 13 | 43.3 | 29 | 96.7 | 24 | 80.0 | 14 | 46.7 |
| Rhode Island | 12 | 2 | 16.7 | 10 | 83.3 | 3 | 25.0 | 11 | 91.7 | 9 | 75.0 | 3 | 25.0 |
| Vermont | 16 | 6 | 37.5 | 13 | 81.3 | 8 | 50.0 | 15 | 93.8 | 9 | 56.3 | 6 | 37.5 |
| CENSUS DIVISION 2, MIDDLE ATLANTIC | 442 | 101 | 22.9 | 380 | 86.0 | 109 | 24.7 | 399 | 90.3 | 266 | 60.2 | 235 | 53.2 |
| New Jersey | 72 | 13 | 18.1 | 62 | 86.1 | 19 | 26.4 | 67 | 93.1 | 50 | 69.4 | 47 | 65.3 |
| New York | 180 | 54 | 30.0 | 155 | 86.1 | 53 | 29.4 | 158 | 87.8 | 116 | 64.4 | 75 | 41.7 |
| Pennsylvania | 190 | 34 | 17.9 | 163 | 85.8 | 37 | 19.5 | 174 | 91.6 | 100 | 52.6 | 113 | 59.5 |
| CENSUS DIVISION 3, SOUTH ATLANTIC | 714 | 154 | 21.6 | 605 | 84.7 | 173 | 24.2 | 606 | 84.9 | 377 | 52.8 | 347 | 48.6 |
| Delaware | 8 | 6 | 75.0 | 7 | 87.5 | 1 | 12.5 | 7 | 87.5 | 6 | 75.0 | 3 | 37.5 |
| District of Columbia | 13 | 6 | 46.2 | 10 | 76.9 | 4 | 30.8 | 12 | 92.3 | 9 | 69.2 | 10 | 76.9 |
| Florida | 158 | 30 | 19.0 | 141 | 89.2 | 49 | 31.0 | 132 | 83.5 | 85 | 53.8 | 91 | 57.6 |
| Georgia | 147 | 33 | 22.4 | 124 | 84.4 | 29 | 19.7 | 113 | 76.9 | 62 | 42.2 | 61 | 41.5 |
| Maryland | 61 | 13 | 21.3 | 49 | 80.3 | 19 | 31.1 | 59 | 96.7 | 36 | 59.0 | 33 | 54.1 |
| North Carolina | 111 | 20 | 18.0 | 98 | 88.3 | 30 | 27.0 | 101 | 91.0 | 61 | 55.0 | 55 | 49.5 |
| South Carolina | 67 | 10 | 14.9 | 54 | 80.6 | 8 | 11.9 | 51 | 76.1 | 38 | 56.7 | 16 | 23.9 |
| Virginia | 84 | 16 | 19.0 | 71 | 84.5 | 20 | 23.8 | 76 | 90.5 | 49 | 58.3 | 54 | 64.3 |
| West Virginia | 65 | 20 | 30.8 | 51 | 78.5 | 13 | 20.0 | 55 | 84.6 | 31 | 47.7 | 24 | 36.9 |
| CENSUS DIVISION 4, EAST NORTH CENTRAL | 749 | 246 | 32.8 | 636 | 84.9 | 278 | 37.1 | 622 | 83.0 | 398 | 53.1 | 389 | 51.9 |
| Illinois | 186 | 81 | 43.5 | 168 | 90.3 | 52 | 28.0 | 157 | 84.4 | 99 | 53.2 | 99 | 53.2 |
| Indiana | 107 | 20 | 18.7 | 88 | 82.2 | 31 | 29.0 | 94 | 87.9 | 59 | 55.1 | 56 | 52.3 |
| Michigan | 154 | 41 | 26.6 | 130 | 84.4 | 74 | 48.1 | 131 | 85.1 | 83 | 53.9 | 88 | 57.1 |
| Ohio | 161 | 47 | 29.2 | 144 | 89.4 | 53 | 32.9 | 153 | 95.0 | 97 | 60.2 | 77 | 47.8 |
| Wisconsin | 141 | 57 | 40.4 | 106 | 75.2 | 68 | 48.2 | 87 | 61.7 | 60 | 42.6 | 69 | 48.9 |
| CENSUS DIVISION 5, EAST SOUTH CENTRAL | 438 | 132 | 30.1 | 354 | 80.8 | 41 | 9.4 | 247 | 56.4 | 166 | 37.9 | 114 | 26.0 |
| Alabama | 97 | 28 | 28.9 | 83 | 85.6 | 9 | 9.3 | 70 | 72.2 | 40 | 41.2 | 27 | 27.8 |
| Kentucky | 102 | 23 | 22.5 | 91 | 89.2 | 16 | 15.7 | 80 | 78.4 | 46 | 45.1 | 37 | 36.3 |
| Mississippi | 104 | 64 | 61.5 | 77 | 74.0 | 7 | 6.7 | 2 | 1.9 | 28 | 26.9 | 4 | 3.8 |
| Tennessee | 135 | 17 | 12.6 | 103 | 76.3 | 9 | 6.7 | 95 | 70.4 | 52 | 38.5 | 46 | 34.1 |
| CENSUS DIVISION 6, WEST NORTH CENTRAL | 695 | 213 | 30.6 | 510 | 73.4 | 119 | 17.1 | 472 | 67.9 | 208 | 29.9 | 262 | 37.7 |
| Iowa | 125 | 81 | 64.8 | 104 | 83.2 | 26 | 20.8 | 97 | 77.6 | 38 | 30.4 | 52 | 41.6 |
| Kansas | 145 | 14 | 9.7 | 91 | 62.8 | 10 | 6.9 | 78 | 53.8 | 33 | 22.8 | 54 | 37.2 |
| Minnesota | 117 | 40 | 34.2 | 89 | 76.1 | 29 | 24.8 | 90 | 76.9 | 39 | 33.3 | 40 | 34.2 |
| Missouri | 143 | 30 | 21.0 | 111 | 77.6 | 31 | 21.7 | 113 | 79.0 | 59 | 41.3 | 67 | 46.9 |
| Nebraska | 75 | 18 | 24.0 | 55 | 73.3 | 8 | 10.7 | 45 | 60.0 | 14 | 18.7 | 22 | 29.3 |
| North Dakota | 32 | 21 | 65.6 | 19 | 59.4 | 5 | 15.6 | 24 | 75.0 | 11 | 34.4 | 10 | 31.3 |
| South Dakota | 58 | 9 | 15.5 | 41 | 70.7 | 10 | 17.2 | 25 | 43.1 | 14 | 24.1 | 17 | 29.3 |
| CENSUS DIVISION 7, WEST SOUTH CENTRAL | 784 | 269 | 34.3 | 559 | 71.3 | 112 | 14.3 | 499 | 63.6 | 270 | 34.4 | 329 | 42.0 |
| Arkansas | 104 | 16 | 15.4 | 80 | 76.9 | 13 | 12.5 | 63 | 60.6 | 37 | 35.6 | 34 | 32.7 |
| Louisiana | 111 | 18 | 16.2 | 84 | 75.7 | 23 | 20.7 | 70 | 63.1 | 40 | 36.0 | 48 | 43.2 |
| Oklahoma | 108 | 43 | 39.8 | 75 | 69.4 | 19 | 17.6 | 72 | 66.7 | 31 | 28.7 | 46 | 42.6 |
| Texas | 461 | 192 | 41.6 | 320 | 69.4 | 57 | 12.4 | 294 | 63.8 | 162 | 35.1 | 201 | 43.6 |
| CENSUS DIVISION 8, MOUNTAIN | 320 | 129 | 40.3 | 270 | 84.4 | 77 | 24.1 | 228 | 71.3 | 132 | 41.3 | 145 | 45.3 |
| Arizona | 55 | 19 | 34.5 | 48 | 87.3 | 14 | 25.5 | 49 | 89.1 | 25 | 45.5 | 40 | 72.7 |
| Colorado | 56 | 48 | 85.7 | 51 | 91.1 | 13 | 23.2 | 40 | 71.4 | 26 | 46.4 | 30 | 53.6 |
| Idaho | 30 | 6 | 20.0 | 27 | 90.0 | 4 | 13.3 | 23 | 76.7 | 11 | 36.7 | 9 | 30.0 |
| Montana | 54 | 16 | 29.6 | 38 | 70.4 | 10 | 18.5 | 35 | 64.8 | 17 | 31.5 | 15 | 27.8 |
| Nevada | 22 | 3 | 13.6 | 16 | 72.7 | 9 | 40.9 | 14 | 63.6 | 9 | 40.9 | 9 | 40.9 |
| New Mexico | 34 | 6 | 17.6 | 29 | 85.3 | 10 | 29.4 | 16 | 47.1 | 10 | 29.4 | 13 | 38.2 |
| Utah | 41 | 15 | 36.6 | 36 | 87.8 | 13 | 31.7 | 33 | 80.5 | 25 | 61.0 | 16 | 39.0 |
| Wyoming | 28 | 16 | 57.1 | 25 | 89.3 | 4 | 14.3 | 18 | 64.3 | 9 | 32.1 | 13 | 46.4 |
| CENSUS DIVISION 9, PACIFIC | 576 | 164 | 28.5 | 381 | 66.1 | 140 | 24.3 | 359 | 62.3 | 204 | 35.4 | 194 | 33.7 |
| Alaska | 15 | 2 | 13.3 | 14 | 93.3 | 1 | 6.7 | 10 | 66.7 | 5 | 33.3 | 6 | 40.0 |
| California | 402 | 60 | 14.9 | 227 | 56.5 | 89 | 22.1 | 222 | 55.2 | 125 | 31.1 | 116 | 28.9 |
| Hawaii | 18 | 2 | 11.1 | 12 | 66.7 | 3 | 16.7 | 14 | 77.8 | 6 | 33.3 | 10 | 55.6 |
| Oregon | 59 | 42 | 71.2 | 59 | 100.0 | 17 | 28.8 | 49 | 83.1 | 33 | 55.9 | 31 | 52.5 |
| Washington | 82 | 58 | 70.7 | 69 | 84.1 | 30 | 36.6 | 64 | 78.0 | 35 | 42.7 | 31 | 37.8 |

# Table 8



MSAs

## Metropolitan Statistical Areas

According to the U.S. Office of Management and Budget, an MSA is a geographical designation that represents an integrated social and economic unit with a large population nucleus. Under these standards, an area qualifies for recognition as an MSA if there is a city within the area of at least 50,000 population or an urban area of at least 50,000 with a total metropolitan population of at least 100,000. MSAs are defined as entire counties. In addition to the county containing the main city, an MSA also includes additional counties having strong economic and social ties to the central county. Such counties must have a specified level of commuting to the central counties and must meet certain standards regarding metropolitan character, such as population density.

When an MSA encompasses two or more central cities, up to three cities may be specified in the MSA title. They will be listed in order of population size. When a single central city exists, the MSA is named for that particular city. The official MSA title will also include a list of each of the states it covers. A MSA may extend beyond a single state.

This publication includes the most current MSAs as defined by the Office of Management and Budget.

# TABLE 8

# U.S. CENSUS DIVISION 1, NEW ENGLAND

*U.S. Community Hospitals*
*(Nonfederal, short-term general and other special hospitals)*

## 2003 Utilization, Personnel and Finances



| CLASSIFICATION | Hospitals | Beds | Admissions | Inpatient Days | Adjusted Patient Days | Average Daily Census | Adjusted Average Daily Census | Average Stay (days) | Surgical Operations | NEWBORNS | | OUTPATIENT VISITS | |
|---|---|---|---|---|---|---|---|---|---|---|---|---|---|
| | | | | | | | | | | Bassinets | Births | Emergency | Total |
| UNITED STATES | 4,895 | 813,307 | 34,782,742 | 196,649,769 | 326,299,942 | 538,797 | 894,019 | 5.7 | 27,106,538 | 59,662 | 3,915,842 | 111,069,871 | 563,186,046 |
| Nonmetropolitan | 2,166 | 168,374 | 5,368,552 | 35,076,707 | 73,724,487 | 96,136 | 202,034 | 6.5 | 4,592,380 | 13,462 | 530,805 | 23,720,395 | 117,598,717 |
| Metropolitan | 2,729 | 644,933 | 29,414,190 | 161,573,062 | 252,575,455 | 442,661 | 691,985 | 5.5 | 22,514,158 | 46,200 | 3,385,037 | 87,349,476 | 445,587,329 |
| CENSUS DIVISION 1, NEW ENGLAND | 203 | 33,600 | 1,598,123 | 8,854,347 | 17,033,225 | 24,258 | 46,674 | 5.5 | 1,490,958 | 2,605 | 169,753 | 6,275,074 | 37,815,707 |
| Nonmetropolitan | 77 | 6,403 | 264,961 | 1,474,430 | 3,425,728 | 4,039 | 9,388 | 5.6 | 277,829 | 646 | 28,540 | 1,382,054 | 7,855,586 |
| Metropolitan | 126 | 27,197 | 1,333,162 | 7,379,917 | 13,607,497 | 20,219 | 37,286 | 5.5 | 1,213,129 | 1,959 | 141,213 | 4,893,020 | 29,960,121 |
| Connecticut | 34 | 7,185 | 372,630 | 2,029,059 | 3,292,592 | 5,558 | 9,022 | 5.4 | 305,871 | 536 | 43,131 | 1,372,015 | 6,862,798 |
| Nonmetropolitan | 6 | 453 | 26,269 | 112,272 | 234,049 | 307 | 641 | 4.3 | 27,237 | 46 | 2,611 | 167,641 | 803,178 |
| Metropolitan | 28 | 6,732 | 346,361 | 1,916,787 | 3,058,543 | 5,251 | 8,381 | 5.5 | 278,634 | 490 | 40,520 | 1,204,374 | 6,059,620 |
| Bridgeport | 4 | 881 | 45,265 | 233,688 | 359,991 | 640 | 986 | 5.2 | 30,496 | 82 | 5,247 | 181,089 | 535,637 |
| Danbury | 2 | 340 | 19,598 | 86,077 | 166,559 | 236 | 457 | 4.4 | 18,600 | 36 | 2,754 | 82,783 | 308,976 |
| Hartford | 10 | 2,401 | 118,778 | 751,267 | 1,206,217 | 2,058 | 3,306 | 6.3 | 112,413 | 143 | 13,159 | 408,535 | 2,706,931 |
| New Haven-Meriden | 5 | 1,512 | 74,596 | 420,957 | 594,101 | 1,153 | 1,627 | 5.6 | 51,267 | 64 | 7,134 | 221,106 | 829,630 |
| New London-Norwich | 2 | 417 | 25,897 | 120,109 | 206,922 | 329 | 567 | 4.6 | 22,523 | 46 | 2,827 | 80,243 | 467,937 |
| Stamford-Norwalk | 3 | 744 | 37,687 | 189,507 | 320,878 | 520 | 879 | 5.0 | 26,702 | 59 | 6,893 | 115,632 | 818,098 |
| Waterbury | 2 | 437 | 24,540 | 115,182 | 203,875 | 315 | 559 | 4.7 | 16,633 | 60 | 2,506 | 114,986 | 392,411 |
| Maine | 37 | 3,702 | 148,517 | 816,332 | 1,618,630 | 2,238 | 4,436 | 5.5 | 160,726 | 303 | 13,263 | 710,201 | 3,925,464 |
| Nonmetropolitan | 29 | 2,041 | 69,656 | 396,898 | 939,472 | 1,088 | 2,575 | 5.7 | 89,825 | 198 | 6,326 | 449,571 | 2,420,841 |
| Metropolitan | 8 | 1,661 | 78,861 | 419,434 | 679,158 | 1,150 | 1,861 | 5.3 | 70,901 | 105 | 6,937 | 260,630 | 1,504,623 |
| Bangor | 2 | 417 | 20,592 | 106,304 | 175,683 | 292 | 482 | 5.2 | 24,087 | 20 | 1,626 | 68,624 | 466,972 |
| Lewiston-Auburn | 2 | 360 | 14,484 | 79,044 | 140,632 | 216 | 385 | 5.5 | 10,078 | 36 | 1,352 | 70,308 | 378,158 |
| Portland | 3 | 805 | 39,779 | 216,563 | 323,093 | 594 | 885 | 5.4 | 32,316 | 42 | 3,575 | 104,079 | 570,316 |
| Portsmouth-Rochester | 1 | 79 | 4,006 | 17,523 | 39,750 | 48 | 109 | 4.4 | 4,420 | 7 | 384 | 17,619 | 89,177 |
| Massachusetts | 79 | 16,001 | 784,618 | 4,372,515 | 8,584,973 | 11,980 | 23,523 | 5.6 | 696,404 | 1,149 | 80,016 | 2,929,681 | 19,633,146 |
| Nonmetropolitan | 11 | 1,412 | 74,255 | 373,806 | 796,270 | 1,024 | 2,182 | 5.0 | 59,836 | 167 | 10,258 | 314,183 | 1,732,366 |
| Metropolitan | 68 | 14,589 | 710,363 | 3,998,709 | 7,788,703 | 10,956 | 21,341 | 5.6 | 636,568 | 982 | 69,758 | 2,615,498 | 17,900,780 |
| Barnstable-Yarmouth | 1 | 223 | 17,080 | 68,128 | 147,539 | 187 | 404 | 4.0 | 21,957 | 10 | 990 | 80,379 | 392,102 |
| Boston | 37 | 8,415 | 410,895 | 2,375,992 | 4,695,609 | 6,510 | 12,866 | 5.8 | 361,578 | 506 | 39,124 | 1,355,172 | 10,884,946 |
| Brockton | 2 | 481 | 25,706 | 121,661 | 243,145 | 333 | 666 | 4.7 | 14,176 | 36 | 2,190 | 115,643 | 408,288 |
| Fitchburg-Leominster | 2 | 232 | 14,193 | 62,182 | 162,806 | 171 | 447 | 4.4 | 9,859 | 21 | 1,832 | 78,884 | 407,900 |
| Lawrence | 5 | 590 | 27,731 | 143,403 | 299,443 | 393 | 821 | 5.2 | 24,803 | 63 | 3,096 | 132,972 | 485,348 |
| Lowell | 2 | 339 | 16,857 | 71,577 | 190,755 | 196 | 523 | 4.2 | 22,296 | 39 | 2,741 | 88,611 | 513,202 |
| Pittsfield | 1 | 290 | 12,977 | 77,109 | 156,880 | 211 | 430 | 5.9 | 13,589 | 20 | 788 | 51,020 | 143,526 |
| Providence-Fall River-Warwick | 3 | 1,033 | 48,720 | 276,790 | 468,199 | 759 | 1,282 | 5.7 | 57,235 | 95 | 4,808 | 238,077 | 1,155,541 |
| Springfield | 9 | 1,715 | 70,319 | 463,953 | 799,688 | 1,271 | 2,191 | 6.6 | 60,880 | 96 | 7,445 | 264,553 | 2,122,694 |
| Worcester | 6 | 1,271 | 65,885 | 337,914 | 624,639 | 925 | 1,711 | 5.1 | 50,195 | 96 | 6,744 | 210,187 | 1,387,233 |
| New Hampshire | 28 | 2,796 | 117,814 | 637,803 | 1,435,748 | 1,746 | 3,935 | 5.4 | 121,330 | 299 | 13,634 | 547,870 | 3,071,130 |
| Nonmetropolitan | 18 | 1,414 | 59,373 | 347,455 | 829,344 | 951 | 2,273 | 5.9 | 59,153 | 142 | 5,353 | 245,759 | 1,699,752 |
| Metropolitan | 10 | 1,382 | 58,441 | 290,348 | 606,404 | 795 | 1,662 | 5.0 | 62,177 | 157 | 8,281 | 302,111 | 1,371,378 |
| Lawrence | 2 | 162 | 4,386 | 33,169 | 76,135 | 91 | 208 | 7.6 | 6,225 | 10 | 482 | 28,191 | 259,654 |
| Manchester | 2 | 469 | 19,802 | 98,999 | 167,982 | 271 | 461 | 5.0 | 14,379 | 34 | 2,821 | 74,686 | 330,524 |
| Nashua | 2 | 313 | 14,080 | 64,298 | 162,343 | 176 | 445 | 4.6 | 10,021 | 63 | 2,096 | 76,212 | 384,259 |
| Portsmouth-Rochester | 4 | 438 | 20,173 | 93,882 | 199,944 | 257 | 548 | 4.7 | 31,552 | 50 | 2,882 | 123,022 | 396,941 |
| Rhode Island | 11 | 2,410 | 122,692 | 657,057 | 1,219,980 | 1,800 | 3,343 | 5.4 | 137,271 | 179 | 13,681 | 463,961 | 2,111,605 |
| Nonmetropolitan | 1 | 148 | 6,316 | 30,004 | 81,035 | 91 | 222 | 5.2 | 9,765 | 12 | 643 | 31,451 | 108,957 |
| Metropolitan | 10 | 2,262 | 116,376 | 623,993 | 1,138,945 | 1,709 | 3,121 | 5.4 | 127,506 | 167 | 13,038 | 432,510 | 2,002,648 |
| New London-Norwich | 1 | 125 | 4,637 | 23,178 | 40,427 | 64 | 111 | 5.0 | 9,929 | 18 | 415 | 30,000 | 450,000 |
| Providence-Fall River-Warwick | 9 | 2,137 | 111,739 | 600,815 | 1,098,518 | 1,645 | 3,010 | 5.4 | 117,577 | 149 | 12,623 | 402,510 | 1,552,648 |
| Vermont | 14 | 1,506 | 51,852 | 341,581 | 881,302 | 936 | 2,415 | 6.6 | 69,356 | 139 | 6,028 | 251,346 | 2,211,564 |
| Nonmetropolitan | 12 | 935 | 29,092 | 210,935 | 545,558 | 578 | 1,495 | 7.3 | 32,013 | 81 | 3,349 | 173,449 | 1,090,492 |
| Metropolitan | 2 | 571 | 22,760 | 130,646 | 335,744 | 358 | 920 | 5.7 | 37,343 | 58 | 2,679 | 77,897 | 1,121,072 |
| Burlington | 2 | 571 | 22,760 | 130,646 | 335,744 | 358 | 920 | 5.7 | 37,343 | 58 | 2,679 | 77,897 | 1,121,072 |

 

# U.S. CENSUS DIVISION 1, NEW ENGLAND

*U.S. Community Hospitals*
*(Nonfederal, short-term general and other special hospitals)*

## 2003 Utilization, Personnel and Finances

| FULL-TIME EQUIVALENT PERSONNEL | | | | | FULL-TIME EQUIV. TRAINEES | | | EXPENSES | | | | | | |
|---|---|---|---|---|---|---|---|---|---|---|---|---|---|---|
| | | | | | | | | LABOR | | | | TOTAL | | |
| Physicians and Dentists | Registered Nurses | Licensed Practical Nurses | Other Salaried Personnel | Total Personnel | Medical and Dental Residents | Other Trainees | Total Trainees | Payroll (in thousands) | Employee Benefits (in thousands) | Total (in thousands) | Percent of Total | Amount (in thousands) | Adjusted per Admission | Adjusted per Inpatient Day |
| 71,335 | 1,021,346 | 126,328 | 2,889,619 | 4,108,628 | 77,813 | 7,954 | 85,767 | $187,822,974 | $45,438,505 | $233,261,475 | 51.8 | $450,124,257 | $7,796.41 | $1,379.48 |
| 8,445 | 147,570 | 37,579 | 485,049 | 678,643 | 1,775 | 600 | 2,375 | 25,551,777 | 6,425,000 | 31,976,774 | 53.8 | 59,444,378 | 5,305.04 | 806.30 |
| 62,890 | 873,776 | 88,749 | 2,404,570 | 3,429,985 | 76,038 | 7,354 | 83,392 | 162,271,198 | 39,013,505 | 201,284,701 | 51.5 | 390,679,879 | 8,396.37 | 1,546.78 |
| 7,781 | 52,350 | 3,228 | 169,538 | 232,897 | 6,614 | 741 | 7,355 | 11,525,278 | 2,639,146 | 14,164,426 | 52.9 | 26,783,737 | 8,448.96 | 1,572.44 |
| 764 | 9,254 | 727 | 28,548 | 39,293 | 567 | 10 | 577 | 1,853,384 | 437,051 | 2,290,438 | 55.6 | 4,121,326 | 6,713.73 | 1,203.05 |
| 7,017 | 43,096 | 2,501 | 140,990 | 193,604 | 6,047 | 731 | 6,778 | 9,671,895 | 2,202,095 | 11,873,988 | 52.4 | 22,662,411 | 8,865.67 | 1,665.44 |
| 804 | 11,661 | 552 | 33,971 | 46,988 | 1,165 | 177 | 1,342 | 2,509,385 | 606,651 | 3,116,035 | 56.2 | 5,543,272 | 8,800.67 | 1,683.56 |
| 45 | 698 | 72 | 2,313 | 3,128 | 0 | 1 | 1 | 166,896 | 43,725 | 210,622 | 57.5 | 366,207 | 6,655.17 | 1,564.66 |
| 759 | 10,963 | 480 | 31,658 | 43,860 | 1,165 | 176 | 1,341 | 2,342,488 | 562,926 | 2,905,413 | 56.1 | 5,177,064 | 9,006.05 | 1,692.66 |
| 120 | 1,085 | 61 | 3,458 | 4,724 | 116 | 1 | 117 | 247,170 | 66,278 | 313,449 | 52.9 | 592,140 | 8,407.86 | 1,644.88 |
| 11 | 537 | 24 | 1,901 | 2,473 | 56 | 0 | 56 | 143,906 | 41,234 | 185,140 | 55.3 | 334,641 | 8,834.93 | 2,009.14 |
| 261 | 4,033 | 138 | 12,819 | 17,251 | 118 | 131 | 249 | 871,905 | 199,510 | 1,071,413 | 58.9 | 1,819,034 | 8,742.83 | 1,508.05 |
| 104 | 2,731 | 102 | 5,782 | 8,719 | 652 | 24 | 676 | 504,952 | 123,567 | 628,519 | 54.6 | 1,150,573 | 10,891.35 | 1,936.66 |
| 48 | 731 | 69 | 2,019 | 2,867 | 11 | 4 | 15 | 149,790 | 37,269 | 187,058 | 54.1 | 346,079 | 7,743.48 | 1,672.51 |
| 111 | 1,204 | 67 | 3,477 | 4,859 | 101 | 4 | 105 | 269,307 | 56,496 | 325,804 | 52.6 | 618,847 | 9,581.01 | 1,928.61 |
| 104 | 642 | 19 | 2,202 | 2,967 | 111 | 12 | 123 | 155,458 | 38,572 | 194,030 | 61.5 | 315,751 | 7,249.63 | 1,548.75 |
| 703 | 5,749 | 373 | 16,102 | 22,927 | 245 | 60 | 305 | 985,243 | 243,737 | 1,228,982 | 53.6 | 2,291,787 | 7,774.70 | 1,415.88 |
| 272 | 2,747 | 236 | 8,478 | 11,733 | 3 | 2 | 5 | 464,887 | 110,490 | 575,380 | 55.9 | 1,029,812 | 6,233.47 | 1,096.16 |
| 431 | 3,002 | 137 | 7,624 | 11,194 | 242 | 58 | 300 | 520,356 | 133,247 | 653,602 | 51.8 | 1,261,974 | 9,739.86 | 1,858.15 |
| 120 | 903 | 29 | 1,892 | 2,944 | 24 | 0 | 24 | 156,175 | 37,676 | 193,851 | 52.5 | 368,909 | 10,711.64 | 2,099.85 |
| 112 | 545 | 40 | 1,412 | 2,109 | 18 | 0 | 18 | 79,472 | 19,460 | 98,931 | 42.9 | 230,441 | 8,943.96 | 1,638.61 |
| 183 | 1,392 | 63 | 3,889 | 5,527 | 200 | 58 | 258 | 252,128 | 66,920 | 319,049 | 54.2 | 588,138 | 9,757.41 | 1,820.34 |
| 16 | 162 | 5 | 431 | 614 | 0 | 0 | 0 | 32,581 | 9,190 | 41,771 | 56.1 | 74,487 | 8,197.08 | 1,873.88 |
| 5,031 | 25,475 | 1,468 | 88,422 | 120,396 | 3,855 | 487 | 4,342 | 5,762,958 | 1,230,224 | 6,993,180 | 49.9 | 14,000,780 | 8,648.20 | 1,630.85 |
| 131 | 2,220 | 79 | 6,268 | 8,698 | 219 | 7 | 226 | 472,604 | 99,506 | 572,109 | 53.4 | 1,072,039 | 6,593.43 | 1,346.33 |
| 4,900 | 23,255 | 1,389 | 82,154 | 111,698 | 3,636 | 480 | 4,116 | 5,290,353 | 1,130,718 | 6,421,071 | 49.7 | 12,928,740 | 8,877.61 | 1,659.93 |
| 26 | 416 | 14 | 1,147 | 1,603 | 0 | 0 | 0 | 99,212 | 28,521 | 127,732 | 51.7 | 247,184 | 6,682.62 | 1,675.38 |
| 4,315 | 15,545 | 835 | 55,210 | 75,905 | 3,350 | 478 | 3,828 | 3,509,867 | 727,622 | 4,237,490 | 46.5 | 9,109,780 | 10,631.32 | 1,940.06 |
| 42 | 537 | 6 | 1,744 | 2,329 | 0 | 0 | 0 | 121,589 | 22,498 | 144,087 | 58.1 | 248,035 | 4,835.84 | 1,020.11 |
| 12 | 370 | 27 | 1,198 | 1,607 | 0 | 0 | 0 | 72,842 | 14,775 | 87,617 | 56.1 | 156,051 | 4,191.19 | 958.51 |
| 48 | 735 | 36 | 2,096 | 2,915 | 0 | 0 | 0 | 150,889 | 30,238 | 181,128 | 58.1 | 311,675 | 5,295.83 | 1,040.85 |
| 9 | 409 | 48 | 1,576 | 2,042 | 0 | 0 | 0 | 93,609 | 18,398 | 112,007 | 54.3 | 206,417 | 4,616.07 | 1,082.10 |
| 26 | 450 | 47 | 1,195 | 1,718 | 11 | 1 | 12 | 89,229 | 20,703 | 109,932 | 54.9 | 200,257 | 7,584.93 | 1,276.50 |
| 54 | 1,291 | 106 | 4,259 | 5,710 | 0 | 0 | 0 | 292,757 | 71,972 | 364,730 | 81.5 | 447,430 | 5,352.54 | 955.64 |
| 338 | 1,822 | 97 | 8,321 | 10,578 | 268 | 0 | 268 | 446,740 | 95,984 | 542,724 | 53.6 | 1,012,677 | 7,454.93 | 1,266.34 |
| 30 | 1,680 | 173 | 5,408 | 7,291 | 7 | 1 | 8 | 413,619 | 100,005 | 513,624 | 51.9 | 989,233 | 7,943.48 | 1,583.69 |
| 207 | 4,492 | 229 | 13,683 | 18,611 | 345 | 0 | 345 | 885,278 | 221,389 | 1,106,668 | 55.5 | 1,994,794 | 7,592.48 | 1,389.38 |
| 175 | 2,565 | 144 | 7,759 | 10,643 | 345 | 0 | 345 | 504,315 | 118,292 | 622,608 | 56.5 | 1,102,048 | 7,930.97 | 1,328.82 |
| 32 | 1,927 | 85 | 5,924 | 7,968 | 0 | 0 | 0 | 380,963 | 103,097 | 484,060 | 54.2 | 892,746 | 7,212.48 | 1,472.20 |
| 0 | 171 | 5 | 610 | 786 | 0 | 0 | 0 | 38,746 | 7,645 | 46,390 | 53.2 | 87,194 | 8,118.65 | 1,145.26 |
| 3 | 646 | 25 | 1,810 | 2,484 | 0 | 0 | 0 | 123,659 | 40,421 | 164,080 | 54.9 | 299,103 | 8,770.83 | 1,780.57 |
| 15 | 365 | 33 | 1,392 | 1,805 | 0 | 0 | 0 | 92,659 | 22,710 | 115,369 | 59.0 | 195,422 | 5,525.23 | 1,203.76 |
| 14 | 745 | 22 | 2,112 | 2,893 | 0 | 0 | 0 | 125,899 | 32,321 | 158,221 | 50.9 | 311,027 | 7,139.05 | 1,555.57 |
| 488 | 3,147 | 273 | 10,634 | 14,542 | 741 | 1 | 742 | 857,176 | 213,260 | 1,070,435 | 55.1 | 1,941,065 | 8,504.94 | 1,591.06 |
| 0 | 129 | 10 | 434 | 573 | 0 | 0 | 0 | 32,268 | 6,274 | 38,542 | 48.7 | 79,070 | 5,107.87 | 975.75 |
| 488 | 3,018 | 263 | 10,200 | 13,969 | 741 | 1 | 742 | 824,908 | 206,986 | 1,031,893 | 55.4 | 1,861,995 | 8,752.12 | 1,634.84 |
| 6 | 113 | 15 | 319 | 453 | 2 | 0 | 2 | 28,430 | 6,841 | 35,271 | 53.5 | 65,939 | 8,152.67 | 1,631.06 |
| 482 | 2,905 | 248 | 9,881 | 13,516 | 739 | 1 | 740 | 796,478 | 200,145 | 996,622 | 55.5 | 1,796,057 | 8,775.81 | 1,634.98 |
| 548 | 1,826 | 333 | 6,726 | 9,433 | 263 | 16 | 279 | 525,239 | 123,886 | 649,126 | 64.1 | 1,012,040 | 7,467.06 | 1,148.35 |
| 141 | 895 | 186 | 3,296 | 4,518 | 0 | 0 | 0 | 212,412 | 58,764 | 271,177 | 57.4 | 472,150 | 6,163.44 | 865.44 |
| 407 | 931 | 147 | 3,430 | 4,915 | 263 | 16 | 279 | 312,827 | 65,122 | 377,949 | 70.0 | 539,890 | 9,161.70 | 1,608.04 |
| 407 | 931 | 147 | 3,430 | 4,915 | 263 | 16 | 279 | 312,827 | 65,122 | 377,949 | 70.0 | 539,890 | 9,161.70 | 1,608.04 |

# TABLE 8

## U.S. CENSUS DIVISION 2, MIDDLE ATLANTIC

*U.S. Community Hospitals*
*(Nonfederal, short-term general and other special hospitals)*

## 2003 Utilization, Personnel and Finances

| CLASSIFICATION | Hospitals | Beds | Admissions | Inpatient Days | Adjusted Patient Days | Average Daily Census | Adjusted Average Daily Census | Average Stay (days) | Surgical Operations | NEWBORNS | | OUTPATIENT VISITS | |
|---|---|---|---|---|---|---|---|---|---|---|---|---|---|
| | | | | | | | | | | Bassinets | Births | Emergency | Total |
| UNITED STATES | 4,895 | 813,307 | 34,782,742 | 196,649,769 | 326,299,942 | 538,797 | 894,019 | 5.7 | 27,106,538 | 59,662 | 3,915,842 | 111,069,871 | 563,186,046 |
| Nonmetropolitan | 2,166 | 168,374 | 5,368,552 | 35,076,707 | 73,724,487 | 96,136 | 202,034 | 6.5 | 4,592,380 | 13,462 | 530,805 | 23,720,395 | 117,598,717 |
| Metropolitan | 2,729 | 644,933 | 29,414,190 | 161,573,062 | 252,575,455 | 442,661 | 691,985 | 5.5 | 22,514,158 | 46,200 | 3,385,037 | 87,349,476 | 445,587,329 |
| CENSUS DIVISION 2, MIDDLE ATLANTIC | 486 | 128,420 | 5,430,928 | 34,910,712 | 53,882,747 | 95,644 | 147,617 | 6.4 | 4,209,158 | 7,846 | 504,382 | 15,567,144 | 96,207,625 |
| Nonmetropolitan | 80 | 10,606 | 343,935 | 2,485,250 | 5,201,683 | 6,807 | 14,249 | 7.2 | 336,894 | 747 | 28,401 | 1,531,625 | 9,771,597 |
| Metropolitan | 406 | 117,814 | 5,086,993 | 32,425,462 | 48,681,064 | 88,837 | 133,368 | 6.4 | 3,872,264 | 7,099 | 475,981 | 14,035,519 | 86,436,028 |
| New Jersey | 78 | 22,807 | 1,107,659 | 6,154,335 | 8,429,982 | 16,861 | 23,098 | 5.6 | 716,802 | 1,741 | 113,420 | 2,922,644 | 14,686,429 |
| Metropolitan | 78 | 22,807 | 1,107,659 | 6,154,335 | 8,429,982 | 16,861 | 23,098 | 5.6 | 716,802 | 1,741 | 113,420 | 2,922,644 | 14,686,429 |
| Atlantic-Cape May | 5 | 1,014 | 49,618 | 263,892 | 381,801 | 723 | 1,047 | 5.3 | 25,412 | 73 | 3,891 | 166,186 | 551,998 |
| Bergen-Passaic | 10 | 3,487 | 190,341 | 940,767 | 1,285,879 | 2,578 | 3,523 | 4.9 | 107,396 | 244 | 18,190 | 369,221 | 3,989,769 |
| Jersey City | 7 | 1,644 | 67,253 | 415,690 | 583,430 | 1,139 | 1,599 | 6.2 | 41,880 | 134 | 6,775 | 184,561 | 963,825 |
| Middlesex-Somerset-Hunterdon | 7 | 2,208 | 113,160 | 655,729 | 861,975 | 1,796 | 2,362 | 5.8 | 59,742 | 233 | 14,873 | 311,479 | 1,459,524 |
| Monmouth-Ocean | 10 | 2,783 | 147,286 | 811,815 | 1,064,081 | 2,224 | 2,915 | 5.5 | 98,654 | 211 | 13,944 | 402,614 | 1,494,600 |
| Newark | 21 | 7,230 | 311,871 | 1,900,342 | 2,594,642 | 5,207 | 7,109 | 6.1 | 217,075 | 495 | 31,888 | 799,116 | 3,529,455 |
| Philadelphia | 11 | 2,688 | 146,939 | 732,835 | 1,030,895 | 2,007 | 2,824 | 5.0 | 102,655 | 182 | 16,037 | 417,546 | 1,428,370 |
| Trenton | 6 | 1,296 | 61,239 | 325,192 | 468,685 | 891 | 1,284 | 5.3 | 45,389 | 127 | 5,724 | 183,335 | 1,037,764 |
| Vineland-Millville-Bridgeton | 1 | 457 | 19,952 | 108,073 | 158,594 | 296 | 435 | 5.4 | 18,599 | 42 | 2,098 | 88,586 | 231,124 |
| New York | 207 | 64,705 | 2,499,137 | 18,455,619 | 28,482,449 | 50,560 | 78,030 | 7.4 | 1,994,417 | 3,695 | 253,244 | 7,483,787 | 48,235,916 |
| Nonmetropolitan | 37 | 5,114 | 134,903 | 1,268,070 | 2,621,744 | 3,473 | 7,183 | 9.4 | 128,831 | 341 | 12,512 | 694,046 | 4,549,214 |
| Metropolitan | 170 | 59,591 | 2,364,234 | 17,187,549 | 25,860,705 | 47,087 | 70,847 | 7.3 | 1,865,586 | 3,354 | 240,732 | 6,789,741 | 43,686,702 |
| Albany-Schenectady-Troy | 13 | 2,909 | 112,992 | 772,276 | 1,341,322 | 2,116 | 3,676 | 6.8 | 97,008 | 139 | 9,773 | 368,484 | 2,319,377 |
| Binghamton | 2 | 665 | 27,230 | 155,340 | 358,300 | 425 | 982 | 5.7 | 35,429 | 36 | 2,608 | 87,801 | 1,286,730 |
| Buffalo-Niagara Falls | 14 | 5,182 | 162,298 | 1,306,706 | 2,037,677 | 3,580 | 5,583 | 8.1 | 163,332 | 301 | 15,117 | 499,254 | 2,672,429 |
| Dutchess County | 3 | 650 | 29,438 | 176,758 | 238,630 | 484 | 654 | 6.0 | 19,791 | 46 | 3,296 | 90,884 | 479,169 |
| Elmira | 2 | 489 | 15,224 | 136,482 | 239,318 | 373 | 656 | 9.0 | 10,224 | 20 | 1,458 | 48,817 | 363,048 |
| Glens Falls | 1 | 342 | 13,093 | 74,192 | 158,686 | 203 | 435 | 5.7 | 15,185 | 25 | 1,398 | 44,829 | 533,410 |
| Jamestown | 4 | 586 | 15,399 | 122,869 | 236,931 | 336 | 649 | 8.0 | 21,885 | 68 | 1,355 | 63,576 | 448,574 |
| Nassau-Suffolk | 25 | 8,410 | 385,508 | 2,680,803 | 3,601,170 | 7,344 | 9,865 | 7.0 | 340,185 | 581 | 41,545 | 943,766 | 5,069,219 |
| New York | 76 | 32,972 | 1,326,890 | 9,833,632 | 14,177,034 | 26,942 | 38,837 | 7.4 | 916,049 | 1,578 | 134,298 | 3,781,553 | 22,636,566 |
| Newburgh | 4 | 871 | 39,451 | 213,670 | 355,238 | 586 | 973 | 5.4 | 32,707 | 46 | 4,127 | 139,988 | 418,509 |
| Rochester | 12 | 3,176 | 115,883 | 837,326 | 1,638,331 | 2,295 | 4,488 | 7.2 | 112,384 | 272 | 13,582 | 373,156 | 4,978,096 |
| Syracuse | 9 | 2,201 | 83,666 | 573,128 | 936,321 | 1,569 | 2,565 | 6.9 | 71,825 | 170 | 9,067 | 235,801 | 1,494,959 |
| Utica-Rome | 5 | 1,138 | 37,162 | 304,367 | 541,747 | 834 | 1,484 | 8.2 | 29,582 | 72 | 3,108 | 111,832 | 986,616 |
| Pennsylvania | 201 | 40,908 | 1,824,132 | 10,300,758 | 16,970,316 | 28,223 | 46,489 | 5.6 | 1,497,939 | 2,410 | 137,718 | 5,160,713 | 33,285,280 |
| Nonmetropolitan | 43 | 5,492 | 209,032 | 1,217,180 | 2,579,939 | 3,334 | 7,066 | 5.8 | 208,063 | 406 | 15,889 | 837,579 | 5,222,383 |
| Metropolitan | 158 | 35,416 | 1,615,100 | 9,083,578 | 14,390,377 | 24,889 | 39,423 | 5.6 | 1,289,876 | 2,004 | 121,829 | 4,323,134 | 28,062,897 |
| Allentown-Bethlehem-Easton | 8 | 1,982 | 102,877 | 532,706 | 846,430 | 1,460 | 2,319 | 5.2 | 80,427 | 110 | 8,574 | 280,999 | 1,753,265 |
| Altoona | 5 | 469 | 24,193 | 128,373 | 241,565 | 352 | 661 | 5.3 | 32,037 | 29 | 2,113 | 67,965 | 716,585 |
| Erie | 6 | 1,170 | 40,535 | 212,244 | 318,151 | 581 | 872 | 5.2 | 20,526 | 61 | 3,676 | 129,763 | 405,470 |
| Harrisburg-Lebanon-Carlisle | 7 | 1,885 | 88,176 | 495,777 | 751,561 | 1,357 | 2,058 | 5.6 | 70,196 | 92 | 7,769 | 246,669 | 1,613,816 |
| Johnstown | 6 | 837 | 35,138 | 178,117 | 348,339 | 487 | 954 | 5.1 | 43,469 | 44 | 2,052 | 112,136 | 797,399 |
| Lancaster | 4 | 1,034 | 45,108 | 219,514 | 371,496 | 601 | 1,019 | 4.9 | 57,818 | 63 | 5,440 | 117,878 | 1,396,360 |
| Philadelphia | 52 | 13,599 | 645,255 | 3,682,304 | 5,422,287 | 10,093 | 14,857 | 5.7 | 462,414 | 823 | 49,154 | 1,648,427 | 9,248,196 |
| Pittsburgh | 40 | 8,916 | 407,690 | 2,297,962 | 3,714,648 | 6,297 | 10,175 | 5.6 | 343,228 | 421 | 24,816 | 1,020,099 | 6,649,242 |
| Reading | 3 | 978 | 41,245 | 234,409 | 391,323 | 643 | 1,072 | 5.7 | 32,038 | 62 | 3,803 | 124,622 | 1,041,863 |
| Scranton--Wilkes-Barre--Hazleton | 16 | 2,578 | 95,018 | 607,556 | 1,012,331 | 1,664 | 2,773 | 6.4 | 59,328 | 177 | 6,401 | 273,339 | 2,008,672 |
| Sharon | 3 | 550 | 24,193 | 123,118 | 273,906 | 337 | 750 | 5.1 | 19,529 | 44 | 1,431 | 79,870 | 615,452 |
| State College | 2 | 253 | 10,526 | 56,953 | 93,470 | 156 | 257 | 5.4 | 12,860 | 3 | 1,288 | 38,983 | 217,518 |
| Williamsport | 2 | 438 | 14,501 | 107,183 | 239,545 | 293 | 656 | 7.4 | 30,756 | 22 | 1,226 | 70,713 | 552,641 |
| York | 4 | 727 | 40,645 | 207,362 | 365,325 | 568 | 1,000 | 5.1 | 25,250 | 53 | 4,086 | 111,671 | 1,046,418 |

 

*U.S. Community Hospitals*
*(Nonfederal, short-term general and other special hospitals)*

## 2003 Utilization, Personnel and Finances

| FULL-TIME EQUIVALENT PERSONNEL | | | | | FULL-TIME EQUIV. TRAINEES | | | EXPENSES | | | | | | |
|---|---|---|---|---|---|---|---|---|---|---|---|---|---|---|
| | | | | | | | | LABOR | | | | TOTAL | | |
| Physicians and Dentists | Registered Nurses | Licensed Practical Nurses | Other Salaried Personnel | Total Personnel | Medical and Dental Residents | Other Trainees | Total Trainees | Payroll (in thousands) | Employee Benefits (in thousands) | Total (in thousands) | Percent of Total | Amount (in thousands) | Adjusted per Admission | Adjusted per Inpatient Day |
| 71,335 | 1,021,346 | 126,328 | 2,889,619 | 4,108,628 | 77,813 | 7,954 | 85,767 | $187,822,974 | $45,438,505 | $233,261,475 | 51.8 | $450,124,257 | $7,796.41 | $1,379.48 |
| 8,445 | 147,570 | 37,579 | 485,049 | 678,643 | 1,775 | 600 | 2,375 | 25,551,777 | 6,425,000 | 31,976,774 | 53.8 | 59,444,378 | 5,305.04 | 806.30 |
| 62,890 | 873,776 | 88,749 | 2,404,570 | 3,429,985 | 76,038 | 7,354 | 83,392 | 162,271,198 | 39,013,505 | 201,284,701 | 51.5 | 390,679,879 | 8,396.37 | 1,546.78 |
| 16,431 | 157,801 | 16,198 | 467,703 | 658,133 | 23,347 | 1,178 | 24,525 | 32,806,019 | 8,113,969 | 40,919,975 | 53.8 | 76,052,323 | 9,020.25 | 1,411.44 |
| 904 | 9,392 | 2,360 | 31,913 | 44,569 | 378 | 331 | 709 | 1,717,986 | 421,879 | 2,139,862 | 53.9 | 3,972,997 | 5,415.94 | 763.79 |
| 15,527 | 148,409 | 13,838 | 435,790 | 613,564 | 22,969 | 847 | 23,816 | 31,088,033 | 7,692,090 | 38,780,113 | 53.8 | 72,079,325 | 9,363.73 | 1,480.64 |
| 2,002 | 28,733 | 2,042 | 80,653 | 113,430 | 2,400 | 59 | 2,459 | 6,054,246 | 1,430,409 | 7,484,656 | 55.0 | 13,616,126 | 8,971.91 | 1,615.20 |
| 2,002 | 28,733 | 2,042 | 80,653 | 113,430 | 2,400 | 59 | 2,459 | 6,054,246 | 1,430,409 | 7,484,656 | 55.0 | 13,616,126 | 8,971.91 | 1,615.20 |
| 50 | 1,451 | 131 | 3,634 | 5,266 | 32 | 0 | 32 | 262,378 | 84,465 | 346,844 | 58.5 | 592,691 | 8,384.01 | 1,552.36 |
| 375 | 5,048 | 116 | 13,988 | 19,527 | 307 | 14 | 321 | 1,040,381 | 243,283 | 1,283,664 | 53.8 | 2,387,407 | 9,253.16 | 1,856.63 |
| 93 | 1,537 | 138 | 4,165 | 5,933 | 59 | 3 | 62 | 343,643 | 78,268 | 421,911 | 52.9 | 797,274 | 8,378.59 | 1,366.53 |
| 271 | 3,325 | 195 | 8,521 | 12,312 | 317 | 0 | 317 | 735,458 | 164,774 | 900,232 | 57.7 | 1,560,014 | 10,379.75 | 1,809.81 |
| 139 | 3,359 | 278 | 9,221 | 12,997 | 248 | 10 | 258 | 690,198 | 170,752 | 860,950 | 53.5 | 1,608,272 | 8,384.10 | 1,511.42 |
| 550 | 7,919 | 565 | 23,563 | 32,597 | 1,146 | 17 | 1,163 | 1,863,588 | 437,180 | 2,300,767 | 55.4 | 4,151,391 | 9,717.79 | 1,599.99 |
| 405 | 3,880 | 282 | 10,881 | 15,448 | 238 | 12 | 250 | 684,955 | 142,474 | 827,430 | 52.5 | 1,575,975 | 7,597.91 | 1,528.74 |
| 117 | 1,728 | 159 | 5,090 | 7,094 | 53 | 3 | 56 | 335,900 | 81,643 | 417,543 | 56.7 | 736,898 | 8,396.16 | 1,572.27 |
| 2 | 486 | 178 | 1,590 | 2,256 | 0 | 0 | 0 | 97,746 | 27,570 | 125,315 | 60.8 | 206,205 | 7,042.76 | 1,300.21 |
| 9,798 | 74,720 | 8,101 | 236,636 | 329,255 | 14,406 | 360 | 14,766 | 17,684,899 | 4,539,435 | 22,224,330 | 55.6 | 39,939,711 | 10,334.59 | 1,402.26 |
| 432 | 3,777 | 1,039 | 14,419 | 19,667 | 84 | 1 | 85 | 788,878 | 185,051 | 973,928 | 57.5 | 1,693,595 | 5,854.74 | 645.98 |
| 9,366 | 70,943 | 7,062 | 222,217 | 309,588 | 14,322 | 359 | 14,681 | 16,896,021 | 4,354,385 | 21,250,402 | 55.6 | 38,246,116 | 10,697.04 | 1,478.93 |
| 251 | 3,444 | 435 | 10,448 | 14,578 | 242 | 21 | 263 | 565,916 | 124,100 | 690,016 | 50.8 | 1,358,400 | 7,224.15 | 1,012.73 |
| 88 | 814 | 78 | 2,798 | 3,778 | 72 | 0 | 72 | 165,696 | 50,258 | 215,953 | 53.0 | 407,172 | 6,294.78 | 1,136.40 |
| 376 | 4,996 | 485 | 14,666 | 20,523 | 259 | 45 | 304 | 762,718 | 229,588 | 992,305 | 47.1 | 2,106,459 | 8,278.94 | 1,033.76 |
| 24 | 882 | 49 | 1,830 | 2,785 | 12 | 5 | 17 | 158,568 | 36,458 | 195,026 | 54.5 | 357,565 | 9,073.41 | 1,498.41 |
| 56 | 489 | 106 | 1,547 | 2,198 | 0 | 0 | 0 | 88,303 | 22,842 | 111,145 | 61.0 | 182,334 | 6,555.00 | 761.89 |
| 51 | 373 | 175 | 1,536 | 2,135 | 0 | 0 | 0 | 83,157 | 16,739 | 99,895 | 60.2 | 165,915 | 5,924.69 | 1,045.56 |
| 18 | 506 | 112 | 1,479 | 2,115 | 3 | 0 | 3 | 71,784 | 19,587 | 91,370 | 57.6 | 158,639 | 4,751.23 | 669.56 |
| 1,500 | 11,498 | 760 | 31,508 | 45,266 | 1,770 | 39 | 1,809 | 2,761,726 | 724,063 | 3,485,788 | 57.6 | 6,055,955 | 11,596.47 | 1,681.66 |
| 6,176 | 39,179 | 3,152 | 128,436 | 176,943 | 11,038 | 248 | 11,286 | 10,564,174 | 2,699,477 | 13,263,650 | 55.9 | 23,721,829 | 12,292.84 | 1,673.26 |
| 26 | 922 | 80 | 2,848 | 3,876 | 0 | 0 | 0 | 192,424 | 53,660 | 246,084 | 59.9 | 411,012 | 6,266.19 | 1,157.01 |
| 621 | 3,940 | 614 | 13,447 | 18,622 | 573 | 1 | 574 | 790,654 | 191,506 | 982,160 | 56.9 | 1,726,538 | 7,803.14 | 1,053.84 |
| 116 | 2,745 | 735 | 7,974 | 11,570 | 323 | 0 | 323 | 498,599 | 141,375 | 639,974 | 54.5 | 1,174,418 | 8,693.86 | 1,254.29 |
| 63 | 1,155 | 281 | 3,700 | 5,199 | 30 | 0 | 30 | 192,301 | 44,733 | 237,036 | 56.5 | 419,880 | 6,387.95 | 775.05 |
| 4,631 | 54,348 | 6,055 | 150,414 | 215,448 | 6,541 | 759 | 7,300 | 9,066,874 | 2,144,124 | 11,210,989 | 49.8 | 22,496,486 | 7,378.35 | 1,325.64 |
| 472 | 5,615 | 1,321 | 17,494 | 24,902 | 294 | 330 | 624 | 929,108 | 236,828 | 1,165,934 | 51.2 | 2,279,402 | 5,130.25 | 883.51 |
| 4,159 | 48,733 | 4,734 | 132,920 | 190,546 | 6,247 | 429 | 6,676 | 8,137,766 | 1,907,296 | 10,045,055 | 49.7 | 20,217,084 | 7,761.84 | 1,404.90 |
| 293 | 3,405 | 255 | 8,157 | 12,110 | 319 | 50 | 369 | 471,060 | 119,380 | 590,439 | 50.4 | 1,170,795 | 7,265.12 | 1,383.22 |
| 24 | 761 | 133 | 1,746 | 2,664 | 16 | 0 | 16 | 115,895 | 29,623 | 145,518 | 51.7 | 281,207 | 5,948.95 | 1,164.10 |
| 103 | 1,371 | 94 | 3,055 | 4,623 | 78 | 0 | 78 | 165,600 | 39,669 | 205,268 | 47.3 | 434,129 | 7,170.12 | 1,364.54 |
| 547 | 2,849 | 417 | 8,786 | 12,599 | 509 | 97 | 606 | 484,271 | 101,833 | 586,105 | 52.4 | 1,117,939 | 8,340.46 | 1,487.49 |
| 45 | 1,059 | 182 | 3,212 | 4,498 | 62 | 0 | 62 | 151,435 | 42,450 | 193,883 | 49.2 | 393,772 | 5,623.79 | 1,130.43 |
| 105 | 1,428 | 224 | 4,344 | 6,101 | 54 | 0 | 54 | 269,415 | 59,029 | 328,444 | 52.9 | 621,299 | 7,981.74 | 1,672.42 |
| 2,198 | 19,264 | 1,229 | 50,177 | 72,868 | 3,450 | 218 | 3,668 | 3,501,949 | 806,052 | 4,307,999 | 49.4 | 8,722,172 | 9,048.28 | 1,608.58 |
| 622 | 12,459 | 851 | 34,810 | 48,742 | 1,421 | 48 | 1,469 | 1,911,823 | 440,395 | 2,352,215 | 47.5 | 4,949,899 | 7,342.93 | 1,332.54 |
| 90 | 1,172 | 248 | 3,422 | 4,932 | 79 | 0 | 79 | 218,345 | 52,917 | 271,263 | 55.3 | 490,819 | 7,027.15 | 1,254.25 |
| 45 | 2,426 | 558 | 6,688 | 9,717 | 63 | 0 | 63 | 390,308 | 99,348 | 489,656 | 49.1 | 997,345 | 6,016.47 | 985.20 |
| 28 | 697 | 113 | 2,042 | 2,880 | 11 | 3 | 14 | 101,645 | 25,825 | 127,470 | 54.1 | 235,583 | 4,352.90 | 860.09 |
| 2 | 249 | 57 | 698 | 1,006 | 0 | 0 | 0 | 42,521 | 10,288 | 52,810 | 56.7 | 93,161 | 5,133.71 | 996.70 |
| 5 | 563 | 88 | 1,809 | 2,465 | 19 | 0 | 19 | 87,068 | 23,065 | 110,133 | 55.0 | 200,403 | 5,971.32 | 836.60 |
| 52 | 1,030 | 285 | 3,974 | 5,341 | 166 | 13 | 179 | 226,431 | 57,421 | 283,852 | 55.8 | 508,560 | 6,844.32 | 1,392.08 |

MSAs

# Table 8

## U.S. CENSUS DIVISION 3, SOUTH ATLANTIC

*U.S. Community Hospitals*
*(Nonfederal, short-term general and other special hospitals)*

## 2003 Utilization, Personnel and Finances

| CLASSIFICATION | Hospitals | Beds | Admissions | Inpatient Days | Adjusted Patient Days | Average Daily Census | Adjusted Average Daily Census | Average Stay (days) | Surgical Operations | NEWBORNS | | OUTPATIENT VISITS | |
|---|---|---|---|---|---|---|---|---|---|---|---|---|---|
| | | | | | | | | | | Bassinets | Births | Emergency | Total |
| UNITED STATES | 4,895 | 813,307 | 34,782,742 | 196,649,769 | 326,299,942 | 538,797 | 894,019 | 5.7 | 27,106,538 | 59,662 | 3,915,842 | 111,069,871 | 563,186,046 |
| Nonmetropolitan | 2,166 | 168,374 | 5,368,552 | 35,076,707 | 73,724,487 | 96,136 | 202,034 | 6.5 | 4,592,380 | 13,462 | 530,805 | 23,720,395 | 117,598,717 |
| Metropolitan | 2,729 | 644,933 | 29,414,190 | 161,573,062 | 252,575,455 | 442,661 | 691,985 | 5.5 | 22,514,158 | 46,200 | 3,385,037 | 87,349,476 | 445,587,329 |
| CENSUS DIVISION 3, SOUTH ATLANTIC | 731 | 151,754 | 6,646,826 | 37,810,333 | 61,356,767 | 103,595 | 168,130 | 5.7 | 5,315,757 | 10,428 | 695,242 | 22,063,587 | 83,896,160 |
| Nonmetropolitan | 289 | 32,595 | 1,144,205 | 7,506,867 | 14,452,338 | 20,571 | 39,614 | 6.6 | 956,526 | 2,344 | 102,753 | 5,013,898 | 19,084,890 |
| Metropolitan | 442 | 119,159 | 5,502,621 | 30,303,466 | 46,904,429 | 83,024 | 128,516 | 5.5 | 4,359,231 | 8,084 | 592,489 | 17,049,689 | 64,811,270 |
| Delaware | 6 | 2,051 | 97,074 | 606,183 | 957,751 | 1,660 | 2,624 | 6.2 | 94,600 | 106 | 11,837 | 300,450 | 2,021,860 |
| Nonmetropolitan | 2 | 437 | 13,834 | 129,381 | 238,148 | 354 | 653 | 9.4 | 16,076 | 27 | 1,724 | 54,054 | 425,326 |
| Metropolitan | 4 | 1,614 | 83,240 | 476,802 | 719,603 | 1,306 | 1,971 | 5.7 | 78,524 | 79 | 10,113 | 246,396 | 1,596,534 |
| Dover | 1 | 325 | 16,761 | 84,299 | 155,053 | 231 | 425 | 5.0 | 17,680 | 29 | 2,033 | 61,530 | 356,946 |
| Wilmington-Newark | 3 | 1,289 | 66,479 | 392,503 | 564,550 | 1,075 | 1,546 | 5.9 | 60,844 | 50 | 8,080 | 184,866 | 1,239,588 |
| District of Columbia | 10 | 3,375 | 134,685 | 905,107 | 1,324,321 | 2,479 | 3,628 | 6.7 | 105,550 | 200 | 14,137 | 359,624 | 1,588,276 |
| Metropolitan | 10 | 3,375 | 134,685 | 905,107 | 1,324,321 | 2,479 | 3,628 | 6.7 | 105,550 | 200 | 14,137 | 359,624 | 1,588,276 |
| Washington | 10 | 3,375 | 134,685 | 905,107 | 1,324,321 | 2,479 | 3,628 | 6.7 | 105,550 | 200 | 14,137 | 359,624 | 1,588,276 |
| Florida | 203 | 50,687 | 2,296,184 | 11,966,726 | 17,857,216 | 32,797 | 48,954 | 5.2 | 1,475,371 | 2,730 | 197,538 | 6,668,184 | 22,023,554 |
| Nonmetropolitan | 33 | 2,711 | 108,319 | 488,321 | 871,705 | 1,349 | 2,413 | 4.5 | 71,245 | 145 | 5,984 | 419,701 | 1,390,150 |
| Metropolitan | 170 | 47,976 | 2,187,865 | 11,478,405 | 16,985,511 | 31,448 | 46,541 | 5.2 | 1,404,126 | 2,585 | 191,554 | 6,248,483 | 20,633,404 |
| Daytona Beach | 7 | 1,554 | 67,668 | 328,489 | 534,238 | 899 | 1,463 | 4.9 | 39,621 | 62 | 3,985 | 305,280 | 889,129 |
| Fort Lauderdale | 17 | 4,921 | 232,398 | 1,180,363 | 1,735,455 | 3,233 | 4,754 | 5.1 | 124,551 | 224 | 21,420 | 642,440 | 2,010,920 |
| Fort Myers-Cape Coral | 5 | 1,735 | 75,868 | 369,163 | 553,668 | 1,011 | 1,517 | 4.9 | 48,606 | 115 | 6,851 | 167,296 | 628,166 |
| Fort Pierce-Port St. Lucie | 3 | 847 | 41,702 | 204,918 | 292,233 | 562 | 801 | 4.9 | 32,934 | 66 | 3,379 | 126,155 | 179,913 |
| Fort Walton Beach | 3 | 422 | 19,157 | 90,831 | 134,206 | 249 | 367 | 4.7 | 16,405 | 32 | 1,758 | 75,780 | 197,017 |
| Gainesville | 4 | 1,139 | 54,513 | 297,389 | 400,900 | 815 | 1,098 | 5.5 | 38,096 | 45 | 5,030 | 119,911 | 829,014 |
| Jacksonville | 11 | 3,092 | 149,804 | 800,518 | 1,245,923 | 2,192 | 3,415 | 5.3 | 123,106 | 238 | 15,201 | 502,434 | 1,653,766 |
| Lakeland-Winter Haven | 4 | 1,190 | 63,790 | 290,980 | 410,580 | 797 | 1,125 | 4.6 | 32,177 | 59 | 5,910 | 221,446 | 548,276 |
| Melbourne-Titusville-Palm Bay | 5 | 1,188 | 59,584 | 278,288 | 460,070 | 763 | 1,261 | 4.7 | 28,586 | 72 | 3,749 | 131,290 | 611,005 |
| Miami | 26 | 7,210 | 318,063 | 1,892,790 | 2,765,655 | 5,187 | 7,579 | 6.0 | 188,681 | 414 | 24,705 | 783,535 | 2,885,915 |
| Naples | 1 | 539 | 31,454 | 143,585 | 185,230 | 393 | 507 | 4.6 | 13,639 | 34 | 3,602 | 109,831 | 227,329 |
| Ocala | 2 | 610 | 36,245 | 114,791 | 159,741 | 315 | 437 | 3.2 | 21,307 | 38 | 2,476 | 128,083 | 202,090 |
| Orlando | 13 | 6,725 | 291,008 | 1,740,614 | 2,514,801 | 4,770 | 6,892 | 6.0 | 170,427 | 365 | 30,254 | 838,109 | 2,379,996 |
| Panama City | 2 | 547 | 26,142 | 126,547 | 200,514 | 347 | 549 | 4.8 | 24,023 | 38 | 2,557 | 87,600 | 282,620 |
| Pensacola | 6 | 1,442 | 59,353 | 321,043 | 500,420 | 880 | 1,372 | 5.4 | 45,911 | 67 | 4,843 | 211,875 | 986,814 |
| Punta Gorda | 3 | 722 | 27,779 | 138,499 | 201,609 | 379 | 553 | 5.0 | 23,410 | 10 | 1,101 | 55,175 | 179,014 |
| Sarasota-Bradenton | 7 | 1,899 | 81,831 | 406,831 | 577,368 | 1,114 | 1,582 | 5.0 | 54,267 | 70 | 5,784 | 250,552 | 900,501 |
| Tallahassee | 4 | 833 | 36,229 | 195,390 | 301,956 | 536 | 828 | 5.4 | 25,621 | 56 | 4,850 | 100,701 | 354,811 |
| Tampa-St. Petersburg-Clearwater | 33 | 8,387 | 366,365 | 1,810,077 | 2,654,882 | 4,959 | 7,275 | 4.9 | 258,796 | 418 | 31,747 | 1,011,067 | 3,550,395 |
| West Palm Beach-Boca Raton | 14 | 2,974 | 148,912 | 747,299 | 1,156,062 | 2,047 | 3,166 | 5.0 | 93,962 | 162 | 12,352 | 379,923 | 1,136,713 |
| Georgia | 146 | 24,624 | 925,681 | 6,024,083 | 10,910,976 | 16,503 | 29,894 | 6.5 | 784,509 | 2,075 | 133,692 | 3,542,261 | 12,849,345 |
| Nonmetropolitan | 83 | 9,441 | 260,148 | 2,223,859 | 4,692,368 | 6,091 | 12,855 | 8.5 | 203,500 | 659 | 30,677 | 1,201,327 | 3,818,310 |
| Metropolitan | 63 | 15,183 | 665,533 | 3,800,224 | 6,218,608 | 10,412 | 17,039 | 5.7 | 581,009 | 1,416 | 103,015 | 2,340,934 | 9,031,035 |
| Albany | 2 | 610 | 22,573 | 116,782 | 225,638 | 320 | 618 | 5.2 | 21,227 | 66 | 2,698 | 78,819 | 620,744 |
| Athens | 2 | 617 | 24,495 | 152,296 | 242,357 | 417 | 664 | 6.2 | 35,650 | 36 | 3,298 | 92,481 | 327,318 |
| Atlanta | 36 | 8,847 | 413,887 | 2,314,037 | 3,739,540 | 6,339 | 10,246 | 5.6 | 333,223 | 843 | 73,851 | 1,489,128 | 5,242,820 |
| Augusta-Aiken | 6 | 1,481 | 58,348 | 328,459 | 517,782 | 900 | 1,419 | 5.6 | 60,637 | 128 | 6,735 | 199,793 | 1,086,567 |
| Chattanooga | 2 | 307 | 7,185 | 79,566 | 151,744 | 218 | 416 | 11.1 | 7,965 | 15 | 854 | 34,973 | 114,129 |
| Columbus | 4 | 1,025 | 33,664 | 206,849 | 353,970 | 507 | 969 | 6.1 | 27,426 | 72 | 4,101 | 131,929 | 351,158 |
| Macon | 7 | 1,176 | 55,410 | 273,434 | 440,959 | 750 | 1,209 | 4.9 | 58,220 | 167 | 6,115 | 166,446 | 709,328 |
| Savannah | 4 | 1,120 | 49,971 | 328,801 | 546,618 | 901 | 1,498 | 6.6 | 36,661 | 89 | 5,363 | 147,365 | 578,971 |

MSAs

# TABLE 8

# U.S. CENSUS DIVISION 3, SOUTH ATLANTIC

*U.S. Community Hospitals*
*(Nonfederal, short-term general and other special hospitals)*

## 2003 Utilization, Personnel and Finances



| FULL-TIME EQUIVALENT PERSONNEL | | | | | FULL-TIME EQUIV. TRAINEES | | | EXPENSES | | | | | | |
|---|---|---|---|---|---|---|---|---|---|---|---|---|---|---|
| | | | | | | | | LABOR | | | | TOTAL | | |
| Physicians and Dentists | Registered Nurses | Licensed Practical Nurses | Other Salaried Personnel | Total Personnel | Medical and Dental Residents | Other Trainees | Total Trainees | Payroll (in thousands) | Employee Benefits (in thousands) | Total (in thousands) | Percent of Total | Amount (in thousands) | Adjusted per Admission | Adjusted per Inpatient Day |
| 71,335 | 1,021,346 | 126,328 | 2,889,619 | 4,108,628 | 77,813 | 7,954 | 85,767 | $187,822,974 | $45,438,505 | $233,261,475 | 51.8 | $450,124,257 | $7,796.41 | $1,379.48 |
| 8,445 | 147,570 | 37,579 | 485,049 | 678,643 | 1,775 | 600 | 2,375 | 25,551,777 | 6,425,000 | 31,976,774 | 53.8 | 59,444,378 | 5,305.04 | 806.30 |
| 62,890 | 873,776 | 88,749 | 2,404,570 | 3,429,985 | 76,038 | 7,354 | 83,392 | 162,271,198 | 39,013,505 | 201,284,701 | 51.5 | 390,679,879 | 8,396.37 | 1,546.78 |
| 7,940 | 194,588 | 22,679 | 513,990 | 739,197 | 10,845 | 968 | 11,813 | 32,658,662 | 7,522,116 | 40,180,788 | 51.0 | 78,776,238 | 7,376.11 | 1,283.90 |
| 1,103 | 29,922 | 7,165 | 92,504 | 130,694 | 466 | 46 | 512 | 4,904,163 | 1,222,276 | 6,126,437 | 53.2 | 11,518,398 | 5,393.24 | 796.99 |
| 6,837 | 164,666 | 15,514 | 421,486 | 608,503 | 10,379 | 922 | 11,301 | 27,754,499 | 6,299,840 | 34,054,351 | 50.6 | 67,257,840 | 7,871.75 | 1,433.93 |
| 246 | 3,101 | 274 | 10,613 | 14,234 | 237 | 0 | 237 | 646,022 | 175,872 | 821,894 | 56.9 | 1,444,199 | 9,447.61 | 1,507.91 |
| 21 | 503 | 37 | 1,726 | 2,287 | 9 | 0 | 9 | 92,665 | 20,752 | 113,417 | 51.4 | 220,822 | 8,426.72 | 927.25 |
| 225 | 2,598 | 237 | 8,887 | 11,947 | 228 | 0 | 228 | 553,357 | 155,120 | 708,477 | 57.9 | 1,223,377 | 9,658.83 | 1,700.07 |
| 9 | 590 | 66 | 1,538 | 2,203 | 0 | 0 | 0 | 88,329 | 28,433 | 116,762 | 57.3 | 203,945 | 6,615.37 | 1,315.33 |
| 216 | 2,008 | 171 | 7,349 | 9,744 | 228 | 0 | 228 | 465,028 | 126,687 | 591,715 | 58.0 | 1,019,432 | 10,637.92 | 1,805.74 |
| 839 | 4,695 | 263 | 13,004 | 18,801 | 1,220 | 70 | 1,290 | 1,119,218 | 187,610 | 1,306,827 | 54.1 | 2,415,900 | 12,273.36 | 1,824.26 |
| 839 | 4,695 | 263 | 13,004 | 18,801 | 1,220 | 70 | 1,290 | 1,119,218 | 187,610 | 1,306,827 | 54.1 | 2,415,900 | 12,273.36 | 1,824.26 |
| 839 | 4,695 | 263 | 13,004 | 18,801 | 1,220 | 70 | 1,290 | 1,119,218 | 187,610 | 1,306,827 | 54.1 | 2,415,900 | 12,273.36 | 1,824.26 |
| 1,661 | 59,896 | 6,695 | 155,195 | 223,447 | 2,302 | 326 | 2,628 | 9,959,032 | 2,360,139 | 12,319,182 | 49.7 | 24,774,273 | 7,210.15 | 1,387.35 |
| 66 | 2,412 | 604 | 6,925 | 10,007 | 5 | 1 | 6 | 372,589 | 91,833 | 464,422 | 50.0 | 928,207 | 4,958.64 | 1,064.82 |
| 1,595 | 57,484 | 6,091 | 148,270 | 213,440 | 2,297 | 325 | 2,622 | 9,586,443 | 2,268,307 | 11,854,760 | 49.7 | 23,846,066 | 7,339.88 | 1,403.91 |
| 47 | 1,650 | 191 | 4,213 | 6,101 | 42 | 1 | 43 | 272,093 | 69,675 | 341,770 | 47.2 | 723,453 | 6,542.00 | 1,354.18 |
| 143 | 5,811 | 540 | 12,367 | 18,861 | 79 | 10 | 89 | 927,509 | 203,868 | 1,131,379 | 50.1 | 2,260,154 | 6,575.47 | 1,302.34 |
| 135 | 1,905 | 232 | 5,743 | 8,015 | 32 | 3 | 35 | 341,680 | 68,684 | 410,364 | 54.4 | 754,458 | 6,619.45 | 1,362.65 |
| 10 | 987 | 73 | 2,141 | 3,211 | 0 | 0 | 0 | 157,767 | 44,379 | 202,146 | 50.1 | 403,771 | 6,745.36 | 1,381.67 |
| 1 | 504 | 70 | 884 | 1,459 | 1 | 0 | 1 | 54,677 | 14,439 | 69,116 | 46.4 | 148,879 | 5,180.57 | 1,109.33 |
| 23 | 1,680 | 113 | 4,359 | 6,175 | 15 | 1 | 16 | 281,496 | 62,708 | 344,205 | 46.1 | 747,344 | 10,042.38 | 1,864.16 |
| 23 | 4,589 | 181 | 11,477 | 16,270 | 35 | 23 | 58 | 640,047 | 169,895 | 809,943 | 47.6 | 1,701,786 | 7,224.24 | 1,365.88 |
| 23 | 1,424 | 319 | 4,602 | 6,368 | 0 | 25 | 25 | 249,671 | 51,119 | 300,791 | 52.5 | 573,423 | 6,357.03 | 1,396.62 |
| 109 | 1,349 | 142 | 4,121 | 5,721 | 111 | 8 | 119 | 284,564 | 68,758 | 353,321 | 50.4 | 701,157 | 7,039.16 | 1,524.02 |
| 381 | 9,600 | 930 | 23,164 | 34,075 | 1,272 | 221 | 1,493 | 1,846,562 | 414,974 | 2,261,537 | 50.3 | 4,492,010 | 9,636.01 | 1,624.21 |
| 3 | 782 | 65 | 2,139 | 2,989 | 0 | 0 | 0 | 120,916 | 24,665 | 145,581 | 49.0 | 296,859 | 7,315.95 | 1,602.65 |
| 0 | 937 | 40 | 2,397 | 3,374 | 0 | 0 | 0 | 128,113 | 32,331 | 160,444 | 52.0 | 308,426 | 6,190.93 | 1,930.79 |
| 191 | 7,519 | 717 | 22,539 | 30,966 | 306 | 7 | 313 | 1,285,024 | 353,360 | 1,638,385 | 51.7 | 3,166,863 | 7,537.24 | 1,259.29 |
| 5 | 667 | 134 | 1,402 | 2,208 | 0 | 1 | 1 | 90,983 | 21,410 | 112,394 | 47.3 | 237,648 | 5,758.36 | 1,185.19 |
| 98 | 1,852 | 197 | 4,565 | 6,712 | 0 | 0 | 0 | 230,730 | 49,473 | 280,204 | 44.8 | 625,790 | 6,753.25 | 1,250.53 |
| 17 | 619 | 92 | 1,593 | 2,321 | 18 | 2 | 20 | 99,804 | 24,889 | 124,694 | 49.5 | 252,058 | 6,218.44 | 1,250.23 |
| 27 | 2,361 | 353 | 5,703 | 8,444 | 14 | 2 | 16 | 328,704 | 79,365 | 408,069 | 49.0 | 833,182 | 7,164.32 | 1,443.07 |
| 46 | 1,071 | 168 | 2,529 | 3,814 | 31 | 0 | 31 | 172,222 | 40,705 | 212,927 | 53.3 | 399,826 | 7,164.31 | 1,324.12 |
| 287 | 8,762 | 1,172 | 24,003 | 34,224 | 315 | 20 | 335 | 1,520,694 | 349,353 | 1,870,048 | 49.2 | 3,803,370 | 7,066.31 | 1,432.59 |
| 26 | 3,415 | 362 | 8,329 | 12,132 | 26 | 1 | 27 | 553,185 | 124,256 | 677,442 | 47.9 | 1,415,609 | 6,138.33 | 1,224.51 |
| 1,129 | 29,420 | 4,691 | 79,648 | 114,888 | 1,025 | 104 | 1,129 | 4,729,585 | 1,109,447 | 5,839,032 | 51.3 | 11,386,865 | 7,135.72 | 1,043.62 |
| 247 | 6,873 | 2,335 | 23,227 | 32,682 | 113 | 9 | 122 | 1,163,017 | 279,968 | 1,442,987 | 53.0 | 2,720,257 | 5,312.72 | 579.72 |
| 882 | 22,547 | 2,356 | 56,421 | 82,206 | 912 | 95 | 1,007 | 3,566,568 | 829,480 | 4,396,045 | 50.7 | 8,666,608 | 7,997.03 | 1,393.66 |
| 46 | 762 | 82 | 2,231 | 3,121 | 81 | 6 | 87 | 125,719 | 33,136 | 158,855 | 41.4 | 383,838 | 8,774.85 | 1,701.12 |
| 7 | 847 | 49 | 2,460 | 3,363 | 0 | 0 | 0 | 147,549 | 38,471 | 186,020 | 57.5 | 323,398 | 8,145.83 | 1,334.39 |
| 303 | 14,081 | 1,290 | 33,601 | 49,275 | 165 | 74 | 239 | 2,219,835 | 486,925 | 2,706,758 | 50.2 | 5,395,716 | 8,086.22 | 1,442.88 |
| 361 | 2,137 | 323 | 5,903 | 8,724 | 405 | 0 | 405 | 325,062 | 99,398 | 424,460 | 50.9 | 834,423 | 8,962.37 | 1,611.53 |
| 1 | 217 | 98 | 904 | 1,220 | 0 | 0 | 0 | 42,360 | 9,918 | 52,279 | 57.3 | 91,274 | 6,644.85 | 601.50 |
| 2 | 902 | 183 | 2,952 | 4,039 | 38 | 0 | 38 | 150,976 | 34,770 | 185,745 | 47.9 | 388,179 | 6,827.53 | 1,096.64 |
| 41 | 2,034 | 173 | 4,498 | 6,746 | 127 | 15 | 142 | 277,487 | 72,450 | 349,937 | 53.1 | 658,953 | 7,218.79 | 1,494.36 |
| 121 | 1,567 | 158 | 3,872 | 5,718 | 96 | 0 | 96 | 277,579 | 54,412 | 331,991 | 56.2 | 590,828 | 7,571.32 | 1,080.88 |

*Table continues*

## TABLE 8

# U.S. CENSUS DIVISION 3, SOUTH ATLANTIC CONTINUED

*U.S. Community Hospitals*
*(Nonfederal, short-term general and other special hospitals)*

## 2003 Utilization, Personnel and Finances

| CLASSIFICATION | Hospitals | Beds | Admissions | Inpatient Days | Adjusted Patient Days | Average Daily Census | Adjusted Average Daily Census | Average Stay (days) | Surgical Operations | NEWBORNS Bassinets | NEWBORNS Births | OUTPATIENT VISITS Emergency | OUTPATIENT VISITS Total |
|---|---|---|---|---|---|---|---|---|---|---|---|---|---|
| Maryland | 51 | 11,613 | 645,158 | 3,167,111 | 4,838,739 | 8,675 | 13,260 | 4.9 | 533,408 | 947 | 65,861 | 2,079,674 | 6,522,366 |
| Nonmetropolitan | 10 | 1,031 | 51,565 | 274,106 | 453,938 | 749 | 1,245 | 5.3 | 46,960 | 79 | 4,397 | 202,823 | 1,264,435 |
| Metropolitan | 41 | 10,582 | 593,593 | 2,893,005 | 4,384,801 | 7,926 | 12,015 | 4.9 | 486,448 | 868 | 61,464 | 1,876,851 | 5,257,931 |
| Baltimore | 23 | 6,889 | 383,782 | 1,900,157 | 2,858,019 | 5,206 | 7,831 | 5.0 | 319,209 | 488 | 33,620 | 1,123,146 | 3,280,670 |
| Cumberland | 2 | 418 | 17,028 | 109,748 | 204,472 | 301 | 561 | 6.4 | 10,075 | 12 | 1,062 | 57,737 | 321,931 |
| Hagerstown | 1 | 287 | 15,232 | 74,981 | 142,975 | 205 | 392 | 4.9 | 10,557 | 41 | 1,802 | 61,831 | 213,631 |
| Washington | 14 | 2,866 | 168,896 | 779,848 | 1,134,210 | 2,137 | 3,107 | 4.6 | 139,114 | 315 | 24,356 | 604,166 | 1,305,724 |
| Wilmington-Newark | 1 | 122 | 8,655 | 28,271 | 45,125 | 77 | 124 | 3.3 | 7,493 | 12 | 624 | 29,971 | 135,975 |
| North Carolina | 113 | 23,285 | 987,209 | 6,053,100 | 10,308,296 | 16,585 | 28,245 | 6.1 | 852,249 | 1,608 | 110,364 | 3,433,432 | 14,540,747 |
| Nonmetropolitan | 62 | 7,688 | 288,519 | 1,855,830 | 3,458,566 | 5,086 | 9,472 | 6.4 | 238,144 | 589 | 26,976 | 1,276,616 | 4,711,494 |
| Metropolitan | 51 | 15,597 | 698,690 | 4,197,270 | 6,849,730 | 11,499 | 18,773 | 6.0 | 614,105 | 1,019 | 83,388 | 2,156,816 | 9,829,253 |
| Asheville | 2 | 821 | 36,821 | 203,867 | 280,578 | 559 | 769 | 5.5 | 39,698 | 32 | 3,496 | 86,376 | 425,284 |
| Charlotte-Gastonia-Rock Hill | 12 | 3,213 | 157,403 | 931,303 | 1,586,264 | 2,551 | 4,347 | 5.9 | 142,885 | 278 | 21,659 | 549,138 | 2,512,978 |
| Fayetteville | 1 | 537 | 28,586 | 159,863 | 239,283 | 438 | 656 | 5.6 | 26,612 | 60 | 3,886 | 99,438 | 399,606 |
| Goldsboro | 1 | 256 | 12,128 | 63,010 | 96,554 | 173 | 265 | 5.2 | 11,885 | 30 | 1,398 | 43,258 | 146,653 |
| Greensboro—Winston-Salem—High Point | 12 | 4,106 | 161,942 | 1,066,458 | 1,774,294 | 2,921 | 4,863 | 6.6 | 112,981 | 202 | 17,270 | 454,864 | 1,405,456 |
| Greenville | 1 | 720 | 33,752 | 208,223 | 278,022 | 570 | 762 | 6.2 | 26,412 | 42 | 3,231 | 63,384 | 256,347 |
| Hickory-Morganton-Lenoir | 5 | 1,136 | 37,995 | 275,910 | 497,714 | 756 | 1,365 | 7.3 | 35,844 | 72 | 3,882 | 190,065 | 611,153 |
| Jacksonville | 1 | 133 | 7,903 | 29,366 | 54,971 | 80 | 151 | 3.7 | 5,663 | 23 | 1,202 | 37,103 | 109,114 |
| Raleigh-Durham-Chapel Hill | 11 | 3,440 | 164,762 | 956,836 | 1,554,274 | 2,623 | 4,258 | 5.8 | 164,724 | 205 | 21,860 | 448,094 | 3,429,200 |
| Rocky Mount | 2 | 431 | 19,138 | 97,760 | 160,222 | 267 | 439 | 5.1 | 12,606 | 31 | 1,861 | 74,053 | 217,186 |
| Wilmington | 3 | 804 | 38,260 | 204,674 | 327,554 | 561 | 898 | 5.3 | 34,795 | 44 | 3,643 | 111,043 | 316,276 |
| South Carolina | 61 | 11,115 | 506,488 | 2,949,736 | 4,626,788 | 8,076 | 12,676 | 5.8 | 468,877 | 847 | 48,497 | 1,807,580 | 7,401,406 |
| Nonmetropolitan | 26 | 3,263 | 127,200 | 760,102 | 1,307,246 | 2,080 | 3,581 | 6.0 | 112,492 | 300 | 11,267 | 563,054 | 1,447,154 |
| Metropolitan | 35 | 7,852 | 379,288 | 2,189,634 | 3,319,542 | 5,996 | 9,095 | 5.8 | 356,385 | 547 | 37,230 | 1,244,526 | 5,954,252 |
| Augusta-Aiken | 2 | 309 | 12,629 | 58,475 | 89,972 | 160 | 247 | 4.6 | 8,274 | 18 | 867 | 53,775 | 62,425 |
| Charleston-North Charleston | 7 | 1,586 | 79,751 | 447,289 | 693,306 | 1,224 | 1,900 | 5.6 | 83,681 | 112 | 8,229 | 262,366 | 1,307,930 |
| Charlotte-Gastonia-Rock Hill | 1 | 237 | 16,054 | 76,862 | 107,082 | 211 | 293 | 4.8 | 14,485 | 37 | 2,115 | 48,765 | 155,209 |
| Columbia | 5 | 1,631 | 83,556 | 480,243 | 676,565 | 1,316 | 1,854 | 5.7 | 67,405 | 105 | 8,336 | 190,502 | 1,683,252 |
| Florence | 4 | 837 | 38,999 | 226,981 | 325,451 | 622 | 891 | 5.8 | 40,009 | 24 | 2,097 | 115,119 | 361,734 |
| Greenville-Spartanburg-Anderson | 12 | 2,445 | 115,494 | 668,115 | 1,037,785 | 1,829 | 2,843 | 5.8 | 103,365 | 183 | 11,951 | 408,921 | 1,883,497 |
| Myrtle Beach | 3 | 571 | 25,054 | 165,173 | 284,742 | 452 | 780 | 6.6 | 23,590 | 48 | 2,469 | 118,242 | 358,523 |
| Sumter | 1 | 236 | 7,751 | 66,496 | 104,639 | 182 | 287 | 8.6 | 15,576 | 20 | 1,166 | 46,836 | 141,682 |
| Virginia | 84 | 17,225 | 758,258 | 4,367,997 | 7,223,111 | 11,971 | 19,787 | 5.8 | 722,658 | 1,428 | 92,014 | 2,759,886 | 11,191,378 |
| Nonmetropolitan | 34 | 3,959 | 150,525 | 839,838 | 1,548,195 | 2,302 | 4,241 | 5.6 | 139,928 | 314 | 12,301 | 676,048 | 2,968,810 |
| Metropolitan | 50 | 13,266 | 607,733 | 3,528,159 | 5,674,916 | 9,669 | 15,546 | 5.8 | 582,730 | 1,114 | 79,713 | 2,083,838 | 8,222,568 |
| Charlottesville | 2 | 687 | 36,727 | 184,880 | 335,790 | 507 | 920 | 5.0 | 46,620 | 45 | 3,045 | 90,729 | 1,421,619 |
| Danville | 1 | 350 | 11,865 | 71,983 | 117,503 | 197 | 322 | 6.1 | 9,028 | 20 | 1,112 | 37,291 | 104,019 |
| Johnson City-Kingsport-Bristol | 1 | 135 | 4,956 | 19,853 | 45,123 | 54 | 124 | 4.0 | 8,507 | 12 | 644 | 30,324 | 97,190 |
| Lynchburg | 2 | 984 | 28,221 | 290,248 | 444,000 | 796 | 1,217 | 10.3 | 24,415 | 48 | 2,582 | 88,888 | 156,227 |
| Norfolk-Virginia Beach-Newport News | 16 | 3,412 | 158,660 | 943,767 | 1,632,330 | 2,583 | 4,470 | 5.9 | 151,298 | 295 | 19,720 | 661,481 | 2,440,010 |
| Richmond-Petersburg | 11 | 3,369 | 141,011 | 857,503 | 1,247,914 | 2,351 | 3,418 | 6.1 | 132,932 | 251 | 14,811 | 478,681 | 1,617,706 |
| Roanoke | 2 | 1,228 | 50,446 | 306,352 | 445,588 | 840 | 1,221 | 6.1 | 50,981 | 67 | 3,842 | 164,289 | 683,277 |
| Washington | 15 | 3,101 | 175,847 | 853,573 | 1,406,668 | 2,341 | 3,854 | 4.9 | 158,949 | 376 | 33,957 | 532,155 | 1,702,520 |
| West Virginia | 57 | 7,779 | 296,089 | 1,770,200 | 3,309,569 | 4,849 | 9,062 | 6.0 | 278,535 | 487 | 21,302 | 1,112,496 | 5,757,228 |
| Nonmotropolitan | 39 | 4,065 | 144,095 | 935,430 | 1,882,172 | 2,560 | 5,154 | 6.5 | 128,181 | 231 | 9,427 | 620,275 | 3,059,211 |
| Metropolitan | 18 | 3,714 | 151,994 | 834,860 | 1,427,397 | 2,289 | 3,908 | 5.5 | 150,354 | 256 | 11,875 | 492,221 | 2,698,017 |
| Charleston | 5 | 1,249 | 55,222 | 286,537 | 461,906 | 784 | 1,265 | 5.2 | 62,888 | 62 | 4,112 | 155,597 | 826,013 |
| Cumberland | 1 | 32 | 1,195 | 3,954 | 11,490 | 11 | 31 | 3.3 | 1,760 | 0 | 0 | 10,718 | 45,385 |
| Huntington-Ashland | 3 | 702 | 34,358 | 178,648 | 264,262 | 490 | 724 | 5.2 | 24,627 | 55 | 3,079 | 107,055 | 447,896 |
| Parkersburg-Marietta | 3 | 542 | 21,132 | 113,882 | 195,253 | 313 | 535 | 5.4 | 20,147 | 54 | 1,656 | 74,132 | 411,669 |
| Steubenville-Weirton | 1 | 238 | 8,234 | 42,394 | 90,309 | 116 | 247 | 5.1 | 5,423 | 21 | 433 | 28,045 | 183,370 |
| Washington | 2 | 204 | 9,847 | 45,437 | 93,379 | 125 | 255 | 4.6 | 12,192 | 30 | 1,091 | 51,922 | 198,328 |
| Wheeling | 3 | 747 | 22,006 | 164,008 | 310,798 | 450 | 851 | 7.5 | 23,317 | 34 | 1,504 | 64,752 | 585,356 |



 

# U.S. CENSUS DIVISION 3, SOUTH ATLANTIC CONTINUED

*U.S. Community Hospitals*
*(Nonfederal, short-term general and other special hospitals)*

## 2003 Utilization, Personnel and Finances

| FULL-TIME EQUIVALENT PERSONNEL | | | | | FULL-TIME EQUIV. TRAINEES | | | EXPENSES | | | | | | |
|---|---|---|---|---|---|---|---|---|---|---|---|---|---|---|
| | | | | | | | | LABOR | | | | TOTAL | | |
| Physicians and Dentists | Registered Nurses | Licensed Practical Nurses | Other Salaried Personnel | Total Personnel | Medical and Dental Residents | Other Trainees | Total Trainees | Payroll (in thousands) | Employee Benefits (in thousands) | Total (in thousands) | Percent of Total | Amount (in thousands) | Adjusted per Admission | Adjusted per Inpatient Day |
| 1,604 | 17,623 | 734 | 49,768 | 69,729 | 1,287 | 220 | 1,507 | 3,251,273 | 663,210 | 3,914,483 | 51.5 | 7,601,418 | 7,625.22 | 1,570.95 |
| 46 | 1,270 | 133 | 4,217 | 5,666 | 0 | 9 | 9 | 232,841 | 56,314 | 289,155 | 52.4 | 551,828 | 6,167.68 | 1,215.65 |
| 1,558 | 16,353 | 601 | 45,551 | 64,063 | 1,287 | 211 | 1,498 | 3,018,432 | 606,896 | 3,625,328 | 51.4 | 7,049,590 | 7,768.93 | 1,607.73 |
| 1,479 | 11,535 | 394 | 32,059 | 45,467 | 1,245 | 186 | 1,431 | 2,110,907 | 416,006 | 2,526,912 | 50.6 | 4,992,892 | 8,545.64 | 1,746.98 |
| 19 | 490 | 33 | 1,473 | 2,015 | 0 | 24 | 24 | 77,253 | 23,401 | 100,654 | 56.5 | 178,092 | 5,507.03 | 870.98 |
| 10 | 414 | 45 | 1,258 | 1,727 | 0 | 0 | 0 | 74,980 | 21,394 | 96,374 | 59.3 | 162,512 | 5,595.17 | 1,136.64 |
| 45 | 3,780 | 112 | 10,192 | 14,129 | 42 | 1 | 43 | 728,343 | 140,161 | 868,504 | 52.7 | 1,648,741 | 6,649.57 | 1,453.65 |
| 5 | 134 | 17 | 569 | 725 | 0 | 0 | 0 | 26,949 | 5,935 | 32,884 | 48.8 | 67,353 | 4,875.36 | 1,492.59 |
| 861 | 32,532 | 2,499 | 86,767 | 122,659 | 1,793 | 122 | 1,915 | 5,385,491 | 1,238,852 | 6,624,345 | 53.6 | 12,369,932 | 7,326.97 | 1,200.00 |
| 236 | 8,124 | 1,145 | 24,378 | 33,883 | 29 | 17 | 46 | 1,253,954 | 309,697 | 1,563,647 | 55.1 | 2,835,783 | 5,300.37 | 819.93 |
| 625 | 24,408 | 1,354 | 62,389 | 88,776 | 1,764 | 105 | 1,869 | 4,131,537 | 929,155 | 5,060,698 | 53.1 | 9,534,148 | 8,267.14 | 1,391.90 |
| 30 | 1,309 | 81 | 3,365 | 4,785 | 0 | 0 | 0 | 221,505 | 52,890 | 274,395 | 51.3 | 534,745 | 10,432.84 | 1,905.87 |
| 124 | 5,810 | 177 | 13,983 | 20,094 | 26 | 0 | 26 | 970,717 | 230,694 | 1,201,411 | 50.9 | 2,360,223 | 8,473.43 | 1,487.91 |
| 46 | 766 | 134 | 2,583 | 3,529 | 0 | 0 | 0 | 162,016 | 37,283 | 199,299 | 55.3 | 360,605 | 8,427.72 | 1,507.02 |
| 0 | 269 | 26 | 975 | 1,270 | 0 | 0 | 0 | 52,730 | 15,868 | 68,599 | 59.8 | 114,760 | 6,175.21 | 1,188.56 |
| 125 | 5,734 | 395 | 14,742 | 20,996 | 630 | 64 | 694 | 866,774 | 200,962 | 1,067,738 | 53.6 | 1,993,301 | 7,373.53 | 1,123.43 |
| 8 | 1,332 | 42 | 3,692 | 5,074 | 390 | 10 | 400 | 202,745 | 50,971 | 253,716 | 51.0 | 497,003 | 11,028.34 | 1,787.64 |
| 60 | 1,125 | 91 | 3,173 | 4,449 | 8 | 2 | 10 | 179,714 | 40,773 | 220,486 | 53.1 | 415,390 | 6,045.11 | 834.59 |
| 4 | 208 | 23 | 583 | 818 | 0 | 0 | 0 | 30,513 | 6,662 | 37,176 | 52.8 | 70,466 | 4,763.12 | 1,281.87 |
| 220 | 6,145 | 279 | 14,708 | 21,352 | 652 | 27 | 679 | 1,149,895 | 219,146 | 1,369,044 | 54.4 | 2,516,876 | 9,336.25 | 1,619.33 |
| 1 | 521 | 29 | 1,533 | 2,084 | 0 | 0 | 0 | 83,507 | 23,231 | 106,739 | 57.4 | 185,819 | 5,898.26 | 1,159.76 |
| 7 | 1,189 | 77 | 3,052 | 4,325 | 58 | 2 | 60 | 211,420 | 50,675 | 262,095 | 54.0 | 484,960 | 7,810.09 | 1,480.55 |
| 693 | 15,899 | 2,402 | 39,536 | 58,530 | 913 | 0 | 913 | 2,482,838 | 607,098 | 3,089,938 | 49.3 | 6,271,306 | 7,910.21 | 1,355.43 |
| 110 | 3,012 | 737 | 9,178 | 13,037 | 30 | 0 | 30 | 504,414 | 127,784 | 632,203 | 52.3 | 1,208,755 | 5,553.82 | 924.66 |
| 583 | 12,887 | 1,665 | 30,358 | 45,493 | 883 | 0 | 883 | 1,978,424 | 479,314 | 2,457,735 | 48.5 | 5,062,551 | 8,801.86 | 1,525.08 |
| 0 | 235 | 83 | 543 | 861 | 0 | 0 | 0 | 47,967 | 5,195 | 53,162 | 40.9 | 129,945 | 6,601.87 | 1,444.28 |
| 8 | 2,942 | 276 | 5,418 | 8,644 | 563 | 0 | 563 | 451,399 | 102,633 | 554,031 | 48.6 | 1,139,754 | 9,256.06 | 1,643.94 |
| 1 | 400 | 5 | 803 | 1,209 | 0 | 0 | 0 | 57,844 | 19,133 | 76,978 | 42.0 | 183,317 | 8,196.25 | 1,711.94 |
| 113 | 2,841 | 249 | 7,067 | 10,270 | 211 | 0 | 211 | 403,234 | 92,903 | 496,137 | 45.4 | 1,092,341 | 9,239.83 | 1,614.54 |
| 22 | 1,341 | 605 | 3,337 | 5,305 | 25 | 0 | 25 | 186,676 | 43,595 | 230,270 | 48.4 | 476,085 | 8,471.57 | 1,462.85 |
| 431 | 4,063 | 321 | 10,753 | 15,568 | 84 | 0 | 84 | 684,085 | 177,733 | 861,817 | 51.6 | 1,668,667 | 9,142.83 | 1,607.91 |
| 8 | 753 | 101 | 1,582 | 2,444 | 0 | 0 | 0 | 99,043 | 26,847 | 125,889 | 51.1 | 246,134 | 6,024.42 | 864.41 |
| 0 | 312 | 25 | 855 | 1,192 | 0 | 0 | 0 | 48,177 | 11,274 | 59,451 | 47.1 | 126,308 | 10,355.66 | 1,207.08 |
| 572 | 23,141 | 3,304 | 56,214 | 83,231 | 1,631 | 105 | 1,736 | 3,765,372 | 800,199 | 4,565,569 | 49.5 | 9,225,810 | 7,261.13 | 1,277.26 |
| 156 | 3,873 | 1,040 | 11,266 | 16,335 | 20 | 2 | 22 | 657,844 | 160,527 | 818,370 | 53.7 | 1,524,437 | 5,414.70 | 984.65 |
| 416 | 19,268 | 2,264 | 44,948 | 66,896 | 1,611 | 103 | 1,714 | 3,107,528 | 639,672 | 3,747,199 | 48.7 | 7,701,372 | 7,786.73 | 1,357.09 |
| 19 | 1,740 | 143 | 3,660 | 5,562 | 662 | 0 | 662 | 279,210 | 64,717 | 343,927 | 47.8 | 719,774 | 10,386.65 | 2,143.52 |
| 1 | 282 | 46 | 974 | 1,303 | 0 | 0 | 0 | 54,710 | 10,228 | 64,939 | 51.9 | 125,241 | 6,466.39 | 1,065.85 |
| 11 | 187 | 49 | 344 | 591 | 0 | 0 | 0 | 21,577 | 6,662 | 28,239 | 51.8 | 54,507 | 4,839.04 | 1,207.96 |
| 33 | 1,057 | 158 | 2,475 | 3,723 | 12 | 0 | 12 | 147,421 | 34,454 | 181,875 | 59.3 | 306,472 | 7,319.25 | 690.25 |
| 91 | 4,852 | 671 | 13,039 | 18,653 | 63 | 0 | 63 | 803,045 | 155,823 | 958,868 | 47.9 | 2,001,317 | 7,218.77 | 1,226.05 |
| 57 | 4,575 | 689 | 9,661 | 14,982 | 664 | 100 | 764 | 679,042 | 130,963 | 810,005 | 46.8 | 1,730,428 | 8,401.93 | 1,386.66 |
| 110 | 1,707 | 211 | 3,785 | 5,813 | 153 | 2 | 155 | 263,127 | 54,163 | 317,289 | 46.2 | 687,246 | 9,239.04 | 1,542.34 |
| 94 | 4,868 | 297 | 11,010 | 16,269 | 57 | 1 | 58 | 859,396 | 182,661 | 1,042,057 | 50.2 | 2,076,388 | 7,168.44 | 1,476.10 |
| 335 | 8,281 | 1,817 | 23,245 | 33,678 | 437 | 21 | 458 | 1,319,831 | 379,688 | 1,699,518 | 51.7 | 3,286,535 | 5,976.74 | 993.04 |
| 221 | 3,855 | 1,134 | 11,587 | 16,797 | 260 | 8 | 268 | 626,837 | 175,401 | 802,236 | 52.5 | 1,528,308 | 5,332.17 | 811.99 |
| 114 | 4,426 | 683 | 11,658 | 16,881 | 177 | 13 | 190 | 692,994 | 204,287 | 897,282 | 51.0 | 1,758,227 | 6,678.47 | 1,231.77 |
| 24 | 1,741 | 194 | 4,341 | 6,300 | 137 | 0 | 137 | 271,677 | 78,874 | 350,552 | 47.8 | 733,694 | 8,172.59 | 1,588.41 |
| 0 | 32 | 9 | 144 | 185 | 0 | 0 | 0 | 5,136 | 951 | 6,087 | 44.6 | 13,647 | 3,930.68 | 1,187.76 |
| 1 | 902 | 160 | 2,274 | 3,337 | 0 | 0 | 0 | 142,409 | 51,603 | 194,012 | 54.1 | 358,634 | 6,886.60 | 1,357.11 |
| 5 | 527 | 127 | 1,492 | 2,151 | 0 | 12 | 12 | 81,986 | 21,893 | 103,879 | 51.5 | 201,830 | 5,432.71 | 1,033.69 |
| 6 | 259 | 25 | 579 | 869 | 0 | 0 | 0 | 33,314 | 8,514 | 41,828 | 53.7 | 77,864 | 4,439.25 | 862.20 |
| 10 | 211 | 44 | 769 | 1,034 | 0 | 0 | 0 | 44,312 | 13,363 | 57,674 | 56.8 | 101,505 | 4,927.19 | 1,087.02 |
| 68 | 754 | 124 | 2,059 | 3,005 | 40 | 1 | 41 | 114,160 | 29,090 | 143,250 | 52.8 | 271,053 | 6,354.98 | 872.12 |

# U.S. CENSUS DIVISION 4, EAST NORTH CENTRAL

*U.S. Community Hospitals*
*(Nonfederal, short-term general and other special hospitals)*

## 2003 Utilization, Personnel and Finances



| CLASSIFICATION | Hospitals | Beds | Admissions | Inpatient Days | Adjusted Patient Days | Average Daily Census | Adjusted Average Daily Census | Average Stay (days) | Surgical Operations | NEWBORNS | | OUTPATIENT VISITS | |
|---|---|---|---|---|---|---|---|---|---|---|---|---|---|
| | | | | | | | | | | Bassinets | Births | Emergency | Total |
| UNITED STATES | 4,895 | 813,307 | 34,782,742 | 196,649,769 | 326,299,942 | 538,797 | 894,019 | 5.7 | 27,106,538 | 59,662 | 3,915,842 | 111,069,871 | 563,186,046 |
| Nonmetropolitan | 2,166 | 168,374 | 5,368,552 | 35,076,707 | 73,724,487 | 96,136 | 202,034 | 6.5 | 4,592,380 | 13,462 | 530,805 | 23,720,395 | 117,598,717 |
| Metropolitan | 2,729 | 644,933 | 29,414,190 | 161,573,062 | 252,575,455 | 442,661 | 691,985 | 5.5 | 22,514,158 | 46,200 | 3,385,037 | 87,349,476 | 445,587,329 |
| CENSUS DIVISION 4, EAST NORTH CENTRAL | 732 | 127,610 | 5,520,916 | 29,253,281 | 53,334,567 | 80,161 | 146,111 | 5.3 | 4,754,024 | 10,551 | 600,200 | 18,517,606 | 111,235,691 |
| Nonmetropolitan | 290 | 23,567 | 782,938 | 4,654,498 | 11,455,356 | 12,760 | 31,380 | 5.9 | 801,095 | 2,177 | 81,199 | 3,694,773 | 21,753,227 |
| Metropolitan | 442 | 104,043 | 4,737,978 | 24,598,783 | 41,879,211 | 67,401 | 114,731 | 5.2 | 3,952,929 | 8,374 | 519,001 | 14,822,833 | 89,482,464 |
| Illinois | 192 | 35,048 | 1,594,007 | 8,174,779 | 13,663,355 | 22,398 | 37,426 | 5.1 | 1,130,538 | 2,821 | 177,192 | 4,867,066 | 27,225,201 |
| Nonmetropolitan | 72 | 5,927 | 187,304 | 1,176,112 | 2,616,112 | 3,223 | 7,165 | 6.3 | 155,112 | 416 | 15,928 | 798,452 | 4,503,881 |
| Metropolitan | 120 | 29,121 | 1,406,703 | 6,998,667 | 11,047,243 | 19,175 | 30,261 | 5.0 | 975,426 | 2,405 | 161,264 | 4,068,614 | 22,721,320 |
| Bloomington-Normal | 2 | 395 | 16,105 | 66,735 | 114,517 | 183 | 314 | 4.1 | 12,541 | 33 | 2,397 | 60,386 | 316,505 |
| Champaign-Urbana | 2 | 580 | 24,740 | 159,868 | 215,952 | 438 | 591 | 6.5 | 18,366 | 32 | 3,157 | 84,050 | 178,882 |
| Chicago | 85 | 21,411 | 1,092,089 | 5,335,466 | 8,196,364 | 14,618 | 22,451 | 4.9 | 690,438 | 1,828 | 128,887 | 3,017,959 | 16,863,460 |
| Davenport-Moline-Rock Island | 4 | 543 | 26,208 | 129,805 | 242,716 | 355 | 665 | 5.0 | 20,651 | 83 | 2,501 | 88,765 | 354,371 |
| Decatur | 2 | 494 | 21,009 | 110,374 | 251,176 | 302 | 688 | 5.3 | 22,538 | 36 | 1,726 | 65,721 | 395,708 |
| Kankakee | 2 | 445 | 20,458 | 99,375 | 174,503 | 273 | 479 | 4.9 | 21,049 | 41 | 1,570 | 66,819 | 472,113 |
| Peoria-Pekin | 5 | 1,332 | 52,302 | 290,914 | 494,975 | 798 | 1,356 | 5.6 | 48,239 | 76 | 5,193 | 175,136 | 1,563,765 |
| Rockford | 5 | 940 | 44,398 | 214,178 | 341,990 | 586 | 937 | 4.8 | 32,206 | 76 | 4,738 | 141,811 | 716,569 |
| Springfield | 2 | 1,023 | 42,133 | 218,397 | 325,235 | 598 | 891 | 5.2 | 47,031 | 60 | 3,683 | 101,455 | 580,978 |
| St. Louis | 11 | 1,958 | 67,261 | 373,555 | 689,815 | 1,024 | 1,889 | 5.6 | 62,367 | 140 | 7,412 | 266,512 | 1,278,969 |
| Indiana | 112 | 18,932 | 712,151 | 3,997,353 | 7,383,923 | 10,953 | 20,233 | 5.6 | 653,550 | 1,603 | 81,200 | 2,492,597 | 14,997,896 |
| Nonmetropolitan | 45 | 3,637 | 127,663 | 598,541 | 1,473,881 | 1,642 | 4,041 | 4.7 | 172,736 | 425 | 14,441 | 624,955 | 3,743,896 |
| Metropolitan | 67 | 15,295 | 584,488 | 3,398,812 | 5,910,042 | 9,311 | 16,192 | 5.8 | 480,814 | 1,178 | 66,759 | 1,867,642 | 11,254,000 |
| Bloomington | 1 | 811 | 18,445 | 220,325 | 314,480 | 604 | 862 | 11.9 | 11,616 | 40 | 1,913 | 57,980 | 345,397 |
| Cincinnati | 1 | 87 | 4,517 | 19,915 | 46,386 | 55 | 127 | 4.4 | 6,338 | 11 | 565 | 17,596 | 125,443 |
| Elkhart-Goshen | 2 | 421 | 18,921 | 93,915 | 173,261 | 258 | 474 | 5.0 | 16,331 | 40 | 3,018 | 76,658 | 259,015 |
| Evansville-Henderson | 6 | 1,225 | 42,573 | 293,600 | 437,240 | 804 | 1,197 | 6.9 | 21,285 | 43 | 4,376 | 113,090 | 552,593 |
| Fort Wayne | 10 | 1,780 | 64,610 | 359,345 | 630,005 | 984 | 1,725 | 5.6 | 50,482 | 179 | 8,232 | 213,889 | 754,890 |
| Gary | 8 | 2,529 | 99,165 | 533,075 | 858,527 | 1,460 | 2,353 | 5.4 | 61,862 | 239 | 8,672 | 260,725 | 1,296,057 |
| Indianapolis | 19 | 5,143 | 202,685 | 1,197,484 | 2,155,724 | 3,279 | 5,907 | 5.9 | 174,631 | 383 | 23,384 | 669,549 | 5,147,812 |
| Kokomo | 4 | 462 | 13,398 | 87,845 | 213,530 | 241 | 585 | 6.6 | 16,245 | 33 | 1,637 | 51,493 | 887,051 |
| Lafayette | 2 | 476 | 19,601 | 96,140 | 176,435 | 263 | 483 | 4.9 | 15,533 | 34 | 3,330 | 81,655 | 307,905 |
| Louisville | 6 | 651 | 27,302 | 130,629 | 277,850 | 359 | 762 | 4.8 | 31,762 | 43 | 2,682 | 105,626 | 530,623 |
| Muncie | 1 | 393 | 18,368 | 98,600 | 183,473 | 270 | 503 | 5.4 | 18,308 | 20 | 1,639 | 46,468 | 337,892 |
| South Bend | 3 | 771 | 32,092 | 158,578 | 248,621 | 435 | 682 | 4.9 | 30,006 | 57 | 5,025 | 96,975 | 263,661 |
| Terre Haute | 4 | 546 | 22,811 | 109,361 | 194,510 | 299 | 532 | 4.8 | 26,415 | 56 | 2,286 | 75,938 | 445,661 |
| Michigan | 144 | 25,820 | 1,168,359 | 6,223,908 | 11,820,384 | 17,055 | 32,388 | 5.3 | 1,148,122 | 2,047 | 128,886 | 3,990,117 | 27,175,040 |
| Nonmetropolitan | 59 | 4,474 | 148,259 | 872,268 | 2,477,039 | 2,392 | 6,788 | 5.9 | 174,388 | 392 | 15,465 | 708,720 | 5,220,357 |
| Metropolitan | 85 | 21,346 | 1,020,100 | 5,351,640 | 9,343,345 | 14,663 | 25,600 | 5.2 | 973,734 | 1,655 | 113,421 | 3,281,397 | 21,954,683 |
| Ann Arbor | 8 | 1,756 | 90,616 | 458,229 | 808,397 | 1,256 | 2,214 | 5.1 | 107,939 | 107 | 10,250 | 291,790 | 3,631,199 |
| Benton Harbor | 2 | 414 | 17,685 | 72,159 | 139,075 | 198 | 381 | 4.1 | 14,765 | 51 | 2,029 | 76,437 | 372,373 |
| Detroit | 40 | 10,587 | 538,660 | 2,744,314 | 4,662,789 | 7,518 | 12,777 | 5.1 | 510,015 | 828 | 57,001 | 1,666,886 | 9,431,317 |
| Flint | 3 | 1,207 | 64,818 | 329,671 | 527,691 | 903 | 1,446 | 5.1 | 46,372 | 89 | 6,629 | 212,722 | 1,942,059 |
| Grand Rapids-Muskegon-Holland | 11 | 2,640 | 112,972 | 604,278 | 1,113,861 | 1,656 | 3,052 | 5.3 | 119,834 | 305 | 16,793 | 403,432 | 2,064,085 |
| Jackson | 2 | 476 | 16,447 | 76,441 | 166,327 | 209 | 456 | 4.6 | 10,426 | 24 | 1,947 | 49,061 | 330,190 |
| Kalamazoo-Battle Creek | 8 | 1,445 | 60,359 | 357,110 | 687,940 | 979 | 1,884 | 5.9 | 53,817 | 117 | 7,054 | 220,730 | 1,415,228 |
| Lansing-East Lansing | 5 | 1,120 | 49,999 | 301,986 | 590,793 | 827 | 1,618 | 6.0 | 44,497 | 56 | 6,036 | 182,055 | 1,350,098 |
| Saginaw-Bay City-Midland | 6 | 1,693 | 68,544 | 407,452 | 646,472 | 1,117 | 1,772 | 5.9 | 66,069 | 78 | 5,682 | 178,284 | 1,418,134 |

 

# TABLE 8

## U.S. CENSUS DIVISION 4, EAST NORTH CENTRAL

*U.S. Community Hospitals*
*(Nonfederal, short-term general and other special hospitals)*

## 2003 Utilization, Personnel and Finances

MSAs

| FULL-TIME EQUIVALENT PERSONNEL | | | | | FULL-TIME EQUIV. TRAINEES | | | EXPENSES | | | | | | |
|---|---|---|---|---|---|---|---|---|---|---|---|---|---|---|
| | | | | | | | | LABOR | | | | TOTAL | | |
| Physicians and Dentists | Registered Nurses | Licensed Practical Nurses | Other Salaried Personnel | Total Personnel | Medical and Dental Residents | Other Trainees | Total Trainees | Payroll (in thousands) | Employee Benefits (in thousands) | Total (in thousands) | Percent of Total | Amount (in thousands) | Adjusted per Admission | Adjusted per Inpatient Day |
| 71,335 | 1,021,346 | 126,328 | 2,889,619 | 4,108,628 | 77,813 | 7,954 | 85,767 | $187,822,974 | $45,438,505 | $233,261,475 | 51.8 | $450,124,257 | $7,796.41 | $1,379.48 |
| 8,445 | 147,570 | 37,579 | 485,049 | 678,643 | 1,775 | 600 | 2,375 | 25,551,777 | 6,425,000 | 31,976,774 | 53.8 | 59,444,378 | 5,305.04 | 806.30 |
| 62,890 | 873,776 | 88,749 | 2,404,570 | 3,429,985 | 76,038 | 7,354 | 83,392 | 162,271,198 | 39,013,505 | 201,284,701 | 51.5 | 390,679,879 | 8,396.37 | 1,546.78 |
| | | | | | | | | | | | | | | |
| 15,087 | 173,001 | 16,054 | 505,202 | 709,344 | 16,748 | 1,754 | 18,502 | 31,611,772 | 7,765,965 | 39,377,738 | 51.8 | 76,040,358 | 7,596.68 | 1,425.72 |
| 1,566 | 23,880 | 4,314 | 81,551 | 111,311 | 126 | 123 | 249 | 4,304,130 | 1,192,955 | 5,497,086 | 54.3 | 10,120,931 | 5,407.84 | 883.51 |
| 13,521 | 149,121 | 11,740 | 423,651 | 598,033 | 16,622 | 1,631 | 18,253 | 27,307,642 | 6,573,011 | 33,880,652 | 51.4 | 65,919,428 | 8,100.04 | 1,574.04 |
| 4,711 | 46,980 | 3,280 | 135,573 | 190,544 | 4,822 | 228 | 5,050 | 8,611,450 | 2,038,661 | 10,650,115 | 52.1 | 20,458,311 | 7,739.44 | 1,497.31 |
| 278 | 5,334 | 1,093 | 17,522 | 24,227 | 38 | 3 | 41 | 859,790 | 235,428 | 1,095,222 | 53.5 | 2,047,297 | 5,010.16 | 782.57 |
| 4,433 | 41,646 | 2,187 | 118,051 | 166,317 | 4,784 | 225 | 5,009 | 7,751,660 | 1,803,232 | 9,554,893 | 51.9 | 18,411,014 | 8,238.49 | 1,666.57 |
| 56 | 434 | 37 | 1,647 | 2,174 | 3 | 0 | 3 | 84,183 | 21,575 | 105,758 | 49.3 | 214,685 | 7,761.28 | 1,874.70 |
| 0 | 647 | 30 | 2,093 | 2,770 | 14 | 0 | 14 | 103,827 | 25,695 | 129,523 | 45.6 | 283,998 | 8,301.13 | 1,315.10 |
| 3,920 | 32,435 | 1,326 | 89,478 | 127,159 | 4,359 | 196 | 4,555 | 6,137,035 | 1,380,484 | 7,517,515 | 52.2 | 14,388,739 | 8,508.49 | 1,755.50 |
| 36 | 653 | 45 | 2,314 | 3,048 | 0 | 0 | 0 | 117,608 | 28,818 | 146,427 | 52.2 | 280,753 | 5,849.27 | 1,156.72 |
| 42 | 503 | 167 | 2,163 | 2,875 | 14 | 0 | 14 | 103,989 | 26,851 | 130,840 | 49.8 | 262,677 | 5,472.66 | 1,045.79 |
| 31 | 591 | 67 | 1,802 | 2,491 | 1 | 0 | 1 | 90,123 | 24,390 | 114,513 | 49.4 | 231,944 | 6,430.92 | 1,329.17 |
| 171 | 2,136 | 80 | 5,273 | 7,660 | 180 | 0 | 180 | 335,680 | 86,752 | 422,432 | 51.5 | 819,533 | 9,116.97 | 1,655.71 |
| 139 | 1,488 | 98 | 4,015 | 5,740 | 0 | 28 | 28 | 270,467 | 70,426 | 340,893 | 52.5 | 649,356 | 9,140.72 | 1,898.76 |
| 1 | 965 | 159 | 3,379 | 4,504 | 204 | 0 | 204 | 215,177 | 58,292 | 273,469 | 47.1 | 580,797 | 9,267.55 | 1,785.78 |
| 37 | 1,794 | 178 | 5,887 | 7,896 | 9 | 1 | 10 | 293,571 | 79,950 | 373,523 | 53.5 | 698,530 | 5,538.79 | 1,012.63 |
| 1,293 | 23,183 | 3,020 | 67,350 | 94,846 | 750 | 210 | 960 | 4,076,005 | 1,057,025 | 5,133,025 | 51.4 | 9,985,287 | 7,434.77 | 1,352.30 |
| 310 | 4,078 | 810 | 14,381 | 19,579 | 8 | 17 | 25 | 717,760 | 196,847 | 914,605 | 54.8 | 1,669,578 | 5,423.37 | 1,132.78 |
| 983 | 19,105 | 2,210 | 52,969 | 75,267 | 742 | 193 | 935 | 3,358,245 | 860,178 | 4,218,420 | 50.7 | 8,315,710 | 8,032.93 | 1,407.05 |
| 70 | 645 | 45 | 1,876 | 2,636 | 113 | 6 | 119 | 94,352 | 22,703 | 117,054 | 51.2 | 228,750 | 8,688.80 | 727.39 |
| 0 | 99 | 25 | 436 | 560 | 0 | 2 | 2 | 22,874 | 6,410 | 29,285 | 57.1 | 51,292 | 4,875.17 | 1,105.76 |
| 31 | 667 | 49 | 1,802 | 2,549 | 0 | 1 | 1 | 106,416 | 37,078 | 143,494 | 52.3 | 274,481 | 7,764.45 | 1,584.21 |
| 132 | 1,270 | 130 | 3,917 | 5,449 | 118 | 22 | 140 | 222,114 | 56,097 | 278,212 | 52.1 | 534,111 | 8,198.18 | 1,221.55 |
| 13 | 2,220 | 219 | 4,852 | 7,304 | 0 | 0 | 0 | 341,950 | 90,154 | 432,105 | 49.6 | 870,547 | 7,568.06 | 1,381.81 |
| 193 | 2,489 | 249 | 7,695 | 10,626 | 62 | 35 | 97 | 514,332 | 139,009 | 653,340 | 52.5 | 1,245,623 | 7,769.94 | 1,450.88 |
| 423 | 7,686 | 987 | 21,181 | 30,277 | 350 | 100 | 450 | 1,386,658 | 327,751 | 1,714,407 | 49.9 | 3,436,662 | 9,391.17 | 1,594.20 |
| 17 | 523 | 56 | 1,694 | 2,290 | 0 | 0 | 0 | 87,765 | 23,879 | 111,644 | 53.5 | 208,806 | 6,321.13 | 977.88 |
| 10 | 512 | 75 | 1,792 | 2,389 | 0 | 23 | 23 | 98,079 | 31,038 | 129,116 | 54.2 | 238,234 | 6,471.46 | 1,350.26 |
| 15 | 708 | 122 | 2,317 | 3,162 | 0 | 0 | 0 | 128,864 | 27,841 | 156,705 | 53.9 | 290,562 | 4,773.33 | 1,045.75 |
| 29 | 507 | 48 | 1,321 | 1,905 | 24 | 4 | 28 | 80,086 | 23,005 | 103,091 | 47.4 | 217,560 | 6,365.31 | 1,185.79 |
| 21 | 1,072 | 38 | 2,341 | 3,472 | 58 | 0 | 58 | 167,900 | 43,990 | 211,890 | 47.5 | 446,037 | 8,846.95 | 1,794.04 |
| 29 | 707 | 167 | 1,745 | 2,648 | 17 | 0 | 17 | 106,855 | 31,223 | 138,077 | 50.6 | 273,046 | 6,618.97 | 1,403.76 |
| 3,124 | 35,165 | 2,981 | 110,208 | 151,478 | 4,203 | 197 | 4,400 | 6,935,664 | 1,692,448 | 8,628,111 | 52.8 | 16,333,925 | 7,440.43 | 1,381.84 |
| 492 | 4,743 | 1,013 | 17,683 | 23,931 | 37 | 6 | 43 | 943,173 | 255,353 | 1,198,527 | 55.4 | 2,162,698 | 5,697.91 | 873.10 |
| 2,632 | 30,422 | 1,968 | 92,525 | 127,547 | 4,166 | 191 | 4,357 | 5,992,491 | 1,437,095 | 7,429,584 | 52.4 | 14,171,228 | 7,804.68 | 1,516.72 |
| 119 | 3,716 | 218 | 9,977 | 14,030 | 1,070 | 10 | 1,080 | 685,902 | 192,181 | 878,083 | 51.8 | 1,696,687 | 10,518.11 | 2,098.83 |
| 5 | 509 | 64 | 1,890 | 2,468 | 0 | 0 | 0 | 93,776 | 28,228 | 122,003 | 56.3 | 216,650 | 6,359.73 | 1,557.80 |
| 1,786 | 14,916 | 555 | 45,282 | 62,539 | 2,416 | 155 | 2,571 | 3,032,128 | 652,950 | 3,685,077 | 51.5 | 7,157,057 | 7,756.44 | 1,534.93 |
| 98 | 1,961 | 182 | 4,352 | 6,593 | 334 | 3 | 337 | 356,724 | 87,058 | 443,782 | 54.7 | 810,695 | 7,788.10 | 1,536.31 |
| 242 | 3,401 | 320 | 11,782 | 15,745 | 105 | 22 | 127 | 658,940 | 163,137 | 822,077 | 52.8 | 1,557,114 | 6,827.14 | 1,397.94 |
| 13 | 379 | 51 | 1,706 | 2,149 | 0 | 0 | 0 | 91,875 | 22,405 | 114,280 | 54.8 | 208,377 | 5,818.96 | 1,252.82 |
| 102 | 1,943 | 131 | 6,299 | 8,475 | 0 | 0 | 0 | 368,690 | 102,992 | 471,682 | 52.4 | 900,414 | 8,086.85 | 1,308.86 |
| 155 | 1,625 | 90 | 4,799 | 6,669 | 205 | 0 | 205 | 335,907 | 89,466 | 425,373 | 57.2 | 744,108 | 7,417.79 | 1,259.51 |
| 112 | 1,972 | 357 | 6,438 | 8,879 | 36 | 1 | 37 | 368,550 | 98,679 | 467,227 | 53.1 | 880,125 | 7,459.07 | 1,361.43 |

*Table continues*

# U.S. CENSUS DIVISION 4, EAST NORTH CENTRAL CONTINUED

*U.S. Community Hospitals*
*(Nonfederal, short-term general and other special hospitals)*

## 2003 Utilization, Personnel and Finances



| | | | | | | | | | | NEWBORNS | | OUTPATIENT VISITS | |
|---|---|---|---|---|---|---|---|---|---|---|---|---|---|
| CLASSIFICATION | Hospitals | Beds | Admissions | Inpatient Days | Adjusted Patient Days | Average Daily Census | Adjusted Average Daily Census | Average Stay (days) | Surgical Operations | Bassinets | Births | Emergency | Total |
| Ohio | 163 | 32,981 | 1,457,933 | 7,501,323 | 13,602,698 | 20,554 | 37,263 | 5.1 | 1,215,557 | 2,765 | 147,253 | 5,354,136 | 30,022,353 |
| Nonmetropolitan | 50 | 4,429 | 178,409 | 833,308 | 1,891,052 | 2,284 | 5,177 | 4.7 | 170,559 | 552 | 21,221 | 1,017,664 | 4,869,269 |
| Metropolitan | 113 | 28,552 | 1,279,524 | 6,668,015 | 11,711,646 | 18,270 | 32,086 | 5.2 | 1,044,998 | 2,213 | 126,032 | 4,336,472 | 25,153,084 |
| Akron | 7 | 1,825 | 90,240 | 466,803 | 759,205 | 1,279 | 2,080 | 5.2 | 69,137 | 126 | 8,277 | 309,761 | 1,613,404 |
| Canton-Massillon | 5 | 1,445 | 57,296 | 325,676 | 559,536 | 893 | 1,534 | 5.7 | 51,063 | 111 | 5,089 | 198,321 | 1,325,816 |
| Cincinnati | 13 | 3,217 | 170,884 | 782,560 | 1,317,499 | 2,146 | 3,610 | 4.6 | 130,039 | 259 | 19,273 | 510,456 | 2,476,817 |
| Cleveland-Lorain-Elyria | 30 | 7,634 | 335,987 | 1,931,868 | 3,504,066 | 5,293 | 9,600 | 5.7 | 320,344 | 502 | 28,385 | 1,010,154 | 8,445,507 |
| Columbus | 14 | 4,478 | 207,029 | 1,004,866 | 1,758,612 | 2,754 | 4,817 | 4.9 | 149,933 | 366 | 25,595 | 780,050 | 3,604,983 |
| Dayton-Springfield | 11 | 2,818 | 129,292 | 656,987 | 1,148,878 | 1,799 | 3,148 | 5.1 | 112,171 | 268 | 13,553 | 443,678 | 2,435,709 |
| Hamilton-Middletown | 4 | 690 | 34,140 | 139,612 | 262,968 | 382 | 720 | 4.1 | 24,047 | 65 | 4,278 | 152,635 | 428,612 |
| Lima | 3 | 658 | 27,627 | 134,360 | 258,092 | 368 | 708 | 4.9 | 16,857 | 70 | 2,769 | 115,833 | 703,991 |
| Mansfield | 3 | 516 | 20,733 | 111,445 | 220,670 | 305 | 604 | 5.4 | 13,563 | 51 | 1,778 | 95,726 | 310,219 |
| Parkersburg-Marietta | 2 | 222 | 8,371 | 35,528 | 84,186 | 97 | 231 | 4.2 | 13,392 | 21 | 680 | 38,157 | 228,078 |
| Steubenville-Weirton | 1 | 338 | 12,543 | 71,644 | 142,985 | 196 | 392 | 5.7 | 6,692 | 17 | 393 | 55,888 | 203,276 |
| Toledo | 10 | 2,753 | 100,830 | 558,285 | 915,654 | 1,528 | 2,507 | 5.5 | 78,241 | 203 | 9,307 | 348,078 | 1,814,476 |
| Wheeling | 3 | 289 | 8,903 | 70,538 | 141,104 | 193 | 387 | 7.9 | 7,343 | 10 | 432 | 30,358 | 273,427 |
| Youngstown-Warren | 7 | 1,669 | 75,649 | 377,843 | 638,191 | 1,037 | 1,748 | 5.0 | 52,176 | 144 | 6,223 | 247,377 | 1,288,769 |
| Wisconsin | 121 | 14,829 | 588,466 | 3,355,918 | 6,864,207 | 9,201 | 18,801 | 5.7 | 606,257 | 1,315 | 65,669 | 1,813,690 | 11,815,201 |
| Nonmetropolitan | 64 | 5,100 | 141,303 | 1,174,269 | 2,997,272 | 3,219 | 8,209 | 8.3 | 128,300 | 392 | 14,144 | 544,982 | 3,415,824 |
| Metropolitan | 57 | 9,729 | 447,163 | 2,181,649 | 3,866,935 | 5,982 | 10,592 | 4.9 | 477,957 | 923 | 51,525 | 1,268,708 | 8,399,377 |
| Appleton-Oshkosh-Neenah | 6 | 745 | 35,503 | 146,956 | 295,888 | 403 | 811 | 4.1 | 54,979 | 103 | 4,993 | 101,146 | 408,062 |
| Duluth-Superior | 1 | 31 | 686 | 2,144 | 8,942 | 6 | 24 | 3.1 | 1,423 | 0 | 0 | 10,729 | 53,450 |
| Eau Claire | 5 | 594 | 22,371 | 116,377 | 235,300 | 319 | 645 | 5.2 | 15,942 | 47 | 2,071 | 66,154 | 362,128 |
| Green Bay | 4 | 644 | 29,434 | 123,867 | 231,718 | 340 | 634 | 4.2 | 38,582 | 69 | 4,210 | 122,304 | 526,577 |
| Janesville-Beloit | 3 | 394 | 14,385 | 91,294 | 180,210 | 250 | 493 | 6.3 | 17,173 | 31 | 1,995 | 62,363 | 959,887 |
| Kenosha | 2 | 220 | 11,406 | 49,447 | 114,211 | 135 | 312 | 4.3 | 11,256 | 37 | 1,642 | 52,736 | 313,795 |
| La Crosse | 2 | 484 | 22,323 | 92,935 | 155,384 | 255 | 426 | 4.2 | 19,584 | 46 | 2,176 | 41,899 | 217,375 |
| Madison | 4 | 1,177 | 58,516 | 294,722 | 450,977 | 808 | 1,236 | 5.0 | 104,801 | 79 | 6,650 | 114,509 | 898,129 |
| Milwaukee-Waukesha | 19 | 4,241 | 200,521 | 984,285 | 1,680,299 | 2,698 | 4,603 | 4.9 | 162,999 | 379 | 21,649 | 542,291 | 3,827,408 |
| Minneapolis-St. Paul | 4 | 116 | 4,694 | 14,965 | 35,286 | 42 | 97 | 3.2 | 5,520 | 22 | 701 | 17,296 | 85,109 |
| Racine | 3 | 438 | 19,755 | 115,373 | 224,948 | 316 | 616 | 5.8 | 16,238 | 45 | 2,242 | 73,243 | 487,638 |
| Sheboygan | 3 | 392 | 12,240 | 85,475 | 161,334 | 235 | 442 | 7.0 | 17,812 | 37 | 1,735 | 39,529 | 175,526 |
| Wausau | 1 | 253 | 15,329 | 63,809 | 92,438 | 175 | 253 | 4.2 | 11,648 | 28 | 1,461 | 24,509 | 84,293 |

# TABLE 8

## U.S. CENSUS DIVISION 4, EAST NORTH CENTRAL CONTINUED

*U.S. Community Hospitals*
*(Nonfederal, short-term general and other special hospitals)*

## 2003 Utilization, Personnel and Finances

| FULL-TIME EQUIVALENT PERSONNEL | | | | | FULL-TIME EQUIV. TRAINEES | | | EXPENSES | | | | | | |
|---|---|---|---|---|---|---|---|---|---|---|---|---|---|---|
| | | | | | | | | LABOR | | | | TOTAL | | |
| Physicians and Dentists | Registered Nurses | Licensed Practical Nurses | Other Salaried Personnel | Total Personnel | Medical and Dental Residents | Other Trainees | Total Trainees | Payroll (in thousands) | Employee Benefits (in thousands) | Total (in thousands) | Percent of Total | Amount (in thousands) | Adjusted per Admission | Adjusted per Inpatient Day |
| 5,035 | 49,800 | 5,429 | 135,636 | 195,900 | 6,301 | 858 | 7,159 | 8,572,354 | 2,070,726 | 10,643,082 | 52.0 | 20,465,149 | 7,623.08 | 1,504.49 |
| 205 | 5,730 | 988 | 17,765 | 24,688 | 43 | 12 | 55 | 939,378 | 284,973 | 1,224,354 | 53.7 | 2,278,571 | 5,357.42 | 1,204.92 |
| 4,830 | 44,070 | 4,441 | 117,871 | 171,212 | 6,258 | 846 | 7,104 | 7,632,976 | 1,785,752 | 9,418,728 | 51.8 | 18,186,579 | 8,049.58 | 1,552.86 |
| 222 | 3,380 | 460 | 8,058 | 12,120 | 377 | 1 | 378 | 522,515 | 118,413 | 640,927 | 53.5 | 1,197,551 | 7,976.65 | 1,577.38 |
| 56 | 1,924 | 320 | 5,293 | 7,593 | 91 | 6 | 97 | 297,903 | 74,016 | 371,919 | 53.1 | 700,313 | 7,145.39 | 1,251.60 |
| 519 | 5,636 | 185 | 14,524 | 20,864 | 859 | 158 | 1,017 | 860,149 | 184,623 | 1,044,772 | 47.2 | 2,214,411 | 7,625.44 | 1,680.77 |
| 1,839 | 10,676 | 1,404 | 33,351 | 47,270 | 2,116 | 63 | 2,179 | 2,507,835 | 567,057 | 3,074,893 | 55.5 | 5,536,689 | 9,024.93 | 1,580.08 |
| 1,772 | 6,690 | 283 | 18,779 | 27,524 | 1,845 | 605 | 2,450 | 1,133,238 | 261,693 | 1,394,929 | 46.1 | 3,027,303 | 8,197.54 | 1,721.42 |
| 44 | 4,141 | 344 | 12,896 | 17,425 | 401 | 0 | 401 | 757,608 | 170,132 | 927,740 | 53.7 | 1,726,739 | 7,587.53 | 1,502.98 |
| 2 | 1,187 | 77 | 2,176 | 3,442 | 0 | 1 | 1 | 136,422 | 29,687 | 166,110 | 49.4 | 336,279 | 5,160.51 | 1,278.78 |
| 19 | 918 | 182 | 2,572 | 3,691 | 2 | 0 | 2 | 151,880 | 47,765 | 199,646 | 52.4 | 380,925 | 7,174.80 | 1,475.93 |
| 6 | 597 | 148 | 1,786 | 2,537 | 0 | 0 | 0 | 105,302 | 37,624 | 142,925 | 54.3 | 263,195 | 6,534.63 | 1,192.71 |
| 3 | 261 | 61 | 758 | 1,083 | 4 | 0 | 4 | 47,366 | 14,798 | 62,164 | 54.5 | 114,146 | 5,756.24 | 1,355.88 |
| 11 | 461 | 38 | 1,207 | 1,717 | 0 | 0 | 0 | 57,115 | 22,550 | 79,665 | 55.0 | 144,759 | 5,782.71 | 1,012.40 |
| 178 | 5,666 | 494 | 9,510 | 15,848 | 423 | 8 | 431 | 638,090 | 149,557 | 787,648 | 51.4 | 1,532,315 | 9,499.02 | 1,673.47 |
| 20 | 317 | 68 | 815 | 1,220 | 0 | 0 | 0 | 40,177 | 9,650 | 49,827 | 56.6 | 88,027 | 4,853.47 | 623.85 |
| 139 | 2,216 | 377 | 6,146 | 8,878 | 140 | 4 | 144 | 377,376 | 98,187 | 475,563 | 51.5 | 923,925 | 7,242.10 | 1,447.73 |
| | | | | | | | | | | | | | | |
| 924 | 17,873 | 1,344 | 56,435 | 76,576 | 672 | 261 | 933 | 3,416,300 | 907,106 | 4,323,405 | 49.1 | 8,797,686 | 7,694.82 | 1,281.68 |
| 281 | 3,995 | 410 | 14,200 | 18,886 | 0 | 85 | 85 | 844,030 | 220,353 | 1,064,378 | 54.2 | 1,962,787 | 5,605.07 | 654.86 |
| 643 | 13,878 | 934 | 42,235 | 57,690 | 672 | 176 | 848 | 2,572,270 | 686,753 | 3,259,027 | 47.7 | 6,834,898 | 8,617.46 | 1,767.52 |
| 18 | 949 | 89 | 2,730 | 3,786 | 0 | 1 | 1 | 193,712 | 47,782 | 241,495 | 54.0 | 447,462 | 6,211.30 | 1,512.27 |
| 0 | 23 | 4 | 103 | 130 | 0 | 0 | 0 | 6,963 | 2,070 | 9,034 | 65.6 | 13,774 | 4,814.35 | 1,540.36 |
| 2 | 677 | 43 | 2,219 | 2,941 | 0 | 29 | 29 | 117,575 | 29,726 | 147,301 | 56.9 | 258,899 | 6,190.06 | 1,100.29 |
| 63 | 1,347 | 125 | 3,552 | 5,087 | 0 | 1 | 1 | 224,769 | 51,709 | 276,478 | 53.2 | 519,651 | 9,261.46 | 2,242.60 |
| 204 | 466 | 36 | 1,519 | 2,225 | 19 | 0 | 19 | 91,804 | 26,418 | 118,223 | 37.3 | 317,316 | 11,277.92 | 1,760.81 |
| 26 | 277 | 25 | 1,206 | 1,534 | 0 | 2 | 2 | 73,113 | 19,499 | 92,612 | 52.5 | 176,417 | 6,701.00 | 1,544.66 |
| 147 | 714 | 81 | 2,476 | 3,418 | 24 | 0 | 24 | 101,509 | 33,762 | 135,271 | 47.3 | 286,046 | 7,690.22 | 1,840.89 |
| 13 | 1,894 | 65 | 5,782 | 7,754 | 474 | 89 | 563 | 378,122 | 114,759 | 492,882 | 52.1 | 945,745 | 10,815.32 | 2,097.10 |
| 153 | 6,029 | 358 | 17,514 | 24,054 | 152 | 6 | 158 | 1,128,303 | 295,676 | 1,423,980 | 44.1 | 3,226,145 | 9,322.66 | 1,919.98 |
| 0 | 138 | 6 | 463 | 607 | 0 | 0 | 0 | 26,627 | 5,210 | 31,837 | 48.6 | 65,531 | 5,822.39 | 1,857.14 |
| 13 | 703 | 63 | 2,336 | 3,115 | 3 | 25 | 28 | 104,047 | 27,309 | 131,356 | 49.9 | 263,470 | 6,815.59 | 1,171.25 |
| 2 | 309 | 25 | 1,126 | 1,462 | 0 | 0 | 0 | 56,709 | 14,537 | 71,246 | 53.2 | 133,988 | 5,817.24 | 830.50 |
| 2 | 352 | 14 | 1,209 | 1,577 | 0 | 23 | 23 | 69,016 | 18,295 | 87,312 | 48.4 | 180,453 | 8,125.96 | 1,952.15 |

# TABLE 8

# U.S. CENSUS DIVISION 5, EAST SOUTH CENTRAL

*U.S. Community Hospitals*
*(Nonfederal, short-term general and other special hospitals)*

## 2003 Utilization, Personnel and Finances

| CLASSIFICATION | Hospitals | Beds | Admissions | Inpatient Days | Adjusted Patient Days | Average Daily Census | Adjusted Average Daily Census | Average Stay (days) | Surgical Operations | NEWBORNS | | OUTPATIENT VISITS | |
|---|---|---|---|---|---|---|---|---|---|---|---|---|---|
| | | | | | | | | | | Bassinets | Births | Emergency | Total |
| UNITED STATES | 4,895 | 813,307 | 34,782,742 | 196,649,769 | 326,299,942 | 538,797 | 894,019 | 5.7 | 27,106,538 | 59,662 | 3,915,842 | 111,069,871 | 563,186,046 |
| Nonmetropolitan | 2,166 | 168,374 | 5,368,552 | 35,076,707 | 73,724,487 | 96,136 | 202,034 | 6.5 | 4,592,380 | 13,462 | 530,805 | 23,720,395 | 117,598,717 |
| Metropolitan | 2,729 | 644,933 | 29,414,190 | 161,573,062 | 252,575,455 | 442,661 | 691,985 | 5.5 | 22,514,158 | 46,200 | 3,385,037 | 87,349,476 | 445,587,329 |
| CENSUS DIVISION 5, EAST SOUTH CENTRAL | 427 | 63,959 | 2,538,273 | 14,171,337 | 23,910,416 | 38,844 | 65,535 | 5.6 | 1,967,954 | 4,446 | 228,955 | 8,827,897 | 31,597,702 |
| Nonmetropolitan | 258 | 24,731 | 809,628 | 4,859,214 | 9,411,345 | 13,332 | 25,811 | 6.0 | 580,376 | 1,685 | 65,146 | 3,622,524 | 11,671,184 |
| Metropolitan | 169 | 39,228 | 1,728,645 | 9,312,123 | 14,499,071 | 25,512 | 39,724 | 5.4 | 1,387,578 | 2,761 | 163,809 | 5,205,373 | 19,926,518 |
| Alabama | 107 | 15,666 | 708,995 | 3,547,203 | 5,579,420 | 9,713 | 15,293 | 5.0 | 533,892 | 1,300 | 57,580 | 2,145,885 | 8,899,175 |
| Nonmetropolitan | 50 | 3,814 | 140,445 | 667,949 | 1,263,929 | 1,829 | 3,468 | 4.8 | 103,445 | 321 | 10,761 | 647,075 | 2,227,037 |
| Metropolitan | 57 | 11,852 | 568,550 | 2,879,254 | 4,315,491 | 7,884 | 11,825 | 5.1 | 430,447 | 979 | 46,819 | 1,498,810 | 6,672,138 |
| Anniston | 3 | 447 | 22,733 | 92,307 | 145,074 | 253 | 398 | 4.1 | 13,938 | 38 | 1,678 | 95,423 | 227,359 |
| Auburn-Opelika | 1 | 273 | 15,945 | 77,600 | 132,799 | 213 | 364 | 4.9 | 10,512 | 36 | 1,428 | 39,365 | 90,681 |
| Birmingham | 17 | 4,347 | 199,161 | 1,047,205 | 1,472,811 | 2,868 | 4,037 | 5.3 | 162,113 | 221 | 14,657 | 474,243 | 2,643,817 |
| Decatur | 4 | 558 | 20,232 | 84,278 | 130,932 | 231 | 358 | 4.2 | 12,844 | 42 | 1,988 | 64,739 | 260,699 |
| Dothan | 3 | 657 | 36,593 | 160,961 | 268,301 | 441 | 736 | 4.4 | 32,553 | 65 | 2,629 | 97,752 | 670,600 |
| Florence | 3 | 552 | 25,511 | 114,425 | 179,052 | 314 | 491 | 4.5 | 20,137 | 60 | 1,873 | 70,466 | 200,332 |
| Gadsden | 2 | 415 | 22,223 | 118,677 | 175,514 | 325 | 480 | 5.3 | 16,199 | 33 | 1,678 | 54,117 | 106,535 |
| Huntsville | 4 | 973 | 50,784 | 247,240 | 402,112 | 677 | 1,101 | 4.9 | 41,418 | 84 | 4,723 | 164,328 | 669,874 |
| Mobile | 10 | 1,975 | 89,793 | 512,734 | 797,121 | 1,403 | 2,184 | 5.7 | 65,691 | 244 | 8,136 | 238,486 | 901,595 |
| Montgomery | 8 | 1,033 | 49,086 | 236,395 | 357,020 | 646 | 978 | 4.8 | 34,290 | 112 | 5,019 | 92,826 | 444,856 |
| Tuscaloosa | 2 | 622 | 36,489 | 187,432 | 254,755 | 513 | 698 | 5.1 | 20,752 | 44 | 3,010 | 107,065 | 455,790 |
| Kentucky | 103 | 14,940 | 600,454 | 3,394,239 | 5,972,225 | 9,300 | 16,359 | 5.7 | 540,303 | 1,007 | 52,813 | 2,137,500 | 8,543,109 |
| Nonmetropolitan | 71 | 7,572 | 273,076 | 1,593,578 | 3,016,487 | 4,366 | 8,261 | 5.8 | 200,519 | 508 | 21,178 | 1,112,430 | 4,484,912 |
| Metropolitan | 32 | 7,368 | 327,378 | 1,800,661 | 2,955,738 | 4,934 | 8,098 | 5.5 | 339,784 | 499 | 31,635 | 1,025,070 | 4,058,197 |
| Cincinnati | 5 | 892 | 44,133 | 205,307 | 362,064 | 562 | 991 | 4.7 | 30,130 | 87 | 4,952 | 192,891 | 715,549 |
| Clarksville-Hopkinsville | 1 | 139 | 6,312 | 29,091 | 58,453 | 80 | 160 | 4.6 | 5,797 | 18 | 730 | 27,014 | 83,285 |
| Evansville-Henderson | 1 | 209 | 7,480 | 37,083 | 63,647 | 102 | 174 | 5.0 | 7,875 | 12 | 799 | 20,320 | 117,232 |
| Huntington-Ashland | 2 | 750 | 28,765 | 171,769 | 299,923 | 471 | 822 | 6.0 | 40,217 | 25 | 1,354 | 96,655 | 381,595 |
| Lexington | 12 | 1,871 | 81,287 | 427,715 | 708,676 | 1,173 | 1,942 | 5.3 | 80,473 | 133 | 8,709 | 262,065 | 1,153,777 |
| Louisville | 10 | 3,162 | 140,494 | 840,833 | 1,322,765 | 2,303 | 3,625 | 6.0 | 156,093 | 190 | 13,255 | 366,257 | 1,364,591 |
| Owensboro | 1 | 345 | 18,907 | 88,863 | 140,210 | 243 | 384 | 4.7 | 19,199 | 34 | 1,836 | 59,868 | 242,168 |
| Mississippi | 92 | 13,040 | 415,909 | 2,696,522 | 4,601,699 | 7,403 | 12,634 | 6.5 | 265,824 | 834 | 39,540 | 1,597,509 | 3,998,966 |
| Nonmetropolitan | 73 | 7,899 | 225,107 | 1,601,012 | 2,987,175 | 4,402 | 8,210 | 7.1 | 134,549 | 498 | 19,915 | 986,983 | 2,296,719 |
| Metropolitan | 19 | 5,141 | 190,802 | 1,095,510 | 1,614,524 | 3,001 | 4,424 | 5.7 | 131,275 | 336 | 19,625 | 610,526 | 1,702,247 |
| Biloxi-Gulfport-Pascagoula | 6 | 1,409 | 52,068 | 284,473 | 428,440 | 778 | 1,175 | 5.5 | 42,345 | 122 | 4,345 | 211,433 | 851,487 |
| Hattiesburg | 2 | 748 | 33,180 | 165,097 | 248,626 | 453 | 681 | 5.0 | 15,298 | 35 | 3,565 | 109,918 | 192,855 |
| Jackson | 10 | 2,785 | 95,423 | 583,753 | 850,760 | 1,600 | 2,330 | 6.1 | 68,860 | 146 | 10,134 | 255,685 | 624,415 |
| Memphis | 1 | 199 | 10,131 | 62,187 | 86,698 | 170 | 238 | 6.1 | 4,772 | 33 | 1,581 | 33,490 | 33,490 |
| Tennessee | 125 | 20,313 | 812,915 | 4,533,373 | 7,757,072 | 12,428 | 21,249 | 5.6 | 627,935 | 1,305 | 79,022 | 2,947,003 | 10,156,452 |
| Nonmetropolitan | 64 | 5,446 | 171,000 | 996,675 | 2,143,754 | 2,735 | 5,872 | 5.8 | 141,863 | 358 | 13,292 | 876,036 | 2,662,516 |
| Metropolitan | 61 | 14,867 | 641,915 | 3,536,698 | 5,613,318 | 9,693 | 15,377 | 5.5 | 486,072 | 947 | 65,730 | 2,070,967 | 7,493,936 |
| Chattanooga | 6 | 1,664 | 68,417 | 354,215 | 537,121 | 970 | 1,471 | 5.2 | 60,550 | 59 | 5,948 | 211,341 | 858,803 |
| Clarksville-Hopkinsville | 1 | 201 | 10,377 | 44,726 | 84,537 | 123 | 232 | 4.3 | 6,047 | 16 | 1,360 | 44,692 | 140,671 |
| Jackson | 2 | 733 | 31,476 | 186,044 | 297,956 | 510 | 817 | 5.9 | 25,975 | 44 | 3,433 | 86,677 | 179,831 |
| Johnson City-Kingsport-Bristol | 11 | 1,897 | 68,452 | 387,654 | 686,872 | 1,063 | 1,881 | 5.7 | 47,498 | 136 | 5,305 | 270,008 | 1,003,708 |
| Knoxville | 10 | 2,461 | 113,667 | 610,585 | 1,003,017 | 1,675 | 2,748 | 5.4 | 90,268 | 172 | 11,169 | 433,592 | 1,472,956 |
| Memphis | 13 | 3,626 | 154,557 | 974,619 | 1,415,705 | 2,668 | 3,877 | 6.3 | 94,107 | 246 | 17,753 | 468,026 | 1,435,218 |
| Nashville | 18 | 4,285 | 194,969 | 978,855 | 1,588,110 | 2,684 | 4,351 | 5.0 | 161,627 | 274 | 20,762 | 556,631 | 2,402,749 |

# TABLE 8

## U.S. CENSUS DIVISION 5, EAST SOUTH CENTRAL

*U.S. Community Hospitals*
*(Nonfederal, short-term general and other special hospitals)*

## 2003 Utilization, Personnel and Finances

| FULL-TIME EQUIVALENT PERSONNEL | | | | | FULL-TIME EQUIV. TRAINEES | | | EXPENSES | | | | | | |
|---|---|---|---|---|---|---|---|---|---|---|---|---|---|---|
| | | | | | | | | LABOR | | | | TOTAL | | |
| Physicians and Dentists | Registered Nurses | Licensed Practical Nurses | Other Salaried Personnel | Total Personnel | Medical and Dental Residents | Other Trainees | Total Trainees | Payroll (in thousands) | Employee Benefits (in thousands) | Total (in thousands) | Percent of Total | Amount (in thousands) | Adjusted per Admission | Adjusted per Inpatient Day |
| 71,335 | 1,021,346 | 126,328 | 2,889,619 | 4,108,628 | 77,813 | 7,954 | 85,767 | $187,822,974 | $45,438,505 | $233,261,475 | 51.8 | $450,124,257 | $7,796.41 | $1,379.48 |
| 8,445 | 147,570 | 37,579 | 485,049 | 678,643 | 1,775 | 600 | 2,375 | 25,551,777 | 6,425,000 | 31,976,774 | 53.8 | 59,444,378 | 5,305.04 | 806.30 |
| 62,890 | 873,776 | 88,749 | 2,404,570 | 3,429,985 | 76,038 | 7,354 | 83,392 | 162,271,198 | 39,013,505 | 201,284,701 | 51.5 | 390,679,879 | 8,396.37 | 1,546.78 |
| 1,962 | 70,336 | 13,108 | 188,491 | 273,897 | 2,303 | 727 | 3,030 | 10,526,875 | 2,519,287 | 13,046,161 | 49.5 | 26,377,671 | 6,143.41 | 1,103.19 |
| 797 | 18,828 | 6,045 | 57,377 | 83,047 | 72 | 18 | 90 | 2,907,135 | 731,112 | 3,638,246 | 51.9 | 7,011,334 | 4,466.29 | 744.99 |
| 1,165 | 51,508 | 7,063 | 131,114 | 190,850 | 2,231 | 709 | 2,940 | 7,619,740 | 1,788,175 | 9,407,915 | 48.6 | 19,366,338 | 7,109.99 | 1,335.70 |
| 603 | 18,833 | 3,366 | 49,426 | 72,228 | 857 | 78 | 935 | 2,531,543 | 594,699 | 3,126,246 | 48.0 | 6,507,393 | 5,728.53 | 1,166.32 |
| 83 | 2,879 | 808 | 7,967 | 11,737 | 11 | 5 | 16 | 383,951 | 92,833 | 476,785 | 51.1 | 932,452 | 3,424.96 | 737.74 |
| 520 | 15,954 | 2,558 | 41,459 | 60,491 | 846 | 73 | 919 | 2,147,591 | 501,867 | 2,649,461 | 47.5 | 5,574,941 | 6,454.64 | 1,291.84 |
| 3 | 542 | 113 | 1,117 | 1,775 | 12 | 0 | 12 | 56,319 | 13,910 | 70,229 | 50.0 | 140,390 | 3,835.89 | 967.71 |
| 7 | 416 | 50 | 1,385 | 1,858 | 0 | 0 | 0 | 69,559 | 14,299 | 83,858 | 52.3 | 160,337 | 5,875.93 | 1,207.36 |
| 242 | 5,950 | 875 | 16,002 | 23,069 | 441 | 30 | 471 | 792,451 | 183,583 | 976,034 | 42.6 | 2,292,192 | 7,984.70 | 1,556.34 |
| 22 | 471 | 83 | 1,351 | 1,927 | 35 | 2 | 37 | 77,897 | 17,942 | 95,839 | 50.7 | 189,158 | 6,001.60 | 1,444.71 |
| 29 | 824 | 318 | 2,982 | 4,153 | 0 | 0 | 0 | 133,848 | 28,835 | 162,683 | 50.0 | 325,649 | 5,301.23 | 1,213.75 |
| 8 | 754 | 164 | 1,532 | 2,458 | 3 | 3 | 6 | 72,903 | 24,054 | 96,957 | 54.1 | 179,280 | 4,432.03 | 1,001.27 |
| 3 | 516 | 87 | 1,008 | 1,614 | 1 | 0 | 1 | 62,195 | 15,418 | 77,613 | 44.7 | 173,450 | 5,277.01 | 988.24 |
| 41 | 1,653 | 169 | 3,473 | 5,336 | 0 | 0 | 0 | 218,214 | 53,640 | 271,854 | 49.6 | 548,029 | 6,559.13 | 1,362.88 |
| 84 | 2,620 | 320 | 6,682 | 9,706 | 307 | 6 | 313 | 354,182 | 87,447 | 441,629 | 51.7 | 854,197 | 6,312.99 | 1,071.60 |
| 74 | 1,372 | 212 | 3,729 | 5,387 | 47 | 5 | 52 | 174,138 | 39,316 | 213,455 | 49.6 | 430,746 | 5,528.34 | 1,206.50 |
| 7 | 836 | 167 | 2,198 | 3,208 | 0 | 27 | 27 | 135,886 | 23,424 | 159,310 | 56.6 | 281,512 | 5,663.31 | 1,105.03 |
| 466 | 16,978 | 3,082 | 45,049 | 65,575 | 66 | 36 | 102 | 2,620,220 | 625,354 | 3,245,570 | 49.1 | 6,606,931 | 6,093.15 | 1,106.28 |
| 300 | 6,740 | 2,066 | 20,061 | 29,167 | 38 | 6 | 44 | 1,052,518 | 272,640 | 1,325,156 | 51.4 | 2,578,594 | 4,818.25 | 854.83 |
| 166 | 10,238 | 1,016 | 24,988 | 36,408 | 28 | 30 | 58 | 1,567,701 | 352,714 | 1,920,414 | 47.7 | 4,028,337 | 7,335.59 | 1,362.89 |
| 59 | 1,185 | 136 | 2,789 | 4,169 | 24 | 10 | 34 | 203,445 | 47,670 | 251,116 | 52.3 | 480,537 | 6,032.28 | 1,327.22 |
| 0 | 143 | 37 | 438 | 618 | 0 | 0 | 0 | 22,487 | 5,596 | 28,083 | 43.7 | 64,281 | 5,068.27 | 1,099.70 |
| 9 | 254 | 31 | 845 | 1,139 | 0 | 0 | 0 | 35,404 | 11,447 | 46,851 | 60.0 | 78,035 | 6,078.47 | 1,226.06 |
| 27 | 732 | 144 | 2,272 | 3,175 | 3 | 0 | 3 | 124,662 | 37,000 | 161,662 | 49.0 | 329,766 | 6,290.12 | 1,099.50 |
| 17 | 3,063 | 186 | 6,254 | 9,520 | 1 | 0 | 1 | 400,715 | 90,694 | 491,408 | 48.1 | 1,022,350 | 7,351.71 | 1,442.62 |
| 50 | 4,335 | 415 | 11,152 | 15,952 | 0 | 20 | 20 | 712,405 | 143,705 | 856,109 | 45.7 | 1,875,280 | 8,422.66 | 1,417.70 |
| 4 | 526 | 67 | 1,238 | 1,835 | 0 | 0 | 0 | 68,583 | 16,603 | 85,185 | 47.8 | 178,087 | 5,969.67 | 1,270.15 |
| 468 | 11,413 | 2,256 | 32,460 | 46,597 | 392 | 6 | 398 | 1,684,322 | 405,165 | 2,089,488 | 51.5 | 4,056,825 | 5,908.79 | 881.59 |
| 327 | 5,546 | 1,618 | 17,185 | 24,676 | 19 | 6 | 25 | 860,201 | 213,167 | 1,073,370 | 52.0 | 2,065,591 | 5,132.88 | 691.49 |
| 141 | 5,867 | 638 | 15,275 | 21,921 | 373 | 0 | 373 | 824,120 | 191,998 | 1,016,118 | 51.0 | 1,991,234 | 7,007.64 | 1,233.33 |
| 53 | 1,850 | 128 | 3,839 | 5,870 | 0 | 0 | 0 | 242,911 | 56,481 | 299,393 | 53.5 | 559,990 | 7,123.92 | 1,307.04 |
| 44 | 775 | 121 | 2,744 | 3,684 | 0 | 0 | 0 | 120,251 | 29,736 | 149,987 | 56.5 | 265,468 | 5,317.97 | 1,067.74 |
| 44 | 3,036 | 355 | 8,080 | 11,515 | 373 | 0 | 373 | 425,977 | 96,899 | 522,875 | 48.7 | 1,073,656 | 7,587.57 | 1,262.00 |
| 0 | 206 | 34 | 612 | 852 | 0 | 0 | 0 | 34,981 | 8,882 | 43,863 | 47.6 | 92,121 | 6,522.29 | 1,062.55 |
| 425 | 23,112 | 4,404 | 61,556 | 89,497 | 988 | 607 | 1,595 | 3,690,791 | 894,069 | 4,584,857 | 49.8 | 9,206,522 | 6,638.70 | 1,186.86 |
| 87 | 3,663 | 1,553 | 12,164 | 17,467 | 4 | 1 | 5 | 610,464 | 152,473 | 762,935 | 53.2 | 1,434,696 | 3,985.40 | 669.24 |
| 338 | 19,449 | 2,851 | 49,392 | 72,030 | 984 | 606 | 1,590 | 3,080,327 | 741,596 | 3,821,922 | 49.2 | 7,771,826 | 7,568.92 | 1,384.53 |
| 51 | 2,119 | 238 | 5,697 | 8,105 | 136 | 2 | 138 | 338,525 | 80,861 | 419,386 | 53.4 | 784,750 | 7,499.66 | 1,461.03 |
| 4 | 301 | 68 | 696 | 1,069 | 0 | 0 | 0 | 40,818 | 9,971 | 50,789 | 54.8 | 92,667 | 4,724.54 | 1,096.17 |
| 2 | 857 | 200 | 2,766 | 3,825 | 0 | 0 | 0 | 147,169 | 38,625 | 185,794 | 53.1 | 350,155 | 6,955.66 | 1,175.19 |
| 3 | 1,809 | 348 | 4,819 | 6,979 | 0 | 50 | 50 | 278,387 | 65,262 | 343,649 | 46.3 | 741,503 | 6,256.62 | 1,079.54 |
| 102 | 3,092 | 530 | 9,735 | 13,459 | 101 | 60 | 161 | 506,760 | 124,156 | 630,916 | 47.4 | 1,329,820 | 7,208.91 | 1,325.82 |
| 79 | 5,251 | 662 | 11,938 | 17,930 | 229 | 485 | 714 | 824,717 | 193,428 | 1,018,145 | 49.3 | 2,066,790 | 9,179.00 | 1,459.90 |
| 97 | 6,020 | 805 | 13,741 | 20,663 | 518 | 9 | 527 | 943,950 | 229,293 | 1,173,243 | 48.8 | 2,406,141 | 7,424.85 | 1,515.10 |

MSAs

# TABLE 8

## U.S. CENSUS DIVISION 6, WEST NORTH CENTRAL

*U.S. Community Hospitals*
*(Nonfederal, short-term general and other special hospitals)*

## 2003 Utilization, Personnel and Finances

MSAs

| CLASSIFICATION | Hospitals | Beds | Admissions | Inpatient Days | Adjusted Patient Days | Average Daily Census | Adjusted Average Daily Census | Average Stay (days) | Surgical Operations | NEWBORNS | | OUTPATIENT VISITS | |
|---|---|---|---|---|---|---|---|---|---|---|---|---|---|
| | | | | | | | | | | Bassinets | Births | Emergency | Total |
| UNITED STATES | 4,895 | 813,307 | 34,782,742 | 196,649,769 | 326,299,942 | 538,797 | 894,019 | 5.7 | 27,106,538 | 59,662 | 3,915,842 | 111,069,871 | 563,186,046 |
| Nonmetropolitan | 2,166 | 168,374 | 5,368,552 | 35,076,707 | 73,724,487 | 96,136 | 202,034 | 6.5 | 4,592,380 | 13,462 | 530,805 | 23,720,395 | 117,598,717 |
| Metropolitan | 2,729 | 644,933 | 29,414,190 | 161,573,062 | 252,575,455 | 442,661 | 691,985 | 5.5 | 22,514,158 | 46,200 | 3,385,037 | 87,349,476 | 445,587,329 |
| CENSUS DIVISION 6, WEST NORTH CENTRAL | 675 | 72,821 | 2,543,012 | 16,336,089 | 30,757,528 | 44,762 | 84,275 | 6.4 | 2,054,194 | 5,195 | 269,860 | 7,227,615 | 47,564,307 |
| Nonmetropolitan | 496 | 32,033 | 727,247 | 6,818,047 | 15,018,026 | 18,691 | 41,153 | 9.4 | 645,262 | 2,475 | 73,539 | 2,636,133 | 19,120,857 |
| Metropolitan | 179 | 40,788 | 1,815,765 | 9,518,042 | 15,739,502 | 26,071 | 43,122 | 5.2 | 1,408,932 | 2,720 | 196,321 | 4,591,482 | 28,443,450 |
| Iowa | 116 | 11,002 | 363,008 | 2,369,769 | 5,021,857 | 6,498 | 13,764 | 6.5 | 373,046 | 782 | 37,936 | 1,066,268 | 9,735,379 |
| Nonmetropolitan | 95 | 5,680 | 138,840 | 1,186,776 | 2,941,128 | 3,258 | 8,061 | 8.5 | 154,827 | 418 | 12,814 | 497,665 | 4,389,664 |
| Metropolitan | 21 | 5,322 | 224,168 | 1,182,993 | 2,080,729 | 3,240 | 5,703 | 5.3 | 218,219 | 364 | 25,122 | 568,603 | 5,345,715 |
| Cedar Rapids | 2 | 731 | 27,814 | 156,349 | 304,122 | 428 | 834 | 5.6 | 39,901 | 54 | 3,425 | 86,462 | 584,522 |
| Davenport-Moline-Rock Island | 2 | 515 | 20,954 | 113,646 | 185,087 | 311 | 507 | 5.4 | 14,212 | 32 | 2,685 | 64,363 | 220,192 |
| Des Moines | 6 | 1,401 | 69,569 | 338,222 | 536,526 | 927 | 1,470 | 4.9 | 49,607 | 111 | 8,736 | 168,523 | 1,662,649 |
| Dubuque | 2 | 447 | 15,305 | 83,169 | 142,607 | 228 | 390 | 5.4 | 16,863 | 42 | 1,595 | 44,434 | 135,441 |
| Iowa City | 2 | 882 | 32,413 | 217,294 | 364,082 | 595 | 998 | 6.7 | 28,733 | 38 | 2,781 | 54,107 | 1,112,473 |
| Omaha | 2 | 312 | 12,412 | 55,780 | 93,945 | 153 | 258 | 4.5 | 11,566 | 22 | 1,108 | 41,835 | 171,540 |
| Sioux City | 2 | 468 | 21,919 | 106,314 | 167,994 | 291 | 461 | 4.9 | 17,934 | 30 | 2,517 | 50,249 | 449,198 |
| Waterloo-Cedar Falls | 3 | 566 | 23,782 | 112,219 | 286,366 | 307 | 785 | 4.7 | 39,403 | 35 | 2,275 | 58,630 | 1,009,700 |
| Kansas | 134 | 10,554 | 331,244 | 2,148,111 | 4,007,937 | 5,889 | 10,982 | 6.5 | 252,472 | 778 | 39,341 | 945,208 | 5,950,038 |
| Nonmetropolitan | 107 | 5,821 | 129,651 | 1,113,079 | 2,345,389 | 3,054 | 6,426 | 8.6 | 98,366 | 465 | 12,000 | 402,749 | 3,048,879 |
| Metropolitan | 27 | 4,733 | 201,593 | 1,035,032 | 1,662,548 | 2,835 | 4,556 | 5.1 | 154,106 | 313 | 27,341 | 542,459 | 2,901,159 |
| Kansas City | 14 | 2,070 | 89,237 | 446,790 | 743,272 | 1,223 | 2,036 | 5.0 | 80,465 | 155 | 13,631 | 234,862 | 1,502,388 |
| Lawrence | 1 | 108 | 6,915 | 28,635 | 77,067 | 78 | 211 | 4.1 | 4,969 | 13 | 1,110 | 28,788 | 152,190 |
| Topeka | 3 | 663 | 25,840 | 123,162 | 228,986 | 338 | 628 | 4.8 | 19,964 | 36 | 3,084 | 87,833 | 435,574 |
| Wichita | 9 | 1,892 | 79,601 | 436,445 | 613,223 | 1,196 | 1,681 | 5.5 | 48,708 | 109 | 9,516 | 190,976 | 811,007 |
| Minnesota | 131 | 16,439 | 614,867 | 4,113,264 | 7,681,842 | 11,269 | 21,049 | 6.7 | 463,903 | 1,315 | 68,492 | 1,581,734 | 9,184,368 |
| Nonmetropolitan | 86 | 6,743 | 126,941 | 1,639,113 | 3,619,336 | 4,491 | 9,920 | 12.9 | 117,390 | 465 | 15,451 | 499,390 | 2,938,143 |
| Metropolitan | 45 | 9,696 | 487,926 | 2,474,151 | 4,062,506 | 6,778 | 11,129 | 5.1 | 346,513 | 850 | 53,041 | 1,082,344 | 6,246,225 |
| Duluth-Superior | 8 | 1,297 | 45,348 | 314,791 | 549,513 | 863 | 1,506 | 6.9 | 42,181 | 89 | 3,442 | 100,060 | 529,166 |
| Grand Forks | 2 | 293 | 2,434 | 79,356 | 253,806 | 217 | 695 | 32.6 | 2,256 | 13 | 175 | 3,400 | 94,950 |
| Minneapolis-St. Paul | 28 | 6,061 | 341,610 | 1,494,085 | 2,342,249 | 4,093 | 6,416 | 4.4 | 251,157 | 650 | 44,721 | 827,868 | 4,816,768 |
| Rochester | 3 | 1,195 | 73,412 | 355,532 | 519,157 | 974 | 1,421 | 4.8 | 36,943 | 47 | 2,161 | 98,489 | 533,293 |
| St. Cloud | 4 | 850 | 25,122 | 230,387 | 397,781 | 631 | 1,091 | 9.2 | 13,976 | 51 | 2,542 | 52,527 | 272,048 |
| Missouri | 119 | 19,346 | 831,210 | 4,342,987 | 7,735,027 | 11,897 | 21,185 | 5.2 | 598,437 | 1,291 | 78,564 | 2,624,926 | 15,668,704 |
| Nonmetropolitan | 58 | 4,475 | 171,870 | 866,203 | 1,890,549 | 2,374 | 5,175 | 5.0 | 130,434 | 437 | 16,222 | 757,436 | 4,891,931 |
| Metropolitan | 61 | 14,871 | 659,340 | 3,476,784 | 5,844,478 | 9,523 | 16,010 | 5.3 | 468,003 | 854 | 62,342 | 1,867,490 | 10,776,773 |
| Columbia | 4 | 918 | 34,342 | 192,278 | 286,270 | 526 | 785 | 5.6 | 26,205 | 38 | 3,331 | 63,628 | 761,901 |
| Joplin | 4 | 780 | 36,394 | 175,253 | 321,417 | 480 | 880 | 4.8 | 22,714 | 52 | 3,282 | 141,539 | 877,165 |
| Kansas City | 21 | 3,734 | 151,608 | 860,361 | 1,469,740 | 2,357 | 4,026 | 5.7 | 111,763 | 217 | 15,949 | 516,352 | 2,357,136 |
| Springfield | 3 | 1,358 | 65,107 | 320,799 | 625,622 | 879 | 1,714 | 4.9 | 48,944 | 78 | 6,224 | 163,003 | 1,447,249 |
| St. Joseph | 1 | 460 | 17,491 | 71,715 | 107,846 | 196 | 295 | 4.1 | 6,366 | 20 | 1,447 | 82,867 | 493,760 |
| St. Louis | 28 | 7,621 | 354,398 | 1,856,378 | 3,033,583 | 5,085 | 8,310 | 5.2 | 252,011 | 449 | 32,109 | 900,101 | 4,839,562 |
| Nebraska | 85 | 7,467 | 211,567 | 1,593,254 | 2,946,949 | 4,362 | 8,073 | 7.5 | 205,294 | 585 | 25,796 | 532,934 | 3,676,098 |
| Nonmetropolitan | 72 | 4,187 | 84,144 | 855,953 | 1,859,170 | 2,344 | 5,094 | 10.2 | 84,040 | 376 | 9,497 | 230,800 | 2,095,287 |
| Metropolitan | 13 | 3,280 | 127,423 | 737,301 | 1,087,779 | 2,018 | 2,979 | 5.8 | 120,654 | 209 | 16,299 | 302,134 | 1,580,811 |
| Lincoln | 3 | 959 | 40,482 | 259,447 | 334,966 | 710 | 917 | 6.4 | 27,807 | 57 | 4,648 | 84,856 | 438,151 |
| Omaha | 10 | 2,321 | 86,941 | 477,854 | 752,813 | 1,308 | 2,062 | 5.5 | 92,847 | 152 | 11,651 | 217,278 | 1,142,660 |
| North Dakota | 40 | 3,595 | 88,132 | 774,175 | 1,568,591 | 2,123 | 4,299 | 8.8 | 76,294 | 201 | 9,143 | 261,714 | 1,812,996 |
| Nonmetropolitan | 34 | 2,235 | 33,296 | 475,211 | 1,028,897 | 1,303 | 2,820 | 14.3 | 28,239 | 124 | 3,143 | 132,592 | 805,414 |
| Metropolitan | 6 | 1,360 | 54,836 | 298,964 | 539,694 | 820 | 1,479 | 5.5 | 48,055 | 77 | 6,000 | 129,122 | 1,007,582 |
| Bismarck | 2 | 475 | 18,593 | 93,257 | 182,543 | 256 | 500 | 5.0 | 18,205 | 15 | 1,707 | 32,352 | 635,263 |
| Fargo-Moorhead | 2 | 532 | 24,091 | 119,876 | 170,399 | 329 | 467 | 5.0 | 20,427 | 39 | 2,959 | 54,894 | 266,985 |
| Grand Forks | 2 | 353 | 12,152 | 85,831 | 186,752 | 235 | 512 | 7.1 | 9,423 | 23 | 1,334 | 41,876 | 105,334 |
| South Dakota | 50 | 4,418 | 102,984 | 994,529 | 1,795,325 | 2,724 | 4,923 | 9.7 | 84,748 | 243 | 10,588 | 214,831 | 1,536,724 |
| Nonmetropolitan | 44 | 2,892 | 42,505 | 681,712 | 1,333,557 | 1,867 | 3,657 | 16.0 | 31,366 | 190 | 4,412 | 115,501 | 951,539 |
| Metropolitan | 6 | 1,526 | 60,479 | 312,817 | 461,768 | 857 | 1,266 | 5.2 | 53,382 | 53 | 6,176 | 99,330 | 585,185 |
| Rapid City | 1 | 372 | 17,054 | 88,991 | 133,788 | 244 | 367 | 5.2 | 8,246 | 15 | 2,052 | 45,503 | 166,582 |
| Sioux Falls | 5 | 1,154 | 43,425 | 223,826 | 327,980 | 613 | 899 | 5.2 | 45,136 | 38 | 4,124 | 53,827 | 418,603 |

# U.S. CENSUS DIVISION 6, WEST NORTH CENTRAL

*U.S. Community Hospitals*
*(Nonfederal, short-term general and other special hospitals)*

## 2003 Utilization, Personnel and Finances

| FULL-TIME EQUIVALENT PERSONNEL | | | | | FULL-TIME EQUIV. TRAINEES | | | EXPENSES | | | | | | |
|---|---|---|---|---|---|---|---|---|---|---|---|---|---|---|
| | | | | | | | | LABOR | | | | TOTAL | | |
| Physicians and Dentists | Registered Nurses | Licensed Practical Nurses | Other Salaried Personnel | Total Personnel | Medical and Dental Residents | Other Trainees | Total Trainees | Payroll (in thousands) | Employee Benefits (in thousands) | Total (in thousands) | Percent of Total | Amount (in thousands) | Adjusted per Admission | Adjusted per Inpatient Day |
| 71,335 | 1,021,346 | 126,328 | 2,889,619 | 4,108,628 | 77,813 | 7,954 | 85,767 | $187,822,974 | $45,438,505 | $233,261,475 | 51.8 | $450,124,257 | $7,796.41 | $1,379.48 |
| 8,445 | 147,570 | 37,579 | 485,049 | 678,643 | 1,775 | 600 | 2,375 | 25,551,777 | 6,425,000 | 31,976,774 | 53.8 | 59,444,378 | 5,305.04 | 806.30 |
| 62,890 | 873,776 | 88,749 | 2,404,570 | 3,429,985 | 76,038 | 7,354 | 83,392 | 162,271,198 | 39,013,505 | 201,284,701 | 51.5 | 390,679,879 | 8,396.37 | 1,546.78 |
| 5,499 | 79,392 | 11,558 | 237,592 | 334,041 | 3,050 | 278 | 3,328 | 14,563,436 | 3,344,116 | 17,907,538 | 53.1 | 33,732,352 | 7,304.58 | 1,096.72 |
| 1,631 | 22,792 | 6,320 | 80,992 | 111,735 | 76 | 12 | 88 | 3,969,915 | 918,084 | 4,887,988 | 55.0 | 8,882,566 | 5,471.88 | 591.46 |
| 3,868 | 56,600 | 5,238 | 156,600 | 222,306 | 2,974 | 266 | 3,240 | 10,593,521 | 2,426,032 | 13,019,550 | 52.4 | 24,849,786 | 8,298.03 | 1,578.82 |
| 878 | 12,449 | 1,334 | 38,033 | 52,694 | 564 | 23 | 587 | 2,053,479 | 504,459 | 2,557,938 | 53.5 | 4,779,866 | 6,468.93 | 951.81 |
| 265 | 4,929 | 836 | 16,335 | 22,365 | 22 | 0 | 22 | 756,449 | 180,194 | 936,644 | 54.4 | 1,720,943 | 5,021.92 | 585.13 |
| 613 | 7,520 | 498 | 21,698 | 30,329 | 542 | 23 | 565 | 1,297,030 | 324,265 | 1,621,294 | 53.0 | 3,058,923 | 7,720.46 | 1,470.12 |
| 4 | 973 | 93 | 2,406 | 3,476 | 0 | 16 | 16 | 129,464 | 35,535 | 164,999 | 50.5 | 326,698 | 6,103.77 | 1,074.23 |
| 12 | 612 | 37 | 1,697 | 2,358 | 5 | 0 | 5 | 96,896 | 24,156 | 121,052 | 46.0 | 263,434 | 7,650.40 | 1,423.30 |
| 303 | 2,140 | 65 | 6,529 | 9,037 | 147 | 0 | 147 | 403,141 | 92,288 | 495,428 | 54.8 | 904,056 | 8,143.62 | 1,685.02 |
| 10 | 521 | 19 | 1,320 | 1,870 | 0 | 0 | 0 | 67,389 | 14,717 | 82,106 | 50.8 | 161,773 | 6,013.85 | 1,134.39 |
| 106 | 1,537 | 5 | 4,494 | 6,142 | 387 | 7 | 394 | 288,444 | 85,891 | 374,336 | 54.2 | 690,959 | 12,671.41 | 1,897.81 |
| 5 | 349 | 27 | 825 | 1,206 | 0 | 0 | 0 | 56,900 | 12,667 | 69,568 | 53.4 | 130,330 | 6,240.36 | 1,387.30 |
| 68 | 680 | 68 | 1,991 | 2,807 | 0 | 0 | 0 | 109,875 | 28,539 | 138,414 | 52.6 | 263,284 | 7,497.56 | 1,567.23 |
| 105 | 708 | 184 | 2,436 | 3,433 | 3 | 0 | 3 | 144,919 | 30,472 | 175,391 | 55.1 | 318,389 | 5,323.51 | 1,111.82 |
| 560 | 9,944 | 1,411 | 29,321 | 41,236 | 125 | 28 | 153 | 1,667,197 | 363,492 | 2,030,686 | 53.2 | 3,816,799 | 6,348.82 | 952.31 |
| 199 | 4,010 | 863 | 13,587 | 18,659 | 3 | 7 | 10 | 633,854 | 135,186 | 769,037 | 56.1 | 1,369,780 | 5,147.67 | 584.03 |
| 361 | 5,934 | 548 | 15,734 | 22,577 | 122 | 21 | 143 | 1,033,343 | 228,306 | 1,261,649 | 51.6 | 2,447,019 | 7,302.68 | 1,471.85 |
| 125 | 2,801 | 123 | 7,083 | 10,132 | 2 | 6 | 8 | 470,529 | 107,939 | 578,468 | 51.0 | 1,134,459 | 7,313.57 | 1,526.30 |
| 17 | 235 | 29 | 617 | 898 | 0 | 0 | 0 | 39,460 | 7,534 | 46,994 | 52.5 | 89,581 | 4,813.32 | 1,162.37 |
| 159 | 930 | 269 | 2,797 | 4,155 | 0 | 0 | 0 | 191,585 | 39,401 | 230,986 | 58.8 | 392,724 | 7,930.30 | 1,715.06 |
| 60 | 1,968 | 127 | 5,237 | 7,392 | 120 | 15 | 135 | 331,769 | 73,433 | 405,201 | 48.8 | 830,255 | 7,423.93 | 1,353.92 |
| 1,199 | 17,890 | 2,826 | 51,606 | 73,521 | 597 | 104 | 701 | 3,874,807 | 936,902 | 4,811,704 | 56.5 | 8,522,794 | 8,042.26 | 1,109.47 |
| 299 | 3,796 | 1,461 | 14,498 | 20,054 | 6 | 3 | 9 | 812,088 | 189,925 | 1,002,008 | 57.1 | 1,755,648 | 6,155.35 | 485.07 |
| 900 | 14,094 | 1,365 | 37,108 | 53,467 | 591 | 101 | 692 | 3,062,720 | 746,977 | 3,809,696 | 56.3 | 6,767,146 | 8,737.12 | 1,665.76 |
| 121 | 1,076 | 253 | 3,058 | 4,508 | 2 | 1 | 3 | 272,007 | 76,570 | 348,577 | 57.6 | 605,371 | 8,178.92 | 1,101.65 |
| 4 | 86 | 69 | 427 | 586 | 0 | 0 | 0 | 20,307 | 3,972 | 24,279 | 62.0 | 39,178 | 5,011.93 | 154.36 |
| 628 | 10,208 | 635 | 26,494 | 37,965 | 478 | 77 | 555 | 2,270,996 | 520,971 | 2,791,966 | 56.6 | 4,934,221 | 9,091.57 | 2,106.62 |
| 122 | 1,788 | 138 | 3,948 | 5,996 | 94 | 23 | 117 | 348,910 | 84,318 | 433,228 | 51.7 | 837,702 | 7,762.83 | 1,613.58 |
| 25 | 936 | 270 | 3,181 | 4,412 | 17 | 0 | 17 | 150,499 | 61,146 | 211,646 | 60.4 | 350,673 | 8,337.84 | 881.57 |
| 1,781 | 25,159 | 3,455 | 74,036 | 104,431 | 1,678 | 91 | 1,769 | 4,453,342 | 983,898 | 5,437,235 | 50.1 | 10,852,259 | 7,368.75 | 1,403.00 |
| 462 | 4,686 | 1,560 | 16,431 | 23,139 | 41 | 0 | 41 | 817,352 | 197,864 | 1,015,212 | 51.7 | 1,962,473 | 5,297.90 | 1,038.04 |
| 1,319 | 20,473 | 1,895 | 57,605 | 81,292 | 1,637 | 91 | 1,728 | 3,635,990 | 786,034 | 4,422,023 | 49.7 | 8,889,786 | 8,064.65 | 1,521.06 |
| 9 | 1,181 | 213 | 3,826 | 5,229 | 289 | 0 | 289 | 192,910 | 55,271 | 248,180 | 46.1 | 538,758 | 10,345.22 | 1,881.99 |
| 189 | 1,020 | 181 | 3,514 | 4,904 | 13 | 0 | 13 | 218,267 | 44,635 | 262,901 | 56.0 | 469,418 | 7,023.53 | 1,460.46 |
| 254 | 4,980 | 439 | 12,129 | 17,802 | 158 | 77 | 235 | 876,342 | 186,569 | 1,062,911 | 51.2 | 2,076,490 | 8,421.71 | 1,412.83 |
| 148 | 2,179 | 213 | 7,787 | 10,327 | 23 | 1 | 24 | 401,383 | 91,542 | 492,925 | 49.4 | 997,259 | 7,936.49 | 1,594.03 |
| 34 | 566 | 51 | 1,541 | 2,192 | 56 | 5 | 61 | 103,409 | 25,403 | 128,812 | 50.4 | 255,533 | 9,714.98 | 2,369.43 |
| 685 | 10,547 | 798 | 28,808 | 40,838 | 1,098 | 8 | 1,106 | 1,843,679 | 382,614 | 2,226,294 | 48.9 | 4,552,327 | 7,783.35 | 1,500.64 |
| 379 | 7,511 | 1,414 | 22,827 | 32,131 | 29 | 32 | 61 | 1,275,394 | 305,233 | 1,580,629 | 51.4 | 3,072,367 | 8,051.93 | 1,042.56 |
| 182 | 2,822 | 963 | 10,235 | 14,202 | 3 | 2 | 5 | 496,348 | 119,437 | 615,786 | 55.2 | 1,115,857 | 5,963.86 | 600.19 |
| 197 | 4,689 | 451 | 12,592 | 17,929 | 26 | 30 | 56 | 779,047 | 185,796 | 964,843 | 49.3 | 1,956,510 | 10,060.94 | 1,798.63 |
| 60 | 1,480 | 217 | 4,308 | 6,065 | 0 | 0 | 0 | 242,664 | 63,508 | 306,172 | 54.3 | 563,415 | 10,068.36 | 1,682.01 |
| 137 | 3,209 | 234 | 8,284 | 11,864 | 26 | 30 | 56 | 536,383 | 122,288 | 658,671 | 47.3 | 1,393,095 | 10,057.94 | 1,850.52 |
| 479 | 2,905 | 804 | 10,779 | 14,967 | 43 | 0 | 43 | 623,579 | 115,945 | 739,522 | 54.9 | 1,347,844 | 7,262.37 | 859.27 |
| 164 | 1,146 | 413 | 4,850 | 6,573 | 1 | 0 | 1 | 215,335 | 41,467 | 256,800 | 56.4 | 455,466 | 5,531.53 | 442.67 |
| 315 | 1,759 | 391 | 5,929 | 8,394 | 42 | 0 | 42 | 408,244 | 74,478 | 482,722 | 54.1 | 892,378 | 8,642.64 | 1,653.49 |
| 146 | 600 | 141 | 2,231 | 3,118 | 0 | 0 | 0 | 146,551 | 22,925 | 169,476 | 56.7 | 298,748 | 8,177.49 | 1,636.59 |
| 0 | 804 | 177 | 1,572 | 2,553 | 42 | 0 | 42 | 121,878 | 20,970 | 142,848 | 44.0 | 324,550 | 9,540.26 | 1,904.65 |
| 169 | 355 | 73 | 2,126 | 2,723 | 0 | 0 | 0 | 139,816 | 30,583 | 170,398 | 63.3 | 269,079 | 8,228.48 | 1,440.84 |
| 223 | 3,534 | 314 | 10,990 | 15,061 | 14 | 0 | 14 | 615,638 | 134,187 | 749,824 | 55.9 | 1,340,422 | 7,520.24 | 746.62 |
| 60 | 1,403 | 224 | 5,056 | 6,743 | 0 | 0 | 0 | 238,490 | 54,012 | 292,501 | 58.2 | 502,399 | 5,617.28 | 376.74 |
| 163 | 2,131 | 90 | 5,934 | 8,318 | 14 | 0 | 14 | 377,148 | 80,175 | 457,323 | 54.6 | 838,024 | 9,436.78 | 1,814.82 |
| 11 | 550 | 60 | 1,757 | 2,378 | 14 | 0 | 14 | 103,457 | 17,149 | 120,606 | 51.3 | 235,019 | 9,166.47 | 1,756.65 |
| 152 | 1,581 | 30 | 4,177 | 5,940 | 0 | 0 | 0 | 273,691 | 63,026 | 336,717 | 55.8 | 603,005 | 9,546.50 | 1,838.54 |

# TABLE 8

# U.S. CENSUS DIVISION 7, WEST SOUTH CENTRAL

*U.S. Community Hospitals*
*(Nonfederal, short-term general and other special hospitals)*

## 2003 Utilization, Personnel and Finances

| CLASSIFICATION | Hospitals | Beds | Admissions | Inpatient Days | Adjusted Patient Days | Average Daily Census | Adjusted Average Daily Census | Average Stay (days) | Surgical Operations | NEWBORNS | | OUTPATIENT VISITS | |
|---|---|---|---|---|---|---|---|---|---|---|---|---|---|
| | | | | | | | | | | Bassinets | Births | Emergency | Total |
| UNITED STATES | 4,895 | 813,307 | 34,782,742 | 196,649,769 | 326,299,942 | 538,797 | 894,019 | 5.7 | 27,106,538 | 59,662 | 3,915,842 | 111,069,871 | 563,186,046 |
| Nonmetropolitan | 2,166 | 168,374 | 5,368,552 | 35,076,707 | 73,724,487 | 96,136 | 202,034 | 6.5 | 4,592,380 | 13,462 | 530,805 | 23,720,395 | 117,598,717 |
| Metropolitan | 2,729 | 644,933 | 29,414,190 | 161,573,062 | 252,575,455 | 442,661 | 691,985 | 5.5 | 22,514,158 | 46,200 | 3,385,037 | 87,349,476 | 445,587,329 |
| CENSUS DIVISION 7, WEST SOUTH CENTRAL | 737 | 96,130 | 4,078,542 | 21,638,131 | 34,031,057 | 59,279 | 93,234 | 5.3 | 2,857,084 | 7,555 | 518,123 | 13,452,657 | 53,591,125 |
| Nonmetropolitan | 333 | 18,314 | 656,757 | 3,174,426 | 6,151,895 | 8,690 | 16,856 | 4.8 | 421,631 | 1,537 | 59,228 | 2,778,944 | 11,850,587 |
| Metropolitan | 404 | 77,816 | 3,421,785 | 18,463,705 | 27,879,162 | 50,589 | 76,378 | 5.4 | 2,435,453 | 6,018 | 458,895 | 10,673,713 | 41,740,538 |
| Arkansas | 88 | 9,909 | 388,046 | 2,088,391 | 3,494,152 | 5,730 | 9,574 | 5.4 | 268,834 | 762 | 38,892 | 1,251,391 | 4,582,352 |
| Nonmetropolitan | 56 | 4,214 | 146,923 | 801,558 | 1,520,122 | 2,200 | 4,163 | 5.5 | 91,512 | 308 | 12,436 | 552,613 | 1,963,243 |
| Metropolitan | 32 | 5,695 | 241,123 | 1,286,833 | 1,974,030 | 3,530 | 5,411 | 5.3 | 177,322 | 454 | 26,456 | 698,778 | 2,619,109 |
| Fayetteville-Springdale-Rogers | 8 | 860 | 42,535 | 182,515 | 286,239 | 501 | 783 | 4.3 | 29,813 | 84 | 6,257 | 159,266 | 274,357 |
| Fort Smith | 5 | 853 | 34,497 | 191,938 | 274,111 | 530 | 754 | 5.6 | 36,618 | 67 | 3,569 | 119,648 | 295,690 |
| Jonesboro | 3 | 476 | 23,007 | 122,064 | 195,604 | 334 | 536 | 5.3 | 16,450 | 32 | 2,008 | 61,404 | 246,224 |
| Little Rock-North Little Rock | 14 | 3,008 | 124,613 | 702,346 | 1,075,947 | 1,924 | 2,949 | 5.6 | 84,372 | 235 | 12,685 | 302,030 | 1,608,853 |
| Memphis | 1 | 121 | 3,821 | 19,827 | 31,480 | 54 | 86 | 5.2 | 3,585 | 11 | 699 | 22,101 | 44,464 |
| Pine Bluff | 1 | 377 | 12,650 | 68,143 | 110,649 | 187 | 303 | 5.4 | 6,484 | 25 | 1,238 | 34,329 | 149,521 |
| Louisiana | 127 | 17,829 | 690,246 | 3,872,912 | 6,094,152 | 10,605 | 16,698 | 5.6 | 425,841 | 1,190 | 63,923 | 2,498,935 | 10,824,010 |
| Nonmetropolitan | 49 | 2,903 | 101,726 | 532,570 | 948,409 | 1,456 | 2,599 | 5.2 | 54,275 | 177 | 7,542 | 490,798 | 1,533,221 |
| Metropolitan | 78 | 14,926 | 588,520 | 3,340,342 | 5,145,743 | 9,149 | 14,099 | 5.7 | 371,566 | 1,013 | 56,381 | 2,008,137 | 9,290,789 |
| Alexandria | 5 | 705 | 34,184 | 173,048 | 281,924 | 475 | 771 | 5.1 | 20,616 | 65 | 3,190 | 121,761 | 398,106 |
| Baton Rouge | 9 | 1,930 | 83,488 | 472,846 | 741,069 | 1,295 | 2,031 | 5.7 | 55,068 | 125 | 9,949 | 253,396 | 854,928 |
| Houma | 5 | 653 | 29,421 | 132,565 | 227,804 | 363 | 624 | 4.5 | 19,590 | 70 | 3,350 | 136,992 | 428,093 |
| Lafayette | 13 | 1,617 | 60,877 | 326,544 | 516,440 | 894 | 1,416 | 5.4 | 45,380 | 98 | 6,595 | 211,286 | 727,514 |
| Lake Charles | 7 | 857 | 35,713 | 173,822 | 302,238 | 476 | 827 | 4.9 | 19,269 | 65 | 2,538 | 100,126 | 425,987 |
| Monroe | 5 | 1,021 | 42,516 | 240,566 | 361,533 | 658 | 991 | 5.7 | 22,122 | 94 | 3,651 | 112,881 | 430,391 |
| New Orleans | 24 | 5,738 | 215,647 | 1,317,204 | 1,979,316 | 3,608 | 5,423 | 6.1 | 133,640 | 362 | 19,628 | 806,900 | 5,155,928 |
| Shreveport-Bossier City | 10 | 2,405 | 86,674 | 503,747 | 735,419 | 1,380 | 2,016 | 5.8 | 55,881 | 134 | 7,480 | 264,795 | 869,842 |
| Oklahoma | 108 | 11,018 | 449,936 | 2,380,232 | 3,761,712 | 6,515 | 10,307 | 5.3 | 297,393 | 831 | 44,736 | 1,386,848 | 5,489,728 |
| Nonmetropolitan | 67 | 3,830 | 137,568 | 671,220 | 1,255,588 | 1,833 | 3,441 | 4.9 | 85,638 | 379 | 12,820 | 524,907 | 2,078,385 |
| Metropolitan | 41 | 7,188 | 312,368 | 1,709,012 | 2,506,124 | 4,682 | 6,866 | 5.5 | 211,755 | 452 | 31,916 | 861,941 | 3,411,343 |
| Enid | 2 | 309 | 12,004 | 82,417 | 116,894 | 225 | 320 | 6.9 | 6,215 | 16 | 1,086 | 31,002 | 198,704 |
| Fort Smith | 1 | 25 | 713 | 2,431 | 12,667 | 7 | 35 | 3.4 | 184 | 1 | 6 | 16,449 | 16,533 |
| Lawton | 2 | 445 | 15,045 | 91,722 | 157,604 | 251 | 432 | 6.1 | 9,769 | 37 | 1,469 | 51,854 | 174,024 |
| Oklahoma City | 20 | 3,686 | 163,844 | 887,364 | 1,280,314 | 2,430 | 3,508 | 5.4 | 110,143 | 266 | 16,237 | 474,516 | 1,617,667 |
| Tulsa | 16 | 2,723 | 120,762 | 645,078 | 938,645 | 1,769 | 2,571 | 5.3 | 85,444 | 132 | 13,118 | 288,120 | 1,404,415 |
| Texas | 414 | 57,374 | 2,550,314 | 13,296,596 | 20,681,041 | 36,429 | 56,655 | 5.2 | 1,865,016 | 4,772 | 370,572 | 8,315,483 | 32,695,035 |
| Nonmetropolitan | 161 | 7,367 | 270,540 | 1,169,078 | 2,427,776 | 3,201 | 6,653 | 4.3 | 190,206 | 673 | 26,430 | 1,210,626 | 6,275,738 |
| Metropolitan | 253 | 50,007 | 2,279,774 | 12,127,518 | 18,253,265 | 33,228 | 50,002 | 5.3 | 1,674,810 | 4,099 | 344,142 | 7,104,857 | 26,419,297 |
| Abilene | 2 | 535 | 23,227 | 124,828 | 195,683 | 342 | 536 | 5.4 | 13,509 | 46 | 2,705 | 65,826 | 319,449 |
| Amarillo | 3 | 875 | 41,561 | 203,606 | 290,442 | 557 | 795 | 4.9 | 29,522 | 54 | 4,539 | 103,870 | 374,612 |
| Austin-San Marcos | 16 | 2,448 | 110,181 | 605,678 | 980,214 | 1,660 | 2,686 | 5.5 | 100,929 | 238 | 23,076 | 493,647 | 1,274,950 |
| Beaumont-Port Arthur | 10 | 1,412 | 58,195 | 323,785 | 482,529 | 886 | 1,323 | 5.6 | 38,792 | 90 | 5,214 | 153,662 | 578,970 |
| Brazoria | 3 | 234 | 9,022 | 35,699 | 88,018 | 98 | 241 | 4.0 | 8,595 | 32 | 1,195 | 53,835 | 171,459 |
| Brownsville-Harlingen-San Benito | 5 | 975 | 49,259 | 226,898 | 310,381 | 622 | 850 | 4.6 | 25,136 | 85 | 8,957 | 99,712 | 262,410 |
| Bryan-College Station | 2 | 398 | 20,817 | 94,441 | 142,153 | 259 | 390 | 4.5 | 15,264 | 60 | 3,327 | 65,430 | 248,458 |
| Corpus Christi | 6 | 1,635 | 72,953 | 404,776 | 590,988 | 1,109 | 1,619 | 5.6 | 50,950 | 148 | 9,606 | 190,864 | 639,207 |
| Dallas | 46 | 8,311 | 396,848 | 2,040,204 | 3,003,894 | 5,592 | 8,229 | 5.1 | 278,390 | 743 | 67,275 | 1,382,445 | 4,535,785 |
| El Paso | 8 | 1,649 | 77,896 | 385,929 | 567,563 | 1,058 | 1,556 | 5.0 | 40,373 | 202 | 15,410 | 231,898 | 1,125,444 |
| Fort Worth-Arlington | 26 | 3,957 | 191,425 | 983,989 | 1,519,528 | 2,697 | 4,166 | 5.1 | 157,539 | 397 | 31,363 | 702,660 | 2,362,379 |
| Galveston-Texas City | 3 | 992 | 43,553 | 235,256 | 398,958 | 644 | 1,092 | 5.4 | 23,982 | 47 | 6,699 | 107,040 | 962,723 |
| Houston | 52 | 11,469 | 503,897 | 2,917,251 | 4,291,440 | 7,992 | 11,753 | 5.8 | 375,895 | 833 | 73,567 | 1,427,136 | 6,047,290 |
| Killeen-Temple | 4 | 899 | 36,154 | 190,882 | 463,156 | 523 | 1,268 | 5.3 | 30,297 | 40 | 3,976 | 111,637 | 1,733,110 |
| Laredo | 2 | 492 | 23,973 | 123,723 | 191,058 | 339 | 523 | 5.2 | 17,844 | 69 | 6,413 | 63,535 | 240,788 |
| Longview-Marshall | 4 | 717 | 28,309 | 136,922 | 238,554 | 376 | 653 | 4.8 | 20,277 | 64 | 3,534 | 135,671 | 298,380 |
| Lubbock | 5 | 1,417 | 58,165 | 311,272 | 447,683 | 853 | 1,226 | 5.4 | 40,735 | 55 | 5,314 | 121,746 | 485,062 |
| McAllen-Edinburg-Mission | 7 | 1,405 | 76,428 | 376,101 | 484,105 | 1,030 | 1,326 | 4.9 | 37,686 | 114 | 15,682 | 128,241 | 337,190 |
| Odessa-Midland | 4 | 811 | 32,833 | 169,372 | 263,359 | 463 | 721 | 5.2 | 26,894 | 72 | 5,761 | 121,685 | 363,597 |
| San Angelo | 2 | 385 | 18,877 | 88,151 | 149,780 | 241 | 410 | 4.7 | 18,229 | 37 | 2,114 | 64,683 | 181,021 |
| San Antonio | 23 | 4,965 | 236,589 | 1,217,919 | 1,752,531 | 3,337 | 4,802 | 5.1 | 189,009 | 423 | 32,320 | 653,735 | 1,916,169 |
| Sherman-Denison | 3 | 607 | 25,679 | 140,024 | 216,083 | 383 | 592 | 5.5 | 25,328 | 46 | 2,281 | 176,418 | 342,267 |
| Texarkana | 4 | 575 | 28,527 | 155,122 | 224,499 | 425 | 614 | 5.4 | 14,400 | 46 | 2,298 | 102,234 | 355,811 |
| Tyler | 5 | 958 | 47,852 | 256,449 | 370,461 | 703 | 1,015 | 5.4 | 29,138 | 49 | 3,418 | 128,485 | 626,707 |
| Victoria | 2 | 607 | 21,626 | 97,721 | 148,587 | 268 | 407 | 4.5 | 18,785 | 48 | 2,088 | 55,562 | 166,307 |
| Waco | 2 | 825 | 26,982 | 181,440 | 287,026 | 497 | 786 | 6.7 | 26,157 | 51 | 3,721 | 92,928 | 302,759 |
| Wichita Falls | 4 | 454 | 18,946 | 100,080 | 154,592 | 274 | 423 | 5.3 | 21,152 | 12 | 2,289 | 70,272 | 166,993 |

# TABLE 8

# U.S. CENSUS DIVISION 7, WEST SOUTH CENTRAL

*U.S. Community Hospitals*
*(Nonfederal, short-term general and other special hospitals)*

## 2003 Utilization, Personnel and Finances

| FULL-TIME EQUIVALENT PERSONNEL | | | | | FULL-TIME EQUIV. TRAINEES | | | EXPENSES | | | | | | |
|---|---|---|---|---|---|---|---|---|---|---|---|---|---|---|
| | | | | | | | | LABOR | | | | TOTAL | | |
| Physicians and Dentists | Registered Nurses | Licensed Practical Nurses | Other Salaried Personnel | Total Personnel | Medical and Dental Residents | Other Trainees | Total Trainees | Payroll (in thousands) | Employee Benefits (in thousands) | Total (in thousands) | Percent of Total | Amount (in thousands) | Adjusted per Admission | Adjusted per Inpatient Day |
| 71,335 | 1,021,346 | 126,328 | 2,889,619 | 4,108,628 | 77,813 | 7,954 | 85,767 | $187,822,974 | $45,438,505 | $233,261,475 | 51.8 | $450,124,257 | $7,796.41 | $1,379.48 |
| 8,445 | 147,570 | 37,579 | 485,049 | 678,643 | 1,775 | 600 | 2,375 | 25,551,777 | 6,425,000 | 31,976,774 | 53.8 | 59,444,378 | 5,305.04 | 806.30 |
| 62,890 | 873,776 | 88,749 | 2,404,570 | 3,429,985 | 76,038 | 7,354 | 83,392 | 162,271,198 | 39,013,505 | 201,284,701 | 51.5 | 390,679,879 | 8,396.37 | 1,546.78 |
| 2,962 | 108,870 | 24,011 | 309,889 | 445,732 | 3,999 | 1,312 | 5,311 | 18,519,744 | 4,171,693 | 22,691,443 | 49.1 | 46,189,639 | 7,047.92 | 1,357.28 |
| 497 | 14,357 | 7,371 | 49,239 | 71,464 | 16 | 3 | 19 | 2,355,572 | 549,909 | 2,905,490 | 52.8 | 5,506,747 | 4,237.15 | 895.13 |
| 2,465 | 94,513 | 16,640 | 260,650 | 374,268 | 3,983 | 1,309 | 5,292 | 16,164,172 | 3,621,784 | 19,785,953 | 48.6 | 40,682,892 | 7,743.19 | 1,459.26 |
| 311 | 10,813 | 3,272 | 29,078 | 43,474 | 11 | 1 | 12 | 1,591,135 | 365,829 | 1,956,963 | 49.6 | 3,947,108 | 5,916.56 | 1,129.63 |
| 186 | 3,508 | 1,726 | 10,635 | 16,055 | 0 | 0 | 0 | 521,226 | 124,809 | 646,033 | 52.4 | 1,233,662 | 4,226.78 | 811.55 |
| 125 | 7,305 | 1,546 | 18,443 | 27,419 | 11 | 1 | 12 | 1,069,909 | 241,020 | 1,310,930 | 48.3 | 2,713,446 | 7,230.82 | 1,374.57 |
| 48 | 1,124 | 264 | 2,945 | 4,381 | 0 | 0 | 0 | 155,003 | 32,836 | 187,839 | 48.0 | 391,528 | 5,805.92 | 1,367.84 |
| 1 | 979 | 275 | 2,724 | 3,979 | 0 | 0 | 0 | 139,844 | 37,288 | 177,132 | 49.5 | 357,636 | 7,047.15 | 1,304.71 |
| 2 | 587 | 244 | 1,410 | 2,243 | 0 | 0 | 0 | 69,527 | 16,979 | 86,506 | 41.2 | 209,844 | 5,527.02 | 1,072.80 |
| 70 | 4,178 | 621 | 10,203 | 15,072 | 11 | 1 | 12 | 639,523 | 141,443 | 780,966 | 49.1 | 1,589,583 | 8,257.53 | 1,477.38 |
| 3 | 100 | 44 | 296 | 443 | 0 | 0 | 0 | 18,312 | 2,410 | 20,722 | 49.8 | 41,645 | 6,864.11 | 1,322.89 |
| 1 | 337 | 98 | 865 | 1,301 | 0 | 0 | 0 | 47,700 | 10,066 | 57,765 | 46.9 | 123,210 | 5,998.24 | 1,113.52 |
| 929 | 18,047 | 3,719 | 54,771 | 77,466 | 608 | 123 | 731 | 2,911,861 | 652,811 | 3,564,675 | 49.7 | 7,170,688 | 6,509.20 | 1,176.65 |
| 111 | 2,401 | 816 | 8,001 | 11,329 | 8 | 3 | 11 | 359,610 | 77,138 | 436,749 | 54.1 | 807,321 | 4,320.14 | 851.24 |
| 818 | 15,646 | 2,903 | 46,770 | 66,137 | 600 | 120 | 720 | 2,552,250 | 575,673 | 3,127,926 | 49.2 | 6,363,367 | 6,956.40 | 1,236.63 |
| 52 | 816 | 150 | 2,335 | 3,353 | 23 | 9 | 32 | 132,704 | 32,241 | 164,944 | 47.5 | 347,393 | 6,397.77 | 1,232.22 |
| 99 | 2,022 | 379 | 6,399 | 8,899 | 29 | 9 | 38 | 361,998 | 72,343 | 434,342 | 50.7 | 857,016 | 6,545.05 | 1,156.46 |
| 21 | 659 | 115 | 2,250 | 3,045 | 0 | 0 | 0 | 120,629 | 29,662 | 150,291 | 50.2 | 299,643 | 5,903.36 | 1,315.35 |
| 56 | 1,596 | 443 | 4,630 | 6,725 | 20 | 16 | 36 | 241,156 | 54,399 | 295,555 | 47.3 | 624,780 | 6,504.40 | 1,209.78 |
| 25 | 844 | 173 | 2,462 | 3,504 | 10 | 1 | 11 | 117,371 | 27,868 | 145,240 | 50.8 | 286,134 | 4,512.58 | 946.72 |
| 93 | 1,059 | 194 | 2,976 | 4,322 | 65 | 2 | 67 | 172,933 | 41,171 | 214,104 | 49.8 | 430,137 | 6,820.64 | 1,189.76 |
| 231 | 6,460 | 999 | 19,009 | 26,699 | 279 | 54 | 333 | 1,082,728 | 242,758 | 1,325,488 | 48.2 | 2,751,529 | 8,431.94 | 1,390.14 |
| 241 | 2,190 | 450 | 6,709 | 9,590 | 174 | 29 | 203 | 322,732 | 75,232 | 397,962 | 51.9 | 766,736 | 5,902.38 | 1,042.58 |
| 477 | 10,423 | 2,778 | 34,622 | 48,300 | 197 | 59 | 256 | 1,780,166 | 390,365 | 2,170,532 | 49.0 | 4,427,836 | 6,084.85 | 1,177.08 |
| 157 | 2,891 | 1,399 | 10,401 | 14,848 | 8 | 0 | 8 | 483,031 | 115,696 | 598,728 | 53.4 | 1,121,580 | 4,286.19 | 893.27 |
| 320 | 7,532 | 1,379 | 24,221 | 33,452 | 189 | 59 | 248 | 1,297,135 | 274,669 | 1,571,804 | 47.5 | 3,306,256 | 7,094.83 | 1,319.27 |
| 14 | 254 | 70 | 925 | 1,263 | 0 | 0 | 0 | 48,086 | 6,985 | 55,070 | 45.0 | 122,346 | 7,252.74 | 1,046.64 |
| 0 | 10 | 8 | 168 | 186 | 0 | 0 | 0 | 3,676 | 505 | 4,182 | 53.8 | 7,779 | 2,094.05 | 614.15 |
| 64 | 248 | 231 | 1,582 | 2,125 | 0 | 0 | 0 | 76,198 | 18,234 | 94,432 | 44.8 | 210,631 | 8,093.72 | 1,336.46 |
| 210 | 4,111 | 638 | 12,750 | 17,709 | 66 | 0 | 66 | 698,325 | 155,077 | 853,403 | 47.8 | 1,784,867 | 7,446.63 | 1,394.09 |
| 32 | 2,909 | 432 | 8,796 | 12,169 | 123 | 59 | 182 | 470,849 | 93,868 | 564,717 | 47.8 | 1,180,632 | 6,569.54 | 1,257.80 |
| 1,245 | 69,587 | 14,242 | 191,418 | 276,492 | 3,183 | 1,129 | 4,312 | 12,236,582 | 2,762,689 | 14,999,273 | 48.9 | 30,644,007 | 7,552.95 | 1,481.74 |
| 43 | 5,557 | 3,430 | 20,202 | 29,232 | 0 | 0 | 0 | 991,705 | 232,267 | 1,223,980 | 52.2 | 2,344,184 | 4,191.88 | 965.57 |
| 1,202 | 64,030 | 10,812 | 171,216 | 247,260 | 3,183 | 1,129 | 4,312 | 11,244,877 | 2,530,422 | 13,775,293 | 48.7 | 28,299,823 | 8,090.28 | 1,550.40 |
| 3 | 729 | 224 | 1,784 | 2,740 | 0 | 26 | 26 | 101,156 | 19,869 | 121,025 | 50.5 | 239,779 | 6,602.57 | 1,225.34 |
| 12 | 1,274 | 223 | 2,621 | 4,130 | 0 | 0 | 0 | 164,080 | 39,378 | 203,458 | 45.9 | 443,282 | 7,357.26 | 1,526.23 |
| 62 | 3,113 | 447 | 7,702 | 11,324 | 98 | 0 | 98 | 545,136 | 94,654 | 639,789 | 49.1 | 1,302,942 | 7,216.47 | 1,329.24 |
| 1 | 1,551 | 358 | 3,565 | 5,475 | 0 | 0 | 0 | 223,200 | 50,468 | 273,668 | 49.2 | 556,790 | 6,213.76 | 1,153.90 |
| 0 | 185 | 53 | 605 | 843 | 0 | 0 | 0 | 35,711 | 8,180 | 43,891 | 49.9 | 87,932 | 3,895.09 | 999.02 |
| 21 | 817 | 332 | 2,388 | 3,558 | 27 | 4 | 31 | 180,358 | 49,521 | 229,879 | 49.7 | 462,426 | 6,751.34 | 1,489.87 |
| 0 | 473 | 164 | 1,503 | 2,140 | 0 | 0 | 0 | 74,888 | 20,015 | 94,904 | 49.3 | 192,500 | 6,142.31 | 1,354.17 |
| 6 | 1,801 | 389 | 4,743 | 6,939 | 104 | 9 | 113 | 275,471 | 60,727 | 336,198 | 46.2 | 727,252 | 6,875.59 | 1,230.57 |
| 221 | 12,630 | 1,149 | 28,449 | 42,449 | 1,306 | 185 | 1,491 | 2,114,028 | 445,684 | 2,559,711 | 48.6 | 5,268,684 | 8,710.41 | 1,753.95 |
| 1 | 1,806 | 183 | 5,236 | 7,226 | 0 | 0 | 0 | 308,190 | 72,550 | 380,740 | 44.8 | 849,078 | 7,355.66 | 1,496.01 |
| 41 | 5,679 | 968 | 14,053 | 20,741 | 248 | 0 | 248 | 972,107 | 210,618 | 1,182,725 | 48.6 | 2,433,176 | 7,984.17 | 1,601.27 |
| 0 | 1,458 | 170 | 3,545 | 5,173 | 556 | 0 | 556 | 265,600 | 63,623 | 329,223 | 53.9 | 610,675 | 8,360.95 | 1,530.68 |
| 625 | 15,589 | 1,966 | 45,021 | 63,201 | 473 | 647 | 1,120 | 3,108,374 | 748,954 | 3,857,325 | 50.1 | 7,706,515 | 10,069.87 | 1,795.79 |
| 0 | 1,153 | 382 | 5,145 | 6,680 | 305 | 249 | 554 | 359,433 | 85,141 | 444,574 | 58.5 | 760,309 | 9,339.14 | 1,641.58 |
| 0 | 472 | 86 | 1,629 | 2,187 | 0 | 0 | 0 | 81,960 | 16,661 | 98,620 | 47.0 | 209,678 | 5,660.71 | 1,097.46 |
| 0 | 894 | 117 | 2,114 | 3,125 | 0 | 3 | 3 | 120,699 | 31,189 | 151,889 | 50.2 | 302,285 | 6,107.87 | 1,267.15 |
| 8 | 1,616 | 343 | 4,205 | 6,172 | 0 | 0 | 0 | 251,280 | 58,973 | 310,254 | 47.7 | 650,416 | 7,642.33 | 1,452.85 |
| 0 | 1,559 | 328 | 3,269 | 5,156 | 0 | 0 | 0 | 226,292 | 33,600 | 259,892 | 44.9 | 579,282 | 5,760.16 | 1,196.60 |
| 1 | 889 | 215 | 2,514 | 3,619 | 0 | 2 | 2 | 141,030 | 52,280 | 193,310 | 48.2 | 400,741 | 7,871.57 | 1,521.65 |
| 0 | 407 | 139 | 1,387 | 1,933 | 0 | 0 | 0 | 69,764 | 18,314 | 88,078 | 48.7 | 180,854 | 5,636.88 | 1,207.46 |
| 75 | 5,555 | 1,169 | 15,969 | 22,768 | 42 | 4 | 46 | 936,187 | 183,289 | 1,119,475 | 44.3 | 2,527,602 | 7,340.13 | 1,442.26 |
| 4 | 596 | 172 | 2,056 | 2,828 | 1 | 0 | 1 | 107,084 | 22,307 | 129,391 | 49.1 | 263,427 | 6,644.30 | 1,219.10 |
| 0 | 795 | 216 | 1,535 | 2,546 | 0 | 0 | 0 | 100,506 | 22,693 | 123,199 | 45.7 | 269,398 | 6,296.25 | 1,199.99 |
| 107 | 1,320 | 392 | 5,595 | 7,414 | 23 | 0 | 23 | 234,182 | 67,707 | 301,888 | 45.1 | 669,650 | 9,605.12 | 1,807.61 |
| 0 | 532 | 146 | 1,216 | 1,894 | 0 | 0 | 0 | 68,931 | 16,465 | 85,396 | 54.5 | 156,665 | 4,764.91 | 1,054.37 |
| 14 | 678 | 215 | 2,020 | 2,927 | 0 | 0 | 0 | 105,070 | 20,579 | 125,649 | 47.9 | 262,098 | 6,071.72 | 913.15 |
| 0 | 459 | 266 | 1,347 | 2,072 | 0 | 0 | 0 | 74,158 | 16,983 | 91,142 | 48.9 | 186,389 | 6,103.29 | 1,205.68 |

MSAs

# TABLE 8

## U.S. CENSUS DIVISION 8, MOUNTAIN

*U.S. Community Hospitals*
*(Nonfederal, short-term general and other special hospitals)*

## 2003 Utilization, Personnel and Finances

| | | | | | | | | | | NEWBORNS | | OUTPATIENT VISITS | |
|---|---|---|---|---|---|---|---|---|---|---|---|---|---|
| CLASSIFICATION | Hospitals | Beds | Admissions | Inpatient Days | Adjusted Patient Days | Average Daily Census | Adjusted Average Daily Census | Average Stay (days) | Surgical Operations | Bassinets | Births | Emergency | Total |
| UNITED STATES | 4,895 | 813,307 | 34,782,742 | 196,649,769 | 326,299,942 | 538,797 | 894,019 | 5.7 | 27,106,538 | 59,662 | 3,915,842 | 111,069,871 | 563,186,046 |
| Nonmetropolitan | 2,166 | 168,374 | 5,368,552 | 35,076,707 | 73,724,487 | 96,136 | 202,034 | 6.5 | 4,592,380 | 13,462 | 530,805 | 23,720,395 | 117,598,717 |
| Metropolitan | 2,729 | 644,933 | 29,414,190 | 161,573,062 | 252,575,455 | 442,661 | 691,985 | 5.5 | 22,514,158 | 46,200 | 3,385,037 | 87,349,476 | 445,587,329 |
| CENSUS DIVISION 8, MOUNTAIN | 348 | 42,159 | 1,936,327 | 9,825,461 | 16,365,518 | 26,918 | 44,832 | 5.1 | 1,394,850 | 3,734 | 298,539 | 6,191,190 | 31,401,603 |
| Nonmetropolitan | 205 | 11,858 | 352,615 | 2,344,119 | 4,960,358 | 6,424 | 13,590 | 6.6 | 292,313 | 1,106 | 52,997 | 1,626,954 | 8,948,696 |
| Metropolitan | 143 | 30,301 | 1,583,712 | 7,481,342 | 11,405,160 | 20,494 | 31,242 | 4.7 | 1,102,537 | 2,628 | 245,542 | 4,564,236 | 22,452,907 |
| Arizona | 61 | 10,801 | 603,310 | 2,669,152 | 3,984,431 | 7,314 | 10,913 | 4.4 | 382,257 | 951 | 87,912 | 1,781,590 | 6,706,717 |
| Nonmetropolitan | 15 | 858 | 40,082 | 173,504 | 388,448 | 477 | 1,063 | 4.3 | 32,553 | 81 | 5,957 | 190,850 | 1,230,331 |
| Metropolitan | 46 | 9,943 | 563,228 | 2,495,648 | 3,595,983 | 6,837 | 9,850 | 4.4 | 349,704 | 870 | 81,955 | 1,590,740 | 5,476,386 |
| Flagstaff | 2 | 267 | 12,444 | 58,751 | 94,006 | 161 | 257 | 4.7 | 8,214 | 34 | 1,790 | 38,029 | 94,292 |
| Las Vegas | 3 | 361 | 19,359 | 97,485 | 150,615 | 267 | 412 | 5.0 | 13,377 | 25 | 2,016 | 75,384 | 225,972 |
| Phoenix-Mesa | 31 | 7,004 | 396,983 | 1,768,920 | 2,495,308 | 4,847 | 6,835 | 4.5 | 229,845 | 638 | 61,536 | 1,084,757 | 3,583,597 |
| Tucson | 9 | 2,034 | 117,884 | 506,087 | 754,696 | 1,386 | 2,068 | 4.3 | 89,155 | 154 | 13,178 | 338,630 | 1,442,352 |
| Yuma | 1 | 277 | 16,558 | 64,405 | 101,358 | 176 | 278 | 3.9 | 9,113 | 19 | 3,435 | 53,940 | 130,173 |
| Colorado | 68 | 9,479 | 443,773 | 2,252,174 | 3,796,587 | 6,166 | 10,400 | 5.1 | 306,193 | 851 | 65,907 | 1,384,544 | 6,987,293 |
| Nonmetropolitan | 36 | 1,635 | 46,465 | 315,911 | 761,362 | 863 | 2,086 | 6.8 | 44,119 | 161 | 7,443 | 229,309 | 1,399,550 |
| Metropolitan | 32 | 7,844 | 397,308 | 1,936,263 | 3,035,225 | 5,303 | 8,314 | 4.9 | 262,074 | 690 | 58,464 | 1,155,235 | 5,587,743 |
| Boulder-Longmont | 3 | 458 | 29,969 | 117,718 | 214,388 | 322 | 588 | 3.9 | 19,986 | 62 | 5,557 | 102,731 | 673,239 |
| Colorado Springs | 2 | 868 | 49,896 | 217,611 | 353,630 | 596 | 969 | 4.4 | 31,303 | 129 | 7,654 | 183,439 | 594,184 |
| Denver | 18 | 4,538 | 237,722 | 1,175,531 | 1,797,594 | 3,220 | 4,924 | 4.9 | 156,707 | 363 | 34,914 | 585,593 | 2,613,266 |
| Fort Collins-Loveland | 3 | 445 | 23,950 | 101,125 | 168,839 | 277 | 462 | 4.2 | 15,733 | 55 | 3,753 | 64,173 | 472,777 |
| Grand Junction | 3 | 716 | 17,799 | 150,665 | 239,189 | 413 | 654 | 8.5 | 13,910 | 18 | 1,868 | 92,052 | 624,324 |
| Greeley | 1 | 276 | 15,721 | 65,752 | 99,173 | 180 | 272 | 4.2 | 8,119 | 18 | 2,396 | 44,471 | 269,757 |
| Pueblo | 2 | 543 | 22,251 | 107,861 | 162,412 | 295 | 445 | 4.8 | 16,316 | 45 | 2,322 | 82,776 | 340,196 |
| Idaho | 39 | 3,412 | 135,920 | 698,748 | 1,325,067 | 1,917 | 3,629 | 5.1 | 103,656 | 276 | 19,796 | 468,818 | 2,769,604 |
| Nonmetropolitan | 33 | 2,036 | 67,827 | 401,539 | 816,216 | 1,102 | 2,235 | 5.9 | 53,522 | 168 | 9,687 | 269,647 | 1,358,450 |
| Metropolitan | 6 | 1,376 | 68,093 | 297,209 | 508,851 | 815 | 1,394 | 4.4 | 50,134 | 108 | 10,109 | 199,171 | 1,411,154 |
| Boise City | 5 | 1,048 | 58,764 | 234,042 | 406,873 | 642 | 1,115 | 4.0 | 45,151 | 92 | 8,310 | 165,573 | 1,201,625 |
| Pocatello | 1 | 328 | 9,329 | 63,167 | 101,978 | 173 | 279 | 6.8 | 4,983 | 16 | 1,799 | 33,598 | 209,529 |
| Montana | 53 | 4,326 | 107,024 | 1,049,607 | 1,964,422 | 2,877 | 5,384 | 9.8 | 73,990 | 253 | 10,301 | 301,772 | 2,737,734 |
| Nonmetropolitan | 48 | 2,872 | 50,642 | 694,646 | 1,364,405 | 1,904 | 3,741 | 13.7 | 33,148 | 172 | 5,071 | 194,677 | 1,196,855 |
| Metropolitan | 5 | 1,454 | 56,382 | 354,961 | 600,017 | 973 | 1,643 | 6.3 | 40,842 | 81 | 5,230 | 107,095 | 1,540,879 |
| Billings | 2 | 618 | 26,511 | 165,707 | 333,455 | 454 | 913 | 6.3 | 20,271 | 36 | 2,263 | 44,299 | 1,128,029 |
| Great Falls | 1 | 490 | 14,155 | 115,926 | 154,915 | 318 | 424 | 8.2 | 8,460 | 24 | 1,421 | 30,180 | 122,790 |
| Missoula | 2 | 346 | 15,716 | 73,328 | 111,647 | 201 | 306 | 4.7 | 12,111 | 21 | 1,546 | 32,616 | 290,060 |
| Nevada | 25 | 4,282 | 212,821 | 1,111,624 | 1,606,470 | 3,046 | 4,401 | 5.2 | 138,400 | 245 | 30,801 | 626,686 | 2,283,973 |
| Nonmetropolitan | 9 | 470 | 14,669 | 88,620 | 186,235 | 244 | 510 | 6.0 | 11,710 | 40 | 2,073 | 89,463 | 378,913 |
| Metropolitan | 16 | 3,812 | 198,152 | 1,023,004 | 1,420,235 | 2,802 | 3,891 | 5.2 | 126,690 | 205 | 28,728 | 537,223 | 1,905,060 |
| Las Vegas | 11 | 2,795 | 158,704 | 804,708 | 1,101,370 | 2,205 | 3,018 | 5.1 | 94,882 | 144 | 22,108 | 414,291 | 1,336,110 |
| Reno | 5 | 1,017 | 39,448 | 218,296 | 318,865 | 597 | 873 | 5.5 | 31,808 | 61 | 6,620 | 122,932 | 568,950 |
| New Mexico | 37 | 3,680 | 165,709 | 780,895 | 1,392,314 | 2,137 | 3,813 | 4.7 | 132,597 | 336 | 27,950 | 675,058 | 4,502,569 |
| Nonmetropolitan | 22 | 1,624 | 59,534 | 252,467 | 517,311 | 689 | 1,416 | 4.2 | 50,936 | 187 | 9,239 | 320,123 | 1,550,753 |
| Metropolitan | 15 | 2,056 | 106,175 | 528,428 | 875,003 | 1,448 | 2,397 | 5.0 | 81,661 | 149 | 18,711 | 354,935 | 2,951,816 |
| Albuquerque | 11 | 1,449 | 78,137 | 410,157 | 656,992 | 1,124 | 1,800 | 5.2 | 55,171 | 83 | 13,182 | 234,605 | 2,491,483 |
| Las Cruces | 2 | 314 | 15,766 | 68,914 | 133,714 | 189 | 366 | 4.4 | 15,189 | 33 | 3,549 | 47,566 | 240,414 |
| Santa Fe | 2 | 293 | 12,272 | 49,357 | 84,297 | 135 | 231 | 4.0 | 11,301 | 33 | 1,980 | 72,764 | 219,919 |
| Utah | 42 | 4,406 | 215,158 | 921,001 | 1,622,005 | 2,523 | 4,443 | 4.3 | 215,667 | 643 | 49,824 | 740,160 | 4,545,669 |
| Nonmetropolitan | 21 | 993 | 38,692 | 155,037 | 369,083 | 426 | 1,010 | 4.0 | 37,012 | 158 | 9,529 | 181,509 | 1,163,534 |
| Metropolitan | 21 | 3,413 | 176,466 | 765,964 | 1,252,922 | 2,097 | 3,433 | 4.3 | 178,655 | 485 | 40,295 | 558,651 | 3,382,135 |
| Flagstaff | 1 | 38 | 344 | 1,064 | 2,808 | 3 | 8 | 3.1 | 1,202 | 5 | 95 | 2,527 | 13,226 |
| Provo-Orem | 5 | 656 | 33,851 | 132,012 | 204,477 | 362 | 560 | 3.9 | 30,260 | 111 | 9,952 | 113,303 | 618,240 |
| Salt Lake City-Ogden | 15 | 2,719 | 142,271 | 632,888 | 1,045,637 | 1,732 | 2,865 | 4.4 | 147,193 | 369 | 30,248 | 442,821 | 2,750,669 |
| Wyoming | 23 | 1,773 | 52,612 | 342,260 | 674,222 | 938 | 1,849 | 6.5 | 42,090 | 179 | 6,048 | 212,562 | 868,044 |
| Nonmetropolitan | 21 | 1,370 | 34,704 | 262,395 | 557,298 | 719 | 1,529 | 7.6 | 29,313 | 139 | 3,998 | 151,376 | 670,310 |
| Metropolitan | 2 | 403 | 17,908 | 79,865 | 116,924 | 219 | 320 | 4.5 | 12,777 | 40 | 2,050 | 61,186 | 197,734 |
| Casper | 1 | 205 | 9,199 | 37,652 | 54,759 | 103 | 150 | 4.1 | 5,245 | 24 | 940 | 32,533 | 64,897 |
| Cheyenne | 1 | 198 | 8,709 | 42,213 | 62,165 | 116 | 170 | 4.8 | 7,532 | 16 | 1,110 | 28,653 | 132,837 |

# TABLE 8

# U.S. CENSUS DIVISION 8, MOUNTAIN

*U.S. Community Hospitals*
*(Nonfederal, short-term general and other special hospitals)*

## 2003 Utilization, Personnel and Finances

| FULL-TIME EQUIVALENT PERSONNEL | | | | | FULL-TIME EQUIV. TRAINEES | | | EXPENSES | | | | | | |
|---|---|---|---|---|---|---|---|---|---|---|---|---|---|---|
| | | | | | | | | LABOR | | | | TOTAL | | |
| Physicians and Dentists | Registered Nurses | Licensed Practical Nurses | Other Salaried Personnel | Total Personnel | Medical and Dental Residents | Other Trainees | Total Trainees | Payroll (in thousands) | Employee Benefits (in thousands) | Total (in thousands) | Percent of Total | Amount (in thousands) | Adjusted per Admission | Adjusted per Inpatient Day |
| 71,335 | 1,021,346 | 126,328 | 2,889,619 | 4,108,628 | 77,813 | 7,954 | 85,767 | $187,822,974 | $45,438,505 | $233,261,475 | 51.8 | $450,124,257 | $7,796.41 | $1,379.48 |
| 8,445 | 147,570 | 37,579 | 485,049 | 678,643 | 1,775 | 600 | 2,375 | 25,551,777 | 6,425,000 | 31,976,774 | 53.8 | 59,444,378 | 5,305.04 | 806.30 |
| 62,890 | 873,776 | 88,749 | 2,404,570 | 3,429,985 | 76,038 | 7,354 | 83,392 | 162,271,198 | 39,013,505 | 201,284,701 | 51.5 | 390,679,879 | 8,396.37 | 1,546.78 |
| | | | | | | | | | | | | | | |
| 3,107 | 55,897 | 5,755 | 153,588 | 218,347 | 1,534 | 164 | 1,698 | 9,634,851 | 2,195,119 | 11,829,977 | 50.8 | 23,296,281 | 7,294.06 | 1,423.50 |
| 574 | 10,621 | 1,866 | 34,677 | 47,738 | 21 | 29 | 50 | 1,774,257 | 440,427 | 2,214,684 | 52.8 | 4,195,249 | 5,463.65 | 845.76 |
| 2,533 | 45,276 | 3,889 | 118,911 | 170,609 | 1,513 | 135 | 1,648 | 7,860,594 | 1,754,693 | 9,615,293 | 50.3 | 19,101,032 | 7,873.39 | 1,674.77 |
| | | | | | | | | | | | | | | |
| 692 | 15,155 | 1,188 | 36,759 | 53,794 | 835 | 45 | 880 | 2,477,654 | 556,781 | 3,034,435 | 48.5 | 6,256,631 | 6,974.15 | 1,570.27 |
| 31 | 1,142 | 130 | 3,378 | 4,681 | 0 | 5 | 5 | 182,494 | 45,420 | 227,914 | 51.8 | 439,888 | 5,251.45 | 1,132.42 |
| 661 | 14,013 | 1,058 | 33,381 | 49,113 | 835 | 40 | 875 | 2,295,160 | 511,361 | 2,806,521 | 48.2 | 5,816,743 | 7,151.56 | 1,617.57 |
| 2 | 580 | 12 | 1,527 | 2,121 | 0 | 23 | 23 | 69,731 | 19,893 | 89,625 | 46.4 | 193,295 | 9,722.61 | 2,056.20 |
| 16 | 462 | 82 | 1,335 | 1,895 | 1 | 0 | 1 | 70,904 | 16,897 | 87,801 | 48.9 | 179,441 | 5,960.32 | 1,191.39 |
| 552 | 9,602 | 723 | 21,495 | 32,372 | 759 | 3 | 762 | 1,616,037 | 361,294 | 1,977,331 | 48.3 | 4,094,397 | 7,314.91 | 1,640.84 |
| 91 | 2,943 | 211 | 7,844 | 11,089 | 75 | 14 | 89 | 472,105 | 97,086 | 569,191 | 47.5 | 1,197,397 | 6,743.05 | 1,586.59 |
| 0 | 426 | 30 | 1,180 | 1,636 | 0 | 0 | 0 | 66,383 | 16,190 | 82,573 | 54.2 | 152,213 | 5,841.33 | 1,501.74 |
| | | | | | | | | | | | | | | |
| 672 | 13,815 | 1,011 | 36,957 | 52,455 | 484 | 61 | 545 | 2,519,346 | 539,837 | 3,059,184 | 52.0 | 5,886,658 | 7,936.26 | 1,550.51 |
| 85 | 1,565 | 273 | 5,397 | 7,320 | 0 | 2 | 2 | 288,439 | 73,513 | 361,952 | 53.0 | 682,570 | 6,023.50 | 896.51 |
| 587 | 12,250 | 738 | 31,560 | 45,135 | 484 | 59 | 543 | 2,230,907 | 466,324 | 2,697,232 | 51.8 | 5,204,087 | 8,281.17 | 1,714.56 |
| 34 | 907 | 38 | 2,436 | 3,415 | 0 | 0 | 0 | 161,913 | 33,066 | 194,979 | 55.9 | 348,996 | 6,371.56 | 1,627.87 |
| 22 | 1,345 | 31 | 3,827 | 5,225 | 0 | 8 | 8 | 232,921 | 57,206 | 290,127 | 52.3 | 554,411 | 6,857.36 | 1,567.77 |
| 427 | 7,194 | 444 | 17,187 | 25,252 | 377 | 45 | 422 | 1,322,087 | 254,872 | 1,576,960 | 50.9 | 3,100,938 | 8,438.30 | 1,725.05 |
| 16 | 777 | 45 | 1,961 | 2,799 | 18 | 0 | 18 | 139,026 | 35,673 | 174,699 | 52.9 | 330,324 | 8,635.92 | 1,956.44 |
| 52 | 971 | 65 | 2,762 | 3,850 | 50 | 6 | 56 | 190,823 | 45,981 | 236,804 | 53.9 | 439,149 | 14,707.91 | 1,835.99 |
| 15 | 361 | 15 | 1,425 | 1,816 | 27 | 0 | 27 | 85,066 | 17,441 | 102,507 | 49.0 | 209,134 | 8,819.74 | 2,108.78 |
| 21 | 695 | 100 | 1,962 | 2,778 | 12 | 0 | 12 | 99,070 | 22,087 | 121,156 | 54.8 | 221,136 | 6,601.65 | 1,361.57 |
| | | | | | | | | | | | | | | |
| 160 | 3,992 | 636 | 11,687 | 16,475 | 1 | 0 | 1 | 685,387 | 164,721 | 850,110 | 52.0 | 1,636,080 | 6,340.44 | 1,234.72 |
| 41 | 1,880 | 428 | 5,812 | 8,161 | 0 | 0 | 0 | 313,162 | 78,064 | 391,229 | 51.1 | 764,875 | 5,520.85 | 937.10 |
| 119 | 2,112 | 208 | 5,875 | 8,314 | 1 | 0 | 1 | 372,225 | 86,657 | 458,881 | 52.7 | 871,206 | 7,290.67 | 1,712.10 |
| 119 | 1,872 | 113 | 5,102 | 7,206 | 1 | 0 | 1 | 327,957 | 75,080 | 403,036 | 52.9 | 761,743 | 7,293.94 | 1,872.19 |
| 0 | 240 | 95 | 773 | 1,108 | 0 | 0 | 0 | 44,268 | 11,577 | 55,845 | 51.0 | 109,463 | 7,267.95 | 1,073.39 |
| | | | | | | | | | | | | | | |
| 447 | 3,097 | 661 | 11,082 | 15,287 | 0 | 3 | 3 | 647,303 | 144,865 | 792,168 | 55.0 | 1,440,704 | 7,247.80 | 733.40 |
| 115 | 1,506 | 334 | 5,701 | 7,656 | 0 | 3 | 3 | 272,865 | 65,345 | 338,210 | 55.4 | 610,749 | 5,802.34 | 447.63 |
| 332 | 1,591 | 327 | 5,381 | 7,631 | 0 | 0 | 0 | 374,438 | 79,520 | 453,958 | 54.7 | 829,955 | 8,874.72 | 1,383.22 |
| 255 | 681 | 206 | 2,813 | 3,955 | 0 | 0 | 0 | 202,447 | 43,122 | 245,570 | 56.2 | 436,812 | 8,628.90 | 1,309.96 |
| 7 | 374 | 49 | 1,117 | 1,547 | 0 | 0 | 0 | 66,732 | 15,670 | 82,402 | 53.0 | 155,353 | 8,212.77 | 1,002.83 |
| 70 | 536 | 72 | 1,451 | 2,129 | 0 | 0 | 0 | 105,259 | 20,727 | 125,986 | 53.0 | 237,790 | 9,915.76 | 2,129.84 |
| | | | | | | | | | | | | | | |
| 131 | 5,383 | 521 | 12,883 | 18,918 | 18 | 14 | 32 | 984,708 | 242,822 | 1,227,530 | 47.5 | 2,583,114 | 8,556.28 | 1,607.94 |
| 29 | 433 | 78 | 1,449 | 1,989 | 2 | 6 | 8 | 92,099 | 21,071 | 113,170 | 50.6 | 223,628 | 7,863.98 | 1,200.78 |
| 102 | 4,950 | 443 | 11,434 | 16,929 | 16 | 8 | 24 | 892,608 | 221,750 | 1,114,360 | 47.2 | 2,359,486 | 8,628.27 | 1,661.34 |
| 97 | 3,825 | 353 | 7,696 | 11,971 | 15 | 8 | 23 | 626,625 | 177,181 | 803,807 | 48.0 | 1,673,794 | 7,738.55 | 1,519.74 |
| 5 | 1,125 | 90 | 3,738 | 4,958 | 1 | 0 | 1 | 265,983 | 44,569 | 310,553 | 45.3 | 685,692 | 11,994.55 | 2,150.42 |
| | | | | | | | | | | | | | | |
| 680 | 5,694 | 820 | 19,999 | 27,193 | 27 | 29 | 56 | 963,263 | 205,056 | 1,168,320 | 53.7 | 2,175,581 | 7,223.57 | 1,562.56 |
| 168 | 1,896 | 290 | 6,086 | 8,440 | 15 | 9 | 24 | 282,316 | 68,911 | 351,228 | 53.4 | 657,737 | 5,226.94 | 1,271.45 |
| 512 | 3,798 | 530 | 13,913 | 18,753 | 12 | 20 | 32 | 680,946 | 136,145 | 817,092 | 53.8 | 1,517,844 | 8,656.48 | 1,734.67 |
| 477 | 3,076 | 459 | 11,493 | 15,505 | 5 | 19 | 24 | 552,408 | 98,290 | 650,698 | 52.6 | 1,237,697 | 9,994.49 | 1,883.89 |
| 18 | 381 | 37 | 1,019 | 1,455 | 6 | 1 | 7 | 63,023 | 15,090 | 78,113 | 41.9 | 186,584 | 6,116.52 | 1,395.40 |
| 17 | 341 | 34 | 1,401 | 1,793 | 1 | 0 | 1 | 65,516 | 22,764 | 88,281 | 94.4 | 93,562 | 4,455.54 | 1,109.91 |
| | | | | | | | | | | | | | | |
| 256 | 7,088 | 711 | 19,343 | 27,398 | 165 | 8 | 173 | 1,089,981 | 272,977 | 1,362,961 | 50.8 | 2,682,024 | 6,853.30 | 1,653.52 |
| 38 | 1,092 | 184 | 3,407 | 4,721 | 0 | 0 | 0 | 163,901 | 41,895 | 205,796 | 50.5 | 407,562 | 4,284.67 | 1,104.26 |
| 218 | 5,996 | 527 | 15,936 | 22,677 | 165 | 8 | 173 | 926,080 | 231,082 | 1,157,165 | 50.9 | 2,274,462 | 7,678.10 | 1,815.33 |
| 1 | 24 | 9 | 91 | 125 | 0 | 0 | 0 | 2,771 | 651 | 3,421 | 55.5 | 6,168 | 6,792.93 | 2,196.58 |
| 31 | 1,113 | 70 | 2,353 | 3,567 | 18 | 0 | 18 | 144,352 | 37,523 | 181,876 | 52.4 | 346,841 | 6,343.45 | 1,696.23 |
| 186 | 4,859 | 448 | 13,492 | 18,985 | 147 | 8 | 155 | 778,957 | 192,908 | 971,868 | 50.6 | 1,921,453 | 7,984.70 | 1,837.59 |
| | | | | | | | | | | | | | | |
| 69 | 1,673 | 207 | 4,878 | 6,827 | 4 | 4 | 8 | 267,210 | 68,060 | 335,269 | 52.8 | 635,489 | 6,123.90 | 942.55 |
| 67 | 1,107 | 149 | 3,447 | 4,770 | 4 | 4 | 8 | 178,980 | 46,206 | 225,185 | 55.2 | 408,240 | 5,262.93 | 732.53 |
| 2 | 566 | 58 | 1,431 | 2,057 | 0 | 0 | 0 | 88,229 | 21,854 | 110,084 | 48.4 | 227,249 | 8,672.62 | 1,943.56 |
| 2 | 290 | 5 | 764 | 1,061 | 0 | 0 | 0 | 42,822 | 12,074 | 54,896 | 45.5 | 120,771 | 9,027.61 | 2,205.51 |
| 0 | 276 | 53 | 667 | 996 | 0 | 0 | 0 | 45,408 | 9,780 | 55,188 | 51.8 | 106,477 | 8,302.32 | 1,712.82 |

MSAs

# U.S. CENSUS DIVISION 9, PACIFIC

*U.S. Community Hospitals*
*(Nonfederal, short-term general and other special hospitals)*

## 2003 Utilization, Personnel and Finances



| CLASSIFICATION | Hospitals | Beds | Admissions | Inpatient Days | Adjusted Patient Days | Average Daily Census | Adjusted Average Daily Census | Average Stay (days) | Surgical Operations | NEWBORNS | | OUTPATIENT VISITS | |
|---|---|---|---|---|---|---|---|---|---|---|---|---|---|
| | | | | | | | | | | Bassinets | Births | Emergency | Total |
| UNITED STATES | 4,895 | 813,307 | 34,782,742 | 196,649,769 | 326,299,942 | 538,797 | 894,019 | 5.7 | 27,106,538 | 59,662 | 3,915,842 | 111,069,871 | 563,186,046 |
| Nonmetropolitan | 2,166 | 168,374 | 5,368,552 | 35,076,707 | 73,724,487 | 96,136 | 202,034 | 6.5 | 4,592,380 | 13,462 | 530,805 | 23,720,395 | 117,598,717 |
| Metropolitan | 2,729 | 644,933 | 29,414,190 | 161,573,062 | 252,575,455 | 442,661 | 691,985 | 5.5 | 22,514,158 | 46,200 | 3,385,037 | 87,349,476 | 445,587,329 |
| CENSUS DIVISION 9, PACIFIC | 556 | 96,854 | 4,489,795 | 23,850,078 | 35,628,117 | 65,336 | 97,611 | 5.3 | 3,062,559 | 7,302 | 630,788 | 12,947,101 | 69,876,126 |
| Nonmetropolitan | 138 | 8,267 | 286,266 | 1,759,856 | 3,647,758 | 4,822 | 9,993 | 6.1 | 280,454 | 745 | 39,002 | 1,433,490 | 7,542,093 |
| Metropolitan | 418 | 88,587 | 4,203,529 | 22,090,222 | 31,980,359 | 60,514 | 87,618 | 5.3 | 2,782,105 | 6,557 | 591,786 | 11,513,611 | 62,334,033 |
| Alaska | 19 | 1,456 | 45,982 | 287,351 | 520,543 | 786 | 1,425 | 6.2 | 51,561 | 146 | 7,608 | 213,380 | 1,443,409 |
| Nonmetropolitan | 16 | 758 | 19,107 | 146,852 | 302,455 | 401 | 828 | 7.7 | 19,929 | 85 | 3,055 | 104,547 | 647,684 |
| Metropolitan | 3 | 698 | 26,875 | 140,499 | 218,088 | 385 | 597 | 5.2 | 31,632 | 61 | 4,553 | 108,833 | 795,725 |
| Anchorage | 3 | 698 | 26,875 | 140,499 | 218,088 | 385 | 597 | 5.2 | 31,632 | 61 | 4,553 | 108,833 | 795,725 |
| California | 370 | 74,330 | 3,473,879 | 18,814,783 | 26,602,372 | 51,546 | 72,886 | 5.4 | 2,172,734 | 5,153 | 492,547 | 9,260,312 | 48,036,139 |
| Nonmetropolitan | 40 | 2,251 | 82,996 | 506,933 | 1,031,458 | 1,391 | 2,827 | 6.1 | 87,719 | 195 | 12,310 | 503,425 | 2,710,696 |
| Metropolitan | 330 | 72,079 | 3,390,883 | 18,307,850 | 25,570,914 | 50,155 | 70,059 | 5.4 | 2,085,015 | 4,958 | 480,237 | 8,756,887 | 45,325,443 |
| Bakersfield | 10 | 1,498 | 61,751 | 375,710 | 498,066 | 1,030 | 1,365 | 6.1 | 37,046 | 72 | 11,573 | 164,597 | 562,215 |
| Chico-Paradise | 4 | 450 | 28,786 | 131,220 | 204,046 | 359 | 558 | 4.6 | 18,948 | 40 | 2,776 | 96,055 | 686,654 |
| Fresno | 14 | 2,625 | 125,240 | 717,111 | 1,101,021 | 1,965 | 3,015 | 5.7 | 85,354 | 205 | 22,377 | 323,875 | 2,554,813 |
| Los Angeles-Long Beach | 97 | 23,191 | 1,061,672 | 5,884,255 | 7,919,249 | 16,120 | 21,695 | 5.5 | 606,382 | 1,563 | 146,782 | 2,644,715 | 11,637,919 |
| Merced | 2 | 289 | 11,001 | 49,104 | 81,859 | 134 | 225 | 4.5 | 6,750 | 40 | 2,781 | 47,448 | 186,988 |
| Modesto | 4 | 1,198 | 48,048 | 328,886 | 473,056 | 901 | 1,296 | 6.8 | 34,567 | 74 | 9,043 | 193,534 | 368,031 |
| Oakland | 19 | 5,351 | 265,040 | 1,401,532 | 1,915,091 | 3,838 | 5,248 | 5.3 | 146,699 | 349 | 36,150 | 657,646 | 3,395,960 |
| Orange County | 29 | 5,212 | 271,952 | 1,266,409 | 1,758,191 | 3,469 | 4,816 | 4.7 | 180,108 | 428 | 41,071 | 641,112 | 3,111,654 |
| Redding | 3 | 492 | 20,795 | 130,600 | 196,397 | 358 | 538 | 6.3 | 15,606 | 11 | 2,089 | 61,849 | 207,605 |
| Riverside-San Bernardino | 32 | 6,150 | 342,537 | 1,581,620 | 2,267,592 | 4,332 | 6,215 | 4.6 | 191,599 | 477 | 44,051 | 1,021,942 | 3,155,587 |
| Sacramento | 13 | 3,421 | 178,729 | 900,287 | 1,244,301 | 2,466 | 3,408 | 5.0 | 127,370 | 268 | 22,705 | 359,355 | 2,236,826 |
| Salinas | 4 | 637 | 36,723 | 168,249 | 246,984 | 462 | 677 | 4.6 | 23,472 | 80 | 5,975 | 103,106 | 682,950 |
| San Diego | 19 | 5,827 | 272,967 | 1,508,617 | 2,110,966 | 4,133 | 5,785 | 5.5 | 168,696 | 360 | 38,650 | 513,539 | 2,636,548 |
| San Francisco | 20 | 5,583 | 166,382 | 1,371,855 | 1,861,744 | 3,761 | 5,101 | 8.2 | 115,020 | 159 | 13,393 | 458,348 | 4,987,545 |
| San Jose | 12 | 3,206 | 165,755 | 776,168 | 1,139,276 | 2,127 | 3,121 | 4.7 | 109,871 | 274 | 29,683 | 376,238 | 3,278,662 |
| San Luis Obispo-Atascadero-Paso Robles | 4 | 366 | 19,894 | 85,429 | 132,277 | 233 | 362 | 4.3 | 15,285 | 26 | 1,660 | 87,981 | 389,126 |
| Santa Barbara-Santa Maria-Lompoc | 6 | 900 | 35,139 | 219,389 | 344,628 | 600 | 944 | 6.2 | 26,859 | 86 | 5,964 | 115,126 | 508,570 |
| Santa Cruz-Watsonville | 3 | 368 | 20,991 | 90,974 | 130,451 | 249 | 358 | 4.3 | 13,912 | 37 | 2,097 | 81,417 | 274,809 |
| Santa Rosa | 8 | 824 | 38,902 | 186,580 | 290,882 | 511 | 798 | 4.8 | 31,382 | 83 | 5,945 | 119,167 | 1,223,787 |
| Stockton-Lodi | 7 | 1,080 | 57,519 | 288,610 | 401,615 | 791 | 1,100 | 5.0 | 34,279 | 80 | 9,379 | 208,917 | 1,276,015 |
| Vallejo-Fairfield-Napa | 6 | 946 | 45,609 | 226,313 | 342,094 | 620 | 936 | 5.0 | 25,181 | 63 | 5,888 | 103,333 | 595,206 |
| Ventura | 7 | 1,353 | 61,912 | 349,736 | 504,053 | 958 | 1,382 | 5.6 | 38,164 | 108 | 10,482 | 193,479 | 557,373 |
| Visalia-Tulare-Porterville | 3 | 736 | 32,768 | 188,624 | 274,455 | 517 | 752 | 5.8 | 14,928 | 47 | 6,636 | 135,487 | 631,057 |
| Yolo | 2 | 163 | 7,002 | 22,579 | 46,044 | 62 | 127 | 3.2 | 9,962 | 14 | 908 | 22,662 | 115,688 |
| Yuba City | 2 | 213 | 13,769 | 57,993 | 86,576 | 159 | 237 | 4.2 | 7,575 | 14 | 2,179 | 25,959 | 63,855 |
| Hawaii | 24 | 3,121 | 111,713 | 815,796 | 1,320,919 | 2,235 | 3,621 | 7.3 | 86,735 | 214 | 12,476 | 330,034 | 1,917,741 |
| Nonmetropolitan | 11 | 961 | 29,429 | 269,241 | 445,440 | 739 | 1,222 | 9.1 | 23,036 | 62 | 4,341 | 87,315 | 269,774 |
| Metropolitan | 13 | 2,160 | 82,284 | 546,555 | 875,479 | 1,496 | 2,399 | 6.6 | 63,699 | 152 | 8,135 | 242,719 | 1,647,967 |
| Honolulu | 13 | 2,160 | 82,284 | 546,555 | 875,479 | 1,496 | 2,399 | 6.6 | 63,699 | 152 | 8,135 | 242,719 | 1,647,967 |
| Oregon | 58 | 6,757 | 342,282 | 1,455,069 | 2,609,639 | 3,985 | 7,148 | 4.3 | 310,475 | 722 | 45,704 | 1,113,166 | 8,187,084 |
| Nonmetropolitan | 31 | 1,910 | 87,066 | 371,606 | 789,920 | 1,019 | 2,164 | 4.3 | 77,228 | 205 | 10,255 | 378,259 | 2,053,957 |
| Metropolitan | 27 | 4,847 | 255,216 | 1,083,463 | 1,819,719 | 2,966 | 4,984 | 4.2 | 233,247 | 517 | 35,440 | 704,907 | 6,133,127 |
| Corvalis | 1 | 134 | 7,988 | 27,783 | 47,908 | 76 | 131 | 3.5 | 9,103 | 24 | 1,004 | 17,024 | 212,699 |
| Eugene-Springfield | 4 | 604 | 33,248 | 133,674 | 195,985 | 366 | 536 | 4.0 | 27,380 | 68 | 3,511 | 101,079 | 307,814 |
| Medford-Ashland | 3 | 539 | 23,078 | 95,082 | 150,242 | 260 | 411 | 4.1 | 16,793 | 34 | 2,199 | 63,962 | 838,382 |
| Portland-Vancouver | 15 | 3,050 | 167,660 | 728,023 | 1,255,385 | 1,993 | 3,440 | 4.3 | 163,422 | 321 | 23,759 | 454,995 | 4,295,075 |
| Salem | 4 | 520 | 23,242 | 98,901 | 170,199 | 271 | 466 | 4.3 | 16,549 | 70 | 4,976 | 97,847 | 479,157 |
| Washington | 85 | 11,190 | 515,939 | 2,477,079 | 4,574,644 | 6,784 | 12,531 | 4.8 | 441,054 | 1,067 | 72,453 | 2,030,209 | 10,291,753 |
| Nonmetropolitan | 40 | 2,387 | 67,668 | 465,224 | 1,078,485 | 1,272 | 2,952 | 6.9 | 72,542 | 198 | 9,041 | 359,944 | 1,859,982 |
| Metropolitan | 45 | 8,803 | 448,271 | 2,011,855 | 3,496,159 | 5,512 | 9,579 | 4.5 | 368,512 | 869 | 63,412 | 1,670,265 | 8,431,771 |
| Bellingham | 1 | 226 | 14,248 | 57,736 | 91,246 | 158 | 250 | 4.1 | 8,284 | 30 | 1,944 | 53,676 | 106,536 |
| Bremerton | 1 | 255 | 13,832 | 52,937 | 80,604 | 145 | 221 | 3.8 | 11,597 | 24 | 1,791 | 51,370 | 132,574 |
| Olympia | 2 | 434 | 21,950 | 88,918 | 141,772 | 244 | 388 | 4.1 | 18,708 | 40 | 2,709 | 73,914 | 396,857 |
| Portland-Vancouver | 1 | 336 | 21,101 | 80,743 | 154,730 | 221 | 424 | 3.8 | 14,245 | 50 | 4,655 | 87,766 | 241,373 |
| Richland-Kennewick-Pasco | 4 | 431 | 17,299 | 80,991 | 175,423 | 221 | 480 | 4.7 | 12,763 | 53 | 3,851 | 96,832 | 259,692 |
| Seattle-Bellevue-Everett | 21 | 4,237 | 228,627 | 1,043,037 | 1,861,328 | 2,857 | 5,100 | 4.6 | 187,722 | 463 | 30,616 | 839,969 | 5,115,302 |
| Spokane | 6 | 1,312 | 52,331 | 280,075 | 407,428 | 768 | 1,117 | 5.4 | 51,081 | 85 | 6,222 | 152,115 | 437,536 |
| Tacoma | 5 | 1,059 | 58,444 | 245,982 | 441,277 | 675 | 1,209 | 4.2 | 51,230 | 81 | 7,630 | 205,753 | 1,149,295 |
| Yakima | 4 | 513 | 20,439 | 81,436 | 142,351 | 223 | 390 | 4.0 | 12,882 | 43 | 3,994 | 108,870 | 592,606 |

 

# U.S. CENSUS DIVISION 9, PACIFIC

*U.S. Community Hospitals*
*(Nonfederal, short-term general and other special hospitals)*

## 2003 Utilization, Personnel and Finances

| FULL-TIME EQUIVALENT PERSONNEL | | | | | FULL-TIME EQUIV. TRAINEES | | | EXPENSES | | | | | | |
|---|---|---|---|---|---|---|---|---|---|---|---|---|---|---|
| | | | | | | | | LABOR | | | | TOTAL | | |
| Physicians and Dentists | Registered Nurses | Licensed Practical Nurses | Other Salaried Personnel | Total Personnel | Medical and Dental Residents | Other Trainees | Total Trainees | Payroll (in thousands) | Employee Benefits (in thousands) | Total (in thousands) | Percent of Total | Amount (in thousands) | Adjusted per Admission | Adjusted per Inpatient Day |
| 71,335 | 1,021,346 | 126,328 | 2,889,619 | 4,108,628 | 77,813 | 7,954 | 85,767 | $187,822,974 | $45,438,505 | $233,261,475 | 51.8 | $450,124,257 | $7,796.41 | $1,379.48 |
| 8,445 | 147,570 | 37,579 | 485,049 | 678,643 | 1,775 | 600 | 2,375 | 25,551,777 | 6,425,000 | 31,976,774 | 53.8 | 59,444,378 | 5,305.04 | 806.30 |
| 62,890 | 873,776 | 88,749 | 2,404,570 | 3,429,985 | 76,038 | 7,354 | 83,392 | 162,271,198 | 39,013,505 | 201,284,701 | 51.5 | 390,679,879 | 8,396.37 | 1,546.78 |
| 10,566 | 129,111 | 13,737 | 343,626 | 497,040 | 9,373 | 832 | 10,205 | 25,976,336 | 7,167,093 | 33,143,429 | 52.7 | 62,875,658 | 9,267.23 | 1,764.78 |
| 609 | 8,524 | 1,411 | 28,248 | 38,792 | 53 | 28 | 81 | 1,765,234 | 511,307 | 2,276,543 | 55.3 | 4,114,830 | 6,974.94 | 1,128.04 |
| 9,957 | 120,587 | 12,326 | 315,378 | 458,248 | 9,320 | 804 | 10,124 | 24,211,102 | 6,655,786 | 30,866,886 | 52.5 | 58,760,828 | 9,485.53 | 1,837.40 |
| 289 | 2,129 | 183 | 5,442 | 8,043 | 49 | 30 | 79 | 417,080 | 108,931 | 526,013 | 51.8 | 1,016,056 | 12,370.41 | 1,951.92 |
| 83 | 781 | 128 | 2,678 | 3,670 | 7 | 1 | 8 | 193,549 | 51,337 | 244,887 | 55.4 | 441,865 | 10,931.56 | 1,460.93 |
| 206 | 1,348 | 55 | 2,764 | 4,373 | 42 | 29 | 71 | 223,531 | 57,594 | 281,126 | 49.0 | 574,191 | 13,764.63 | 2,632.84 |
| 206 | 1,348 | 55 | 2,764 | 4,373 | 42 | 29 | 71 | 223,531 | 57,594 | 281,126 | 49.0 | 574,191 | 13,764.63 | 2,632.84 |
| 7,243 | 95,182 | 11,003 | 250,406 | 363,834 | 7,655 | 708 | 8,363 | 19,169,588 | 5,410,407 | 24,579,992 | 52.4 | 46,910,735 | 9,450.73 | 1,763.40 |
| 101 | 2,512 | 515 | 8,026 | 11,154 | 14 | 10 | 24 | 488,380 | 167,491 | 655,872 | 54.0 | 1,215,143 | 7,232.91 | 1,178.08 |
| 7,142 | 92,670 | 10,488 | 242,380 | 352,680 | 7,641 | 698 | 8,339 | 18,681,208 | 5,242,916 | 23,924,120 | 52.4 | 45,695,592 | 9,528.42 | 1,787.01 |
| 55 | 1,394 | 259 | 4,312 | 6,020 | 27 | 20 | 47 | 286,546 | 77,383 | 363,928 | 55.3 | 657,640 | 8,210.34 | 1,320.39 |
| 14 | 700 | 127 | 2,769 | 3,610 | 5 | 1 | 6 | 134,543 | 57,388 | 191,930 | 54.2 | 353,881 | 8,026.70 | 1,734.32 |
| 225 | 3,163 | 477 | 10,114 | 13,979 | 262 | 33 | 295 | 647,148 | 153,999 | 801,148 | 52.9 | 1,513,119 | 7,658.41 | 1,374.29 |
| 3,157 | 28,560 | 3,536 | 73,930 | 109,183 | 3,256 | 112 | 3,368 | 5,617,319 | 1,471,122 | 7,088,435 | 51.1 | 13,877,891 | 9,559.08 | 1,752.43 |
| 18 | 240 | 35 | 778 | 1,071 | 6 | 2 | 8 | 52,049 | 13,318 | 65,367 | 55.2 | 118,473 | 6,631.20 | 1,447.28 |
| 0 | 1,728 | 130 | 3,612 | 5,470 | 0 | 40 | 40 | 255,268 | 86,437 | 341,705 | 51.1 | 668,106 | 10,337.39 | 1,412.32 |
| 375 | 6,239 | 647 | 17,656 | 24,917 | 480 | 51 | 531 | 1,754,602 | 509,252 | 2,263,854 | 56.5 | 4,009,297 | 10,974.24 | 2,093.53 |
| 95 | 6,889 | 716 | 18,951 | 26,651 | 138 | 6 | 144 | 1,271,162 | 333,755 | 1,604,917 | 50.2 | 3,200,048 | 8,432.07 | 1,820.08 |
| 15 | 785 | 87 | 1,583 | 2,470 | 23 | 3 | 26 | 123,878 | 38,289 | 162,167 | 52.5 | 308,763 | 10,925.03 | 1,572.14 |
| 929 | 8,736 | 968 | 20,799 | 31,432 | 704 | 130 | 834 | 1,375,544 | 370,715 | 1,746,259 | 49.4 | 3,533,188 | 7,167.83 | 1,558.12 |
| 237 | 5,826 | 561 | 15,252 | 21,876 | 431 | 17 | 448 | 1,193,015 | 352,129 | 1,545,144 | 53.6 | 2,882,505 | 11,455.06 | 2,316.57 |
| 36 | 985 | 151 | 2,791 | 3,963 | 25 | 12 | 37 | 229,515 | 123,086 | 352,601 | 59.7 | 590,471 | 11,342.34 | 2,390.72 |
| 134 | 7,412 | 677 | 16,585 | 24,808 | 633 | 51 | 684 | 1,270,372 | 326,485 | 1,596,856 | 51.6 | 3,097,577 | 8,250.70 | 1,467.37 |
| 783 | 6,682 | 650 | 15,631 | 23,746 | 631 | 204 | 835 | 1,600,486 | 456,980 | 2,057,469 | 54.3 | 3,788,639 | 15,017.00 | 2,034.99 |
| 786 | 4,782 | 452 | 14,588 | 20,608 | 811 | 2 | 813 | 1,262,532 | 385,651 | 1,648,183 | 52.7 | 3,128,173 | 12,784.02 | 2,745.76 |
| 6 | 485 | 41 | 1,132 | 1,664 | 0 | 0 | 0 | 78,595 | 19,827 | 98,423 | 50.7 | 194,133 | 6,253.49 | 1,467.63 |
| 27 | 978 | 72 | 2,739 | 3,816 | 58 | 0 | 58 | 169,760 | 56,845 | 226,605 | 53.3 | 424,948 | 8,292.63 | 1,233.06 |
| 8 | 430 | 59 | 1,247 | 1,744 | 0 | 0 | 0 | 113,233 | 32,837 | 146,070 | 58.0 | 251,759 | 7,867.71 | 1,929.91 |
| 17 | 1,180 | 124 | 2,731 | 4,052 | 2 | 4 | 6 | 217,241 | 63,893 | 281,134 | 55.3 | 508,819 | 8,216.69 | 1,749.23 |
| 115 | 1,458 | 158 | 4,031 | 5,762 | 92 | 5 | 97 | 276,904 | 82,347 | 359,250 | 53.4 | 672,283 | 8,385.62 | 1,673.95 |
| 22 | 973 | 76 | 2,971 | 4,042 | 10 | 1 | 11 | 225,177 | 66,422 | 291,600 | 51.5 | 566,398 | 8,160.54 | 1,655.68 |
| 64 | 1,742 | 139 | 3,817 | 5,762 | 42 | 3 | 45 | 283,723 | 91,208 | 374,932 | 51.0 | 735,708 | 8,344.95 | 1,459.58 |
| 0 | 817 | 229 | 2,712 | 3,758 | 0 | 0 | 0 | 144,155 | 49,605 | 193,760 | 54.6 | 354,724 | 7,259.72 | 1,292.47 |
| 18 | 214 | 36 | 707 | 975 | 4 | 1 | 5 | 43,841 | 10,510 | 54,351 | 52.9 | 102,744 | 7,136.47 | 2,231.43 |
| 6 | 272 | 81 | 942 | 1,301 | 1 | 0 | 1 | 54,599 | 13,433 | 68,032 | 43.5 | 156,306 | 7,699.41 | 1,805.42 |
| 319 | 3,941 | 488 | 10,583 | 15,331 | 57 | 20 | 77 | 768,656 | 183,678 | 952,335 | 53.4 | 1,783,816 | 9,677.61 | 1,350.44 |
| 36 | 822 | 163 | 2,291 | 3,312 | 13 | 10 | 23 | 150,825 | 43,479 | 194,304 | 56.5 | 343,778 | 6,800.63 | 771.77 |
| 283 | 3,119 | 325 | 8,292 | 12,019 | 44 | 10 | 54 | 617,831 | 140,199 | 758,031 | 52.6 | 1,440,037 | 10,764.78 | 1,644.86 |
| 283 | 3,119 | 325 | 8,292 | 12,019 | 44 | 10 | 54 | 617,831 | 140,199 | 758,031 | 52.6 | 1,440,037 | 10,764.78 | 1,644.86 |
| 1,414 | 11,367 | 675 | 28,592 | 42,048 | 712 | 14 | 726 | 1,999,752 | 570,707 | 2,570,459 | 53.5 | 4,806,544 | 7,848.79 | 1,841.84 |
| 215 | 2,220 | 306 | 7,653 | 10,394 | 13 | 2 | 15 | 472,535 | 134,627 | 607,162 | 55.0 | 1,104,558 | 6,302.15 | 1,398.32 |
| 1,199 | 9,147 | 369 | 20,939 | 31,654 | 699 | 12 | 711 | 1,527,217 | 436,080 | 1,963,297 | 53.0 | 3,701,985 | 8,468.92 | 2,034.37 |
| 22 | 265 | 41 | 894 | 1,222 | 8 | 2 | 10 | 59,663 | 17,549 | 77,213 | 54.5 | 141,747 | 10,290.88 | 2,958.73 |
| 22 | 1,041 | 54 | 2,378 | 3,495 | 0 | 0 | 0 | 169,667 | 47,516 | 217,183 | 53.0 | 409,399 | 8,115.59 | 2,088.93 |
| 20 | 664 | 35 | 1,886 | 2,605 | 8 | 0 | 8 | 117,963 | 44,842 | 162,805 | 53.9 | 302,302 | 8,231.96 | 2,012.10 |
| 1,107 | 6,439 | 183 | 13,528 | 21,257 | 683 | 10 | 693 | 1,032,168 | 286,623 | 1,318,791 | 52.2 | 2,528,441 | 8,567.65 | 2,014.08 |
| 28 | 738 | 56 | 2,253 | 3,075 | 0 | 0 | 0 | 147,756 | 39,550 | 187,305 | 58.5 | 320,097 | 7,794.31 | 1,880.72 |
| 1,301 | 16,492 | 1,388 | 48,603 | 67,784 | 900 | 60 | 960 | 3,621,261 | 893,370 | 4,514,630 | 54.0 | 8,358,508 | 8,871.63 | 1,827.14 |
| 174 | 2,189 | 299 | 7,600 | 10,262 | 6 | 5 | 11 | 459,945 | 114,373 | 574,318 | 56.9 | 1,009,486 | 6,483.37 | 936.02 |
| 1,127 | 14,303 | 1,089 | 41,003 | 57,522 | 894 | 55 | 949 | 3,161,316 | 778,997 | 3,940,312 | 53.6 | 7,349,021 | 9,344.47 | 2,102.03 |
| 12 | 343 | 4 | 1,022 | 1,381 | 0 | 0 | 0 | 73,137 | 18,086 | 91,223 | 55.0 | 165,837 | 7,364.99 | 1,817.48 |
| 0 | 0 | 0 | 1,166 | 1,166 | 0 | 0 | 0 | 68,178 | 20,258 | 88,437 | 67.7 | 130,712 | 6,206.34 | 1,621.65 |
| 18 | 539 | 63 | 1,639 | 2,259 | 18 | 6 | 24 | 114,543 | 31,308 | 145,851 | 54.6 | 267,194 | 7,598.71 | 1,884.67 |
| 36 | 782 | 30 | 1,658 | 2,506 | 21 | 0 | 21 | 125,039 | 33,571 | 158,610 | 55.9 | 283,689 | 7,015.75 | 1,833.45 |
| 16 | 525 | 67 | 1,470 | 2,078 | 1 | 0 | 1 | 100,124 | 22,806 | 122,930 | 51.8 | 237,473 | 6,630.17 | 1,353.72 |
| 871 | 8,008 | 457 | 23,550 | 32,886 | 740 | 26 | 766 | 1,883,112 | 455,864 | 2,338,975 | 53.1 | 4,404,147 | 10,644.70 | 2,366.13 |
| 44 | 1,666 | 145 | 4,229 | 6,084 | 71 | 21 | 92 | 309,507 | 85,230 | 394,737 | 58.2 | 677,866 | 8,771.68 | 1,663.77 |
| 114 | 1,709 | 225 | 4,470 | 6,518 | 38 | 1 | 39 | 375,773 | 83,061 | 458,833 | 50.8 | 903,364 | 8,645.13 | 2,047.16 |
| 16 | 731 | 98 | 1,799 | 2,644 | 5 | 1 | 6 | 111,902 | 28,812 | 140,716 | 50.5 | 278,739 | 7,753.74 | 1,958.11 |

# Statistics for Multihospital Health Care Systems and their Hospitals

The following tables describe multihospital health care systems for all U.S. Hospitals.

Table 1 shows the number of multihospital health care systems by type of control. Table 2 provides a breakdown of the number of systems that own, lease, sponsor or contract manage hospitals within each control category. Table 3 gives the number of hospitals and beds in each control category as well as total hospitals and beds. Finally, Table 4 shows the percentage of hospitals and beds in each control category.

For more information on multihospital health care systems, please write to the Section for Health Care Systems, One North Franklin, Chicago, Illinois 60606–3401 or call 312/422–3000.

**Table 1. Multihospital Health Care Systems, by Type of Organizaton Control**

| Type of Control | Code | Number of Systems |
|---|---|---|
| Catholic (Roman) church–related | CC | 43 |
| Other church–related | CO | 13 |
| Subtotal, church–related | | 56 |
| Other not–for–profit | NP | 223 |
| Subtotal, not–for–profit | | 279 |
| Investor Owned | IO | 55 |
| Federal Government | FG | 5 |
| Total | | 339 |

**Table 2. Multihospital Health Care Systems, by Type of Ownership and Control**

| Type of Ownership | Catholic Church–Related (CC) | Other Church–Related (CO) | Total Church–Related (CC + CO) | Other Not–for–Profit (NP) | Total Not–for–Profit (CC, CO, + NP) | Investor–Owned (IO) | Federal Govern–ment | All Systems |
|---|---|---|---|---|---|---|---|---|
| Systems that only own, lease or sponsor | 35 | 12 | 47 | 191 | 238 | 48 | 5 | 291 |
| Systems that only contract–manage | 0 | 0 | 0 | 1 | 1 | 4 | 0 | 5 |
| Systems that manage, own, lease, or sponsor | 8 | 1 | 9 | 31 | 40 | 3 | 0 | 43 |
| Total | 43 | 13 | 56 | 223 | 279 | 55 | 5 | 339 |

**Table 3. Hospitals and Beds in Multihospital Health Care Systems, by Type of Ownership and Control**

| | Catholic Church–Related (CC) | | Other Church–Related (CO) | | Total Church–Related (CC + CO) | | Other Not–for–Profit (NP) | | Total Not–for–Profit (CC, CO, + NP) | | Investor–Owned (IO) | | Federal Govern–ment | | All Systems | |
|---|---|---|---|---|---|---|---|---|---|---|---|---|---|---|---|---|
| Type of Ownership | H | B | H | B | H | B | H | B | H | B | H | B | H | B | H | B |
| Owned, leased or sponsored | 531 | 111,461 | 111 | 22,316 | 642 | 133,777 | 1,058 | 246,029 | 1,700 | 379,806 | 938 | 125,496 | 246 | 47,942 | 2,884 | 553,244 |
| Contract–managed | 45 | 2,688 | 1 | 268 | 46 | 2,956 | 94 | 7,574 | 140 | 10,530 | 191 | 15,630 | 0 | 0 | 331 | 26,160 |
| Total | 576 | 114,149 | 112 | 22,584 | 688 | 136,403 | 1,152 | 253,603 | 1,840 | 390,006 | 1,129 | 141,126 | 246 | 47,942 | 3,215 | 579,404 |

**H** = *hospitals;* **B** = *beds.*

**Table 4. Hospitals and Beds in Multihospital Health Care Systems, by Type of Ownership and Control as a Percentage of All Systems**

| | Catholic Church–Related (CC) | | Other Church–Related (CO) | | Total Church–Related (CC + CO) | | Other Not–for–Profit (NP) | | Total Not–for–Profit (CC, CO, + NP) | | Investor–Owned (IO) | | Federal Govern–ment | | All Systems | |
|---|---|---|---|---|---|---|---|---|---|---|---|---|---|---|---|---|
| Type of Ownership | H | B | H | B | H | B | H | B | H | B | H | B | H | B | H | B |
| Owned, leased or sponsored | 18.4 | 20.1 | 3.8 | 4.0 | 22.3 | 24.1 | 36.7 | 44.5 | 58.9 | 68.6 | 32.5 | 22.7 | 8.5 | 8.7 | 100.0 | 100.0 |
| Contract–managed | 13.6 | 10.3 | 0.3 | 1.0 | 13.9 | 11.3 | 28.4 | 29.0 | 42.3 | 40.3 | 57.7 | 59.7 | 0.0 | 0.0 | 100.0 | 100.0 |
| Total | 17.9 | 19.7 | 3.5 | 3.9 | 21.4 | 23.6 | 35.8 | 43.8 | 57.2 | 67.3 | 35.1 | 24.4 | 7.7 | 8.3 | 100.0 | 100.0 |

**H** = *hospitals;* **B** = *beds.*
*Please note that figures may not always equal the provided subtotal or total percentages due to rounding.

# Summary of Total United States Registered Hospitals

This summary table reflects the change in the number of Total U.S. Registered Hospitals between fiscal year 2002 and fiscal year 2003.

| 2002 vs 2003 ANNUAL SURVEY DATA | |
|---|---|
| **CLASSIFICATION** | **UNITED STATES** |
| **2002 TOTAL** | **5794** |
| **Deletions** | |
| Status changed from registered to non-registered | 1 |
| Changed to inpatient care other than a hospital | 1 |
| Changed to an outpatient facility | 4 |
| Closed | 33 |
| Demerged/Dissolution | 0 |
| Merged to form a new hospital | 12 |
| Merged into a hospital already on file | 5 |
| Temporarily inactive record/Under construction | 2 |
| **Total Deletions** | **58** |
| **Additions** | |
| Status changed from non-registered to registered | 5 |
| Demerger result | 2 |
| Merger result | 6 |
| Newly added to the registered file | 15 |
| Previously closed/reopened | 0 |
| Changed to hospital from other inpatient care | 0 |
| **Total Additions** | **28** |
| **2003 TOTAL** | **5764** |

# Glossary

*This glossary explains specific terms as they are used in the tables and text of AHA Hospital Statistics*

**Acute long term care:** Providers specialized acute hospital care to medically complex patients who are critically ill, have multisystem complications and/or failure, and require hospitalization averaging 25 days, in a facility offering specialized treatment programs and therapeutic intervention on a 24 hour/7day a week basis.

**Adjusted average daily census:** An estimate of the average number of patients (both inpatients and outpatients) receiving care each day during the reporting period, which is usually 12 months. The figure is derived by dividing the number of inpatient day equivalents (also called adjusted inpatient days) by the number of days in the reporting period.

**Adjusted inpatient days:** An aggregate figure reflecting the number of days of inpatient care, plus an estimate of the volume of outpatient services, expressed in units equivalent to an inpatient day in terms of level of effort. The figure is derived by first multiplying the number of outpatient visits by the ratio of outpatient revenue per outpatient visit to inpatient revenue per inpatient day. The product (which represents the number of patient days attributable to outpatient services) is then added to the number of *inpatient days*. Originally, the purpose of this calculation was to summarize overall productivity and calculate a unit cost that would include both inpatient and outpatient activities.

**Formula 1:**

$$\frac{\text{total expenses}}{\text{inpatient days} + \text{outpatient visits}\left(\dfrac{\text{outpatient revenue per outpatient visit}}{\text{inpatient revenue per inpatient day}}\right)}$$

However, the value of this calculation has changed over the years as the outpatient share of total revenue has grown and third-party payers have exerted a greater influence on pricing.

**Admissions:** The number of patients, excluding newborns, accepted for inpatient service during the reporting period; the number includes patients who visit the emergency room and are later admitted for inpatient service.

**Adult day care program:** Program providing supervision, medical and psychological care, and social activities for older adults who live at home or in another family setting, but cannot be alone or prefer to be with others during the day. May include intake assessment, health monitoring, occupational therapy, personal care, noon meal, and transportation services.

**Airborne infection isolation room:** A single-occupancy room for patient care where environmental factors are controlled in an effort to minimize the transmission of those infectious agents, usually spread person to person by droplet nuclei associated with coughing and inhalation. Such rooms typically have specific ventilation requirements for controlled ventilation, air pressure and filtration.

**Alcoholism-drug abuse or dependency inpatient care:** Provides diagnosis and therapeutic services to patients with alcoholism or other drug dependencies. Includes care for inpatient/residential treatment for patients whose course of treatment involves more intensive care than provided in an outpatient setting or where patient requires supervised withdrawal.

**Alcoholism-drug abuse or dependency outpatient services:** Organized hospital services that provide medical care and/or rehabilitative treatment services to outpatients for whom the primary diagnosis is alcoholism or other chemical dependency.

**Alzheimer Center:** Facility that offers care to persons with Alzheimer's disease and their families through an integrated program of clinical services, research, and education.

**Ambulance services:** Provision of ambulance services to the ill and injured who require medical attention on a scheduled or unscheduled basis.

**Angioplasty:** The reconstruction or restructuring of a blood vessel by operative means or by nonsurgical techniques such as balloon dilation or laser.

**Arthritis treatment center:** Specifically equipped and staffed center for the diagnosis and treatment of arthritis and other joint disorders.

**Assisted living:** A special combination of housing, supportive services, personalized assistance and health care designed to respond to the individual needs of those who need help in activities of daily living and instrumental activities of daily living. Supportive services are available, 24 hours a day, to meet scheduled and unscheduled needs, in a way that promotes maximum independence and dignity for each resident and encourages the involvement of a resident's family, neighbor and friends.

**Auxiliary:** A volunteer community organization formed to assist the hospital in carrying out its purpose and to serve as a link between the institution and the community.

**Average daily census:** The average number of people served on an inpatient basis on a single day during the reporting period; the figure is calculated by dividing the number of inpatient days by the number of days in the reporting period.

**Bariactric/weight control services:** Bariatrics is the medical practice of weight reduction.

**Beds:** Number of beds regularly maintained (set up and staffed for use) for inpatients as of the close of the reporting period. Excludes newborn bassinets.

**Bed-size category:** Hospitals are categorized by the number of beds set up and staffed for use at the end of the reporting period. The eight categories in Hospital Statistics are: 6 to 24 beds; 25 to 49; 50 to 99; 100 to 199; 200 to 299; 300 to 399; 400 to 499; and 500 or more.

**Birthing room-LDR room-LDRP room:** A single-room type of maternity care with a more homelike setting for families than the traditional three-room unit(labor/delivery/recovery) with a separate postpartum area. A birthing room combines labor and delivery in one room. An LDR room accommodates three stages in the birthing process—labor, delivery, and recovery. An LDRP room accommodates all four stages of the birth process—labor, delivery, recovery, and postpartum.

**Births:** Total number of infants born in the hospital during the reporting period. Births do not include infants transferred from other institutions, and are excluded from admission and discharge figures.

**Breast cancer screening/mammograms:** Mammography screening - The use of breast x-ray to detect unsuspected breast cancer in asymptomatic women. Diagnostic mammography - The x-ray imaging of breast tissue in symptomatic women who are considered to have a substantial likelihood of having breast cancer already.

**Burn care:** Provides care to severely burned patients. Severely burned patients are those with any of the following: (1) second-degree burns of more than 25% total body surface area for adults or 20% total body surface area for children: (2) third-degree burns of more than 10% total body surface area; (3) any severe burns of the hands, face, eyes, ears, or feet; or (4) all inhalation injuries, electrical burns, complicated burn injuries involving fractures and other major traumas, and all other poor risk factors.

**Cardiac catheterization laboratory:** Facilities offering special diagnostic procedures for cardiac patients. Available procedures must include, but need not be limited to, introduction of a catheter into the interior of the heart by way of a vein or artery or by direct needle puncture. Procedures must be performed in a laboratory or a special procedure room.

**Cardiac intensive care:** Provides patient care of a more specialized nature than the usual medical and surgical care, on the basis of physicians' orders and approved nursing care plans. The unit is staffed with specially trained nursing personnel and contains monitoring and specialized support or treatment equipment for patients who, because of heart seizure, open-heart surgery, or other life-threatening conditions, require intensified, comprehensive observation and care. May include myocardial infarction, pulmonary care, and heart transplant units.

**Cardiology services:** Services which include the diagnosis and treatment of diseases and disorders involving the heart and circulatory system.

**Case management:** A system of assessment, treatment planning, referral and follow-up that ensures the provision of comprehensive and continuous services and the coordination of payment and reimbursement for care.

**Chaplaincy/pastoral care services:** A service ministering religious activities and providing pastoral counseling to patients, their families, and staff of a health care organization.

**Chemotherapy:** An organized program for the treatment of cancer by the use of drugs or chemicals.

**Children wellness program:** A program that encourages improved health status and a healthful lifestyle of children through health education, exercise, nutrition and health promotion.

**Chiropractic services:** An organized clinical service including spinal manipulation or adjustment and related diagnostic and therapeutic services.

**Closed physician-hospital organization (Closed PHO):** A joint venture between the hospital and physicians who have been selected on the basis of cost-effectiveness and/or high quality. The PHO can act as a unified agent in managed care contracting, own a managed care plan, own and operate ambulatory care centers or ancillary services projects, or provide administrative services to physician members.

**Community hospitals:** All nonfederal, short-term general, and special hospitals whose facilities and services are available to the public. (Special hospitals include obstetrics and gynecology; eye, ear, nose, and throat; rehabilitation; orthopedic; and other individually described specialty services.) Short-term general and special childrens hospitals are also considered to be community hospitals.

A hospital may include a nursing-home-type unit and still be classified as short-term, provided that the majority of its patients are admitted to units where the average length of stay is less than 30 days. Therefore, statistics for community hospitals often include some data about such nursing-home-type units. An example is furnished by Montana, where in 1995 63.6 percent of all hospitals classified as community hospitals include nursing-home-type units. Expense, revenue, utilization, and personnel data for these hospitals include data about their nursing-home-type units. Thus, total admissions to Montana community hospitals in 1995 were 96,154; total inpatient days, 997,759; total expenses, $791,806,393; and total payroll expenses, $352,583,331. If nursing-home-type unit data were excluded, these same items would be 94,034; 457,340; 752,567,865; and $328,911841, respectively.

Note that before 1972, hospital units of institutions such as prison and college infirmaries were included in the category of community hospitals. Including these units made this category equivalent to the short-term general and other special hospitals category. Although these hospital units are few in number and small in size, this change in definition should be taken into consideration when comparing data.

**Community outreach:** A program that systematically interacts with the community to identify those in need of services, alerting persons and their families to the availability of services, locating needed services, and enabling persons to enter the service delivery system.

**Complementary Medicine Services:** Organized hospital services or formal arrangements to providers that provide care or treatment not based solely on traditional western allopathic medical teachings as instructed in most U.S. medical schools. Includes any of the following: acupuncture, chiropractic, homeopathy, osteopathy, diet and lifestyle changes, herbal medicine, message therapy, etc.

**Control:** The type of organization responsible for establishing policy concerning the overall operation of hospitals. The three major categories are government (including federal, state, and local); nongovernment (nonprofit); and investor-owned (for-profit).

**Crisis prevention:** Services provided in order to promote physical and mental well being and the early identification of disease and ill health prior to the onset and recognition of symptoms so as to permit early treatment.

**CT scanner:** Computed tomographic scanner for head or whole body scans.

**Deduction from revenue:** The difference between revenue at full established rates (gross) and the payment actually received from payers (net).

**Dental Services:** An organized dental service or dentists on staff, not necessarily involving special facilities, providing dental or oral services to inpatients or outpatients.

**Diagnostic radioisotope facility:** The use of radioactive isotopes (Radiopharmaceuticals) as tracers or indicators to detect an abnormal condition or disease.

**Electron beam computed tomography (EBCT):** A high tech computed tomography scan used to detect coronary artery disease by measuring coronary calcifications. This imaging procedure uses electron beams which are magnetically steered to produce a visual of the coronary artery and the images are produced faster than conventional CT scans.

**Emergency department:** Hospital facilities for the provision of unscheduled outpatient services to patients whose conditions require immediate care.

**Emergency room visits:** The number of visits to the emergency unit. When emergency outpatients are admitted to the inpatient areas of the hospital, they are counted as emergency room visits and subsequently, as inpatient admissions.

**Enabling services:** A program that is designed to help the patient access health care services by offering any of the following: linguistic services, transportation services, and/or referrals to local social services agencies.

**Enrollment assistance services:** A program that provides enrollment assistance for patients who are potentially eligible for public health insurance programs such as Medicaid, State Children's Health Insurance, or local/state indigent care programs. The specific services offered could include explanation of benefits, assist applicants in completing the application and locating all relevant documents, conduct eligibility interviews, and/or forward applications and documentation to state/local social service or health agency.

**Equity model:** An arrangement that allows established practitioners to become shareholders in a professional corporation in exchange for tangible and intangible assets of their existing practices.

**Expenses:** Includes all expenses for the reporting period including payroll, non-payroll, bad debt, and all nonoperating expenses. *Payroll expenses* include all salaries and wages. *Non-payroll expenses* are all professional fees and those salary expenditures excluded from payroll. *Labor related expenses* are defined as payroll expenses plus employee benefits. *Non-labor related expenses* are all other non-payroll expenses. *Bad debt* has been reclassified from a "reduction in revenue" to an expense in accordance with the revised AICPA Audit Guide. However, for purposes of historical consistency, the expense total that appears throughout *AHA Hospital Statistics does not include "bad debt" as an expense item.* Note: Financial data may not add due to rounding.

**Extracorporeal shock wave lithotripter (ESWL):** A medical device used for treating stones in the kidney or ureter. The device disintegrates kidney stones noninvasively through the transmission of acoustic shock waves directed at the stones.

**Fertility Clinic:** A specialized program set in an infertility center that provides counseling and education as well as advanced reproductive techniques such as: injectable therapy, reproductive surgeries, treatment for endometriosis, male factor infertility, tubal reversals, in vitro fertilization (IVF), donor eggs, and other such services to help patients achieve successful pregnancies.

**Fitness center:** Provides exercise, testing, or evaluation programs and fitness activities to the community and hospital employees.

**Foundation:** A corporation, organized as a hospital affiliate or subsidiary, that purchases both tangible and intangible assets of one or more medical group practices. Physicians remain in a separate corporate entity but sign a professional services agreement with the foundation.

**Gamma knife:** A non-invasive and bloodless procedure which uses a technological device that delivers concentrated gamma radiation to target points selected in the brain and is used for treatment on patients with brain tumors and other brain disorders.

**General medical-surgical care:** Provides acute care to patients in medical and surgical units on the basis of physicians' orders and approved nursing care plans.

**Genetic testing/counseling:** A service equipped with adequate laboratory facilities and directed by a qualified physician to advise parents and prospective parents on potential problems in cases of genetic defects. A genetic test is the analysis of human DNA, RNA, chromosomes, proteins, and certain metabolites in order to detect heritable disease-related genotypes, mutations, phenotypes, or karyotypes for clinical purposes. Genetic tests can have diverse purposes, including the diagnosis of genetic diseases in newborns, children, and adults; the identification of future health risks; the prediction of drug responses; and the assessment of risks to future children.

**Geriatric services:** The branch of medicine dealing with the physiology of aging and the diagnosis and treatment of disease affecting the aged. Services could include: Adult day care; Alzheimer's diagnostic-assessment services; Comprehensive geriatric assessment; Emergency response system; Geriatric acute care unit; and/or Geriatric clinics.

**Government, nonfederal, state, local:** Controlled by an agency of state, county, or city government.

**Gross inpatient revenue:** Revenue from services rendered to inpatients at full established rates (also known as "charges").

**Gross outpatient revenue:** Revenue from services rendered to outpatients at full established rates.

**Group practice without walls:** In this organization, the hospital sponsors the formation of a physician group or provides capital to physicians to establish one. The group shares administrative expenses, although the physicians remain independent practitioners.

**Group Purchasing Organization:** An organization whose primary function is to negotiate contracts for the purpose of purchasing for members of the group or has a central supply site for its members.

**Health fair:** Community health education events that focus on the prevention of disease and promotion of health through such activities as audiovisual exhibits and free diagnostic services.

**Health information center:** Education which is directed at increasing the information of individuals and populations. It is intended to increase the ability to make informed personal, family and community health decisions by providing consumers with informed choices about health matters with the objective of improving health status.

**Health maintenance organization (HMO):** A health care organization that acts as both insurer and provider of comprehensive but specified medical services in return for prospective per capita (capitation) payments.

**Health screening:** A preliminary procedure such as a test or examination to detect the most characteristic sign or signs of a disorder that may require further investigation.

**Hemodialysis:** Provision of equipment and personnel for the treatment of renal insufficiency on an inpatient or outpatient basis.

**HIV-AIDS services:** (could include). *HIV-AIDS unit* - Special unit or team designated and equipped specifically for diagnosis, treatment, continuing care planning, and counseling services for HIV-AIDS patients and their families. *General inpatient care for HIV-AIDS* - Inpatient diagnosis and treatment for human immunodeficiency virus and acquired immunodeficiency syndrome patients, but dedicated unit is not available. *Specialized outpatient program for HIV-AIDS* - Special outpatient program providing diagnostic, treatment, continuing care planning, and counseling for HIV-AIDS patients and their families.

**Home health services:** Service providing nursing, therapy, and health-related homemaker or social services in the patient's home.

**Hospice:** A program providing palliative care, chiefly medical relief of pain and supportive services, addressing the emotional, social, financial, and legal needs of terminally ill patients and their families. Care can be provided in a variety of settings, both inpatient and at home.

**Hospital unit:** The hospital operation, excluding activity pertaining to nursing-home-type unit (as described below), for the following items: Admissions, Beds, FTEs (full-time, part-time, and total), Inpatient Days, Length of Stay, Net Revenue, and Total Expense.

**Hospital unit of institutions:** A hospital unit that is not open to the public and is contained within a nonhospital unit. An example is an infirmary that is contained within a college.

**Hospitals in a network:** Hospitals participating in a group that may include other hospitals, physicians, other providers, insurers, and/or community agencies that work together to coordinate and deliver a broad spectrum of services to the community.

**Hospitals in a system:** Hospitals belonging to a corporate body that owns and/or manages health provider facilities or health-related subsidiaries; the system may also own non-health-related facilities.

**Indemnity fee for service:** The traditional type of health insurance, in which the insured is reimbursed for covered expenses without regard to choice of provider. Payment up to a stated limit may be made either to the individual incurring and claiming the expense, or directly to providers.

**Independent practice association (IPA):** An IPA is a legal entity that holds managed care contracts and contracts with physicians, usually in solo practice, to provide care either on a fee-for-services or capitated basis. The purpose of an IPA is to assist solo physicians in obtaining managed care contracts.

**Inpatient days:** The number of adult and ediatric days of care, excluding newborn days of care, rendered during the entire reporting period.

**Inpatient surgeries:** Surgical services provided to patients who remain in the hospital overnight.

**Insurance product:** In tables 3 through 6, insurance product refers to a hospital-owned insurance product.

**Integrated salary model:** In this arrangement, physicians are salaried by the hospital or other entity of a health system to provide medical services for primary care and specialty care.

**Intensity-Modulated Radiation Therapy (IMRT):** A type of three-dimensional radiation therapy, which improves the targeting of treatment delivery in a way that is likely to decrease damage to normal tissues and allows varying intensities.

**Intermediate nursing care:** Provides health-related services (skilled nursing care and social services) to residents with a variety of physical conditions or functional disabilities. These residents do not require the care provided by a hospital or skilled nursing facility, but do need supervision and support services.

**Investor-owned, for-profit:** Investor-owned, for-profit hospitals are those controlled on a for-profit basis by an individual, partnership, or profit-making corporation.

**Labor-related expenses:** Payroll expenses plus employee benefits. *Non-labor-related expenses refers* to all other nonpayroll expenses, such as interest depreciation, supplies, purchased services, professional fees, and others.

**Length of stay (LOS):** LOS refers to the average number of days a patient stays at the facility. Short-term hospitals are those where the average LOS is less than 30 days. Long-term hospitals are those where the average LOS is 30 days or more. The figure is derived by dividing the number of inpatient days by the number of admissions.

Note that this publication carries two LOS variables: *total facility length of stay and hospital unit length of stay. Total facility* includes admissions and inpatient days from nursing-home-type units under control of the hospital. In *hospital unit length of stay*, nursing home utilization is subtracted.

**Licensed practical nurse (LPN):** A nurse who has graduated from an approved school of practical (vocational) nursing and works under the supervision of registered nurses and/or physicians.

**Long-term:** Hospitals are classified either short-term or long-term according to the average length of stay (LOS). A long-term hospital is one in which the average LOS is 30 days or more.

**Magnetic resonance imaging (MRI):** The use of a uniform magnetic field and radio frequencies to study tissue and structure of the body. This procedure enables the visualization of biochemical activity of the cell in vivo without the use of ionizing radiation, radioisotopic substances, or high-frequency sound.

**Managed care:** A term covering a broad spectrum of arrangements for health care delivery and financing, including managed indemnity plans (MIP), health maintenance organizations (HMO), preferred provider organizations (PPO), point-of-service plans (POS), and direct contracting arrangements between employers and providers.

**Managed care contract:** A contract between the hospital and a managed care organization.

**Management services organization (MSO):** A corporation owned by the hospital or a physician/hospital joint venture that provides management services to one or more medical group practices. As part of a full-service management agreement, the MSO purchases the tangible assets of the practices and leases them back, employs all non-physician staff, and provides all supplies/administrative systems for a fee.

**Meals on wheels:** A hospital sponsored program which delivers meals to people, usually the elderly, who are unable to prepare their own meals. Low cost, nutritional meals are delivered to individuals' homes on a regular basis.

**Medical surgical intensive care:** Provides patient care of a more intensive nature than the usual medical and surgical care, on the basis of physicians' orders and approved nursing care plans. These units are staffed with specially trained nursing personnel and contain monitoring and specialized support equipment for patients who, because of shock, trauma, or other life-threatening conditions, require intensified, comprehensive observation and care. Includes mixed intensive care units.

**Multislice spiral computed tomography (MSCT):** A specialized computed tomography procedure that provides three-dimensional processing and allows narrower and multiple slices with increased spatial resolution and faster scanning times as compared to a regular computed tomography scan.

**Neonatal intensive care:** A unit that must be separate from the newborn nursery providing intensive care to all sick infants including those with the very lowest birth weights (less than 1500 grams). NICU has potential for providing mechanical ventilation, neonatal surgery, and special care for the sickest infants born in the hospital or transferred from another institution. A full-time neonatologist serves as director of the NICU.

**Neonatal intermediate care:** A unit that must be separate from the normal newborn nursery and that provides intermediate and/or recovery care and some specialized services, including immediate resuscitation, intravenous therapy, and capacity for prolonged oxygen therapy and monitoring.

**Net patient revenue:** The estimated net realizable amounts from patients, third-party payers, and others for services rendered. The number includes estimated retroactive adjustments called for by agreements with third-party payers; retroactive adjustments are accrued on an estimated basis in the period the related services are rendered and then adjusted later as final settlements are determined.

**Net total revenue:** Net patient revenue plus all other revenue, including contributions, endowment revenue, governmental grants, and all other payments not made on behalf of individual patients.

**Neurological services:** Services provided by the hospital dealing with the operative and nonoperative management of disorders of the central, peripheral, and autonomic nervous system.

**Nongovernment, nonprofit:** Hospitals that are nongovernment, nonprofit are controlled by not-for-profit organizations, including religious organizations (Catholic hospitals, for example), fraternal societies, and others.

**Nursing-home-type unit/facility:** A unit/facility that primarily offers the following type of services to a majority of all admissions:

- *Skilled nursing*: The provision of medical and nursing care services, health-related services, and social services under the supervision of a registered nurse on a 24-hour basis.
- *Intermediate care*: The provision, on a regular basis, of health-related care and services to individuals who do not require the degree of care or treatment that a skilled nursing unit is designed to provide.
- *Personal care*: The provision of general supervision and direct personal care services for residents who require assistance in activities of daily living but who do not need nursing services or inpatient care. Medical and nursing services are available as needed.
- *Sheltered/residential care*: The provision of general supervision and protective services for residents who do not need nursing services or continuous personal care services in the conduct of daily life. Medical and nursing services are available as needed.

**Nutrition programs:** Those services within a health care facility which are designed to provide inexpensive, nutritionally sound meals to patients.

**Obstetrics:** Levels should be designated: (1) unit provides services for uncomplicated maternity and newborn cases; (2) unit provides services for uncomplicated cases, the majority of complicated problems, and special neonatal services; and (3) unit provides services for all serious illnesses and abnormalities and is supervised by a full-time maternal/fetal specialist.

**Occupational health services:** Includes services designed to protect the safety of employees from hazards in the work environment.

**Oncology services:** An organized program for the treatment of cancer by the use of drugs or chemicals.

**Open heart surgery:** Heart surgery where the chest has been opened and the blood recirculated and oxygenated with the proper equipment and the necessary staff to perform the surgery.

**Open physician hospital organization (Open PHO):** A joint venture between the hospital and all members of the medical staff who wish to participate. The open PHO can act as a unified agent in managed care contracting, own a managed care plan, own and operate ambulatory care centers or ancillary services projects, or provide administrative services to physician members.

**Orthopedic services:** Services provided for the prevention or correction of injuries or disorders of the skeletal system and associated muscles, joints and ligaments.

**Osteopathic hospitals:** Osteopathic medicine is a medical practice based on a theory that diseases are due chiefly to a loss of structural integrity, which can be restored by manipulation of the neuro-muscular and skeletal systems, supplemented by therapeutic measures (such as medicine or surgery).

**Other Intensive Care:** A distinct intensive care unit that is not one of the following types: medical/surgical, cardiac, pediatric and neonatal.

**Other long term care:** Provision of long term care other than skilled nursing care or intermediate care. This can include residential care-elderly housing services for those who do not require daily medical or nursing services, but may require some assistance in the activities of daily living, or sheltered care facilities for developmentally disabled.

**Other special care:** Provides care to patients requiring care more intensive than that provided in the acute area, yet not sufficiently intensive to require admission to an intensive care unit. Patients admitted to this area are usually transferred here from an intensive care unit once their condition has improved. These units are sometimes referred to as definitive observation, step-down, or progressive care units.

**Outpatient care:** Treatment provided to patients who do not remain in the hospital for overnight care. Hospitals may deliver outpatient care on site or through a facility owned and operated by the hospital, but physically separate from the hospital. In addition to treating minor illnesses or injuries, a free-standing center will stabilize seriously ill or injured patients before transporting them to a hospital. Laboratory and radiology services are usually available.

**Outpatient care center (Freestanding):** A facility owned and operated by the hospital, but physically separate from the hospital, that provides various medical treatments on an outpatient basis only. In addition to treating minor illnesses or injuries, the center will stabilize seriously ill or injured patients before transporting them to a hospital. Laboratory and radiology services are usually available.

**Outpatient care center-services (Hospital-based):** Organized hospital health care services offered by appointment on an ambulatory basis. Services may include outpatient surgery, examination, diagnosis, and treatment of a variety of medical conditions on a nonemergency basis, and laboratory and other diagnostic testing as ordered by staff or outside physician referral.

**Outpatient surgeries:** Scheduled surgical services provided to patients who do not remain in the hospital overnight. In the AHA Annual Survey, outpatient surgery may be performed in operating suites also used for inpatient surgery, specially designated surgical suites for outpatient surgery, or procedure rooms within an outpatient care facility.

**Outpatient visit:** A visit by a patient who is not lodged in the hospital while receiving medical, dental, or other services. Each visit an outpatient makes to a discrete unit constitutes one visit regardless of the number of diagnostic and/or therapeutic treatments that the patient receives. Total outpatient visits should include all clinic visits, referred visits, observation services, outpatient surgeries, and emergency room visits.

**Pain management:** A hospital wide formalized program that includes staff education for the management of chronic and acute pain based on guidelines and protocols like those developed by the Agency for Health Care Policy Research, etc.

**Palliative care program:** An organized program providing specialized medical care, drugs or therapies for the management of acute or chronic pain and/or the control of symptoms administered by specially trained physicians and other clinicians; and supportive care services, such as counseling on advanced directives, spiritual care, and social services, to patients with advanced disease and their families.

**Patient education center:** Written goals and objectives for the patient and/or family related to therapeutic regimens, medical procedures, and self care.

**Patient representative services:** Organized hospital services providing personnel through whom patients and staff can seek solutions to institutional problems affecting the delivery of high-quality care and services.

**Payroll expenses:** Includes all salaries and wages. All professional fees and salary expenditures excluded from payroll, such as employee benefits, are defined as nonpayroll expenses and are included in total expenses.

**Pediatric intensive care:** Provides care to pediatric patients that is of a more intensive nature than that usually provided to pediatric patients. The unit is staffed with specially trained personnel and contains monitoring and specialized support equipment for treatment of patients who, because of shock, trauma, or other life-threatening conditions, require intensified, comprehensive observation and care.

**Pediatric medical-surgical care:** Provides acute care to pediatric patients on the basis of physicians' orders and approved nursing care plans.

**Personnel:** Number of persons on the hospital payroll at the end of the reporting period. Personnel are recorded in *Hospital Statistics* as full-time equivalents (FTEs), which are calculated by adding the number of full-time personnel to one-half the number of part-time personnel, excluding medical and dental residents, interns, and other trainees. *Per 100 adjusted census* indicates the ratio of personnel to adjusted average daily census, calculated on a per-100 basis.

**Physical rehabilitation inpatient care:** Provides care encompassing a comprehensive array of restoration services for the disabled and all support services necessary to help patients attain their maximum functional capacity.

**Physical rehabilitation outpatient services:** Outpatient program providing medical, health-related, therapy, social, and/or vocational services to help disabled persons attain or retain their maximum functional capacity.

**Population:** Population refers to the residential population of the United States. This includes both civilian and military personnel. Note that population is being used to calculate the values *for community health indicators per 1000 population.*

**Positron emission tomography scanner (PET):** A nuclear medicine imaging technology which uses radioactive (positron emitting) isotopes created in a cyclotron or generator and computers to produce composite pictures of the brain and heart at work. PET scanning produces sectional images depicting metabolic activity or blood flow rather than anatomy.

**Preferred provider organization (PPO):** A pre-set arrangement in which purchasers and providers agree to furnish specified health services to a group of employees/patients.

**Primary care department:** A unit or clinic within the hospital that provides primary care services (e.g. general pediatric care, general internal medicine, family practice, gynecology) through hospital-salaried medical and/or nursing staff, focusing on evaluating and diagnosing medical problems and providing medical treatment on an outpatient basis.

**Psychiatric child-adolescent services:** Provides care to emotionally disturbed children and adolescents, including those admitted for diagnosis and those admitted for treatment.

**Psychiatric consultation-liaison services:** Provides organized psychiatric consultation/liaison services to nonpsychiatric hospital staff and/or departments on psychological aspects of medical care that may be generic or specific to individual patients.

**Psychiatric education services:** Provides psychiatric educational services to community agencies and workers such as schools, police, courts, public health nurses, welfare agencies, clergy, and so forth. The purpose is to expand the mental health knowledge and competence of personnel not working in the mental health field and to promote good mental health through improved understanding, attitudes, and behavioral patterns.

**Psychiatric emergency services:** Services of facilities available on a 24-hour basis to provide immediate unscheduled out-patient care, diagnosis, evaluation, crisis intervention, and assistance to persons suffering acute emotional or mental distress.

**Psychiatric geriatric services:** Provides care to emotionally disturbed elderly patients, including those admitted for diagnosis and those admitted for treatment.

**Psychiatric inpatient care:** Provides acute or long-term care to emotionally disturbed patients, including patients admitted for diagnosis and those admitted for treatment of psychiatric problems, on the basis of physicians' orders and approved nursing care plans. Long-term care may include intensive supervision to the chronically mentally ill, mentally disordered, or other mentally incompetent persons.

**Psychiatric outpatient services:** Provides medical care, including diagnosis and treatment, of psychiatric outpatients.

**Psychiatric partial hospitalization program:** Organized hospital services of intensive day/evening outpatient services of three hours of more duration, distinguished from other outpatient visits of one hour.

**Radiation therapy:** The branch of medicine concerned with radioactive substances and using various techniques of visualization, with the diagnosis and treatment of disease using any of the various sources of radiant energy. Services could include: megavoltage radiation therapy; radioactive implants; stereotactic radiosurgery; therapeutic radioisotope facility; X-ray radiation therapy.

**Registered nurse (RN):** A nurse who has graduated from an approved school of nursing and who is currently registered by the state. RNs are responsible for the nature and quality of all nursing care that patients receive. In these tables, the number of RNs does not include those registered nurses more appropriately reported in other occupational categories, such as facility administrators, which are listed under *all other personnel* (Tables 1 and 2).

**Rehabilitation services:** A wide array of restoration services for disabled and recuperating patients, including all support services necessary to help them attain their maximum functional capacity.

**Retirement housing:** A facility which provides social activities to senior citizens, usually retired persons, who do not require health care but some short-term skilled nursing care may be provided. A retirement center may furnish housing and may also have acute hospital and long-term care facilities, or it may arrange for acute and long term care through affiliated institutions.

**Rural:** A rural hospital is located outside a metropolitan statistical area (MSA), as designated by the U.S. Office of Management and Budget, which is a geographically defined, integrated social and economic unit with a large population nucleus.

**Single photon emission computerized tomography (SPECT):** A nuclear medicine imaging technology that combines existing technology of gamma camera imaging with computed tomographic imaging technology to provide a more precise and clear image.

**Skilled nursing care:** Provides non-acute medical and skilled nursing care services, therapy, and social services under the supervision of a licensed registered nurse on a 24-hour basis.

**Sleep Center:** Specially equipped and staffed center for the diagnosis and treatment of sleep disorders.

**Social work services** (could include)**:** Organized services that are properly directed and sufficiently staffed by qualified individuals who provide assistance and counseling to patients and their families in dealing with social, emotional, and environmental problems associated with illness or disability, often in the context of financial or discharge planning coordination.

**Sports medicine:** Provision of diagnostic screening and assessment and clinical and rehabilitation services for the prevention and treatment of sports-related injuries.

**Support groups:** A hospital sponsored program which allows a group of individuals with the same or similar problems who meet periodically to share experiences, problems, and solutions in order to support each other.

**Surgical operations:** Those surgical operations, whether major or minor, performed in the operating room(s). A surgical operation involving more than one surgical procedure is still considered only one surgical operation.

**Swing bed services:** A hospital bed that can be used to provide either acute or long-term care depending on community or patient needs. To be eligible a hospital must have a Medicare provider agreement in place, have fewer than 100 beds, be located in a rural area, do not have a 24 hour nursing service waiver in effect, have not been terminated from the program in the prior two years, and meet various service conditions.

**Teen outreach services:** A program focusing on the teenager which encourages an improved health status and a healthful lifestyle including physical, emotional, mental, social, spiritual and economic health through education, exercise, nutrition and health promotion.

**Tobacco treatment/cessation program:** Organized hospital services with the purpose of ending tobacco-use habits of patients addicted to tobacco/nicotine.

**Transplant services:** The branch of medicine that transfers an organ or tissue from one person to another or from one body part to another to replace a diseased structure or to restore function or to change appearance. Services could include: Bone marrow transplant program; kidney transplant; organ transplant (other than kidney); tissue transplant.

**Transportation to health facilities:** A long-term care support service designed to assist the mobility of the elderly. Some programs offer improved financial access by offering reduced rates and barrier-free buses or vans with ramps and lifts to assist the elderly or handicapped; others offer subsidies for public transport systems or operate mini-bus services exclusively for use by senior citizens.

**Trauma center (certified):** A facility to provide emergency and specialized intensive care to critically ill and injured patients. **Level 1:** A regional resource trauma center, which is capable of providing total care for every aspect of injury and plays a leadership role in trauma research and education. **Level 2:** A community trauma center, which is capable of providing trauma care to all but the most severely injured patients who require highly specialized care. **Level 3:** A rural trauma hospital, which is capable of providing care to a large number of injury victims and can resuscitate and stabilize more severely injured patients so that they can be transported to Level 1 or 2 facilities.

**Ultrasound:** The use of acoustic waves above the range of 20,000 cycles per second to visualize internal body structures.

**Urban:** An urban hospital is located inside a Metropolitan Statistical Area (MSA), designated by the U.S. Office of Management and Budget, which is a geographically defined, integrated social and economic unit with a large population base.

**Urgent care center:** A facility that provides care and treatment for problems that are not life-threatening but require attention over the short term. These units function like emergency rooms but are separate from hospitals with which they may have backup affiliation arrangements.

**Volunteer services department:** An organized hospital department responsible for coordinating the services of volunteers working within the institution.

**Women's health center/services:** An area set aside for coordinated education and treatment services specifically for and promoted to women as provided by this special unit. Services may or may not include obstetrics but include a range of services other than OB.

**Wound Management Services:** Services for patients with chronic wounds and nonhealing wounds often resulting from diabetes, poor circulation, improper seating and immunocompromising conditions. The goals are to progress chronic wounds through stages of healing, reduce and eliminate infections, increase physical function to minimize complications from current wounds and prevent future chronic wounds. Wound management services are provided on an inpatient or outpatient basis, depending on the intensity of service needed.

# 2003 AHA Annual Survey
# Health Forum, L.L.C.

AHA ID ____________________

NAME OF HOSPITAL ________________________________

CITY, STATE, ZIP ________________________________

**Please return to:**
**AHA Annual Survey**
**One North Franklin, 29th Floor**
**Chicago, Illinois 60606**

## A. REPORTING PERIOD (please refer to the instructions and definitions at the end of this questionnaire)

Report data for a full 12-month period, preferably your last completed fiscal year (365 days). (Be consistent in using the same reporting period for responses throughout various sections of this survey.)

1. Reporting Period used (beginning and ending date) ...... __ __ / __ __ / __ __ __ __ to __ __ / __ __ / __ __ __ __
   (Month / Day / Year to Month / Day / Year)

2. a. Were you in operation 12 full months at the end of your reporting period ......................... YES ☐ NO ☐

   b. Number of days open during reporting period ....... ________

3. Indicate the beginning of your current fiscal year ......... __ __ / __ __ / __ __ __ __
   (Month / Day / Year)

## B. ORGANIZATIONAL STRUCTURE

1. **CONTROL**

   Indicate the type of organization that is responsible for establishing policy for overall operation of your hospital. CHECK ONLY ONE:

   **Government, nonfederal**
   - ☐ 12 State
   - ☐ 13 County
   - ☐ 14 City
   - ☐ 15 City-County
   - ☐ 16 Hospital district or authority

   **Nongovernment, not-for profit (NFP)**
   - ☐ 21 Church-operated
   - ☐ 23 Other not-for-profit (including NFP Corporation)

   **Investor-owned, for-profit**
   - ☐ 31 Individual
   - ☐ 32 Partnership
   - ☐ 33 Corporation

   **Government, federal**
   - ☐ 41 Air Force
   - ☐ 42 Army
   - ☐ 43 Navy
   - ☐ 44 Public Health Service
   - ☐ 45 Veterans' Affairs
   - ☐ 46 Federal other than 41-45 or 47-48
   - ☐ 47 PHS Indian Service
   - ☐ 48 Department of Justice

2. **SERVICE**

   Indicate the ONE category that BEST describes your hospital or the type of service it provides to the MAJORITY of admissions:
   - ☐ 10 General medical and surgical
   - ☐ 11 Hospital unit of an institution (prison hospital, college infirmary)
   - ☐ 12 Hospital unit within an institution for the mentally retarded
   - ☐ 22 Psychiatric
   - ☐ 33 Tuberculosis and other respiratory diseases
   - ☐ 41 Cancer
   - ☐ 42 Heart
   - ☐ 44 Obstetrics and gynecology
   - ☐ 45 Eye, ear, nose, and throat
   - ☐ 46 Rehabilitation
   - ☐ 47 Orthopedic
   - ☐ 48 Chronic disease
   - ☐ 62 Institution for mentally retarded
   - ☐ 80 Acute Long-Term Care
   - ☐ 82 Alcoholism and other chemical dependency
   - ☐ 49 Other-specify treatment area: ________________

3. **OTHER**

   a. Does your hospital restrict admissions primarily to children? ........................................ YES ☐ NO ☐

   b. Is your hospital primarily osteopathic? ........................................ YES ☐ NO ☐

## B. Organizational Structure (continued)

c. Does the hospital itself operate subsidiary corporations? ........................................................ YES ☐ No ☐

d. Is the hospital contract managed? If yes, please provide the name, city, and state of the organization ... YES ☐ No ☐
Name: ____________________ City: ____________________ State: __________

e. Is the hospital a participant in a network? If yes, please provide the name and telephone number........ YES ☐ No ☐
of the network. If the hospital participates in more than one network, please provide the name, address, city, state and telephone number of the network(s) on page 8, under supplemental information.
Name: ____________________ City: ____________________ State: _____ Telephone__________________

f. Does the hospital participate in a group purchasing arrangement? If yes, please provide the............ YES ☐ No ☐
name, city, and state of the group purchasing organization:

Name: ______________________________ City: ______________________________ State: ______

## C. FACILITIES AND SERVICES

For each service or facility listed below, please check all the categories that describe how each item is provided as of the last day of the reporting period. Check all categories that apply for an item. Leave all categories blank for a facility or service that is not provided. Column 3 refers to the networks that were identified in section B, question 3e.

| | (1) Owned or provided by my hospital or it's subsidiary | (2) Provided by my Health System (in my local community) | (3) Provided by my network (in my local community) | (4) Provided through a formal contractual arrangement or joint venture with another provider that is not in my system or network (in my local community) |
|---|---|---|---|---|
| 1. General medical-surgical care ................ | ☐ (# Beds: _____) | ☐ | ☐ | ☐ |
| 2. Pediatric medical-surgical care .............. | ☐ (# Beds: _____) | ☐ | ☐ | ☐ |
| 3. Obstetrics [Level of unit (1-3): (______).......... | ☐ (# Beds: _____) | ☐ | ☐ | ☐ |
| 4. Medical surgical intensive care .............. | ☐ (# Beds: _____) | ☐ | ☐ | ☐ |
| 5. Cardiac intensive care .......................... | ☐ (# Beds: _____) | ☐ | ☐ | ☐ |
| 6. Neonatal intensive care ........................ | ☐ (# Beds: _____) | ☐ | ☐ | ☐ |
| 7. Neonatal intermediate care ................... | ☐ (# Beds: _____) | ☐ | ☐ | ☐ |
| 8. Pediatric intensive care ........................ | ☐ (# Beds: _____) | ☐ | ☐ | ☐ |
| 9. Burn care .......................................... | ☐ (# Beds: _____) | ☐ | ☐ | ☐ |
| 10. Other special care ............................... | ☐ (# Beds: _____) | ☐ | ☐ | ☐ |
| 11. Other intensive care (specify:_____________) | ☐ (# Beds: _____) | ☐ | ☐ | ☐ |
| 12. Physical rehabilitation ........................... | ☐ (# Beds: _____) | ☐ | ☐ | ☐ |
| 13. Alcoholism-drug abuse or dependency care. | ☐ (# Beds: _____) | ☐ | ☐ | ☐ |
| 14. Psychiatric care .................................. | ☐ (# Beds: _____) | ☐ | ☐ | ☐ |
| 15. Skilled nursing care .............................. | ☐ (# Beds: _____) | ☐ | ☐ | ☐ |
| 16. Intermediate nursing care ....................... | ☐ (# Beds: _____) | ☐ | ☐ | ☐ |
| 17. Acute long term care .............................. | ☐ (# Beds: _____) | ☐ | ☐ | ☐ |
| 18. Other long term care ................................. | ☐ (# Beds: _____) | ☐ | ☐ | ☐ |
| 19. Other care (specify: _________________ ).. | ☐ (# Beds: _____) | ☐ | ☐ | ☐ |

## C. FACILITIES AND SERVICES (continued)

| | (1) Owned or provided by my hospital or it's subsidiary | (2) Provided by my Health System (in my local community) | (3) Provided by my network (in my local community) | (4) Provided through a formal contractual arrangement or joint venture with another provider that is not in my system or network (in my local community) |
|---|---|---|---|---|
| 20. Adult day care program | ☐ | ☐ | ☐ | ☐ |
| 21. Airborne infection isolation room (# rooms________) | ☐ | ☐ | ☐ | ☐ |
| 22. Alcoholism-drug abuse or dependency outpatient services | ☐ | ☐ | ☐ | ☐ |
| 23. Alzheimer Center | ☐ | ☐ | ☐ | ☐ |
| 24. Ambulance services | ☐ | ☐ | ☐ | ☐ |
| 25. Arthritis treatment center | ☐ | ☐ | ☐ | ☐ |
| 26. Assisted living | ☐ | ☐ | ☐ | ☐ |
| 27. Auxiliary | ☐ | ☐ | ☐ | ☐ |
| 28. Bariatric/weight control services | ☐ | ☐ | ☐ | ☐ |
| 29. Birthing room - LDR room -LDRP room | ☐ | ☐ | ☐ | ☐ |
| 30. Breast cancer screening/mammograms | ☐ | ☐ | ☐ | ☐ |
| 31. Cardiology services | ☐ | ☐ | ☐ | ☐ |
| a. Angioplasty | ☐ | ☐ | ☐ | ☐ |
| b. Cardiac catheterization laboratory | ☐ | ☐ | ☐ | ☐ |
| c. Open heart surgery | ☐ | ☐ | ☐ | ☐ |
| 32. Case management | ☐ | ☐ | ☐ | ☐ |
| 33. Chaplaincy/pastoral care services. | ☐ | ☐ | ☐ | ☐ |
| 34. Chemotherapy | ☐ | ☐ | ☐ | ☐ |
| 35. Children wellness program | ☐ | ☐ | ☐ | ☐ |
| 36. Chiropractic services | ☐ | ☐ | ☐ | ☐ |
| 37. Community outreach | ☐ | ☐ | ☐ | ☐ |
| 38. Complementary medicine services | ☐ | ☐ | ☐ | ☐ |
| 39. Crisis prevention | ☐ | ☐ | ☐ | ☐ |
| 40. Dental services | ☐ | ☐ | ☐ | ☐ |
| 41. Emergency services | | | | |
| a. Emergency department | ☐ | ☐ | ☐ | ☐ |
| b. Trauma center (certified) [Level of unit (1-3):] ______ | ☐ | ☐ | ☐ | ☐ |
| 42. Enabling services | ☐ | ☐ | ☐ | ☐ |
| 43. End of life service | | | | |
| a. Hospice program | ☐ | ☐ | ☐ | ☐ |
| b. Pain management program | ☐ | ☐ | ☐ | ☐ |
| c. Palliative care program | ☐ | ☐ | ☐ | ☐ |
| 44. Enrollment assistance services | ☐ | ☐ | ☐ | ☐ |
| 45. Extracorporeal shock wave lithotripter (ESWL) | ☐ | ☐ | ☐ | ☐ |
| 46. Fitness center | ☐ | ☐ | ☐ | ☐ |
| 47. Freestanding outpatient care center | ☐ | ☐ | ☐ | ☐ |
| 48. Geriatric services | ☐ | ☐ | ☐ | ☐ |
| 49. Gamma knife | ☐ | ☐ | ☐ | ☐ |
| 50. Health fair | ☐ | ☐ | ☐ | ☐ |
| 51. Health information center | ☐ | ☐ | ☐ | ☐ |
| 52. Health screenings | ☐ | ☐ | ☐ | ☐ |
| 53. Hemodialysis | ☐ | ☐ | ☐ | ☐ |
| 54. HIV-AIDS services | ☐ | ☐ | ☐ | ☐ |
| 55. Home health services... | ☐ | ☐ | ☐ | ☐ |

## C. FACILITIES AND SERVICES (continued)

| | (1) Owned or provided by my hospital or it's subsidiary | (2) Provided by my Health System (in my local community) | (3) Provided by my network (in my local community) | (4) Provided through a formal contractual arrangement or joint venture with another provider that is not in my system or network (in my local community) |
|---|---|---|---|---|
| 56. Hospital-based outpatient care center-services | ☐ | ☐ | ☐ | ☐ |
| 57. Linguistic/translation services | ☐ | ☐ | ☐ | ☐ |
| 58. Meals on wheels | ☐ | ☐ | ☐ | ☐ |
| 59. Neurological services | ☐ | ☐ | ☐ | ☐ |
| 60. Nutrition programs | ☐ | ☐ | ☐ | ☐ |
| 61. Occupational health services | ☐ | ☐ | ☐ | ☐ |
| 62. Oncology services | ☐ | ☐ | ☐ | ☐ |
| 63. Orthopedic services | ☐ | ☐ | ☐ | ☐ |
| 64. Outpatient surgery | ☐ | ☐ | ☐ | ☐ |
| 65. Patient education center | ☐ | ☐ | ☐ | ☐ |
| 66. Patient representative services | ☐ | ☐ | ☐ | ☐ |
| 67. Physical rehabilitation outpatient services | ☐ | ☐ | ☐ | ☐ |
| 68. Primary care department | ☐ | ☐ | ☐ | ☐ |
| 69. Psychiatric services | | | | |
| a. Psychiatric child-adolescent services | ☐ | ☐ | ☐ | ☐ |
| b. Psychiatric consultation-liaison services | ☐ | ☐ | ☐ | ☐ |
| c. Psychiatric education services | ☐ | ☐ | ☐ | ☐ |
| d. Psychiatric emergency services | ☐ | ☐ | ☐ | ☐ |
| e. Psychiatric geriatric services | ☐ | ☐ | ☐ | ☐ |
| f. Psychiatric outpatient services | ☐ | ☐ | ☐ | ☐ |
| g. Psychiatric partial hospitalization program | ☐ | ☐ | ☐ | ☐ |
| 70. Radiation therapy | ☐ | ☐ | ☐ | ☐ |
| a. Intensity-Modulated Radiation Therapy (IMRT) | ☐ | ☐ | ☐ | ☐ |
| 71. Radiology, diagnostic | | | | |
| a. CT scanner | ☐ | ☐ | ☐ | ☐ |
| b. Diagnostic radioisotope facility | ☐ | ☐ | ☐ | ☐ |
| c. Electron Beam Computed Tomography (EBCT) | ☐ | ☐ | ☐ | ☐ |
| d. Magnetic resonance imaging (MRI) | ☐ | ☐ | ☐ | ☐ |
| e. Multislice spiral computed tomography(MSCT) | ☐ | ☐ | ☐ | ☐ |
| f. Positron emission tomography (PET) | ☐ | ☐ | ☐ | ☐ |
| g. Single photon emission computerized tomography (SPECT). | ☐ | ☐ | ☐ | ☐ |
| h. Ultrasound | ☐ | ☐ | ☐ | ☐ |
| 72. Reproductive health | | | | |
| a. Fertility Clinic | ☐ | ☐ | ☐ | ☐ |
| b. Genetic testing/counseling | ☐ | ☐ | ☐ | ☐ |
| 73. Retirement housing | ☐ | ☐ | ☐ | ☐ |
| 74. Sleep Center | ☐ | ☐ | ☐ | ☐ |
| 75. Social work services | ☐ | ☐ | ☐ | ☐ |
| 76. Sports medicine | ☐ | ☐ | ☐ | ☐ |
| 77. Support groups | ☐ | ☐ | ☐ | ☐ |
| 78. Swing bed services | ☐ | ☐ | ☐ | ☐ |

## C. FACILITIES AND SERVICES (continued)

| | (1) Owned or provided by my hospital or it's subsidiary | (2) Provided by my Health System (in my local community) | (3) Provided by my network (in my local community) | (4) Provided through a formal contractual arrangement or joint venture with another provider that is not in my system or network (in my local community) |
|---|---|---|---|---|
| 79. Teen outreach services | ☐ | ☐ | ☐ | ☐ |
| 80. Tobacco Treatment/Cessation program | ☐ | ☐ | ☐ | ☐ |
| 81. Transplant services | ☐ | ☐ | ☐ | ☐ |
| 82. Transportation to health facilities | ☐ | ☐ | ☐ | ☐ |
| 83. Urgent care center | ☐ | ☐ | ☐ | ☐ |
| 84. Volunteer services department | ☐ | ☐ | ☐ | ☐ |
| 85. Women's health center/services | ☐ | ☐ | ☐ | ☐ |
| 86. Wound Management Services | ☐ | ☐ | ☐ | ☐ |

87. In which of the following physician arrangements does your hospital or system/network participate? Column 3 refers to the networks that were identified in section b, question 3f. For hospital level physician arrangements that are reported in column 1, please report the number of physicians involved.

| | (1) My Hospital | | (2) My Heatlh System | (3) My Health Network |
|---|---|---|---|---|
| a. Independent Practice Association | ☐ | (# of physicians ________) | ☐ | ☐ |
| b. Group practice without walls | ☐ | (# of physicians ________) | ☐ | ☐ |
| c. Open Physician-Hospital Organization (PHO) | ☐ | (# of physicians ________) | ☐ | ☐ |
| d. Closed Physician-Hospital Organization (PHO) | ☐ | (# of physicians ________) | ☐ | ☐ |
| e. Management Service Organization (MSO) | ☐ | (# of physicians ________) | ☐ | ☐ |
| f. Integrated Salary Model | ☐ | (# of physicians ________) | ☐ | ☐ |
| g. Equity Model | ☐ | (# of physicians ________) | ☐ | ☐ |
| h. Foundation | ☐ | (# of physicians ________) | ☐ | ☐ |

Please provide a separate list of the name(s) and address(es) of the hospital's physician arrangements reported in column 1.

88. Does your hospital, health system or health network have an equity interest in any of the following insurance products? (Check all that apply) Contractual relationships with HMOs and PPOs should not be reported here but in Question 88. Column 3 refers to the networks that were identified in section B, question 3f.

| | (1) My Hospital | (2) My Health System | (3) My Health Network | (4) Joint Venture With Insurer |
|---|---|---|---|---|
| a. Health Maintenance Organization | ☐ | ☐ | ☐ | ☐ |
| b. Preferred Provider Organization | ☐ | ☐ | ☐ | ☐ |
| c. Indemnity Fee For Service Plan | ☐ | ☐ | ☐ | ☐ |

89. Does your hospital have a formal written contract that specifies the obligations of each party with:

a. Health maintenance organization (HMO) .............. YES ☐ NO ☐ b. If YES, how many contracts? ________

b. Preferred provider organization (PPO) ................. YES ☐ NO ☐ d. If YES, how many contracts? ________

90a. What percentage of the hospital's net patient revenue is paid on a capitated basis?
If the hospital does not participate in capitated arrangements, please enter "0") ________ %

90b. What percentage of the hospital's net patient revenue is paid on a shared risk basis? ________ %

91. Does your hospital contract directly with employers or a coalition of employers to provide care on a capitated, predetermined, or shared risk basis? ............ YES ☐ NO ☐

92. If your hospital has arrangements to care for a specific group of enrollees in exchange for a capitated payment, how many lives are covered? ________

## D. COMMUNITY ORIENTATION

1. Does your hospital's mission statement include a focus on community benefit? ............................................. YES ☐ NO ☐
2. Does your hospital have a long-term plan for improving the health of its community? ....................................... YES ☐ NO ☐
3. Does your hospital have resources for its community benefit activities? ........................................................ YES ☐ NO ☐
4. Does your hospital work with other providers, public agencies, or community representatives to conduct a health status assessment of the community? ........................................................................................................ YES ☐ NO ☐
5. Does your hospital use health status indicators (such as rates of health problems or surveys of self-reported health) for defined populations to design new services or modify existing services? ......................................... YES ☐ NO ☐

6a. Does your hospital work with other local providers, public agencies, or community representatives to develop a written assessment of the appropriate capacity for health services in the community? ...................................... YES ☐ NO ☐

6b. If yes, have you used the assessment to identify unmet health needs, excess capacity, or duplicative services in the community? ........................................................................................................................ YES ☐ NO ☐

7. Does your hospital work with other providers to collect, track, and communicate clinical and health information across cooperating organizations? .................................................................................................. YES ☐ NO ☐
8. Does your hospital either by itself or in conjunction with others disseminate reports to the community on the quality and costs of health care services? ............................................................................................ YES ☐ NO ☐
9. Does your hospital self-assess against Baldrige like criteria for sustained continuous improvement? ..................... YES ☐ NO ☐
10. Does your hospital gather information on a patient's race/ethnicity at any point during their stay?....... ..................... YES ☐ NO ☐
11. Does your hospital gather information on a patient's primary language at any point during their stay?.........................YES ☐ NO ☐
12. Does your hospital participate in the Quality Initiative?.........................................................................................YES ☐ NO ☐
13. If yes, have you submitted data on: ...........☐ One condition ☐ Two conditions ☐ Three conditions ☐ No data submitted

## E. TOTAL FACILITY BEDS, UTILIZATION, FINANCES, AND STAFFING

Please report beds, utilization, financial, and staffing data for a 12 month period that is consistent with the period reported on page 1. Report financial data for reporting period only. Include within your operations all activities that are wholly owned by the hospital, including subsidiary corporations regardless of where the activity is physically located. Please do not include within your operations distinct and separate divisions that may be owned by your hospital's parent corporation. If final figures are not available, please estimate. Round to the nearest dollar. Report all personnel who were on the payroll and whose payroll expenses are reported in E3f. (Please refer to specific definitions on pages 15-16.)

> Fill out column (2) if hospital owns and operates a nursing home type unit/facility. Column (1) should be the combined total of hospital plus Nursing Home Unit/Facility.

| | (1) Total Facility | (2) Nursing Home Unit/Facility |
|---|---|---|
| **1. BEDS AND UTILIZATION** | | |
| a. Total licensed beds | | |
| b. Beds set up and staffed for use at the end of the reporting period | | |
| c. Bassinets set up and staffed for use at the end of the reporting period | | |
| d. Births (exclude fetal deaths) | | |
| e. Admissions (exclude newborns, include neonatal & swing admissions) | | |
| f. Inpatient days (exclude newborns, include neonatal & swing days) | | |
| g. Emergency room visits | | |
| h. Total outpatient visits (include emergency room visits & outpatient surgeries) | | |
| i. Inpatient surgical operations | | |
| Number of operating rooms | | |
| j. Outpatient surgical operations | | |
| **2. MEDICARE/MEDICAID UTILIZATION** (exclude newborns, include neonatal & swing days and deaths) | | |
| a1. Total Medicare (Title XVIII) inpatient discharges (including Medicare Managed Care) | | |
| a2. How many Medicare inpatient discharges were Medicare Managed Care | | |
| b1. Total Medicare (Title XVIII) inpatient days (including Medicare Managed Care) | | |
| b2. How many Medicare inpatient days were Medicare Managed Care | | |
| c1. Total Medicaid (Title XIX) inpatient discharges (including Medicaid Managed Care) | | |
| c2. How many Medicaid inpatient discharges were Medicaid Managed Care | | |
| d1. Total Medicaid (Title XIX) inpatient days (including Medicaid Managed Care) | | |
| d2. How many Medicaid inpatient days were Medicaid Managed Care | | |
| **3. FINANCIAL** | | |
| * a. Net patient revenue | .00 | .00 |
| * b. Tax appropriations | .00 | |
| * c. Other operating revenue | .00 | |
| * d. Nonoperating revenue | .00 | |
| * e. TOTAL REVENUE (add 3a thru 3d) | .00 | .00 |
| f. PAYROLL EXPENSES (only) | .00 | .00 |
| g. Employee benefits | .00 | .00 |
| h. Depreciation expense (for reporting period only) | .00 | |
| i. Interest expense | .00 | |
| j. TOTAL EXPENSES (Payroll plus all non-payroll expenses, including bad debt) | .00 | .00 |
| ***4. REVENUE BY TYPE** | | |
| a. Total gross inpatient revenue | .00 | |
| b. Total gross outpatient revenue | .00 | |
| c. Total gross patient revenue | .00 | |
| ***5. UNCOMPENSATED CARE** | | |
| a. Bad debt expense | .00 | |
| b. Charity (Revenue forgone at full established rates. Include in gross revenue) | .00 | |

*These data will be treated as confidential and not released without written permission. AHA will, however, share these data with your respective state hospital association and, if requested, with your appropriate metropolitan/regional association. For members of the Catholic Health Association of the United States (CHA), AHA will also share these data with CHA unless there are objections expressed by checking this box ☐.
The state/metropolitan/regional association and CHA may not release these data without written permission from the hospital.

## E. TOTAL FACILITY BEDS, UTILIZATION, FINANCES, AND STAFFING (continued)

***6. REVENUE BY PAYOR (report total facility gross and net figures)**
(E.6a(2a) should include Medicaid disproportionate payments in the net column (2)

| | | (1) Gross | (2) Net |
|---|---|---|---|
| *a. GOVERNMENT | (1) Medicare: | | |
| | a) Routine patient revenue | .00 | .00 |
| | b) Managed care revenue | .00 | .00 |
| | **c) Total (a + b)** | **.00** | **.00** |
| | (2) Medicaid: | | |
| | a) Routine patient revenue | .00 | .00 |
| | b) Managed care revenue | .00 | .00 |
| | **c) Total (a + b)** | **.00** | **.00** |
| | (3) Other government: | .00 | .00 |
| *b. NONGOVERNMENT | (1) Self-pay | .00 | .00 |
| | (2) Third-party payors: | | |
| | a) Managed care (includes HMO and PPO) | .00 | .00 |
| | b) Other third-party payors | .00 | .00 |
| | **c) Total third-party payors (a + b)** | **.00** | **.00** |
| | (3) All Other nongovernment: | .00 | .00 |
| *c. TOTAL | | **.00** | **.00** |

**(Total gross should equal 4c on page 7, total net should equal 3a on page 7.)**

**Are the financial data on pages 7 and 8 from your audited financial statement?** .......................... **YES** ☐ **No** ☐

**7. FIXED ASSETS**

| | | |
|---|---|---|
| a. | Property, plant and equipment at cost | .00 |
| b. | Accumulated depreciation | .00 |
| c. | Net property, plant and equipment (a-b) | .00 |
| **d.** | **Total gross square feet of your physical plant used for or in support of your healthcare activities** | **.00** |

*These data will be treated as confidential and not released without written permission. AHA will, however, share these data with your respective state hospital association and, if requested, with your appropriate metropolitan/regional association. For members of the Catholic Health Association of the United States (CHA), AHA will also share these data with CHA unless there are objections expressed by checking this box ☐.
The state/metropolitan/regional association and CHA may not release these data without written permission from the hospital.

8. **STAFFING**

Report full-time (35 hours or more) and part-time (less than 35 hours) personnel who were on the hospital/facility **payroll at the end of your reporting period.** Include members of religious orders for whom dollar equivalents were reported. Exclude private-duty nurses, volunteers, and all personnel whose salary is financed entirely by outside research grants. Exclude physicians and dentists who are paid on a fee basis. FTE is the total number of hours worked by all employees over the full (12 month) reporting period divided by the normal number of hours worked by a full-time employee for that same time period. For example, if your hospital considers a normal work week for a full-time employee to be 40 hours, a total of 2,080 would be worked over a full year (52 weeks). If the total number of hours worked by all employees on the payroll is 208,000, then the number of Full-Time Equivalents (FTE) is 100 (employees). The FTE calculation for a specific occupational category such as Registered nurses is exactly the same. The calculation for each occupational category should be based on the number of hours worked by staff employed in that specific category.

| | (1) Full-Time (35 hr/wk or more) On Payroll | (2) Part-Time (less than 35 hr/wk) On Payroll | (3) FTE |
|---|---|---|---|
| a. Physicians and dentists | ______ | ______ | ______ |
| b. Medical and dental residents/interns | ______ | ______ | ______ |
| c. Other trainees | ______ | ______ | ______ |
| d. Registered nurses | ______ | ______ | ______ |
| e. Licensed practical (vocational) nurses | ______ | ______ | ______ |
| f. Nursing assistive personnel | ______ | ______ | ______ |
| g. All other personnel | ______ | ______ | ______ |
| h. Total facility personnel (add 8a through 8g) (Should include hospital plus nursing home type unit/facility personnel) | ______ | ______ | ______ |
| i. Nursing home type unit/facility personnel (if applicable - please break out these personnel from the total facility number.) | ______ | ______ | ______ |

j. Do hospitalists provide care for patients in your hospital? .............................................. YES ☐ NO ☐

k. If yes, please report the number of full time and part time hospitalists? ____________Full-time____________Part-time

l. If yes, please select the category below that best describes the employment model for your hospitalists?

☐ Independent provider group ☐ Employed by your hospital

☐ Employed by a physician group ☐ Employed by a university or school program ☐ Other

## SUPPLEMENTAL INFORMATION

1. Does your hospital participate in any joint venture arrangements? ................................ YES ☐ NO ☐

2. Does your hospital provide services through a satellite facility(s)? ................................. YES ☐ NO ☐

3. For the titles listed below, please indicate the name and the exact title of the person who holds the position in the hospital.

| | Name | Title |
|---|---|---|
| a. Chief Financial Officer | ______ | ______ |
| b. Chief Information Officer | ______ | ______ |
| c. Vice President, Strategic Planning | ______ | ______ |
| d. Chief of the Medical Staff | ______ | ______ |

Use this space or an additional sheet if more space is required for comments or to elaborate on any of the information supplied on this survey. Refer to the response by page, section, and item name. Also, use this space to describe your community benefit activities.

As declared previously, hospital specific revenue data are treated as confidential. AHA's policy is not to release these data without written permission from your institution. The AHA will however, share these data with your respective state hospital association and if requested with your appropriate metropolitan/regional association.

On occasion, the AHA is asked to provide these data to external organizations, both public and private, for their use in analyzing crucial health care policy or research issues. The AHA is requesting your permission to allow us to release your confidential data to those requests that we consider legitimate and worthwhile. In every instance of disclosure, the receiving organization will be prohibited from releasing hospital specific information.

**Please indicate below whether or not you agree to these types of disclosure:**

[ ] I hereby grant AHA permission to release my hospital's revenue data to external users that the AHA determines have a legitimate and worthwhile need to gain access to these data subject to the user's agreement with the AHA not to release hospital specific information.

______________________________________________

Chief Executive Officer                    Date

[ ] I do not grant AHA permission to release my confidential data.

______________________________________________

Chief Executive Officer                    Date

**Does your hospital or health system have an Internet or Homepage address?** **Yes** ☐ **No** ☐

**If yes, please provide the address: http://** ______________________________

Thank you for your cooperation in completing this survey. If there are any questions about your responses to this survey, who should be contacted?

| Name (please print) | Title | (Area Code) Telephone Number |
|---|---|---|
| ____/____/____ Date of Completion | Chief Executive Officer | (___)______ Hospital's Main Fax Number |

**NOTE: PLEASE PHOTOCOPY THE INFORMATION FOR YOUR HOSPITAL FILE BEFORE RETURNING THE ORIGINAL FORM TO THE AMERICAN HOSPITAL ASSOCIATION. ALSO, PLEASE FORWARD A PHOTOCOPY OF THE COMPLETED QUESTIONNAIRE TO YOUR STATE HOSPITAL ASSOCIATION.**

**THANK YOU**

# SECTION A
# REPORTING PERIOD
## Instructions

**INSTRUCTIONS AND DEFINITIONS FOR THE 2002 ANNUAL SURVEY**

HOSPITAL. For purposes of this survey, a hospital is defined as the organization or corporate entity licensed or registered as a hospital by a state to provide diagnostic and therapeutic patient services for a variety of medical conditions, both surgical and nonsurgical.

1. **Reporting period used (beginning and ending date):** Record the beginning and ending dates of the reporting period in an eight-digit number: for example, January 1, 2003 should be shown as 01/01/2003. Number of days should equal the time span between the two dates that the hospital was open. If you are reporting for less than 365 days, utilization and finances should be presented for days reported only.
2. **Were you in operation 12 full months at the end of your reporting period?** If you are reporting for less than 365 days, utilization and finances should be presented for days reported only.
3. **Number of days open during reporting period:** Number of days should equal the time span between the two dates that the hospital was open.

# SECTION B
# ORGANIZATIONAL STRUCTURE
## Instructions and Definitions

1. CONTROL
   Check the box to the left of the type of organization that is responsible for establishing policy for overall operation of the hospital.
   **Government, nonfederal.**
   **State.** Controlled by an agency of state government.
   **County.** Controlled by an agency of county government.
   **City.** Controlled by an agency of municipal government.
   **City-County.** Controlled jointly by agencies of municipal and county governments.
   **Hospital district or authority.** Controlled by a political subdivision of a state, county, or city created solely for the purpose of establishing and maintaining medical care or health-related care institutions.
   **Nongovernment, not for profit.** Hospitals controlled by not-for-profit organizations, including religious organizations (Catholic hospitals, for example), community hospitals, cooperative hospitals, hospitals operated by fraternal societies, and so forth.
   **Investor owned, for profit.** Hospitals controlled on a for profit basis by an individual, partnership, or a profit making corporation.
   **Government, federal.** Hospitals controlled by an agency or department of the federal government.
2. SERVICE
   Indicate the ONE category that best describes the type of service that your hospital provides to the majority of admissions.
   **General medical and surgical.** Provides diagnostic and therapeutic services to patients for a variety of medical conditions, both surgical and nonsurgical.
   **Hospital unit of an institution.** Provides diagnostic and therapeutic services to patients in an institution.
   **Hospital unit within an institution for the mentally retarded.** Provides diagnostic and therapeutic services to patients in an institution for the mentally retarded.
   **Psychiatric.** Provides diagnostic and therapeutic services to patients with mental or emotional disorders.
   **Tuberculosis and other respiratory diseases.** Provides medical care and rehabilitative services to patients for whom the primary diagnosis is tuberculosis or other respiratory diseases.
   **Cancer.** Provides medical care to patients for whom the primary diagnosis is cancer.
   **Heart.** Provides diagnosis and treatment of heart disease.
   **Obstetrics and gynecology.** Provides medical and surgical treatment to pregnant women and to mothers following delivery. Also provides diagnostic and therapeutic services to women with diseases or disorders of the reproductive organs.
   **Eye, ear, nose, and throat.** Provides diagnosis and treatment of diseases and injuries of the eyes, ears, nose, and throat.
   **Rehabilitation.** Provides a comprehensive array of restoration services for the disabled and all support services necessary to help them attain their maximum functional capacity.
   **Orthopedic.** Provides corrective treatment of deformities, diseases, and ailments of the locomotive apparatus, especially affecting the limbs, bones, muscles, and joints.
   **Chronic disease.** Provides medical and skilled nursing services to patients with long-term illnesses who are not in an acute phase, but who require an intensity of services not available in nursing homes.
   **Institution for the mentally retarded.** Provides health-related care on a regular basis to patients with psychiatric or developmental impairment who cannot be treated in a skilled nursing unit.
   **Alcoholism and other chemical dependency.** Provides diagnostic and therapeutic services to patients with alcoholism or other drug dependencies.
   **Acute Long Term Care.** Provides high acuity interdisciplinary services to medically complex patients that require more intensive recuperation and care than can be provided in a typical nursing facility.
3. OTHER
   a. **Children admissions.** A hospital whose primary focus is the health and treatment of children and adolescents.
   b. **Osteopathic.** Osteopathic medicine is a medical practice based on a theory that diseases are due chiefly to a loss of structural integrity which can be restored by manipulation of the neuro-muscular and skeletal system, supplemented by therapeutic measures (as use of medicine or surgery).
   c. **Subsidiary.** A company that is wholly controlled by another or one that is more than 50% owned by another organization.
   d. **Contract managed.** General day-to-day management of an entire organization by another organization under a formal contract. Managing organization reports directly to the board of trustees or owners of the managed organization; managed organization retains total legal responsibility and ownership of the facility's assets and liabilities.
   e. **Network.** A group of hospitals, physicians, other providers, insurers and/or community agencies that voluntarily work together to coordinate and deliver health services
   f. **Group Purchasing Organization.** An organization whose primary function is to negotiate contracts for the purpose of purchasing for members of the group or has a central supply site for its members.

## SECTION C
## FACILITIES AND SERVICES
### Definitions

1. **General medical-surgical care.** Provides acute care to patients in medical and surgical units on the basis of physicians' orders and approved nursing care plans.
2. **Pediatric medical-surgical care.** Provides acute care to pediatric patients on the basis of physicians' orders and approved nursing care plans.
3. **Obstetrics.** Levels should be designated: (1) unit provides services for uncomplicated maternity and newborn cases; (2) unit provides services for uncomplicated cases, the majority of complicated problems, and special neonatal services; and (3) unit provides services for all serious illnesses and abnormalities and is supervised by a full-time maternal/fetal specialist.
4. **Medical surgical intensive care.** Provides patient care of a more intensive nature than the usual medical and surgical care, on the basis of physicians' orders and approved nursing care plans. These units are staffed with specially trained nursing personnel and contain monitoring and specialized support equipment for patients who because of shock, trauma or other life-threatening conditions require intensified comprehensive observation and care. Includes mixed intensive care units.
5. **Cardiac intensive care.** Provides patient care of a more specialized nature than the usual medical and surgical care, on the basis of physicians' orders and approved nursing care plans. The unit is staffed with specially trained nursing personnel and contains monitoring and specialized support or treatment equipment for patients who, because of heart seizure, open-heart surgery, or other life-threatening conditions, require intensified, comprehensive observation and care. May include myocardial infarction, pulmonary care, and heart transplant units.
6. **Neonatal intensive care.** A unit that must be separate from the newborn nursery providing intensive care to all sick infants including those with the very lowest birth weights (less than 1500 grams). NICU has potential for providing mechanical ventilation, neonatal surgery, and special care for the sickest infants born in the hospital or transferred from another institution. A full-time neonatologist serves as director of the NICU.
7. **Neonatal intermediate care.** A unit that must be separate from the normal newborn nursery and that provides intermediate and/or recover care and some specialized services, including immediate resuscitation, intravenous therapy, and capacity for prolonged oxygen therapy and monitoring.
8. **Pediatric intensive care.** Provides care to pediatric patients that is of a more intensive nature than that usually provided to pediatric patients. The unit is staffed with specially trained personnel and contains monitoring and specialized support equipment for treatment of patients who, because of shock, trauma, or other life-threatening conditions, require intensified, comprehensive observation and care.
9. **Burn care.** Provides care to severely burned patients. Severely burned patients are those with any of the following: (1) second-degree burns of more than 25% total body surface area for adults or 20% total body surface area for children: (2) third-degree burns of more than 10% total body surface area; (3) any severe burns of the hands, face, eyes, ears, or feet; or (4) all inhalation injuries, electrical burns, complicated burn injuries involving fractures and other major traumas, and all other poor risk factors.
10. **Other special care.** Provides care to patients requiring care more intensive than that provided in the acute area, yet not sufficiently intensive to require admission to an intensive care unit. Patients admitted to this area are usually transferred here from an intensive care unit once their condition has improved. These units are sometimes referred to as definitive observation, step-down, or progressive care units.
11. **Other intensive care.** A specially staffed, specialty equipped, separate section of a hospital dedicated to the observation, care, and treatment of patients with life threatening illnesses, injuries, or complications from which recovery is possible. It provides special expertise and facilities for the support of vital function and utilizes the skill of medical nursing and other staff experienced in the management of these problems.
12. **Physical rehabilitation.** Provides care encompassing a comprehensive array of restoration services for the disabled and all support services necessary to help patients attain their maximum functional capacity.
13. **Alcoholism-drug abuse or dependency care.** Provides diagnosis and therapeutic services to patients with alcoholism or other drug dependencies. Includes care for inpatient/residential treatment for patients whose course of treatment involves more intensive care than provided in an outpatient setting or where patient requires supervised withdrawal.
14. **Psychiatric care.** Provides acute or long-term care to emotionally disturbed patients, including patients admitted for diagnosis and those admitted for treatment of psychiatric problems, on the basis of physicians' orders and approved nursing care plans. Long-term care may include intensive supervision to the chronically mentally ill, mentally disordered, or other mentally incompetent persons.
15. **Skilled nursing care.** Provides non-acute medical and skilled nursing care services, therapy, and social services under the supervision of a licensed registered nurse on a 24-hour basis.
16. **Intermediate nursing care.** Provides health-related services (skilled nursing care and social services) to residents with a variety of physical conditions or functional disabilities. These residents do not require the care provided by a hospital or skilled nursing facility, but do need supervision and support services.
17. **Acute long term care.** Provides specialized acute hospital care to medically complex patients who are critically ill, have multisystem complications and/or failure, and require hospitalization averaging 25 days, in a facility offering specialized treatment programs and therapeutic intervention on a 24 hour/7 day a week basis.
18. **Other long term care.** Provision of long term care other than skilled nursing care or intermediate care. This can include residential care-elderly housing services for those who do not require daily medical or nursing services, but may require some assistance in the activities of daily living, or sheltered care facilities for developmentally disabled.
19. **Other care.** (specify) Any type of care other than those listed above.

**Total beds. The sum of the beds reported in this section should equal what you have reported in Section E for beds set up and staffed.**

20. **Adult day care program.** Program providing supervision, medical and psychological care, and social activities for older adults who live at home or in another family setting, but cannot be alone or prefer to be with others during the day. May include intake assessment, health monitoring, occupational therapy, personal care, noon meal, and transportation services.
21. **Airborne infection isolation room.** A single-occupancy room for patient care where environmental factors are controlled in an effort to minimize the transmission of those infectious agents, usually spread person to person by droplet nuclei associated with coughing and inhalation. Such rooms typically have specific ventilation requirements for controlled ventilation, air pressure and filtration.
22. **Alcoholism-drug abuse or dependency outpatient services.** Organized hospital services that provide medical care and/or rehabilitative treatment services to outpatients for whom the primary diagnosis is alcoholism or other chemical dependency.
23. **Alzheimer Center.** Facility that offers care to persons with Alzheimer's disease and their families through an integrated program of clinical services, research, and education.
24. **Ambulance services.** Provision of ambulance service to the ill and injured who require medical attention on a scheduled and unscheduled basis.
25. **Arthritis treatment center.** Specifically equipped and staffed center for the diagnosis and treatment of arthritis and other joint disorders.
26. **Assisted living.** A special combination of housing, supportive services, personalized assistance and health care designed to respond to the individual needs of those who need help in activities of daily living and instrumental activities of daily living. Supportive services are available, 24 hours a day, to meet scheduled and unscheduled needs, in a way that promotes maximum independence an dignity for each resident and encourages the involvement of a resident's family, neighbor and friends.

27. **Auxiliary.** A volunteer community organization formed to assist the hospital in carrying out its purpose and to serve as a link between the institution and the community.
28. **Bariactric/weight control services.** Bariatrics is the medical practice of weight reduction.
29. **Birthing room/LDR room/LDRP room.** A single-room type of maternity care with a more homelike setting for families than the traditional three-room unit (labor/delivery/recovery) with a separate postpartum area. A birthing room combines labor and delivery in one room. An LDR room accommodates three stages in the birthing process--labor, delivery, and recovery. An LDRP room accommodates all four stages of the birth process--labor, delivery, recovery, and postpartum.
30. **Breast cancer screening/mammograms.** Mammography screening - The use of breast x-ray to detect unsuspected breast cancer in asymptomatic women. Diagnostic mammography - The x-ray imaging of breast tissue in symptomatic women who are considered to have a substantial likelihood of having breast cancer already.
31. **Cardiology services.** Services which include the diagnosis and treatment of diseases and disorders involving the heart and circulatory system.
    a. **Angioplasty.** The reconstruction or restructuring of a blood vessel by operative means or by non-surgical techniques such as balloon dilation or laser.
    b. **Cardiac catheterization laboratory.** Facilities offering special diagnostic procedures for cardiac patients. Available procedures must include, but need not be limited to, introduction of a catheter into the interior of the heart by way of a vein or artery or by direct needle puncture. Procedures must be performed in a laboratory or a special procedure room.
    c. **Open heart surgery.** Heart surgery where the chest has been opened and the blood recirculated and oxygenated with the proper equipment and the necessary staff to perform the surgery.
32. **Case management.** A system of assessment, treatment planning, referral and follow-up that ensures the provision of comprehensive and continuous services and the coordination of payment and reimbursement for care.
33. **Chaplaincy/pastoral care services.** A service ministering religious activities and providing pastoral counseling to patients, their families, and staff of a health care organization.
34. **Chemotherapy.** An organized program for the treatment of cancer by the use of drugs or chemicals.
35. **Children wellness program.** A program that encourages improved health status and a healthful lifestyle of children through health education, exercise, nutrition and health promotion.
36. **Chiropractic services.** An organized clinical service including spinal manipulation or adjustment and related diagnostic and therapeutic services.
37. **Community outreach.** A program that systematically interacts with the community to identify those in need of services, alerting persons and their families to the availability of services, locating needed services, and enabling persons to enter the service delivery system.
38. **Complementary medicine services.** Organized hospital services or formal arrangements to providers that provide care or treatment not based solely on traditional western allopathic medical teachings as instructed in most U.S. medical schools. Includes any of the following: acupuncture, chiropractic, homeopathy, osteopathy, diet and lifestyle changes, herbal medicine, massage therapy, etc.
39. **Crisis prevention.** Services provided in order to promote physical and mental well being and the early identification of disease and ill health prior to the onset and recognition of symptoms so as to permit early treatment.
40. **Dental Services.** An organized dental service or dentists on staff, not necessarily involving special facilities, providing dental or oral services to inpatients or outpatients.
41. **Emergency services**. Health services that are provided after the onset of a medical condition that manifests itself by symptoms of sufficient severity, including severe pain, that the absence of immediate medical attention could reasonably be expected by a prudent layperson, who possesses an average knowledge of health and medicine, to result in placing the patient's health in serious jeopardy.
    a. **Emergency department.** Hospital facilities for the provision of unscheduled outpatient services to patients whose conditions require immediate care.
    b. **Trauma center (certified).** A facility to provide emergency and specialized intensive care to critically ill and injured patients. Level 1: A regional resource trauma center, which is capable of providing total care for every aspect of injury and plays a leadership role in trauma research and education. Level 2: A community trauma center, which is capable of providing trauma care to all but the most severely injured patients who require highly specialized care. Level 3: A rural trauma hospital, which is capable of providing care to a large number of injury victims and can resuscitate and stabilize more severely injured patients so that they can be transported to level 1 or 2 facilities. Please provide explanation on page 15 if necessary.
42. **Enabling services.** A program that is designed to help the patient access health care services by offering any of the following: transportation services, and/or referrals to local social services agencies.
43. **End of life services.** Services offered to patients suffering from chronic, severe, and life-threatening diseases including comprehensive services that give patients and caregivers the resources and the confidence to manage symptoms, avoid emergency room admissions and frequent hospitalization, and remain in familiar and comfortable settings.
    a. **Hospice Program.** A recognized clinical program with specific eligibility criteria that provides palliative medical care focused on relief of pain and symptom control and other services that address the emotional, social, financial and spiritual needs of terminally ill patients and their families. Hospice care can be provided either at home, in a hospital setting, or a free-standing facility.
    b. **Pain management program.** A recognized clinical service or program providing specialized medical care, drugs or therapies for the management of acute or chronic pain and other distressing symptoms, administered by specially trained physicians and other clinicians, to patients suffering from an acute illness of diverse causes.
    c. **Palliative care program.** An organized program providing specialized medical care, drugs or therapies for the management of acute or chronic pain and/or the control of symptoms administered by specially trained physicians and other clinicians; and supportive care services, such as counseling on advanced directives, spiritual care, and social services, to patients with advanced disease and their families.
44. **Enrollment assistance services.** A program that provides enrollment assistance for patients who are potentially eligible for public health insurance programs such as Medicaid, State Children's Health Insurance, or local/state indigent care programs. The specific services offered could include explanation of benefits, assist applicants in completing the application and locating all relevant documents, conduct eligibility interviews, and/or forward applications and documentation to state/local social service or health agency.
45. **Extracorporeal shock wave lithotripter (ESWL).** A medical device used for treating stones in the kidney or urether. The device disintegrates kidney stones noninvasively through the transmission of acoustic shock waves directed at the stones.
46. **Fitness center.** Provides exercise, testing, or evaluation programs and fitness activities to the community and hospital employees.
47. **Freestanding outpatient care center.** A facility owned and operated by the hospital, but physically separate from the hospital, that provides various medical treatments on an outpatient basis only. In addition to treating minor illnesses or injuries, the center will stabilize seriously ill or injured patients before transporting them to a hospital. Laboratory and radiology services are usually available.
48. **Gamma knife.** A non-invasive and bloodless procedure which uses a technological device that delivers concentrated gamma radiation to target points selected in the brain and is used for treatment on patients with brain tumors and other brain disorders.

49. **Geriatric services.** The branch of medicine dealing with the physiology of aging and the diagnosis and treatment of disease affecting the aged. Services could include: Adult day care; Alzheimer's diagnostic-assessment services; Comprehensive geriatric assessment; Emergency response system; Geriatric acute care unit; and/or Geriatric clinics.
50. **Health fair.** Community health education events that focus on the prevention of disease and promotion of health through such activities as audiovisual exhibits and free diagnostic services.
51. **Health information center.** Education which is directed at increasing the information of individuals and populations. It is intended to increase the ability to make informed personal, family and community health decisions by providing consumers with informed choices about health matters with the objective of improving health status.
52. **Health screening.** A preliminary procedure such as a test or examination to detect the most characteristic sign or signs of a disorder that may require further investigation.
53. **Hemodialysis:** Provision of equipment and personnel for the treatment of renal insufficiency on an inpatient or outpatient basis.
54. **HIV-AIDS services** (could include). HIV-AIDS unit-Special unit or team designated and equipped specifically for diagnosis, treatment, continuing care planning, and counseling services for HIV-AIDS patients and their families. General inpatient care for HIV-AIDS-Inpatient diagnosis and treatment for human immunodeficiency virus and acquired immunodeficiency syndrome patients, but dedicated unit is not available. Specialized outpatient program for HIV-AIDS-Special outpatient program providing diagnostic, treatment, continuing care planning, and counseling for HIV-AIDS patients and their families.
55. **Home health services.** Service providing nursing, therapy, and health-related homemaker or social services in the patient's home.
56. **Hospital-based outpatient care center-services.** Organized hospital health care services offered by appointment on an ambulatory basis. Services may include outpatient surgery, examination, diagnosis, and treatment of a variety of medical conditions on a nonemergency basis, and laboratory and other diagnostic testing as ordered by staff or outside physician referral.
57. **Linguistic/translation services.** Services provided by the hospital designed to make health care more accessible to non- English speaking patients and their physicians.
58. **Meals on wheels.** A hospital sponsored program which delivers meals to people, usually the elderly, who are unable to prepare their own meals. Low cost, nutritional meals are delivered to individuals' homes on a regular basis.
59. **Neurological services.** Services provided by the hospital dealing with the operative and nonoperative management of disorders of the central, peripheral, and autonomic nervous system.
60. **Nutrition programs.** Those services within a health care facility which are designed to provide inexpensive, nutritionally sound meals to patients.
61. **Occupational health services.** Includes services designed to protect the safety of employees from hazards in the work environment.
62. **Oncology services.** Inpatient and outpatient services for patients with cancer, including comprehensive care, support and guidance in addition to patient education and prevention, chemotherapy, counseling and other treatment methods.
63. **Orthopedic services.** Services provided for the prevention or correction of injuries or disorders of the skeletal system and associated muscles, joints and ligaments.
64. **Outpatient surgery.** Scheduled surgical services provided to patients who do not remain in the hospital overnight. The surgery may be performed in operating suites also used for inpatient surgery, specially designated surgical suites for outpatient surgery, or procedure rooms within an outpatient care facility.
65. **Patient education center.** Written goals and objectives for the patient and/or family related to therapeutic regimens, medical procedures, and self care.
66. **Patient representative services.** Organized hospital services providing personnel through whom patients and staff can seek solutions to institutional problems affecting the delivery of high-quality care and services.
67. **Physical rehabilitation outpatient services.** Outpatient program providing medical, health-related, therapy, social, and/or vocational services to help disabled persons attain or retain their maximum functional capacity.
68. **Primary care department.** A unit or clinic within the hospital that provides primary care services (e.g. general pediatric care, general internal medicine, family practice, gynecology) through hospital-salaried medical and/or nursing staff, focusing on evaluating and diagnosing medical problems and providing medical treatment on an outpatient basis.
69. **Psychiatric services:** Services provided by the hospital that offer immediate initial evaluation and treatment to patients with mental or emotional disorders.
    a. **Psychiatric child-adolescent services.** Provides care to emotionally disturbed children and adolescents, including those admitted for diagnosis and those admitted for treatment.
    b. **Psychiatric consultation-liaison services.** Provides organized psychiatric consultation/liaison services to nonpsychiatric hospital staff and/or departments on psychological aspects of medical care that may be generic or specific to individual patients.
    c. **Psychiatric education services.** Provides psychiatric educational services to community agencies and workers such as schools, police, courts, public health nurses, welfare agencies, clergy, and so forth. The purpose is to expand the mental health knowledge and competence of personnel not working in the mental health field and to promote good mental health through improved understanding, attitudes, and behavioral patterns.
    d. **Psychiatric emergency services.** Services of facilities available on a 24-hour basis to provide immediate unscheduled out-patient care, diagnosis, evaluation, crisis intervention, and assistance to persons suffering acute emotional or mental distress.
    e. **Psychiatric geriatric services.** Provides care to emotionally disturbed elderly patients, including those admitted for diagnosis and those admitted for treatment.
    f. **Psychiatric outpatient services.** Provides medical care, including diagnosis and treatment, of psychiatric outpatients
    g. **Psychiatric partial hospitalization program.** Organized hospital services of intensive day/evening outpatient services of three hours of more duration, distinguished from other outpatient visits of one hour.
70. **Radiation therapy.** The branch of medicine concerned with radioactive substances and using various techniques of visualization, with the diagnosis and treatment of disease using any of the various sources of radiant energy. Services could include: megavoltage radiation therapy; radioactive implants; stereotactic radiosurgery; therapeutic radioisotope facility; X-ray radiation therapy.
    a. **Intensity-Modulated Radiation Therapy(IMRT).** A type of three-dimensional radiation therapy, which improves the targeting of treatment delivery in a way that is likely to decrease damage to normal tissues and allows varying intensities.
71. **Radiology, diagnostic.** The branch of radiology that deals with the utilization of all modalities of radiant energy in medical Diagnoses and therapeutic procedures using radiologic guidance. This includes, but is not restricted to, imaging techniques and methodologies utilizing radiation emitted by x-ray tubes, radionnuclides, and ultrasonographic devices and the radiofrequency electromagnetic radiation emitted by atoms.
    a. **CT scanner.** Computed tomographic scanner for head or whole body scans.
    b. **Diagnostic radioisotope facility.** The use of radioactive isotopes (Radiopharmaceuticals) as tracers or indicators to detect an abnormal condition or disease.

c. **Electron beam computed tomography (EBCT).** A high tech computed tomography scan used to detect coronary artery disease by measuring coronary calcifications. This imaging procedure uses electron beams which are magnetically steered to produce a visual of the coronary artery and the images are produced faster than conventional CT scans.
d. **Magnetic resonance imaging (MRI).** The use of a uniform magnetic field and radio frequencies to study tissue and structure of the body. This procedure enables the visualization of biochemical activity of the cell in vivo without the use of ionizing radiation, radioisotopic substances, or high-frequency sound.
e. **Multislice spiral computed tomography (MSCT).** A specialized computed tomography procedure that provides three-dimensional processing and allows narrower and multiple slices with increased spatial resolution and faster scanning times as compared to a regular computed tomography scan.
f. **Positron emission tomography (PET).** Positron emission tomography scanner is a nuclear medicine imaging technology which uses radioactive (positron emitting) isotopes created in a cyclotron or generator and computers to produce composite pictures of the brain and heart at work. PET scanning produces sectional images depicting metabolic activity or blood flow rather than anatomy.
g. **Single photon emission computerized tomography (SPECT).** Single photon emission computerized tomography is a nuclear medicine imaging technology that combines existing technology of gamma camera imaging with computed tomographic imaging technology to provide a more precise and clear image.
h. **Ultrasound.** The use of acoustic waves above the range of 20,000 cycles per second to visualize internal body structures.

72. **Reproductive health**
a. **Fertility Clinic.** A specialized program set in an infertility center that provides counseling and education as well as advanced reproductive techniques such as: injectable therapy, reproductive surgeries, treatment for endometriosis, male factor infertility, tubal reversals, in vitro fertilization (IVF), donor eggs, and other such services to help patients achieve successful pregnancies.
a. **Genetic testing/counseling.** A service equipped with adequate laboratory facilities and directed by a qualified physician to advise parents and prospective parents on potential problems in cases of genetic defects. A genetic test is the analysis of human DNA, RNA, chromosomes, proteins, and certain metabolites in order to detect heritable disease-related genotypes, mutations, phenotypes, or karyotypes for clinical purposes. Genetic tests can have diverse purposes, including the diagnosis of genetic diseases in newborns, children, and adults; the identification of future health risks; the prediction of drug responses; and the assessment of risks to future children.

73. **Retirement housing.** A facility that provides social activities to senior citizens, usually retired persons, who do not require health care but some short-term skilled nursing care may be provided. A retirement center may furnish housing and may also have acute hospital and long-term care facilities, or it may arrange for acute and long-term care through affiliated institutions.
74. **Sleep Center.** Specially equipped and staffed center for the diagnosis and treatment of sleep disorders.
75. **Social work services** (could include). Organized services that are properly directed and sufficiently staffed by qualified individuals who provide assistance and counseling to patients and their families in dealing with social, emotional, and environmental problems associated with illness or disability, often in the context of financial or discharge planning coordination.
76. **Sports medicine.** Provision of diagnostic screening and assessment and clinical and rehabilitation services for the prevention and treatment of sports-related injuries.
77. **Support groups.** A hospital sponsored program that allows a group of individuals with the same or similar problems who meet periodically to share experiences, problems, and solutions in order to support each other.
78. **Swing bed services.** A hospital bed that can be used to provide either acute or long-term care depending on community or patient needs. To be eligible a hospital must have a Medicare provider agreement in place, have fewer than 100 beds, be located in a rural area, do not have a 24 hour nursing service waiver in effect, have not been terminated from the program in the prior two years, and meet various service conditions.
79. **Teen outreach services.** A program focusing on the teenager which encourages an improved health status and a healthful lifestyle including physical, emotional, mental, social, spiritual and economic health through education, exercise, nutrition and health promotion.
80. **Tobacco Treatment/Cessation Program.** Organized hospital services with the purpose of ending tobacco-use habits of patients addicted to tobacco/nicotine.
81. **Transplant services.** The branch of medicine that transfers an organ or tissue from one person to another or from one body part to another to replace a diseased structure or to restore function or to change appearance. Services could include: Bone marrow transplant program; kidney transplant; organ transplant (other than kidney); tissue transplant.
82 **Transportation to health facilities.** A long-term care support service designed to assist the mobility of the elderly. Some programs offer improved financial access by offering reduced rates and barrier-free buses or vans with ramps and lifts to assist the elderly or handicapped; others offer subsidies for public transport systems or operate mini-bus services exclusively for use by senior citizens.
83. **Urgent care center.** A facility that provides care and treatment for problems that are not life-threatening but require attention over the short term. These units function like emergency rooms but are separate from hospitals with which they may have backup affiliation arrangements.
84. **Volunteer services department.** An organized hospital department responsible for coordinating the services of volunteers working within the institution.
85. **Women's health center/services.** An area set aside for coordinated education and treatment services specifically for and promoted to women as provided by this special unit. Services may or may not include obstetrics but include a range of services other than OB.
86. **Wound Management Services.** Services for patients with chronic wounds and nonhealing wounds often resulting from diabetes, poor circulation, improper seating and immunocompromising conditions. The goals are to progress chronic wounds through stages of healing, reduce and eliminate infections, increase physical function to minimize complications from current wounds and prevent future chronic wounds. Wound management services are provided on an inpatient or outpatient basis, depending on the intensity of service needed.
87. **Physician arrangements.** An integrated healthcare delivery program implementing physician compensation and incentive systems for managed care services.
a. **Independent practice association (IPA).** AN IPA is a legal entity that holds managed care contracts. The IPA then contracts with physicians, usually in solo practice, to provide care either on a fee-for-services or capitated basis. The purpose of an IPA is to assist solo physicians in obtaining managed care contracts.
b. **Group practice without walls.** Hospital sponsors the formation of, or provides capital to physicians to establish, a "quasi" group to share administrative expenses while remaining independent practitioners.
c. **Open physician-hospital organization (PHO).** A joint venture between the hospital and all members of the medical staff who wish to participate. The PHO can act as a unified agent in managed care contracting, own a managed care plan, own and operate ambulatory care centers or ancillary services projects, or provide administrative services to physician members.
d. **Closed physician-hospital organization (PHO).** A PHO that restricts physician membership to those practitioners who meet criteria for cost effectiveness and/or high quality.

e. **Management services organization (MSO).** A corporation, owned by the hospital or a physician/hospital joint venture, that provides management services to one or more medical group practices. The MSO purchases the tangible assets of the practices and leases them back as part of a full-service management agreement, under which the MSO employs all non-physician staff and provides all supplies/administrative systems for a fee.

f. **Integrated salary model.** Physicians are salaried by the hospital or another entity of a health system to provide medical services for primary care and specialty care.

g. **Equity model.** Allows established practitioners to become shareholders in a professional corporation in exchange for tangible and intangible assets of their existing practices.

h. **Foundation.** A corporation, organized either as a hospital affiliate or subsidiary, which purchases both the tangible and intangible assets of one or more medical group practices. Physicians remain in a separate corporate entity but sign a professional services agreement with the foundation.

**90. Percentage of hospital's net patient revenue.**

a. **Capitation.** An at-risk payment arrangement in which an organization receives a fixed prearranged payment and in turn guarantees to deliver or arrange all medically necessary care required by enrollers in the capitated plan. The fixed amount is specified within contractual agreements between the payor and the involved organization. The fixed payment amount is based on an actuarial assessment of the services required by enrollees and the costs of providing these services, recognizing enrollees adjustment factors such as age, sex, and family size.

b. **Shared risk payments.** A payment arrangement in which a hospital and a managed care organization share the risk of adverse claims experience. Methods for sharing risk could include: capitation with partial refunds or supplements if billed hospital charges or costs differ from capitated payments, and service or discharge-based payments with withholds and bonus payouts that depend on expenditure targets.

## SECTION D
## COMMUNITY ORIENTATION
### Definitions

1. **Mission statement.** A general statement that describes a company's reason for existence, its vision and direction, its areas of expertise and its goals.

5. **Health Status indicators.** A tool used to quantify various aspects of a populations health status.

9. **Self assessment.** An evaluation of an organization's management system through achievements in areas such as: leadership, strategic planning, human resource management, information management, process management, customer focus and satisfaction, and business results.

## SECTION E
## TOTAL FACILITY BEDS, UTILIZATION, FINANCES, AND STAFFING
### Instructions and Definitions

For the purposes of this survey, nursing home type unit/facility provides care for the elderly and chronic care in a non-acute setting in any of the following categories: *Skilled nursing care *Intermediate care *Residential care/elderly housing (*see page 4 definitions)**The nursing home type units/facilities are to be owned an operated by the hospital. Only one legal entity may be vested with title to the physical property or operate under the authority of a duly executed lease of the physical property.**

1a. **Total licensed beds** is the total number of beds authorized by the state licensing (certifying agency).

b. Report the number of **beds** regularly available (those **set up and staffed for use**) at the end of the reporting period. Report only operating beds, not constructed bed capacity. Include all bed facilities that are set up and staffed for use by inpatients who have no other bed facilities, such as pediatric bassinets, isolation units, quiet rooms, and reception and observation units assigned to or reserved for them. Exclude newborn bassinets and bed facilities for patients receiving special procedures for a portion of their stay and who have other bed facilities assigned to or reserved for them. Exclude, for example, labor room, postanesthesia, or postoperative recovery room beds, psychiatric holding beds, and beds that are used only as holding facilities for patients prior to their transfer to another hospital.

c. Report the number of normal newborn **bassinets**. Do not include neonatal intensive care or intermediate care bassinets. These should be reported on page 2, C6 and C7.

d. Total **births** should exclude fetal deaths.

e. Include the number of adult and pediatric **admissions** only (exclude births). This figure should include all patients admitted during the reporting period, including neonatal and swing admissions.

f. Report the number of adult and pediatric days of care rendered during the entire reporting period. Do not include days of care rendered for normal infants born in the hospital, but do include those for their mothers. Include days of care for infants born in the hospital and transferred into a neonatal care unit. Also include swing bed inpatient days. **Inpatient day** of care (also commonly referred to as a **patient day** or a **census day**, or by some federal hospitals as an **occupied bed day**) is a period of service between the census-taking hours on two successive calendar days, the day of discharge being counted only when the patient was admitted the same day.

g. **Emergency room visits** should reflect the number of visits to the emergency unit. Emergency outpatients can be admitted to the inpatient areas of the hospital, but they are still counted as emergency visits and subsequently as inpatient admissions.

h. An **Outpatient visit** is a visit by a patient who is not lodged in the hospital while receiving medical, dental, or other services. Each appearance of an outpatient in each unit constitutes one visit regardless of the number of diagnostic and/or therapeutic treatments that the patient receives. Total outpatient visits should include all clinic visits, referred visits, observation services, outpatient surgeries, home health service visits, and emergency room visits.

**Clinic** visits should reflect total number of visits to each specialized medical unit that is responsible for the diagnosis and treatment of patients on an outpatient, nonemergency basis (i.e., alcoholism, dental, gynecology, etc.). Visits to the satellite clinics and primary group practices should be included if revenue is received by the hospital.

**Referred** visits should reflect total number of outpatient ancillary visits to each specialty unit of the hospital established for providing technical aid used in the diagnosis and treatment of patients. Examples of such units are diagnostic radiology, EKG, pharmacy, etc.

**Observation** services are those services furnished on a hospital's premises, including use of a bed and periodic monitoring by a hospital's nursing or other staff, which are reasonable and necessary to evaluate an outpatient's condition or determine the need for a possible admission to the hospital as an inpatient. Observation services usually do not exceed 24 hours. However, there is no hourly limit on the extent to which they may be used.

**Home health service** visits are visits by home health personnel to a patient's residence.

Also include the number of outpatient surgeries reported on line E1i. and the emergency room visits reported on line E1f.

i-j. Count each patient undergoing surgery as one surgical operation regardless of the number of surgical procedures that were performed while the patient was in the operating or procedure room.

16

i. **Operating room.** A unit/room of a hospital or other health care facility in which surgical procedures requiring anesthesia are performed. For outpatient surgical operations, please record operations performed on patients who do not remain in the hospital overnight. Include all operations whether performed in the inpatient operating rooms or in procedure rooms located in an outpatient facility. Include an endoscopy only when used as an operative tool and not when used for diagnosis alone.

2a2 **Managed Care Medicare Discharges.** A discharge day where a Medicare Managed Care Plan is the source of payment.

2b2 **Managed Care Medicare Inpatient Days.** An inpatient day where a Medicare Managed Care Plan is the source of payment.

2c2 **Managed Care Medicaid Discharges.** A discharge day where a Medicaid Managed Care Plan is the source of payment.

2d2 **Managed Care Medicaid Inpatient Days.** An inpatient day where a Medicaid Managed Care Plan is the source of payment.

3a. **Net patient revenue.** Reported at the estimated net realizable amounts from patients, third-party payors, and others for services rendered, including estimated retroactive adjustments under reimbursement agreements with third-party payors. Retroactive adjustments are accrued on an estimated basis in the period the related services are rendered and adjusted in future periods, as final settlements are determined.

3b. **Tax appropriations.** A predetermined amount set aside by the government from its taxing authority to support the operation of the hospital.

c. **Other operating revenue.** Revenue from services other than health care provided to patients, as well as sales and services to nonpatients. Revenue that arises from the normal day-to-day operations from services other than health care provided to patients. Includes sales and services to nonpatients, and revenue from miscellaneous sources (rental of hospital space, sale of cafeteria meals, gift shop sales). Also include operating gains in this category.

d. Nonoperating revenue. Includes investment income, extraordinary gains and other nonoperating gains.

e. **Total revenue.** Add net patient revenue, tax appropriations, other operating revenue and nonoperating revenue.

f. **Payroll expenses.** Include payroll for all personnel including medical and dental residents/interns and trainees.

g. **Employee benefits.** Includes social security, group insurance, retirement benefits, workman's compensation, unemployment insurance, etc.

h. **Depreciation expense (for reporting period only)** report only the depreciation expense applicable to the reporting period. The amount also Should be included in accumulate ed depreciation(E 7-b).

i. **Interest expense.** Report interest expense for the reporting period only.

j. Total expenses. Includes all payroll and non-payroll expenses (including bad debt) as well as any nonoperating losses (including extraordinary losses).

4a. **Total gross inpatient revenue.** The hospitals full established rates(charges) for all services rendered to inpatients.

4b. **Total gross outpatient revenue**. The hospitals full established rates(charges) for all services rendered to outpatients.

4c. **Total gross patient revenue.** Total gross patient revenue (add total gross inpatient revenue and total gross outpatient revenue).

5. **Compensated care.** Care for which no payment is expected or no charge is made. It is the sum of bad debt and charity care absorbed by a hospital or other health care organization in providing medical care for patients who are uninsured or are unable to pay.

5a. Bad debt expense. The provision for actual or expected uncollectibles resulting from the extension of credit. Because bad debts are reported as an expense and not a deduction from revenue, the gross charges that result in bad debts will remain in net revenue (E3a).

b. **Charity care.** Health services that were never expected to result in cash inflows. Charity care results from a provider's policy to provide health care services free of charge to individuals who meet certain financial criteria. For purposes of this survey, charity care is measured on the basis of revenue forgone, at full established rates.

## E. TOTAL FACILITY BEDS, UTILIZATION, FINANCES, AND STAFFING (continued)

6a1 **Medicare.** Should agree with the Medicare utilization reported in questions E2a and b.

6a1a **Routine patient revenue.** Include traditional Medicare fee-for-service.

6a1c.**Total.** Medicare revenue (add Medicare routine patient revenue and Medicare managed care revenue).

6a2. **Medicaid.** Should agree with Medicaid utilization reported in questions E2c and d.

6a2a.**Routine patient revenue.** Include Medicaid disproportionate payments under Medicaid routine patient care (2a), in the net column (2) .

6a2c.**Total** Medicaid revenue (add Medicaid routine Patient revenue and Medicaid managed care revenue).

6c. **Total** revenue (gross should equal E4c and net should equal E3a).

7. **Fixed Assets.** Represent land and physical properties that are consumed or used in the creation of economic activity by the health care entity. The historical or acquisition costs are used in recording fixed assets. Net plant, property, and equipment represent the original costs of these items less accumulated depreciation and amortization.

7d. **Gross Square Footage:** Include all inpatient, outpatient, office, and support space used for or in support of your health care activities. Exclude exterior, roof, and garage space in the figure.

## STAFFING

**Full-Time Equivalent (FTE)** is the total number of hours worked by all employees over the full (12 month) reporting period divided by the normal number of hours worked by a full-time employee for that same time period. For example, if your hospital considers a normal work week for a full-time employee to be 40 hours, a total of 2,080 would be worked over a full year (52 weeks). If the total number of hours worked by all employees on the payroll is 208,000, then the number of Full-Time Equivalents (FTE) is 100 (employees). The FTE calculation for a specific occupational category such as Registered nurses is exactly the same. The calculation for each occupational category should be based on the number of hours worked by staff employed in that specific category.

8a. **Physicians and dentists.** Include only those physicians and dentists engaged in clinical practice and on the payroll. Those who hold administrative positions should be reported in "All other personnel."

c. **Other trainees.** A trainee is a person who has not completed the necessary requirements for certification or met the qualifications required for full salary under a related occupational category. Exclude medical and dental residents/interns who should be reported on line 7b.

d. **Registered nurses.** Nurses who have graduated from approved schools of nursing and who are currently registered by the state. They are responsible for the nature and quality of all nursing care that patients receive. Do not include any registered nurses more appropriately reported in other occupational categories, such as facility administrators, and therefore listed under "All other personnel."

e. **Licensed practical (vocational) nurses.** Nurses who have graduated from an approved school of practical (vocational) nursing who work under the supervision of registered nurses and/or physicians.

f. **Nursing assistive personnel.** Certified nursing assistant or equivalent unlicensed staff assigned to patient care units and reporting to nursing.

g. **All other personnel.** This should include all other personnel not already accounted for in other categories.

h. **Total facility personnel.** This line is to include the total facility personnel - hospital plus nursing home type unit/facility personnel (for those hospitals that own and operate a nursing home type unit/facility).

i. **Nursing home type unit/facility personnel.** This line should be filled out only by hospitals that own and operate a nursing home type unit/ facility, where only one legal entity is vested with title to the physical property or operates under the authority of a duly executed lease of the physical property. If nursing home type unit/facility personnel are reported on the total facility personnel line, but cannot be broken out, please write "cannot break out" on this line.

j. **Hospitalist.** Physician whose primary professional focus is the care of hospitalized medical patients (through clinical, education, administrative and research activity).

## SUPPLEMENTAL INFORMATION

1. **Does your hospital participate in any joint venture arrangements?** Joint Venture is a contractual arrangement between two or more parties forming an unincorporated business. The participants in the arrangement remain independent and separate outside of the ventures purpose.

2. **Does your hospital provide services through a satellite facility(s)?** Satellite Services are available at a facility geographically remote from the hospital campus.

# NOTES

# NOTES